Handbook of Communication in Oncology and Palliative Care

Edited by:

David W Kissane

Jimmie C. Holland Chair in Psycho-Oncology, Attending Psychiatrist and Chairman, Department of Psychiatry and Behavioral Sciences, Memorial Sloan-Kettering Cancer Center; Professor of Psychiatry, Weill Medical College of Cornell University, New York, NY, USA

Barry D Bultz

Director, Department of Psychosocial Resources, Program Leader: Psychosocial Oncology, Supportive, Pain, Palliative Care, Tom Baker Cancer Centre; Adjunct Professor and Chair, Division of Psychosocial Oncology, Department of Oncology, University of Calgary, Alberta, Canada

Phyllis N Butow

Professor and Co-Director Centre for Medical Psychology and Evidence-based Decision Making (CeMPED); Chair, Psycho-Oncology Co-operative Research Group (PoCog), University of Sydney, New South Wales, Australia

Ilora G Finlay

Professor of Palliative Medicine and Director of postgraduate MSc in Palliative Care Cardiff University; Consultant in Palliative Medicine, Velindre NHS Trust, Cardiff; Palliative Care Strategy Implementation Lead for Wales; Independent Crossbench Member, House of Lords, Westminster, London, UK

OXFORD
UNIVERSITY PRESS

OXFORD

UNIVERSITY PRESS

Great Clarendon Street, Oxford ox2 6dp

Oxford University Press is a department of the University of Oxford.
It furthers the University's objective of excellence in research, scholarship,
and education by publishing worldwide in

Oxford New York

Auckland Cape Town Dar es Salaam Hong Kong Karachi
Kuala Lumpur Madrid Melbourne Mexico City Nairobi
New Delhi Shanghai Taipei Toronto

With offices in

Argentina Austria Brazil Chile Czech Republic France Greece
Guatemala Hungary Italy Japan Poland Portugal Singapore
South Korea Switzerland Thailand Turkey Ukraine Vietnam

Oxford is a registered trade mark of Oxford University Press
in the UK and in certain other countries

Published in the United States
by Oxford University Press Inc., New York

British Library Cataloguing in Publication Data
Data available

Library of Congress Cataloging in Publication Data
Data available

Typeset by Cepha Imaging Private Ltd., Bangalore, India
Printed in Great Britain
on acid-free paper by
CPI Antony Rowe

ISBN 978–0–19–923836–1

10 9 8 7 6 5 4 3 2 1

Royal Liverpool University Hospital – Staff Library

Please return or renew, on or before the last date below. Items may be renewed **twice**, if not reserved for another user. Renewals may be made in person, by telephone: 0151 706 2248 or email: library.service@rlbuht.nhs.uk. There is a charge of 10p per day for late items.

1 1 SEP 2012

Handbook of Communication in Oncology and Palliative Care

Contents

Section D **Communication issues across the disciplines**

Preface

In this era of personalized medicine, tailoring communication to the specific values and preferences of each individual and their family is crucial. Due allowance is needed for age, gender, literacy, ethnicity and culture. Just as pharmacogenomics will lead to medication prescribing that is specific for each person's genetic profile, message framing requires information to be customized both in style and content in a patient-centred manner. Whether communication occurs through electronic media or in the face-to-face consultation, many challenges emerge in adapting information to suit the needs of the individual.

These challenges are amplified when the threat to life associated with a cancer diagnosis, its treatment, recurrent disease, palliative care or survivorship necessitate active coping to achieve an effective adaptation. While psychosocial specialists treat patients with resultant emotional disorders and other complicated forms of adjustment, the whole treatment team in oncology and palliative care is challenged to support the adaptation of the vast majority of patients and their families. Effective communication is at the heart of accomplishing this, using empathy, compassion and skills, which ensure that information is integrated comprehensively and coping is optimized. Fortunately, an emergent and well-developed body of research now provides a strong evidence-base for the teaching of communication skills to the whole treatment team. Our goal in creating this text is to make this knowledge accessible, model the related attitudes and highlight the skills needed clinically to optimize this care delivery.

Our approach has been to recognize that medical and nursing schools teach generic communication skills, but old habits exemplified by the senior medical workforce can potentially undermine what has been learnt. Educationalists have called these effects a 'hidden curriculum'. The teaching of an applied syllabus as trainees enter advanced training in cancer care serves to both reinforce generic skills and to focus each clinician on the difficult challenges specific to their discipline in delivering this specialist care. As national oncology societies, comprehensive cancer centres and national training programmes mandate that clinicians training in oncology and palliative care achieve competence in communication with patients and their families, educational programmes are emerging at national, regional and institutional levels. This handbook offers a comprehensive curriculum for these programmes, enriched by the international contributions from leading researchers and educators of cancer communication skills across the world.

Our target audience includes physicians and surgeons, medical and radiation oncologists, clinical oncologists, palliative care physicians, hospitalists, nurses, psychologists, psychiatrists and social workers, together with the broad range of allied health practitioners and chaplains that form the multidisciplinary team involved in modern medical care. Clinicians in training will find this book of tremendous value, while family physicians and general practitioners, communication researchers, medical schools, healthcare organizations, pharmaceutical companies, advocacy groups and the lay public will be enriched by the science described herein.

As editors, our collaboration reflects the breadth of communication studies in the United States of America, Canada, Australia, Europe and the United Kingdom. Two years of effort has gone into the creation of this handbook, which has been based on tremendous collegiality, goodwill and friendship. We are deeply indebted to our authors for their willingness to share their science, their commitment to scholarship and the clarity of its presentation, and for their excellent chapters.

We express our wholehearted thanks for their generous efforts and professional collaboration with us.

Each editor has been backed fully by their institution and supported by wonderful administrative staff, who have contributed many hours to this handbook. In the United States, special thanks is offered to Emily Poblocki and Laurie Schulman in the Department of Psychiatry and Behavioral Sciences at Memorial Sloan–Kettering Cancer Center, New York; in Canada, to Joshua Lounsberry at the Tom Baker Cancer Center and the Department of Oncology, Faculty of Medicine, University of Calgary, Alberta; in Australia, to staff in the School of Psychology and the Royal Prince Alfred Hospital at the University of Sydney; and in the United Kingdom, to Jo Sulman in the Department of Palliative Medicine at Velindre Hospital, Cardiff. A project of this scope is enormous in its vision and execution. As editors, we are mindful of the gracious patience and steady encouragement we have received from our partners and families. We wholeheartedly thank them for allowing us to commit so much time and energy to this project.

Oxford University Press has been superbly professional and helpful in bringing this labour to fruition. Our deep thanks to the Commissioning Editors Georgia Pinteau and Nicola Ulyatt, who were skillfully aided by Clare Caruna and Eloise Moir-Ford as we compiled the manuscript. Further thanks to the Production Editor Joanna Hardern and her team. Oxford's expertise in bringing together the artwork, typesetting and proof reading has made the journey painless and fulfilling.

Finally, to our readers! Thank you for recognizing the importance of patient-centred care and the seminal role of communication in information delivery, decision-making, competent treatment, compassionate support and healing. We trust that this handbook will help you to personalize and tailor your communication sensitively and effectively.

David W Kissane, MD
Barry D Bultz, PhD
Phyllis N Butow, PhD
Ilora G Finlay, MD

Foreword

Michael Stefanek

Cancer has long been one of the most feared words in the English language. Along with such scourges as leprosy and, most recently, AIDS, it has arguably stirred more anxiety and distress among the public at large, patients, and loved ones than any other disease known to man. Indeed, in my lifetime, there has been much debate about even providing the diagnosis of 'cancer' to patients afflicted with this disease and their caregivers, for fear of significant depression, anxiety and hopelessness. This text, *Handbook of communication in oncology and palliative care*, reminds us of how far we have come in our ability to communicate about this challenging disease and its complex treatment and provides the road for future growth in our fight to prevent, treat, and care for those with a diagnosis of cancer.

The editors of this book are distinguished, outstanding academics and authors, and have a clear sense of the depth and breadth of communication needs across the cancer continuum, and the need to include patients, caregivers, healthcare providers and the public at large. The chapters in this text reflect their understanding that communication is ubiquitous during all phases of the cancer care continuum, from prevention, early detection, treatment, survivorship, to end-of-life care.

The editors and authors clearly operate from a core concept that pulls them together to produce a text so rich in its depth and breadth: *communication is clearly a sine qua non of cancer care*. The contributors to this book demonstrate that they are astutely aware of this fact by providing not only bountiful information on what we know, but clear, crisp thoughts and guidelines on maximizing this communication process for all professionals engaged in the war against cancer, either in the clinical trenches or in the clinical research laboratory.

Over the past decade, there has been a clear overdue interest in how best to communicate about cancer in a host of arenas, including individual patient–physician communication, cultural tailoring of communication messages and the productive use of the internet in the communication process. Funding organizations in the United States, such as the National Cancer Institute, have recognized this interest by creating the Health Communications and Informatics Research Branch, the Office of Cancer Survivorship and the Basic and Biobehavioral Research Branch. These funding sources, along with others nationally and internationally, provide funding for work ranging from basic communication science to applied intervention work with patients and providers. Much of the fruit of this work is reflected directly and indirectly in the pages of this text. This handbook, which promises to be a classic in the cancer communications field, successfully takes what we know about communication as a result of this increased emphasis on communication science and provides a rich clinical context for this work.

This text is unique in the field in providing not only cancer communication in a historical context and providing a theoretical framework for communication skills, but also by addressing key communication issues across disciplines (e.g. surgeons, nurses, social workers). Finally, in addition to the rich clinical context of the contributions, a section of the text is specifically dedicated to research in cancer communication, including the importance of qualitative, quantitative and mixed methods research.

In sum, reducing the burden of cancer is intimately related to our ability to optimize the communication process among healthcare providers, patients, caregivers and those at risk for developing cancer. The contributors to this text are keenly aware of this important relationship.

This text, *Handbook of communication in oncology and palliative care*, is clearly a major step forward in the invaluable synthesis of research and clinical application in the arena of cancer communication. It should be on the shelves of clinicians, researchers and policy-makers alike, as they partner with the editors and authors of this outstanding text in the shared battle against cancer.

Michael Stefanek, PhD
Vice President, Behavioral Research
American Cancer Society

Foreword

Leslie Fallowfield

Enormous advances have been made over the past decade in the diagnosis and treatment of cancer. Many people are living longer and better lives due to advances made in prevention and early detection, surgical techniques and procedures, newer forms of radiotherapy and systemic drug therapies. Exciting, pioneering, new tailored therapies that target specific cells have been made possible by our expanding knowledge of human genomics; perversely this is called personalized medicine, yet the greater our understanding of cancer, the more depersonalized patients can feel and, despite all these laudable therapeutic achievements, communication within oncology remains problematic. There are an increasing number of sad, bad and just plain difficult issues to discuss with patients and their families. Indeed the complexity of modern diagnostics and treatment options can make some medical interviews sound more like medical undergraduate lectures.

Talking about the diagnosis and prognosis to ill and frightened people is never easy but unless patients have grasped the reality of their situation they are unable to make wise decisions about their therapeutic options or provide truly educated consent to clinical trial participation. Healthcare professionals worldwide admit that they have rarely received sufficient training in handling many of these difficult tasks.

Dyadic exchanges between a patient and their doctor or nurse have been the subject of considerable research conducted by several of the authors included in this textbook. The delivery of cancer services has, however, changed dramatically in many parts of the world with some countries providing care via a multidisciplinary team. The putative benefits of such approaches are that all specialities contribute from their own area of expertise to the opinions and decisions made available to a patient. Unfortunately, merely calling something a team does not make it one and many team members struggle when communicating with their colleagues who may be more used to making autocratic management decisions. Furthermore research has shown that communication by different healthcare team members with each other, and then with their patients, is often inconsistent and confusing, causing even more stress for everyone involved. The lack of awareness by individuals of the information-giving roles of others in the multidisciplinary team means that many patients fall between informational gaps, with everyone assuming that someone else has relayed key areas. Psychosocial issues, sexual matters, family history and available clinical trials are the primary issues that are omitted from many consultations.

The near obsessional preoccupation that the media has with items to do with cancer, together with some of the misinformation available from the internet, can add yet another strain on patients struggling to understand their situation and options. There has been an effort to provide patients with easily accessible written information, leaflets and booklets. Many of these are useful and can complement and reinforce the verbal discussions that have occurred; however, research shows that some oncology teams give patients out-of-date material or information that conflicts with that already provided by them, exacerbating confusion and anxiety even further. Furthermore, the utility of written information correlates highly with the socio-educational background of patients, suggesting that verbal communication should, and will always, have more salience.

It is not only patients and their families who suffer in different ways if communication is less than optimal; senior doctors who feel insufficiently trained in communication skills are more likely to evidence symptoms of burnout and to experience lowered levels of job satisfaction. It seems self-evident that an occupation demanding not only high-level technical and intellectual skills but also an ability to impart complex and uncomfortable information with sensitivity and empathy and in a flexible manner appropriate for the individual in front of them, would ensure that its workforce was equipped with excellent training in communication. Although medical and nursing schools worldwide have increased the amount of communication skills in the curricula, some still use inappropriate teaching methods. Fortunately over the past few years there has been an ever increasing literature demonstrating the value to all of evidence-based communication skills programmes and some countries, such as the UK, have incorporated these as part of their Cancer strategies.

The more scholarly approaches into the science of communicating well are tackled masterfully by the editors of this textbook; they have assembled the very best researchers providing an excellent, up-to-date international perspective on communication in cancer. Hopefully this will be used to inform practice in countries where the need for specialist training is still not recognized and help us all to identify aspects of communication that still require a better evidence-base. Good communication is not just about being kind; it is the basis of working scientifically with patients and consequently key to quality cancer care.

Lesley Fallowfield BSc, DPhil, FMedSci
Director
Sussex Psychosocial Oncology Group
Brighton and Sussex Medical School
University of Sussex
United Kingdom

Contributors

Marie Achille
Associate Professor,
Department of Psychology,
Université de Montréal,
Québec, Canada

Ronald D Adelman
Professor of Medicine,
Co-Chief, Division of Geriatrics and
Gerontology,
Director, the Irving Sherwood
Wright Center on Aging,
Co-Director, the Cornell Center for Aging
Research and Clinical Care,
Weill Medical College of Cornell University,
New York, New York, USA

Terrance L Albrecht
Professor and Interim Associate Center
Director, Population Sciences
Interim Program Leader,
Population Studies and Prevention,
Karmanos Cancer Institute;
Department of Oncology,
Wayne State University School of Medicine,
Detroit, Michigan, USA

Robert Arnold
Professor, Leo H. Criep Chair,
Section of Palliative Care and Medical Ethics,
Division of General Internal Medicine,
University of Pittsburgh School of Medicine,
Pittsburgh, Pennsylvania, USA

Anthony Back
Professor, Department of Medicine,
Oncology Division,
University of Washington Medicine,
Seattle, Washington, USA

Walter F Baile
Professor, Behavioral Science; Director,
Program in Interpersonal Communication
and Relationship Enhancement (I*CARE),
The University of Texas M.D. Anderson
Cancer Center
Houston, Texas, USA

Rachel Bell
Clinical Psychologist, Psychiatry Service,
Department of Psychiatry & Behavioral
Sciences,
Memorial Sloan-Kettering Cancer Center,
New York, New York, USA

Jürg Bernhard
Professor, Inselspital,
Bern University Hospital,
Department of Medical Oncology
Bern, Switzerland

Gabriella Bianchi Micheli
Psychologist and Psychotherapist FSP with
specialization in Psycho-oncology FSP,
Servizio di Psichiatria e Psicologia Medica
OSC,
Lugano, Switzerland

Patrick Boland
Attending Orthopedic Surgeon,
Department of Surgery,
Memorial Sloan-Kettering Cancer Center,
New York, New York, USA

Venetia Bourrier
Director of Provincial Oncology Drug
Program,
Cancer Care Manitoba,
Winnipeg, Manitoba, Canada

Frances Boyle
Clinical Lecturer,
Discipline of Medicine,
Royal North Shore Hospital,
The University of Sydney,
Australia

Richard Brown
Assistant Professor,
Department of Social and Behavioral Health,
School of Medicine,
Virginia Commonwealth University,
Richmond, Virginia, USA

Barry D Bultz
Director, Department of Psychosocial Resources,
Program Leader: Psychosocial Oncology, Supportive, Pain, Palliative Care,
Tom Baker Cancer Centre;
Adjunct Professor and Chair,
Division of Psychosocial Oncology,
Department of Oncology,
University of Calgary, Alberta, Canada

Phyllis N Butow
Professor and Co-Director, Centre for Medical Psychology and
Evidence-based Decision Making (CeMPED);
Chair, Psycho-Oncology Co-operative Research Group (PoCoG),
University of Sydney, Sydney, New South Wales, Australia

Carma L Bylund
Director, Communication Skills Training and Research Laboratory,
Assistant Attending Behavioral Scientist,
Behavioral Sciences Service,
Department of Psychiatry & Behavioral Sciences,
Memorial Sloan-Kettering Cancer Center;
Assistant Professor of Psychology in Psychiatry,
Weill Medical College of Cornell University, New York, New York, USA

Linda E Carlson
Linda E. Carlson, Ph.D., R. Psych.
Enbridge Research Chair in Psychosocial Oncology,
Alberta Heritage Foundation for Medical Research Health Scholar,
Associate Professor,
Division of Psychosocial Oncology,
Department of Oncology,
Faculty of Medicine,
Adjunct Associate Professor, Department of Psychology, University of Calgary;
Clinical Psychologist, Department of Psychosocial Resources,
Tom Baker Cancer Centre, Calgary, Alberta, Canada

Jeanne Carter
Assistant Attending Psychologist,
Psychiatry Service, Department of Psychiatry & Behavioral Sciences,
Memorial Sloan-Kettering Cancer Center, New York, New York, USA

Donald J Cegala
Emeritus Professor of Communication and Family Medicine,
The Ohio State University,
Columbus, OH, USA

Peter Chan
Director of Male Reproductive Medicine,
Associate Professor of Urology,
Department of Surgery,
McGill University Health Center,
Montréal, Québec, Canada

Cathy Charles
Professor, Clinical Epidemiology & Biology,
Health Sciences Centre,
McMaster University, Hamilton, Ontario, Canada

Catherine Charleson
Department of Nursing & Supportive Care Research,
Peter MacCallum Cancer Centre,
East Melbourne, Victoria, Australia

Lai Cheng Yew
Specialist Registrar in Clinical Oncology,
Mount Vernon Cancer Centre,
Northwood, Middlesex, UK

Betty Chewning
Associate Professor,
School of Pharmacy, University of Wisconsin
Madison, Wisconsin, USA

Grace Christ
Professor, School of Social Work,
Columbia University,
New York, New York, USA

Josephine M Clayton
Associate Professor, Sydney Medical School,
University of Sydney;
Staff Specialist in Palliative Medicine and
Head of Palliative Care Department, Royal
North Shore Hospital, St Leonard's, Sydney;
Senior Research Member, Centre for Medical
Psychology and Evidence-based Decision
Making (CeMPED), University of Sydney,
St Leonard's, Australia

Kathy Cole-Kelly
Director of Communications,
School of Medicine,
Case Western Reserve University,
Cleveland, Ohio, USA

Kate Collie
Psychologist, Art Therapist, and Assistant
Professor,
Cross Cancer Institute,
University of Alberta, Edmonton, Canada

Laura Cooke
Senior Income Manager,
American Cancer Society,
Philadelphia, Pennsylvania, USA

Nessa Coyle
Nurse Practitioner, Pain & Palliative Care
Service,
Memorial Sloan-Kettering Cancer Center,
New York, New York, USA

Lesley Degner
Distinguished Professor, Faculty of Nursing,
University of Manitoba,
Winnipeg, Manitoba, Canada

Anthony De La Cruz
Clinical Research Nurse,
Urology Outpatient Center,
Memorial Sloan-Kettering Cancer Center,
New York, New York, USA

Liselotte Dietrich
Supervisor, Psychooncology Counsellor,
and Nurse
Herisau, Switzerland

Justine Diggens
Clinical Psychologist,
Department Clinical Psychology,
Peter MacCallum Cancer Centre,
East Melbourne,
Victoria, Australia

Robyn DiMatteo
Professor of Psychology,
College of Arts, Humanities and Social
Sciences, University of California,
Riverside, California, USA

Stewart M Dunn
Professor of Psychological Medicine,
Royal North Shore Hospital,
The University of Sydney,
New South Wales, Australia

Susan S Eggly
Wayne State University
Medicine, Karmanos Cancer Institute,
Detroit, Michigan, USA

Dana Eisenberg
Health Communications Fellow,
National Cancer Institute, and Ohio State
University,
Columbus, Ohio, USA

John Encandela
Assistant Professor of Clinical Epidemiology,
Columbia University Mailman School of
Public Health,
New York, New York, USA
Adjunct Assistant Professor, University of
Pittsburgh,
Grad School of Public Health,
Pittsburgh, Pennsylvania, USA

Alison Evans
Program Manager,
National Breast and Ovarian Cancer Centre,
Surry Hills, New South Wales, Australia

Kimberly Feigin
Assistant Attending Diagnostic Radiologist,
Department of Radiology,
Breast Imaging Section,
Memorial Sloan-Kettering Cancer Center,
New York, New York, USA

Ilora Finlay
Professor of Palliative Medicine and Director
of Postgraduate MSc in palliative care, Cardiff
University; Consultant in Palliative Medicine,
Velindre NHS Trust, Cardiff; Palliative Care
Strategy Implementation Lead for Wales;
Independent Crossbench Member,
House of Lords, Westminster, London, UK

Kelly Fryer-Edwards
Associate Professor,
Department of Medical History & Ethics,
University of Washington,
Seattle, Washington, USA

Sarah Ford
Clinical Psychologist, School of Psychology,
University of Birmingham,
Birmingham, UK

Clara Gaff
Senior Genetic Counsellor, Genetic Health
Service Victoria,
Departments of Paediatrics and Medicine,
Royal Children's Hospital,
The University of Melbourne,
Victoria, Australia

Amiram Gafni
Professor, Department of Clinical
Epidemiology & Biostatistics,
Health Sciences Centre,
McMaster University, Hamilton,
Ontario, Canada

Thomas Gallagher
Associate Professor of Medicine,
Department of Medicine and Department of
Bioethics & Humanities,
University of Washington,
Seattle, Washington, USA

Afaf Girgis
Professor and Director, Centre for Health
Research & Psycho-oncology,
Cancer Council New South Wales,
University of Newcastle & Hunter Medical
Research Institute, New South Wales,
Australia

Michelle G Greene
Professor, Department of Health and
Nutrition Sciences,
Brooklyn College and CUNY
School of Public Health,
New York, New York, USA

Jennifer A Gueguen
Communication Skills Training and Research
Laboratory,
Behavioral Sciences Service,
Department of Psychiatry & Behavioral
Sciences,
Memorial Sloan-Kettering Cancer Center,
New York, New York, USA

Thomas F Hack
Professor, Faculty of Nursing,
University of Manitoba
Clinical Psychologist, CancerCare Manitoba
Winnipeg, Manitoba, Canada

Judith A Hall
Professor and Social Psychologist,
Department of Psychology,
Northeastern University,
Boston, Massachusetts, USA

James Hallenbeck
Director of Palliative Care,
Stanford Comprehensive Cancer Center,
Stanford, California, USA

Diana Harcourt
Reader in Health Psychology,
Co-Director,
Centre for Appearance Research,
Faculty of Applied Sciences,
University of the West of England,
Bristol, UK

Kelly Haskard
Assistant Professor,
Department of Psychiatry,
Texas State at San Marcos,
San Marcos, Texas, USA

Joshua Hauser
Assistant Professor,
MED-Buehler Center on Aging,
Northwestern University,
Chicago, Illinois, USA

Alexandra Heerdt
Attending Breast Surgeon,
Department of Surgery,
Memorial Sloan-Kettering Cancer Center,
New York, New York, USA

Sue Hegarty
Cancer Services Coordinator,
Cancer Information and Support Service,
The Cancer Council,
Victoria, Australia

Paul Heinrich
Creative Director,
Pam McLean Centre,
The University of Sydney,
New South Wales, Australia

Christopher Herbert
Bishop of St Albans,
St Albans, Herts, UK

Marilyn Hundleby
Clinical Psychologist,
Director of the Arts in Medicine Program,
Cross Cancer Institute,
Edmonton, Alberta, Canada

Christoph Hürny
Professor of Psychosocial Medicine,
University of Bern Medical School,
Medical Director, Geriatric Care Hospital,
St Gallen, Switzerland

Paul B Jacobsen
Chair, Department of Health Outcomes and
Behavior
Moffitt Cancer Center,
Tampa, Florida, USA

Michael Jefford
Deputy Head, Department of Medical
Oncology,
Peter MacCallum Cancer Centre;
Clinical Consultant,
Cancer Council Victoria;
Associate Professor of Medicine,
University of Melbourne, Australia

Alexander Kiss
Professor, Universitätsspital Basel,
Psychosomatik,
Basel, Switzerland

David W Kissane
Jimmie C Holland Chair in Psycho-Oncology,
Attending Psychiatrist, and Chairman,
Department of Psychiatry & Behavioral
Sciences, Memorial Sloan-Kettering Cancer
Center; Professor of Psychiatry,
Weill Medical College of Cornell University,
New York, New York, USA

Steven Klimidis
Deputy Director,
Victorian Transcultural Psychiatry Unit,
School of Population Health,
The University of Melbourne,
Victoria, Australia

Christina Klöckner
Psychologist, University of Neuchâtel,
Neuchâtel, Switzerland

Lyuba Konopasek
Assistant Professor of Pediatrics,
NYPH – Cornell Medical Center,
New York, New York, USA

Suzanne Kurtz
Clinical Professor,
Director of Clinical Communication,
College of Veterinary Medicine,
Washington State University,
Pullman, Washington, USA

Tomer T Levin
Assistant Attending Psychiatrist,
Psychiatry Service, Department of
Psychiatry & Behavioral Sciences,
Memorial Sloan-Kettering Cancer Center;
Assistant Professor of Psychiatry, Weill
Medical College of Cornell University,
New York, New York, USA

Laura Liberman
Attending Radiologist, Department of
Radiology,
Breast Imaging Section,
Memorial Sloan-Kettering Cancer Center,
New York, New York, USA

Mack Lipkin
Professor, Department of Medicine,
New York University Medical Center,
New York, New York, USA

Yves Libert
Psychologist, Institut Jules Bordet,
Bruxelles, Belgium

Carrie Lethborg
Senior Social Worker,
Departments of Oncology & Social Work,
St Vincent's Hospital,
The University of Melbourne,
Victoria, Australia

Elizabeth Lobb
Associate Professor,
Calvary Health Care Sydney and Cunningham
Centre for Palliative Care,
Adjunct Associate Professor, Sydney School of
Medicine, The University of Notre Dame,
Australia, Adjunct Associate Professor,
WA Centre for Cancer & Palliative Care,
Curtin University of Technology,
Western Australia, Australia

Matthew Loscalzo
Associate Clinical Professor, Medicine,
Cancer Symptom Control Program,
Rebecca and John Moores UCSD Cancer
Center,
La Jolla, California, USA

Joshua J Lounsberry
Research Coordinator,
Department of Psychosocial Resources,
Tom Baker Cancer Centre, University of
Calgary, Alberta, Canada

Melanie Lovell
Palliative Care Physician, Greenwich Hospital,
Greenwich, New South Wales,
and University of Sydney,
Australia

Barbara Lubrano di Ciccone
Instructor, Psychiatry Service,
Department of Psychiatry & Behavioral
Sciences,
Memorial Sloan-Kettering Cancer Center
New York, New York, USA

Jane Maher
Chief Medical Officer, Consultant Clinical
Oncologist,
Macmillan Cancer Support;
Senior Clinical Lecturer,
University College London,
London, UK

Gregory Makoul
Professor and Director,
Center for Communication and Medicine,
Division of General Internal Medicine,
Northwestern University Feinberg
School of Medicine,
Chicago, Illinois, USA

Rita Marigliani
Consumer Advocate,
Peter MacCallum Cancer Centre,
East Melbourne, Victoria, Australia

Isabelle Merckaert
Psychologist, Institut Jules Bordet,
Bruxelles, Belgium

Harry Minas
Director, Victorian Transcultural
Psychiatry Unit,
St. Vincent's Hospital,
Victoria, Australia

Cynthia W Moore
Clinical Assistant in Psychology,
Massachusetts General Hospital,
Child & Adolescent Psychiatry,
Boston, Massachusetts, USA

Caroline Nehill
Program Manager,
National Breast and Ovarian Cancer Centre,
Surry Hills, New South Wales, Australia

Christian J Nelson
Assistant Attending Psychologist,
Psychiatry Service,
Department of Psychiatry &
Behavioral Sciences,
Memorial Sloan-Kettering Cancer Center;
Assistant Professor of Psychology in
Psychiatry,
Weill Medical College of Cornell University,
New York, New York, USA

Simon Noble
Clinical Senior Lecturer & Honorary
Consultant in Palliative Medicine,
Department of Palliative Medicine,
Royal Gwent Hospital,
Newport, UK

Bernard Park
Assistant Attending Thoracic Surgeon,
Department of Surgery,
Memorial Sloan-Kettering Cancer Center,
New York, New York, USA

Patricia A Parker
Assistant Professor, Department of
Behavioral Science,
University of Texas M.D. Anderson Cancer
Center
Houston, Texas, USA

Steven D Passik
Associate Attending Psychologist,
Psychiatry Service,
Department of Psychiatry & Behavioral
Sciences,
Memorial Sloan-Kettering Cancer Center;
Associate Professor of Psychology, Weill
Medical College of Cornell University,
New York, New York, USA

Nicola J Pease
Consultant,
Palliative Medicine,
Velindre NHS Trust,
Cardiff, Wales, UK

Michelle Pengelly
Oncology Nurse Specialist,
Velindre Hospital, Whitchurch,
Cardiff, UK

VJ Periyakoil
Associate Director,
VA Hospice Care Center,
Palo Alto, California, USA

Jennifer Philip
Consultant, Palliative Care Service,
St Vincent's Hospital,
Fitzroy, Victoria, Australia

Andrea Pusic
Associate Attending, Plastic Surgery Service,
Memorial Sloan-Kettering Cancer Center
New York, New York, USA

Paula Rauch
Director, Parenting at a Challenging Time
Program (PACT),
Massachusetts General Hospital,
Child & Adolescent Psychiatry,
Boston, Massachusetts, USA

Darius Razavi
Head of Psychiatry Department,
St Pierre University Hospital,
l'universite libre de Bruxelles,
Campus du Solbosch,
Bruxelles, Belgium

Felicia Roberts
Associate Professor,
Department of Communication,
Purdue University,
West Lafayette, Indiana, USA

Marcy Rosenbaum
Associate Professor,
Department of Family Medicine,
University of Iowa Hospitals and Clinics,
Iowa City, Iowa, USA

John W Robinson
Department of Psychosocial Resources,
Tom Baker Cancer Centre;
Adjunct Associate Professor,
Department of Oncology and Programme in
Clinical Psychology,
University of Calgary,
Calgary, Alberta, Canada

Deborah Roter
Professor, Health, Behavior, and Society,
Johns Hopkins School of Public Health,
Baltimore, Maryland, USA

Andrew Roth
Attending Psychiatrist, Psychiatry Service,
Department of Psychiatry & Behavioral
Sciences,
Memorial Sloan-Kettering Cancer Center;
Professor of Clinical Psychiatry,
Weill Medical College of Cornell University,
New York, New York, USA

Zeev Rosberger
Director, Louise Granofsky-Psychosocial
Oncology Program,
Segal Cancer Centre,
Jewish General Hospital;
Associate Professor, Departments of
Oncology, Psychology, and Psychiatry,
McGill University,
Montréal, Québec, Canada

John C Ruckdeschel
President and CEO,
Nevada Cancer Institute,
Las Vegas, Nevada, USA

Brent Schacter
Professor, Department of Internal Medicine,
University of Manitoba/CancerCare
Manitoba,
Winnipeg, Manitoba, Canada

Marianne Schmid Mast
Professor, Institut de Psychologie du Travail
et des Organisations,
Neuchâtel, Switzerland

Penelope Schofield
Nursing and Supportive Care Research,
Peter MacCallum Cancer Centre,
East Melbourne, Victoria, Australia

Linda Sheahan
Consultant Physician, Palliative and
Supportive Care,
Peter MacCallum Cancer Centre, East
Melbourne,
Victoria, Australia

Lidia Schapira
Gilette Center for Breast Cancer,
Yawkey Outpatient Center, Massachusetts
General Hospital
Boston, Massachusetts, USA

Laura A Siminoff
Professor and Chair,
Department of Social and Behavioral Health,
Virginia Commonwealth University Medical
Center,
Richmond, Virginia, USA

Peter W Speck
Chaplain and Research Fellow, Kings College,
Romsey, UK

Friedrich Stiefel
Chef de Service de Psychiatrie de Liaison,
Centre Hospitalier Universitaire Vaudois,
Lausanne, Switzerland

Martin Stockler
Associate Professor of Medicine,
Royal Prince Alfred Hospital,
NHMRC Clinical trials,
University of Sydney,
Sydney, New South Wales, Australia

Martin HN Tattersall
Professor of Cancer Medicine,
Cancer Medicine Research and Teaching,
Discipline of Medicine,
University of Sydney,
New South Wales, Australia

Bejoy C Thomas
Department of Psychosocial Oncology,
Tom Baker Cancer Centre,
Calgary, Alberta, Canada

Jane Turner
Senior Lecturer,
Department of Psychiatry,
The University of Queensland,
Brisbane, Australia

Simon Wein
Consultant Physician, Palliative Care Unit,
Davidoff Cancer Center, Rabin Medical
Center,
Petach Tikvah, Israel

Susan Wilkinson
Principal Research Fellow in Palliative Care,
Marie Curie Palliative Care Research Unit,
Royal Free & University College Medical
School,
Hampstead, London, UK

Sandra Winterburn
National Co-Leader, Advanced
Communication
Skills Training Programme (ACST);
Lecturer, School of Nursing and Midwifery,
University of East Anglia, Norwich,
Norwich, UK

Joseph S Weiner
Associate Professor of Clinical Psychiatry and
Medicine,
Albert Einstein College of Medicine,
Chief, Consultation Liaison Psychiatry,
North Shore University Medical Center/
Manhasset,
Manhasset, New York, USA

Brigitta Woessmer
Professor, Abt. Für Psychosomatik,
Universitätsspital, Basel,
Praxis für Psychotherapie, Olten,
Switzerland

Editor details

David Kissane began teaching physician-patient communication skills to Monash University medical students in Australia in the early 1980s and then incorporated experiential training into the subject Psycho-Oncology within the Postgraduate Diplomas of Palliative Medicine and Psycho-Oncology that he initiated in 1996 at the University of Melbourne during his tenure as foundation Professor and Director of Palliative Medicine. He is currently the incumbent in the Jimmie C. Holland Chair of Psycho-Oncology and Chairman of the Department of Psychiatry and Behavioral Sciences at Memorial Sloan-Kettering Cancer Center in New York. He is thus an Attending Psychiatrist at The Memorial Hospital for Cancer and Allied Diseases, and Professor of Psychiatry at the Weill Medical College of Cornell University. Across his 35-year medical career, he has trained in family medicine, psychiatry of the medically ill and palliative medicine. Dr. Kissane is the author of over 175 publications.

Barry Bultz became Director in 1981 of the Department of Psychosocial Resources at the Tom Baker Cancer Center in Calgary, Alberta, where he has subsequently developed and leads one of the first interdisciplinary psychosocial oncology programs in Canada – Psychosocial Oncology, Supportive, Pain and Palliative Care. As a founding member and Past President of the Canadian Association of Psychosocial Oncology (CAPO), he has been an active member of the Canadian Consortium on Communication Skills Training. He is internationally regarded for the concept of emotional distress as the 6th vital sign and chaired the 1st Canadian conference in Psychosocial Oncology in 1985 and the 6th World Congress of Psycho-Oncology in 2003. He is also holds faculty appointments in Oncology, Psychiatry, Surgery and Psychology. He is the author of over 100 scholarly publications and serves on several editorial boards for cancer-related journals.

Phyllis Butow is currently Professor and National Health and Medical Research Council Principal Research Fellow in the School of Psychology, University of Sydney, where she co-directs the Centre for Medical Psychology and Evidence-based Medicine (CeMPED). She has worked in Psycho-Oncology for over 16 years, currently chairs the newly established Australian Psycho-Oncology Co-operative Research Group and has developed an international reputation in Health Communication. She developed a curriculum in communication skills for the University of Sydney medical programme, chairs the National Breast and Ovarian Cancer Centre (NBOCC) Communication Skills Working Party, was a Principal Investigator on one national and one international randomized controlled trial of communication skills training, and has facilitated hundreds of communication skills courses for the NBOCC and the Pam McLean Cancer Communications Centre over the past 10 years. Professor Butow has over 200 publications in peer reviewed journals.

Ilora Finlay is a Consultant in Palliative Medicine at the Velindre NHS Trust, Cardiff. She is also an honorary Professor at Cardiff University and was Vice Dean of the School of Medicine 2000–2005. Professor Finlay currently chairs the Palliative Care Strategy Implementation Board for the Welsh Assembly Government. She has published over 126 papers and seven books and holds senior editorial positions for medical journals such as Lancet Oncology and the Journal of Evaluation in Clinical Practice. In 1996, Baroness Finlay was named Welsh Woman of the Year in recognition for her work in the field of palliative care. In 2001, she was appointed a people's peer in the first open contest for membership of the House of Lords. In establishing the World-renowned Diploma/MSc in Palliative Medicine (Cardiff University), she has trained over 1500 general practitioners and hospital specialists in communication skills through experiential residential programmes, and has developed teaching tools and assessment methods.

Section A

Introduction to communication studies in cancer and palliative medicine

Section Editor: David W Kissane

To set the scene, this first section takes stock of what has happened within cancer communication studies over recent decades and what we have learnt about the art of teaching communication skills. Distinct theoretical models have emerged about training clinicians, alongside our goal about framing information delivery and clinical decision-making in a patient-centred manner. Our behaviour is guided by strong ethical values and is sensitive to any power differential, social inequity, cultural difference or the influence of gender. Much has been learnt about teaching communication to medical students to establish generic communication skills as they launch their medical careers. This book goes on to develop an applied curriculum for the specialist fields of oncology and palliative medicine, while remaining cognizant of the importance of studies that seek to also optimize patient communication in the clinical encounter.

Chapter 1

The history of communication skills knowledge and training

Mack Lipkin

Introduction

This chapter attempts to provide the reader with a concise and personal journey through which I recall how we got to where we are in the field of communication in medicine, which inheres an implicit 'where we are' (1). For our mutual sanity, it does not attempt to be encyclopaedic, comprehensive, or complete; any accuracy it has, derives from the author's experience as a 35-year participant in the field. It attempts to steer between the Scylla of what Dunn describes as 'evidence-based navel gazing' (Chapter 2) and the Charybdis of self-indulgent, evidence-free, charismatic pronouncement. A talented and lucky reader might extract from this chapter an historical sense of why we are where we are, and so have a skeletal perspective from which to hang what follows in the highly focused remaining 61 chapters.

Most of the history of communication skills knowledge and teaching derives from work and studies done in general medicine, or further afield, rather than in cancer care. This chapter includes such material because much of communication knowledge and skills are generic, cross specific applications and content areas like cancer care, and because the most useful conceptual frameworks and approaches began elsewhere and have only partially been rendered cancer-specific. Nevertheless, cancer care has been advanced in attempting, as this book reflects, to codify the processes required to accomplish some key goals: to help patients to accept their diagnosis and prognosis; to accept or reject tests and difficult treatments according to their core preferences; to participate in studies; to enable them to participate meaningfully when curative care is futile; and to facilitate dying with dignity.

The importance of communication in medicine generally was understood by prehistoric human healers. Fabrega emphasizes that even in the smallest social units, such as isolated tribal groups of as few as five, sick people need to show their sickness in order to seek and get help (2). Healers need also to understand their diseases and illnesses, and to plan and execute their healing rituals and treatments (3).

Communication plays an important role in classical accounts of medicine

Hippocrates' first aphorism speaks of compliance, thus:

> Life is short and the art long; the occasion fleeting; experience fallacious, and judgment difficult. The physician must not only be prepared to do what is right himself, but also to make the patient, the attendants, and externals cooperate.

(4, p.292)

Hippocrates speaks about prognosis like someone who lived daily with the dying beyond help:

> ...by foreseeing and foretelling, in the presence of the sick, the present, past, and the future, ...he will be the more readily believed to be acquainted with the circumstances of the sick; so that men will have more confidence to entrust themselves to such a physician.

(4, p.42)

Galen in his account of caring for Marcus Aurelius uses observation and communication to win the Emperor's loyalty and he says the Emperor said of him:

> ...there is one physician who is not hide-bound by rules.... He is the first of Physicians...and of Philosophers. For Marcus [says Galen] had already had experience with many, not only desirous of money, but contentious, vain-glorious, envious and malignant.

(5, pp.51–2)

And so it goes through most of the greatest, Maimonides (6), Paracelsus, Peabody, *ad scholarum infinitum*. In the pre-scientific era, communication had an honoured place in the physician's work.

The stepchild status of communication in medicine: or is it the runt of the litter?

In the course of the gradual empiricism of medicine, the counting of dead bodies leading to vital statistics, the cutting of corpses leading to pathology, which in turn led to understandings of organs and disease specificities, communication remained but a stepchild. On the one hand, it was and is the medium of care, and so as little noticed as water by fish. On the other, ambitious and righteous pioneers, striving to render their approach the orthodox one, tended to overstate the importance of whatever was their focus and to diminish, or even dismiss, the thing not counted (by them) as soft, subjective, trivial, or unnecessary, a still prevalent attitude of reductionist thinkers, who magically believe all levels of science can be reduced to the lowest.

Nor did the shaky nature of the business (up to 1910 or so, according to Henderson, the average patient meeting the average physician lacked an average chance of benefit), the presence in the field of the epidemiologically expected but nonetheless highly visible presence of scoundrels, fakes, and opportunists, and the ubiquity of physicians, including among them the weakest, fail to earn its comeuppance (7). Take Chaucer's Doctour of Phisik:

> In al this world ne was ther noon hym lyk
> To speke of phisik and of surgerye,
> For he was grounded in astronomye;
> He kepte his pacient a ful greet deel
> In hours, by his magik naturel...
> Therefore he loved gold in special.

(8, p.26)

Or consider Moliere's *Médecin Malgré Lui*, a mock doctor full of himself and absurd in spite of himself. Literature, up to this moment, is rife with fictional takes on medicine's and doctors' frailties. So is history, with the *Oxford Illustrated Companion to Medicine* featuring a section on doctor-murderers (9).

As well, the nature of the work leads to doctors playing important literary roles, from Chekov's dyspeptic, yet quiet, hero-victims of life's small inevitabilities, to the bystander in the *Death of Ivan Ilyich*, and to Drs Jekyll, Manette, and Zhivago. The straw-doctor has been the pawn of many from myriad fields, his communication especially vulnerable as the outward manifestation of his being, up to and including current authors on such topics as narrative medicine, medical ethics, or healthcare reform.

Education about communication reflects the greater world

Medical education on the subject of doctor's talk and behaviour reflects this greater world context consistently, from Flexner forward to the present. There is tedious consistency to the critiques of their peers by sensitive physician-authors writing about what is wrong with how doctors work and communicate, and about how they should and might improve. On the one hand, they are illiterate. They don't listen, care, take time, admit error or behave decently; on the other, they are too technical and scientific: they lack art!

So teaching about communication was ignored, left to advocates, seconded to psychiatry, and given short shrift in curricula and in study. At Harvard Medical School in 1966, the introduction to 'taking a history' was bimodal. First, students were given 'a little red book' (not Mao's), with a 'several hours long' laundry list of specialist-asserted 'essential' questions, to be asked in order, on penalty of incompleteness. Second, small groups were told things like, 'Taking a history is like playing music... now, go do it'.

The history of communication teaching and standard dogma (i.e. prevailing views) has evolved through a series of phases: the prehistoric, classical and ancient, rhetorical, exhortative/charismatic, descriptive empirical, experimental empirical and the consensus dulled by the dismal meta-analytic.

The rhetorical phase was marked by authors such as Osler and exemplified by Peabody in his 'The care of the patient' (1927) with its dictum, '...for the secret of the care of patients is in caring for the patient' (10). This phase is dubbed 'rhetorical' because its promulgators tended to great seniority and did not directly involve themselves in the creation or oversight of curriculum to ensure the promulgation of the values and behaviours they advocated from their experiential bases.

What came next? Great clinician-educators, such as William Morgan and George Engel, codified in 1969 an approach described as *The Clinical Approach to the Patient* (11), which embodies the content of 'the little red book', the wisdom of wise, psychoanalytic teachers, such as Sullivan, Frank, and Engel himself, and the implicit charismatic notion, 'do as I do and you will be as good as I am.' Such teachers were like those of prior eras in exhorting students to do well and right. They differed, however, from prior eras in including an overarching approach to care, claiming to set a standard, and finding time in the curriculum to teach the mandated skills. What was lacking from a current perspective were objective data that what they exhorted was of demonstrated value, concerning such outcomes as knowledge gained, skills acquired, skills enduring, and skills applied in practice. As well, communication was embedded in a broader approach and so relegated once again to hind tit, getting the few remaining drops of curricular milk after 'auscultating the heart' and 'examining the retina' had gorged on hours of teaching time about their highly specific skills (and as recent studies have shown, also not positively and durably changing behaviour: the dysfunction of curricular obesity). Down the road, several authors evolved highly specific, but not empirically-derived methods, for talking with cancer patients. Over time, some of these have been partially, although usually not independently, evaluated.

While Morgan and Engel's approach (11) was being published and a powerful, charismatic series of papers was added by Engel (12), a small revolution began unnoticed by the senior exhorters. This was in the systematic examination of actual interviews, pioneered by Korsch and colleagues in 1968 (13). She captured sequential interviews in a paediatrics emergency department and showed what was really happening according to a rudimentary classification scheme.

The bottom line was that the doctors and the parents were speaking different languages, with arbitrary and unpredictable points of intersection. This work permanently changed the communication analysis business.

Prior to that, there was an enormous literary (narratives with embellishments) literature, with the tone set by psychosomaticians like Groddeck and psychoanalysts like Freud, Jung, and their acolytes. For 70 years or so, schools of thought and care were fashioned, based upon interviews, with sequences of them remembered in scholarly tranquillity by towering figures of unassailable authority, whose actual speech and interaction were unavailable for validation, correction, or bias filtration. Of course, there were sporadic recordings made on audio- and video-recorders, often analysed endlessly and tendentiously. But it was the advent of a practical, real, medical world (as opposed to studio or one-way mirror room) taping that permitted the modern era of communication investigations to begin.

Modern communication analysis

The real innovation, which ensured that a valid and reproducible empirical base of information would evolve into semi-quantitative analysis, eventually justifying models and theory, was foreshadowed by Bales who, for sociological research purposes, invented his interactional analysis method (14). In this method, an encounter was captured on tape and then every thought or phrase, technically an *utterance*, was arranged into a set of categories that were mutually exclusive (every utterance went into just one bin) and exhaustive (a bin could be found for every utterance). In the early 70s, Deborah Roter adapted the Bales method to medical interviews, first for her doctoral thesis and subsequently in print (15).

The Roter Interactional Analysis Scheme (RIAS) became the gold standard method of evaluating what is actually happening verbally in interviews (see Chapter 62). Highly reliable, reproducible, and relevant, at higher reproducibility and coding reliability rates than most research or clinical tests, it categorizes every utterance into one of 34 categories that most subsequent authors have found adequate for their thinking and analysis. Since then, Roter and her colleagues have added items and subscales to especially reflect content needs of particular areas, such as the emergency room or palliative care. In 2000, Fallowfield and Ford added the ability to analyse utterances in sequence and for meaning, thus creating an analytic tool (the MIPS, for Medical Interaction Process System) specifically evolved for evaluation of cancer care communication quality and education (16).

Currently, there is a vast array of such instruments that have been created by investigators striving to pin something particular down or simply to do it their way (see Chapter 61). Pendleton characterized these systems as being of five types: sociolinguistic, non-verbal, clinical process, verbal content or evaluative (17). The differing nuances, while permitting researchers finesse and subtlety, renders comparison across studies sometimes thorny. Nevertheless, using such schema, researchers have demonstrated that when communication is done better, health outcomes (such as blood pressure and glycaemic control) and systems outcomes (such as patient and practitioner satisfaction, return visit rate, medical error rates, and malpractice suits) can result in considerable improvement.

Inui and colleagues strikingly critiqued this approach as stripping rich interactions of meaning, reproaching RIAS and related interactional schema as being like a critic who would describe Hamlet as a '...play with 21 principal characters, a ghost, a group of players, ...' and numerous what-ho's (18, 19). This is rather like attacking physics as stripping a rainbow of its colour by describing it as the refraction of light by the atmosphere. Readers of Roter and her followers (20), and users of RIAS and MIPS, will have noted that the attempt to create an empirical, reproducible, and valid method need not preclude awareness or valuing of meaning. What Inui was on to is that studying meaning lags behind other aspects of understanding how doctors and patients ought to talk together to optimize outcomes of their mutual work. In reviewing such systems, Wasserman and Inui asserted that schema such as Roter's ought to:

> ...take into account the salient dimensions of interpersonal communications...characterize information exchange that occurs through several channels: through tone of voice, sighing, pauses...(and) gesture, facial expression...the context...and the sequencing of communication behaviours...and attempt to change behaviour in light of such lessons...

(18)

A tall order not yet fulfilled by a single system. The reader is urged to recall Peabody in considering the application of scientific methods to the processes of medicine and of medical education. He wrote, in 'The care of the patient':

> There is no more contradiction between the science of medicine and the art of medicine than between the science of aeronautics and the art of flying. Good practice presupposes an understanding of the sciences which contribute to the structure of modern medicine, but it is obvious that sound professional training should include a much broader equipment.

(10)

The Lipkin model and the American Academy on Communication in Healthcare

It was in pursuit of such a 'much broader equipment' that in 1979, Lipkin and Putnam initiated the first interest group in the Society of General Internal Medicine (then SREPCIM), which came to be called the 'Task Force on the Doctor and Patient', growing in 1993 into the current American Academy on Communication in Healthcare (AACH). Lipkin, a colleague of George Engel, and Putnam, a collaborator with Bill Stiles in creating an interactional process analytical method, recognized that the then evolving new science required an innovative basis for teaching and practice. They and their colleagues believed that, precisely as in cardiology or chemotherapy, what is said and done by doctors and by teachers of doctors should, where feasible, have an empirical basis, a theoretical structure, sound values, and be taught using demonstrably effective methods.

The 'Task Force on the Doctor and Patient' began to do bootstrap self-education. In 1984, Lipkin *et al.* published a comprehensive curriculum for the medical interview that provided a roadmap for the teaching and research of the group (21). The curriculum had four general objectives: patient-centred interviewing and treatment; an integrated approach to clinical reasoning and patient care; personal development of humanistic values; and psychosocial and psychiatric medicine. Each objective had extensive, empirical (where possible) knowledge, skills and attitudes specified. It discussed teaching strategies, options, and evaluation. Within the same time-frame, two other task force participants, Cohen-Cole and Bird, described three functions of the interview:

(1) gathering information;

(2) developing a relationship; and

(3) communicating information;

noting that specific teachable behaviours could be allocated to each function (22). Regular meetings of this developing, invisible college of interested persons led to a surprising recognition, that even the best teachers and biggest experts needed significant work on their own skills.

In response to this need, Lipkin in 1982 (23) invented a course model that synthesized educational ideas from Engel (12), Freire (24), Rogers (25, 26), and Knowles (27). It used small groups to both learn about personal skills and how to improve them, and how to integrate such learning into the real world and daily practice. It used Rogerian group methods to help the learner overcome any personal barriers to progress, which appeared rooted in his or her own development and psychological structures. It used a task focus to synthesize and foster integration of these learnings. The progress achieved was a method that used specifically appropriate teaching methods to accomplish explicit, higher order learning challenges, and proceeded to help the learner synthesize and integrate these.

In 1983, Novack and Clark initially directed what became a still ongoing annual course on teaching interviewing (28), which spawned similar courses in the United Kingdom, under the auspices of the Medical Interview Teachers Association and now has offshoots in Scandinavia, Switzerland, and Italy. The Lipkin Model has been documented to change knowledge, skills, and attitudes (23); to demonstrate a dose response (29); to change real world behaviour in the short term and durably; to elicit personal growth and transformational experiences in learners (30); and to be applicable across higher order learning situations as in cancer care, substance abuse, disaster response (31), pain management, and education itself (32). It has grown and evolved as the major model of the AACH and many of its trainees. The place of communication teaching in medical school curricula had shifted from being present in roughly 35% of US schools in 1978 to about 75% in 1992 (28).

Cancer research campaign studies in the United Kingdom

In the United Kingdom during the 1980s, Peter Maguire showed that teaching students about communication processes early in medical school changed behaviour, that the changes endured, and that they generalized over time (33). The gap between the experimental, well-taught groups of students and those taught in the usual (charismatic) manner was not only meaningful and significant, but over five years it continued to widen. Maguire's curriculum, however, was rather general, his main technique being focused on feedback, but the rest was undocumented. When tested in varied health practitioners (doctors, nurses, social workers) with cancer care experience, greater patient disclosure of information resulted from the use of empathic statements, open, directive questions, focus on the psychological, and summarizing (34). For this purpose, he developed a new, cancer research campaign rating system (35).

Fallowfield translated the Lipkin Model into the cancer care setting in the United Kingdom, and over the next decade, evolved it in her team's ongoing studies of its effectiveness (29, 36). She set out to use real patient outcomes with practicing cancer specialists. She first showed that her adaptation of the Lipkin Model had a dose-response and worked better in 3-day than in 1.5-day courses (29). She went on to show experimentally in follow-up at one year that cancer doctors made good use of focused questions (34%), open questions (27%), fewer inappropriate interruptions, and more empathic statements (69%), fewer leading questions (24%), and more recognition of non-verbal and affective cues (37). This remains the most powerful rigorously documented result of communication training in medicine.

European and other studies

In Belgium, Razavi's group showed subsequently that some communication skills training outcomes are enhanced by follow-up consolidation workshops (38). In Chapter 55, the Swiss model makes particular use of post-training supervision to consolidate gains in skills. Other approaches have been developed that overlap with those described. For example, in Chapter 54, the 'Oncotalk'

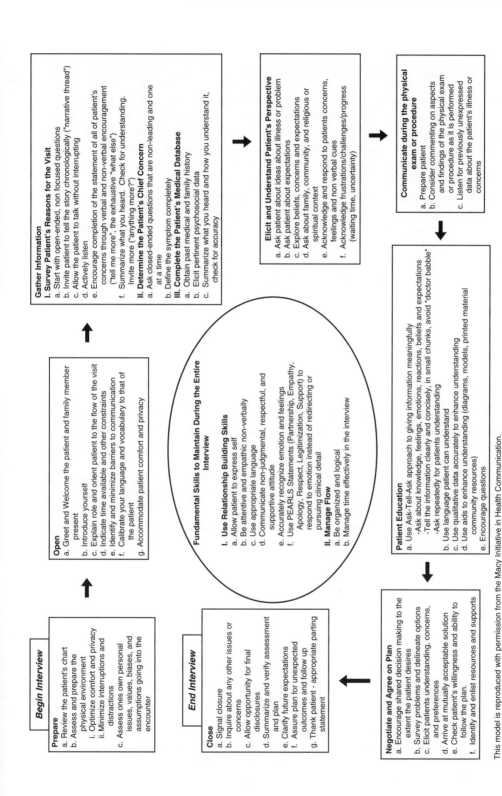

Begin Interview

Prepare
a. Review the patient's chart
b. Assess and prepare the physical environment
   i. Optimize comfort and privacy
   ii. Minimize interruptions and distractions
c. Assess ones own personal issues, values, biases, and assumptions going into the encounter

Open
a. Greet and Welcome the patient and family member present
b. Introduce yourself
c. Explain role and orient patient to the flow of the visit
d. Indicate time available and other constraints
e. Identify and minimize barriers to communication
f. Calibrate your language and vocabulary to that of the patient
g. Accommodate patient comfort and privacy

Gather Information
I. Survey Patient's Reasons for the Visit
a. Start with open-ended, non focused questions
b. Invite patient to tell the story chronologically ("narrative thread")
c. Allow the patient to talk without interrupting
d. Actively listen
e. Encourage completion of the statement of all of patient's concerns through verbal and non-verbal encouragement ("tell me more", the exhaustive "what else")
f. Summarize what you heard. Check for understanding. Invite more ("anything more?")
II. Determine the Patient's Chief Concern
a. Ask closed-ended questions that are non-leading and one at a time
b. Define the symptom completely
III. Complete the Patient's Medical Database
a. Obtain past medical and family history
b. Elicit pertinent psychosocial data
c. Summarize what you heard and how you understand it, check for accuracy

Elicit and Understand Patient's Perspective
a. Ask patient about ideas about illness or problem
b. Ask patient about expectations
c. Explore beliefs, concerns and expectations
d. Ask about family, community, and religious or spiritual context
e. Acknowledge and respond to patients concerns, feelings and non verbal cues
f. Acknowledge frustrations/challenges/progress (waiting time, uncertainty)

Communicate during the physical exam or procedure
a. Prepare patient
b. Consider commenting on aspects and findings of the physical exam or procedure as it is performed
c. Listen for previously unexpressed data about the patient's illness or concerns

Fundamental Skills to Maintain During the Entire Interview

I. Use Relationship Building Skills
a. Allow patient to express self
b. Be attentive and empathic non-verbally
c. Use appropriate language
d. Communicate non-judgmental, respectful, and supportive attitude
e. Accurately recognize emotion and feelings
f. Use PEARLS Statements (Partnership, Empathy, Apology, Respect, Legitimization, Support) to respond to emotion instead of redirecting or pursuing clinical detail

II. Manage Flow
a. Be organized and logical
b. Manage time effectively in the interview

Patient Education
a. Use Ask-Tell-Ask approach to giving information meaningfully
   -Ask about knowledge, feelings, emotions, reactions, beliefs and expectations
   -Tell the information clearly and concisely, in small chunks, avoid "doctor babble"
   -Ask repeatedly for patients understanding
b. Use language patient can understand
c. Use qualitative data accurately to enhance understanding
d. Use aids to enhance understanding (diagrams, models, printed material community resources)
e. Encourage questions

End Interview

Close
a. Signal closure
b. Inquire about any other issues or concerns
c. Allow opportunity for final disclosures
d. Summarize and verify assessment and plan
e. Clarify future expectations
f. Assure plan for unexpected outcomes and follow up
g. Thank patient - appropriate parting statement

Negotiate and Agree on Plan
a. Encourage shared decision making to the extent the patient desires
b. Survey problems and delineate options
c. Elicit patients understanding, concerns, and preferences
d. Arrive at mutually acceptable solution
e. Check patient's willingness and ability to follow the plan.
f. Identify and enlist resources and supports

This model is reproduced with permission from the Macy Initiative in Health Communication.

Fig. 1.1 Structure and sequence of effective doctor–patient communication.

model describes improvement in giving bad news and discussing transitions to palliative care. While showing skills improvement, the use of a non-experimental design and only immediately post-training, standardized patient evaluations limits the validity of claims of superiority of this system.

Rao *et al.* (39) performed a systematic review of 36 randomized controlled trials in which educational interventions were evaluated using objective measures of verbal communication behaviours on physician (18), patient (15), or both (3). This meta-analytic review reduces these rather complex studies to their least common denominator, concluding that higher ratings by physicians occurred when skills practice with feedback occurred and that outcomes included commonly taught behaviours, such as those reported above.

One recent synthesis of communication skills training was expressed in a highly condensed form in the two Kalamazoo consensus statements (40, 41). These were significantly influenced by the more extensive Macy Project in Health Communication (42). In this project, a process of faculty survey, literature review, and expert opinion was used to evolve a set of 60 or so 'competencies' or behaviours, expressed so as to be measurable, believed to be essential for graduating physicians (42). These were organized in a logical schema depicting the flow of the medical interview, as shown in Fig. 1.1. Each of the major headings contains sub-items that are behaviourally expressed, measurable using simple techniques, and empirically derived. A cohort, controlled study demonstrated that this complex set of skills (the evaluation measured some 30, which had been blinded to the curricular designers) could be taught and significantly changed behaviour over a year (43).

Conclusion

By 1993, a consensus was emerging concerning what was empirically validated as the core of teach-worthy communication skills. One example was the Toronto consensus statement (44). In 1995, the AACH published its authoritative reference text, which covered clinical care, education, and research as an exposition of communication training for internal and family medicine (45). Since then, although there have been serial syntheses and consensus efforts (always a moving target), the core principles of communication skills training have remained quite stable, once one translates the babble of new language for common concepts.

Thus, at this point in the evolution of work between doctors and patients, we can fairly say that we know what ought to be done, we can teach it to medical students, residents, and practitioners, and doing so improves important outcomes of care, as well as patient and practitioner satisfaction in their mutual and important work.

References

1. Lipkin M (2008). The medical interview. In: Feldman M, Christiansen J, eds. *Behavioural Medicine*, 3rd edition, pp.1–9. McGraw Hill Medical, New York.
2. Fabrega Jr HF (1999). *Evolution of Sickness and Healing*. University of California Press, Berkeley.
3. Kleinman A, Eisenberg M, Good B (1978). Culture, illness, and care: clinical lessons from anthropologic and cross-cultural research. *Ann Int Med* **88**, 251–58.
4. Hippocrates, Adams F (1849). *The Genuine Works of Hippocrates*. Translated by Francis Adams, Sydenham Society. Kessinger, New York.
5. Clendening L (1942). Galen Prognostics XI. In: Clendening L, ed. *Source Book of Medical History, Compiled with Notes by Logan Clendening*, pp.51–2. Dover, New York.
6. Nuland SB (2005). *Maimonides (Jewish Encounters)*. Schocken, New York.

7. Henderson LJ (1987). Quoted in Stoeckle JD. Encounters between patients and doctors, pp.1–2. MIT Press, Cambridge.

8. Gray D (2003). *The Oxford Companion to Chaucer*. OUP, Oxford.

9. Locke S, Last JM, Dunea G (2001). *Oxford Illustrated Companion to Medicine*. OUP, Oxford.

10. Peabody FW (1927). The care of the patient. *JAMA* **88**, 877–82.

11. Morgan WL, Engel GL (1969). *The Clinical Approach to the Patient*. Saunders, New York.

12. Engel GL (1980). The clinical application of the biopsychosocial model. *Am J Psychiatry* **137**, 107–11.

13. Korsch BM, Gozzi E, Francis F (1968). Gaps in doctor patient communication. *Pediatrics* **42**, 855–71.

14. Bales RF (1950). *Interaction Process Analysis*. Addison Wesley, Cambridge.

15. Roter DL (1977). Patient participation in the patient-provider interaction: the effects of patient question asking on the quality of interaction, satisfaction and compliance. *Health Educ Monogr* **5**, 281–315.

16. Ford S, Hall A, Ratcliff D, *et al.* (2000). The Medical Interaction Process System (MIPS): an instrument for analyzing interviews of oncologists and patients with cancer. *Soc Sci Med* **50**, 553–66.

17. Pendleton D (1983). Doctor-patient communication. A review. In: Pendleton D, Hasler J, eds. *Doctor-patient Communication*. Academic Press, London.

18. Wasserman RC, Inui TS (1983). Systematic analysis of clinician-patient interactions: a critique of recent approaches with suggestions for future research. *Med Care* **21**, 279–312.

19. Inui TS, Carter WB (1985). Problems and prospects for health services research on provider-patient communication. *Med Care*, **23**, 521–38.

20. Stewart M, Roter D (1989). *Communicating with Medical Patients*. Sage, London.

21. Lipkin M, Quill T, Napadano RJ (1984). The medical interview: a core curriculum for residencies in internal medicine. *Ann Int Med* **100**, 277–83.

22. Cohen-Cole SA, Bird J (1991). *The Medical Interview: the Three-Function Approach*. Mosby, St. Louis.

23. Lipkin M, Kaplan C, Clark W, *et al.* (1995). Teaching medical interviewing: the Lipkin Model. In: Lipkin M Jr., Putnam S, Lazare A, eds. *The Medical Interview: Clinical Care, Education and Research*. Springer-Verlag, New York.

24. Freire P (1986). *Pedagogy of the Oppressed*. Continuum, New York.

25. Rogers CR (1970). *On Encounter Groups*. Harper and Row, New York.

26. Rogers CR (1983). *Freedom to Learn for the 80s*. Merrill, Columbus OH.

27. Knowles MS (1980). *The Modern Practice of Adult Education: from Pedagogy to Androgogy*. Adult Education Company, New York.

28. Novack DH, Volk G, Drossman DA, *et al.* (1993). Medical interviewing and interpersonal skills teaching in US medical schools: progress, problems, and promise. *JAMA* **269**, 2101–5.

29. Fallowfield L, Lipkin M, Hall A (1998). Teaching senior oncologists communication skills: results from phase I of a comprehensive longitudinal program in the United Kingdom. *J Clin Onc* **16**, 1961–8.

30. Kern DE, Wright SM, Carrese JA, *et al.* (2001). Personal growth in medical faculty: a qualitative study. *West J Med* **175(2)**, 92–8.

31. Zabar S, Kalet AL, Kachur EK, *et al.* (2004). Practicing bioterrorism-related psychosocial skills with standardized patients. *J Gen Intern Med* **19(s1)**, 109–241.

32. Pololi L, Clay MC, Lipkin Jr M, *et al.* (2001). Reflections on integrating theories of adult education into a medical school faculty development course. *Medical Teacher* **23**, 276–83.

33. Maguire P, Fairbairn S, Fletcher C (1986). Consultation skills of young doctors—benefits of feedback training in interviewing as students persists. *Br Med J* **292**, 1573–8.

34. Maguire P, Faulkner A, Booth K, *et al.* (1996). Helping cancer patients disclose their concerns. *Euro J Cancer* **32A**, 78–81.

35. Maguire P, Booth K (1991). Development of a rating system to assess interaction between cancer patients and health professionals. *Report to the Cancer Research Campaign*. CRC, London.

36. Fallowfield L, Jenkins V, Farewell V, *et al.* (2002). Efficacy of a cancer research UK communication skills training model for oncologists: A randomized controlled trial. *Lancet* **359**, 650–7.

37. Fallowfield L, Jenkins V, Farewell V, *et al.* (2003). Enduring impact of communication skills training: results of a 12-month follow-up. *Br J Cancer* **89**, 1445–9.

38. Merckaert I, Libert Y, Delvaux N, *et al.* (2008). Factors influencing physicians' detection of cancer patients' and relatives' distress: can a communication skills training program improve physicians' detection? *Psycho-Oncology* **17**, 260–9.

39. Rao JK, Anderson LA, Inui TS, *et al.* (2007). Communications interventions make a difference in conversations between physicians and patients. *Medical Care* **45**, 340–9.

40 . Makoul G (2001). Participants in the Bayer-Fetzer Conference on Physician Patient Communication in Medical Communication. Essential elements of communication in medical encounters: the Kalamazoo consensus statement. *Acad Med* **76**, 390–3.

41. Duffy FD, Gordon GH, Whelan G, *et al.* and all the participants in the American Academy on Physician and Patients Conference on Education and Evaluation of Competence in Communication and Interpersonal Skills. (2004) Assessing competence and interpersonal skills. The Kalamazoo II Report. *Acad Med* **79**.

42. Kalet A, Pugnaire MP, Cole-Kelly K, *et al.* (2004). Teaching communication in clinical clerkships: Models from the Macy initiative in health communications. *Acad Med* **79**, 511–20.43.

43. Yedidia MJ, Gillespie CC, Kachur E, *et al.* (2003). Effect of communications training on medical student performance. *JAMA* **290**, 1157–65.

44. Simpson M, Buckman R, Stewart M, *et al.* (1991). Doctor-patient communication: the Toronto consensus statement. *BMJ* **303**, 1385–7.

45. Lipkin Jr M, Putnam S, Lazare A, eds. (1995). *The Medical Interview: Clinical Care, Education and Research.* Springer-Verlag, New York.

Chapter 2

The art of teaching communication skills

Stewart M Dunn

It's easy to criticize us physicians for being paternalistic, for not telling the truth, for sugar-coating reality. But try to imagine what it's like when a young woman with advanced ovarian cancer walks through your door. She is 35 years old and has two kids. More than anything in the world she wants not to die. You tell her the prognosis, and that there is no good therapy for her, and she keeps saying, 'But, doctor, are you telling me there is absolutely no chance I'm going to get better?' You feel yourself back-sliding because you start thinking, 'Gee, how can I speak with that kind of certainty about anything? And how can I deny her even a tiny shred of hope?' That's when a word like 'truth' sort of loses its meaning.
Christakis NA, 2001, p.117.

Introduction

You'll forgive me if I bypass evidence-based navel-gazing about whether communication is important. Good communication in cancer is tough business, not for the faint-hearted. That's why so many times we are just too busy, too distracted, too tired or too afraid to do it well. And, like performing a Chopin Polonaise for a concert audience, it requires knowledge, competence and technical skill, delivered with commitment and passion. Not to mention managing perform-ance anxiety. Of course communication is important. It is an art!

And if communication is an art, it follows that teachers of communication must integrate the artistic components—timing, intuition, creativity—because they are essential drivers of good clinical decision-making. In turn, the art of teaching communication skills, so as to release innate skills, involves finding ways to balance safety with challenge and engagement with objectivity. Actress Megan Cole (who played the role of Dr Vivian Bearing in Margaret Edson's Pulitzer Prize-winning play, *Wit*, and subsequently developed an academic programme for medical profession-als about balancing engagement and attachment) describes it thus:

> When we make conscious choices about our behaviour and have techniques for balancing our involve-ment and non-involvement (which is, of course, what actors do) the fear of losing the Self in the Other is greatly diminished, because we are in control at all times.

(2, pp.38–40)

We make conscious choices…and, most importantly, we foster good relationships. Because, ultimately, good communication is about good relationships! The best doctors and nurses form meaningful relationships with all sorts of patients, under all sorts of situations. Not relationships based on the power of the clinician's personality, as illustrated by Shaw's description of Sir Ralph Bloomfield Bonnington:

> He radiates an enormous self-confidence, cheering, reassuring, healing by the fact that disease or anxiety are incompatible with his welcome presence. Even broken bones, it is said, have been known to unite at the sound of his voice.

(3, p.1339)

On the contrary, great clinical communicators are characterized by relationships that resonate with understanding, sensitivity and flexibility.

Roter and her colleagues waxed axiomatically about the role of emotions in healthcare:

(1) both clinicians and patients have emotions;

(2) both clinicians and patients show emotions; and

(3) both clinicians and patients judge each other's emotions (4).

The ability to judge another's emotional expressions is one of the defining facets of the concept of emotional intelligence and a cornerstone of good communication. Yet medicine has undergone a shift in culture, of which one manifestation is diminished attention to emotion and its role in the healing process.

This chapter explores core questions about teaching communication. Who are the right targets for teaching? How do we engage the people who need most help? What is the role of experience? How do we teach people to recognize and interpret their own emotion? How do we teach people to recognize and interpret emotion in others? How do we encourage people to explore beyond the human barriers that limit open communication?

The art of teaching communication

There are four essential elements to the art of teaching communication: the Task, the Learner, the Teacher and the Strategy. Linked together they look like Fig. 2.1.

The Learner: engaging the right audience at the right time

Who needs communication training? The default answer is, of course, all cancer clinicians. Cancer is a tough business and almost every encounter is fraught with emotion. In 1961, Donald Oken (5) identified the potency of the first experience of breaking bad news for young doctors—and that potency has not diminished 48 years later. In 2001, three out of four US medical trainees reported they first delivered bad news while a student or intern (6); 61% knew the patient for just hours or days; only 59% engaged in any planning; and a senior doctor was present in only 16% of cases. These young doctors rated the importance of skills in delivering bad news highly; they believed such skills can be improved and thought that more guidance should be offered to them during such activity. So the challenge is there to teach everyone.

But you cannot reach everyone; and most often you find yourself teaching the already committed. Reaching the wider community of cancer clinicians and, especially, the poor communicators, is daunting. Appeals to niceness and satisfaction are derided.

> What good are doctors who empathise, smile and maintain eye-contact if they don't know their stuff? How much better to have a brusque expert who can prescribe the right course of action.

(7, p.41)

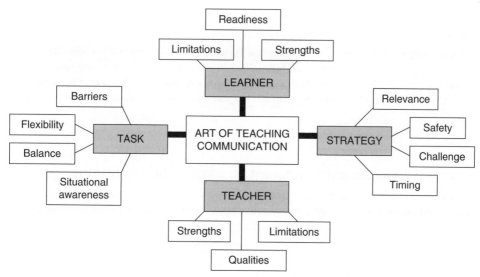

Fig. 2.1 Mind-mapping the art of teaching communication.

Of course, knowledge and competence are prerequisites; but this common and bizarre assumption that competence and compassion are mutually exclusive is consistent with neither anecdote nor evidence. Like great teachers or great concert performers, the best communicators have mastered the tools of trade.

So what will engage busy clinicians to learn more about communication? It does sometimes work to raise the spectre of litigation. A retrospective review of 444 surgical malpractice claims identified inexperience/lack of technical competence (41%) and communication breakdown (24%) as the leading system factors behind surgical error (8). The errant behaviours are well-described. For example, surgeons who convey higher levels of dominance and lower levels of concern or anxiety in their voice tones were much more likely to have been sued than other clinicians (9). In medical student examinations, standardized patients gave higher ratings when students faced them directly, used facilitative nodding, looked at them equally when talking and listening, and spoke at a similar speed and voice volume to them. Importantly, these effects remained significant after controlling for the quality of the interview content (10).

But using the threat of litigation is always a cheap shot at genuine improvement in communication; its legacy, when there is one, is most often plastic copies of learned behaviours. There is no genuineness or art. Moreover, patients see through the façade. A more universal appeal that resonates with busy health professionals, and certainly every cancer clinician, is the appeal to time management. Addressing their need to communicate with sensitivity, and with economy and efficiency, gets doctors' attention! In 2000–01, we conducted a randomized study of prompt sheets in routine oncology consultations (11). The results suggested that addressing the patient's agenda (and, in particular, the emotional agenda) at the start of the consultation, improved patient recall of information, reduced anxiety and shortened the consultation by 3–6 minutes. These are important and attractive outcomes for busy, time-poor clinicians.

We also need to face the sad reality that the art of communication will always elude some practitioners. Froelich in 1966 developed a comprehensive course for second-year medical students using a combination of a programmed manual, role-playing exercises, programmed patients and medical interviewing films, and the writing of medical histories. He concluded that some students were simply lost causes.

> Anyone who has taught in this area recognizes the impossibility of any technic (sic) or method encompassing this Art. No two situations are identical—two personalities are involved and more or less unduplicated case histories. Since this is an Art it can be taught only in sketches, and in the hope that after some hundreds of interviews as a clinical clerk and house officer a technique will evolve. Some never learn!
>
> (12, p.288)

Leaving it to experience: inherent strengths and limitations

It would be comforting to think that experience is a reliable teacher of communication skills or, even more optimistically, that experience generates an appreciation of the art of good clinical communication. Sadly, it appears not. Each of us has a variety of communication skills acquired from childhood—through meaningful interactions with significant others and through millions of trivial exchanges with strangers. Our successes and failures in these interactions leave us with a legacy of communicative strengths and weaknesses that define the limits of our ability to engage openly and transparently with others.

A number of attempts have been made to explore psychological characteristics of both patients and doctors that might be capacity-limiting. One example is Attachment Theory (13). John Bowlby proposed that individuals' early experiences with caregivers become internalized and form cognitive models that determine, for the individual, whether they are worthy of care and whether others can be trusted to provide care. These cognitive models influence the kinds of interactions individuals have with others and their interpretations of these interactions throughout the life-cycle. The relevance to medical practice is unmistakable: doctors must form relationships with patients, with other doctors and with other health professionals.

The dismissing, self-reliant style is reportedly common among medical practitioners and one recent study has shown that *dismissing attachment* in combination with poor patient-provider communication is associated with poorer treatment adherence in patients with diabetes (14). Attachment avoidance also comes at personal cost for the doctor. Insecure, avoidant adults learn to suppress negative thoughts and feelings, but exhibit heightened electrodermal reactivity in stressful situations (15, 16). Cancer clinicians who remain unaware of their own emotional limitations thus have a toxic potential for themselves, their colleagues and those who come under their care.

Where it begins is logically where we should first intervene. Medical students are characteristically anxious about their first approaches to patients on the ward. They feel helpless, voyeuristic and intrusive. Patients want information, assistance or engagement from the student; and the students are at the bottom of the hierarchy in a big teaching hospital. They have no information, feel (quite reasonably) useless, and are scared. We address students' initial fears about approaching patients on the wards by reminding them that they bring four unique 'powers' to the encounter:

1. Ignorance: they have no information about the patient or the disease, and thus they are closer to the patient's knowledge base and able to work collaboratively from that base.

2. No clinical responsibility: patients know they can discuss clinical issues freely with someone who has no authority to make clinical decisions.

3. Strangeness: they are strangers to the patient who can choose to explore deeply personal issues (like: 'how will I tell my children?') with an objective listener.

4. Time: as first-year students, they have more time to sit with patients than they will ever have again in their careers.

When students overcome their need to be busy and helpful (in the practical sense), they begin to appreciate the wisdom of the aphorism, 'Don't just do something, stand there'; they find a role for themselves that makes sense (17). A focus on strengths is a solid basis for developing new skills.

The Task: learning communication at the coalface

As students enter the world of the teaching hospital or community practice, reality takes a different hold. Time becomes the great leveller and any decision that involves more time at the bedside with the patient comes under intense scrutiny. A qualitative study of empathic communication during primary care office visits found that patients seldom verbalize their emotions directly and spontaneously, tending to offer clues instead. In the majority of cases the physicians allowed both clues and direct expressions of affect to pass without acknowledgment.

> The basic empathic skills seem to be recognizing when emotions may be present but not directly expressed, inviting exploration of these unexpressed feelings, and effectively acknowledging these feelings so the patient feels understood. The frequent lack of acknowledgment by physicians of both direct and indirect expressions of affect poses a threat to the patient-physician relationship and warrants further study.

> (18, p.678)

We attempted to quantify these cues and oncologists' responses using transcripts of audiotapes from almost 300 patients with heterogeneous cancers, seeing one of five medical and four radiation oncologists for the first time (19). The doctor's response to informational and emotional cues was coded according to a standardized system. The results were less than inspiring and reflected the pressures on busy oncologists with too many patients and too little time.

Patients asked a median of 11 questions and gave two cues per consultation, usually during treatment discussions. Responses to 72% of informational and 28% of emotional cues were rated appropriate; 15% of informational and 38% of emotional cues were ignored. Gratifyingly, only 3.7% of all cues were postponed and 2.3% of all cues were interrupted by the doctor. So, busy clinicians block emotional cues as a matter of routine. This is no surprise. What is surprising is the analysis of those who did not block: informational and emotional cues were addressed *without lengthening the consultation or increasing patient anxiety.*

Pollak *et al.* (20) analysed a sample of almost 400 clinic transcripts with 51 oncologists and 270 patients. They coded for the presence of empathic opportunities and oncologist responses. In all, 37% of consultations contained at least one empathic opportunity. Oncologists responded with continuers 22% of the time, with females and younger oncologists more likely to respond. So, we have the same problem: for most patients, their emotional overtures go unanswered.

Strategies for teaching young clinicians

Against the background of innate and learned skills that young clinicians bring to medical communication, the art of teaching communication involves two key elements:

◆ Safety: initial interactions with patients need structure and rules so students feel safe to explore, to make mistakes and learn from them; rules can be bent later.

◆ Challenge: situations must be structured so as to engage students at their current level of awareness and skill, and to challenge them both intellectually and emotionally.

From a very small cluster of recent studies, there seems to be an emerging picture of the characteristics of people who demonstrate mastery of communication. Students who excel appear to be instantly recognizable to actor/patients, other students and staff. Austin *et al.* (21), in a study of empathy levels in 273 medical students, found that students who score high on emotional intelligence, and those who are good at reading the emotions of others, are perceived by their peers to be more effective in these groups. Gender, too, plays an important role. Wiskin and colleagues' study of 512 final-year medical students suggests that female students are better at communicating successfully under the stress of examination conditions (22).

Safety and challenge can be augmented by identifying students' innate capacities in problem-solving and working from these strengths. Understanding their own learning styles, for instance, allows students to focus away from their own performance and to attempt different strategies. The original Honey and Mumford classification (23) identified four learning styles: reflector, theorist, pragmatist and activist. While the psychometric properties of the scales remain debatable, they provide one means for clinicians to appreciate the potential for flexibility in responding to patient emotion (24).

The value of this sort of teaching is apparent if one examines what happens when the learning styles of doctor and patient are mismatched. Clack and colleagues found that their sample of 464 doctors differed significantly from UK adult population norms on most of the dimensions of personality measured, including their preferred mode for new learning (25). This suggests potential points for miscommunication in the doctor–patient consultation. Of the UK population, 40% preferred the *reflector* mode and would have only a 1 in 6 chance of seeing a doctor with the same preference. The 31% of doctors with preferences for the *theorist* mode would have only a 1 in 11 chance of a match with the patient. As Clack *et al.* put it:

> If the two individuals involved in the interaction differ to this extent, they are likely to be talking on different wavelengths, resulting in potential misunderstandings unless there is some adjustment or 'flexing' of style.

(25, p.184)

The authors suggest that a lack of accommodation of doctors' interaction styles to these differences may partly explain complaints about poor communication, and patients' lack of understanding and poor compliance. If experienced clinicians learn how to do this through trial and error over many years, perhaps medical students may benefit from learning these differences early in their training, so they develop the ability to adjust their style more quickly.

If learning styles offer insights into how doctors manage patients, they also add to our understanding of how learners respond to teachers. Lewis and Bolden in 1989 showed that the learning styles of hospital tutors and general practitioner trainers were statistically significantly different from those of non-trainer principals and trainees. As you would expect, the tutors and trainers scored much higher on *theorist* styles. Since teachers tend to teach in their preferred learning style, there is often a mismatch with the style of the recipients (26).

The evidence for effective strategies

Communication skills training is not new (27–29). Scientific studies of communication, quite naturally, talk about outcomes and skills that are observable and measurable. But the art of communication does not begin and end with what is measurable—although evidence suggests that those who possess the art are instantly recognizable, i.e. observable. Diligent scientists have exhaustively coded specific measurable behaviours like 'head cock', and this specificity, they argue, holds promise as an evaluation technique and better clarifies which specific behaviours are most critical in influencing patient satisfaction (30).

This confusion between process and outcomes is a core problem for meaningful research into communication training. To capture the artistic qualities of communication and communication training, we need more sensitive measures of process and we need research models beyond the purely quantitative. Small-group teaching is particularly suited for complex skills, such as communication. But, while existing work has identified the basic elements of small-group teaching, few descriptions of higher-order teaching practices exist in the medical literature (31). Ward and Stein concluded that too much teaching emphasis has been placed on content and not enough on the process of the interview (32). They argue that the doctor–patient interaction creates an interpersonal environment that determines how productive the interview will be in terms of generating accurate and natural responses from the patient. Reproducing the outcome behaviours does not generate the underlying process. Actions without objectives are aimless. We hope that models described in this book do much to redress this gap.

Communication skills can be improved by training. There have been two Cochrane reviews. One, cancer-specific, found communication skills do not reliably improve with experience alone and that training programmes were effective in improving some areas of cancer communication skills (33). A second, examining more general patient-centred training, found that interventions to promote patient-centred care within clinical consultations may significantly increase the patient-centredness of care (34). Other systematic reviews confirm that training improves basic communication skills across a broad range of training objectives, including improving the medical interview, assessment of psychological distress, imparting distressing information, counselling, problem solving and assessment of patients' needs for information (35, 36).

Other lengthy interventions confirm the efficacy of skills training but there appears to be a clear deficiency in the transfer of learned communication skills to clinical practice (37–39). What can we do about this? Razavi and his colleagues suggest:

◆ additional training modules;
◆ information about factors, both internal and contextual, that interfere with physicians' implementation of learned skills;
◆ role-playing exercises that focus on assessment and supportive skills.

In addition to this list, we need to address the teaching capabilities of the trainers and investigate the extent to which initial training taps into underlying issues of personal boundaries and emotional engagement. It is unlikely that initial training can be consolidated unless trainees are intensely engaged (40).

The links between research studies need more critical examination. Here is a recent example. Back and colleagues designed a residential communication skills workshop (Oncotalk) about giving bad news and discussing transitions to palliative care for medical oncology fellows (41). The pre-/post-intervention cohort study involved 115 fellows from 62 different institutions during the 3-year study. The primary outcomes were observable changes in participants' communication skills measured during standardized patient assessments (SPA), before and after the workshop. These SPA were audio-recorded and assessed by blinded coders using a validated coding system. Participants acquired a mean of 5.4 new skills in breaking bad news; for example, 16% of participants used the word 'cancer' when giving bad news before the workshop, and 54% used it after the workshop.

One critic of the Oncotalk programme argued that the acquisition of a skills set cannot be concluded to improve communication skills until the skills themselves are shown to be effective at improving the patient experience (42). The efficacy of training, they suggested, would be better demonstrated by examining changes in the participants' real practice, recording encounters in the clinic and using patient satisfaction data as a more representative outcome measure.

Other research already confirms that there is a link between the word 'cancer' and patient outcomes (43). Simply using the word 'cancer' in a questionnaire about cancer adjustment generated anxiety to levels similar to those reported in general medical and surgical patients; however, it did not produce any distortion in reported adjustment. On the other hand, any ambiguity associated with the conditions under which adjustment was assessed, led to distortion and an increase in the patient's reported psychological distress. So there is evidence that changing this specific behaviour is an important outcome for cancer patients. Sadly, however, there is plenty of breathing space between acquiring a skill, like using a specific word, and true competence as a communicator.

Teaching empathic engagement

Since the early 1980s, the American Board of Internal Medicine has required that evidence of a candidate's humanism (i.e. integrity, empathy, compassion and respect for the patient) be provided for board certification. Many eloquent writers (whose wisdom is sadly banished by the rigours of Level 1 evidence-based reviews) have supported this view:

> [Doctors]… have to treat illness rather than disease and need to understand the feelings of regret, guilt, fear, betrayal, loneliness, and other perplexing emotions that turn the same disease into different illnesses in different people.
>
> (44, p.323)

Not surprisingly, physicians appear to be poor judges of emotion. They misread cues of patient distress and tend to rate patients' emotional state and satisfaction with the consultation more negatively than patients. Roter and her colleagues posed important questions: Will greater insight into one's own emotional responses facilitate non-verbal skill acquisition? Is self-awareness related to higher levels of non-verbal sensitivity and emotional intelligence? How might the sensitive and highly emotional issues of transference and counter-transference be best addressed within the training context? How might we best encourage and facilitate emotional self-awareness, without breaching boundaries of privacy and confidentiality?

We are not talking political correctness here. We are talking about a rational, evidence-based approach to the art of teaching communication. Our research, for example, shows that there are times when patients do not necessarily want patient-centred care, and we need to acknowledge flexibility in both patients' needs and our own responses (45).

Empathy is a respectful understanding of what others are experiencing. It is listening with the whole being! We engage with the other person and we give them time and space to express themselves fully and to be understood. Empathy can only occur when we have successfully shed all preconceived ideas and judgments about the other person. For most medical students, this is an inherently painful experience. Young doctors, sadly, lose themselves and their awareness of the power of empathy in the desire to be pragmatically useful. While some people may be more intuitively empathic in their interpersonal style, empathic behaviours can be taught. A model for the evolution of empathy is presented in Fig. 2.2.

Most interactions between patient and professional involve low emotional arousal. However, acute emergencies, diagnosis of life-threatening disease and disease progression confront the health professional with patients in high levels of distress. Fig. 2.2 identifies three categories of professional response when a patient presents with high arousal.

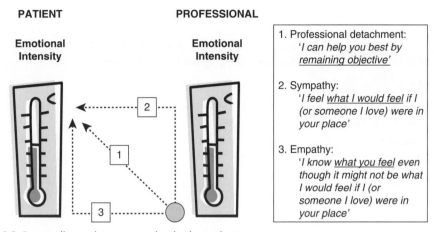

Fig. 2.2 Responding to intense emotion in the patient.

- Pathway 1 involves professional detachment that protects the doctor from becoming caught up in the patient's emotion and allows clear-headed, dispassionate decision-making. It seems self-evident that the anxious patient wants a professional who is competent and rational. The down-side—when things go wrong—is that objectivity can be re-interpreted as a lack of compassion and commitment.

- Pathway 2 describes identification with the subjective experience of the patient, 'putting oneself in the shoes of the patient'. This is sympathy and it arises from one's own life experience and one's ability to imagine how one would feel in the same situation. Medical students experience this personal anguish early in their careers when they confront real-life examples of human suffering. It is potentially burnout territory.

- Pathway 3 is empathy, the accurate appreciation of the patient's experience and emotional state, even though that might be quite different from the professional's personal response to the same situation. This is based on long experience of different people in similar circumstances. It takes time and reflective analysis to acquire.

In this model, the art of communication skills training can then be defined as activities directed at accelerating the progression from pathway 2 to pathway 3 by condensing unstructured life experience into a series of intense structured learning experiences.

The teacher

Teaching about *how to teach* is a glaring omission from most medical curricula; and it will receive limited attention here just as it does in the published literature. Yet it is the cornerstone of medical training. A study of Dutch postgraduate training in general practice (GP) failed to demonstrate acquisition of communication skills of trainees during a 27-month training period, despite the fact that skills like 'exploration of expectations and feelings' were strongly emphasized during the training (46). And why did communication skills not improve? Because the trainers were not much better! The performance of GP trainers was comparable to that of trainees, suggesting that they did not have the capacity to improve trainee performance. The Dutch authors, therefore, recommended communication skills training for the GP instructors if they are to become effective role models. It is time to question the wisdom of the dictum 'see one, do one, teach one' (47).

To finish, here is a quick exercise: think of the best teacher you have ever known. Perhaps someone from your professional education, or perhaps a high school or primary school teacher, a music teacher, a debating or sports coach! What was it that made this teacher outstanding?

Most health professionals cite from the following list of characteristics:

◆ patience;

◆ respect;

◆ humour;

◆ compassion;

◆ feedback;

◆ interaction;

◆ authority and engagement;

◆ enthusiasm and encouragement;

◆ awareness of teaching moments;

◆ emphasis on learning from mistakes;

◆ balance between discipline and enjoyment;

◆ concern with process and perspective, not just content;

◆ commitment to, and confidence in, the learner's experience.

Teaching communication skills is a combination of art and science. And the best teaching of communications skills incorporates all of these elements in the teaching environment. The key elements to new insight are safety and challenge. Trainees must feel safe to reflect on experience, to try different alternatives and to make mistakes, to identify individual barriers and to find new ways to overcome them. Safety comes from being with people who actively encourage the learner; who do not just tolerate error, but actively seek to exploit it to advance learning. Passion is experienced through feedback that captures the essential excitement of human communication, supplemented by a thorough knowledge of evidence-based research.

Teaching communications skills is not about teaching words or actions. It is not about technique, despite the inevitable fact that evaluation of communication skills captures mostly measurable outcomes. It is about teaching understanding of purpose and meaning. Coulehan (48) sets us a potential target for teaching that captures the art of communication: we should strive to impart emotional resilience—characterized by Coulehan as a combination of steadiness (reason and fortitude) and tenderness (humanity and compassion).

> I now understand that detached concern is a risk or failure of medical education, rather than an appropriate goal. Detachment ought to be avoided because it leads to emotional numbness and a general discounting of the affective life. On the contrary, a key feature in professional education ought to be the development of what I have come to call emotional resilience, a resilience that allows one to experience fully the emotional dynamics of patient care as an essential part of—rather than a detriment to—good medical practice.
>
> (48, p. 225)

Conclusion

The art of teaching communication skills for the clinician is about establishing practices that serve the patients' and their families' needs in a manner that is mutually fulfilling for all involved. It requires the tactful use of boundaries that are patrolled and negotiated and, at all times, mindful of the needs of both parties. As a result, a series of conundrums can plague the teaching of communication skills. We do well to be mindful of these:

1. The balance of art and science in clinical communication fluctuates throughout medical training and experience.

2. Communication involves skills, but it is more than behavioural skills, also requiring much practical wisdom.

3. What can be measured is often far removed from the core of effective communication.

4. Flexibility is lost when we act as if communication can be reduced to simple reproducible behaviours.

5. The pressure to publish can generate a pressure to measure so that science dominates a landscape that truly incorporates both science and art.

6. Some aspects of communication are so obvious as to be banal; everyone is an expert.

7. Negotiating the boundaries of engagement and objectivity tests effective communication.

8. Personalities and learning styles common among doctors limit effective communication.

9. Undergraduate teaching operates in a context of open and timeless communication; hospitals, in contrast, demand directed discussion and transitory relationships.

10. Clinical teachers rarely have time or training to rectify poor communication in junior staff.

11. As expertise increases, the esoteric and dynamic nature of decision-making makes its description and measurement extraordinarily difficult.

12. No-one has yet described an effective training programme that captures both the art and the science of communication.

Mindful of these challenges, this book seeks to combine the evidence-base about communication in cancer and palliative care with humanity in its practice. Its goal is to integrate the art with the science. We will let you be the judge.

References

1. Christakis NA (2001). *Death Foretold: Prophecy and Prognosis in Medical Care.* University of Chicago Press, Chicago, p.117.

2. Mulcahy L (2006). *The actor's other career book: using your chops to survive and thrive,* pp.38-40. Allworth Press, New York.

3. Shaw B. (1946). *The Doctor's Dilemma.* Penguin, London, p.104. Quoted in Michael O'Donnell (2006). The night Bernard Shaw taught us a lesson. *BMJ* **333**, 1338–40.

4. Roter DL, Frankel RM, Hall JA, *et al.* (2006). The expression of emotion through nonverbal behavior in medical visits. Mechanisms and outcomes. *J Gen Intern Med* **21**, S28–34.

5. Oken D (1961). What to tell cancer patients. A study of medical attitudes. *JAMA* **175**, 1120–8.

6. Orlander JD, Fincke BG, Hermanns D, *et al.* (2002). Medical residents' first clearly remembered experiences of giving bad news. *J Gen Intern Med* **17**, 825–31.

7. Smithers A (2005). Medical training is heading for disaster. Quoted in Skelton JR (2005) Everything you were afraid to ask about communication skills. *Br J Gen Pract* **55**, 40–6.

8. Rogers SO, Gawande AA, Kwaan M *et al.* (2006). Analysis of surgical errors in closed malpractice claims at 4 liability insurers. *Surgery* **140**, 25–33.

9. Ambady N, Laplante D, Nguyen T, *et al.* (2002). Surgeons' tone of voice: a clue to malpractice history. *Surgery* **132**, 5–9.

10. Ishikawa H, Hashimoto H, Kinoshita M, *et al.* (2006). Evaluating medical students' non-verbal communication during the objective structured clinical examination. *Med Educ* **40**, 1180–7.

11. Brown RF, Butow PN, Dunn SM, *et al.* (2001). Promoting patient participation and shortening cancer consultations: a randomized trial. *Br J Cancer* **85**, 1273–9.

12. Froelich RE (1966). Programmed medical interviewing: a teaching technic. *South Med J* **59**, 281–3.

13. Bowlby J (1973). Separation: anxiety and anger. In: Bowlby J. *Attachment and Loss*, vol 2. Basic Books, New York, pp.1–429.

14. Ciechanowski PS, Katon WJ, Russo JE, *et al.* (2001). The patient–provider relationship: attachment theory and adherence to treatment in diabetes. *Am J Psychiatry* **158**, 29–35.

15. Roisman GI (2007). The psychophysiology of adult attachment relationships: autonomic reactivity in marital and premarital interactions. *Dev Psychol* **43**, 39–53.

16. Diamond LM (2006). Physiological evidence for repressive coping among avoidantly attached adults. *J Soc Pers Relat* **23**, 205–29.

17. Von Roenn JH, von Gunten F (2003). Setting goals to maintain hope. *J Clin Oncol* **21**, 570–4.

18. Suchman AL, Markakis K, Beckman HB, *et al.* (1997). A model of empathic communication in the medical interview. *JAMA* **277**, 678–82.

19. Butow PN, Brown RF, Cogar S, *et al.* (2002). Oncologists' reactions to cancer patients' verbal cues. *Psychooncology* **11**, 47–58.

20. Pollak KI, Arnold RM, Jeffreys AS, *et al.* (2007). Oncologist communication about emotion during visits with patients with advanced cancer. *J Clin Oncol* **25**, 5748–52.

21. Austin EJ, Evans P, Magnus B, *et al.* (2007). A preliminary study of empathy, emotional intelligence and examination performance in MB ChB students. *Med Educ* **41**, 684–9.

22. Wiskin CM, Allan TF, Skelton JR (2004). Gender as a variable in the assessment of final year degree-level communication skills. *Med Educ* **38**, 129–37.

23. Honey P, Mumford A (1992). *The Manual of Learning Styles*, 3rd edn. P Honey, Maidenhead.

24. Lesmes-Anel J, Robinson G, *et al.* (2001). Learning preferences and learning styles: a study of Wessex general practice registrars. *Br J Gen Pract* **51**, 559–64.

25. Clack GB, Allen J, Cooper D, *et al.* (2004). Personality differences between doctors and their patients: implications for the teaching of communication skills. *Med Educ* **38**, 177–86.

26. Lewis AP, Bolden KJ (1989). General practitioners and their learning styles. *J R Coll Gen Pract* **39**, 187–9.

27. Froelich RE (1966). Programmed medical interviewing: a teaching technic. *South Med J* **59**, 281–3.

28. Werner A, Schneider J (1974). Teaching medical students interactional skills. A research-based course in the doctor–patient relationship. *NEJM* **290**, 1232–7.

29. Enelow AJ, Adler LM, Wexler M (1970). Programmed instruction in interviewing: an experiment in medical education. *JAMA* **212**, 1843–6.

30. Sloane PD, Beck R, Kowlowitz V, *et al.* (2004). Behavioral coding for evaluation of medical student communication: Clarification or obfuscation? *Acad Med* **79**, 162–70.

31. Fryer-Edwards K, Arnold RM, Baile W, *et al.* (2006). Reflective teaching practices: an approach to teaching communication skills in a small-group setting. *Acad Med* **81**, 638–44.

32. Ward NG, Stein L (1975). Reducing emotional distance: a new method to teach interviewing skills. *J Med Educ* **50**, 605–14.

33. Fellowes D, Wilkinson S, Moore P (2006). Communication skills training for health care professionals working with cancer patients, their families and/or carers [reviews]. In: *The Cochrane Library*, Issue 1, pp.1–16. Wiley, Chichester.

34. Lewin SA, Skea ZC, Entwistle V, *et al.* (2001). Interventions for providers to promote a patient-centred approach in clinical consultations. *Cochrane Database Syst Rev* **4**, CD003267.

35. Gysels M, Richardson A, Higginson IJ (2004). Communication training for health professionals who care for patients with cancer: a systematic review of effectiveness. *Support Care Cancer* **12**, 692–700.

36. Fallowfield L, Jenkins V, Farewell V, *et al.* (2003). Enduring impact of communication skills training: results of a 12-month follow-up. *Br J Cancer* **89**, 1445–9.

37. Delvaux N, Razavi D, Marchal S, *et al.* (2004). Effects of a 105 hours psychological training program on attitudes, communication skills and occupational stress in oncology: a randomized study. *Br J Cancer* **90**, 106–14.

38. Delvaux N, Merckaert I, Marchal S, *et al.* (2005). Physicians' communication with a cancer patient and a relative: a randomized study assessing the efficacy of consolidation workshops. *Cancer* **103**, **2397–411**.

39. Merckaert I, Libert Y, Delvaux N, *et al.* (2005). Factors that influence physicians' detection of distress in patients with cancer: can a communication skills training program improve physicians' detection? *Cancer* **104**, 411–21.

40. Razavi D. Delvaux N, Marchal S, *et al.* (2000). Testing health care professionals' communication skills: the usefulness of highly emotional standardized role-playing sessions with simulators. *Psychooncology* **9**, 293–302.

41. Back AL, Arnold RM, Baile WF, *et al.* (2007). Efficacy of communication skills training for giving bad news and discussing transitions to palliative care. *Arch Intern Med* **167**, 453–60.

42. Kaushik A, Pothier DD (2007). Learned techniques do not necessarily translate to real change. *Arch Intern Med*, **167**, 2261.

43. Dunn SM, Patterson PU, Butow PN, *et al.* (1993). Cancer by another name: a randomized trial of the effects of euphemism and uncertainty in communicating with cancer patients. *J Clin Oncol* **11**, 989–96.

44. O'Donnell M (2005). Doctors as performance artists. *J R Soc Med* **98**, 323–4.

45. Dowsett SM, Saul JL, Butow PN, *et al.* (2000). Communication styles in the cancer consultation: preferences for a patient-centred approach. *Psychooncology* **9**, 147–56.

46. Kramer AW, Dusman H, Tan LH, *et al.* (2004). Acquisition of communication skills in postgraduate training for general practice. *Med Educ* **38**, 158–67.

47. Giuliano AE (1999). See one, do twenty-five, teach one: the implementation of sentinel node dissection in breast cancer. *Ann Surg Oncol* **6**, 520–1.

48. Coulehan JL (1995). Tenderness and steadiness: emotions in medical practice. *Lit Med* **14**, 222–36.

Chapter 3

Theoretical models of communication skills training

Richard Brown and Carma L Bylund

Introduction

Several models of physician–patient communication that have served as conceptual frameworks for communication skills training have been described over recent years. Studies have explored the efficacy of such training in altering physician behaviours. We begin this chapter with a review of these models and a critique of their strengths and weaknesses. We then focus on a new model of communication skills training, which we have developed at Memorial Sloan-Kettering Cancer Center in an effort to address critiques of these earlier models.

Review of existing models

Our review of the literature indicated six established models of physician–patient communication that have served theoretically to guide communication skills training programmes: the Bayer Institute for Healthcare Communication E4 Model; the Three-Function Model/Brown Interview Checklist; the Calgary–Cambridge Observation Guide; Patient-Centred Clinical Method; SEGUE Framework for Teaching and Assessing Communication Skills; and The Four Habits Model. For each of these, we summarize first the conceptualization of the model and then the way in which its application is assessed.

The Bayer Institute for Healthcare Communication E4 Model (1)

Four important elements of communication lead to the 'find it and fix it' approach underpinning this biomedical model. These four 'Es' are: Engage, Empathize, Educate, and Enlist.

- Engage includes eliciting the patient's story and setting an agenda.
- Empathize ensures awareness and acceptance of the patient's feelings and values, thus being 'present' with the patient.
- Educate seeks to assess the patient's understanding, answer questions and ensure realistic appreciation.
- Finally, Enlist establishes decision-making and encouragement of adherence, keeping the patient's understanding and involvement central.

The Bayer Institute developed a rating scale that codes for the four 'Es' (2). Coders utilize a Likert scale to rate doctor–patient interactions in three domains: physician behaviours, including a measure of empathy, patient behaviours, and combined interactional items.

The Three-Function Model/Brown Interview Checklist (3)

Here there is emphasis on three functions of effective medical interviewing: building the relationship; assessing the patient's problems; and managing the patient's problem.

The relationship is established with basic skills like empathy, support, and respect. Then the physician collects information by non-verbal listening, asking open-ended questions, facilitating, and clarifying. The patient's ideas about aetiology are elicited before the clinician provides the diagnosis, checks understanding, describes treatment goals and plans, and checks willingness to proceed. The Brown Interview Checklist (4) operationalizes the three-function approach (5). This checklist details 32 specific communication behaviours that can be categorized into five areas: opening, exploration of problems, facilitation, relationship skills, and closing. Raters use scales anchored by 'fully employs' and 'does not employ', with 'partially employs' as a mid-point.

The Calgary–Cambridge Observation Guide (6)

This model divides the consultation into five tasks: initiating the session; gathering information; building the relationship; giving information—explanation and planning; and closing the session. Establishing rapport and identifying reasons for attendance initiates the session, then problems are explored to understand the patient's perspective. As the patient is involved more and more, the relationship is built. The process of giving information includes aiding accurate recall, achieving a shared understanding, and planning treatment. The session is closed by summarizing and contracting. An assessment instrument rates tasks on a three-point scale from satisfactory to unsatisfactory (7).

Patient-Centred Clinical Method (8)

The Patient-Centred Clinical Method is based on six interactive components: exploring both the disease and the illness experience; understanding the whole person; finding common ground regarding management; incorporating prevention and health promotion; enhancing the patient–doctor relationship; and being realistic. These six components are 'intricately interwoven' (p.30) with a skilled clinician using patient cues to move flexibly between each element. Measuring use of this method involves coding the first three components. First, raters list the patient's symptoms, expectations, and feelings; the level of exploration or dismissal is assessed. Similarly, any focus on life-cycle, family, and social support is noted. Then problems and management goals are recorded for clarity of expression and patient involvement. The overall emphasis is on mutual discussion and clarification of agreement.

SEGUE framework for teaching and assessing communication skills (9)

The acronym for this approach is derived from the first letter for each step: Set the stage; Elicit information; Give information; Understand the patient's perspective; End the encounter. Within each domain are identified communication tasks. For instance, set the stage includes creating an agenda and making a personal connection. Elicit information seeks the patient's view of the problem, including both physical and psychosocial factors. Giving information includes providing explanations, while understand the patient's perspective acknowledges their accomplishments respectfully. The next steps are reviewed during closure. The SEGUE assessment system codes the 25 communication tasks taught and has demonstrated validity and reliability. Unlike other coding systems, its distinction between discrete and continuous communication tasks is unique. Seventeen discrete items focus on content (e.g. eliciting the patient's view of the problem); eight focus on process and indicate behaviours that should be displayed continuously (e.g. maintain patient's privacy; express concern and empathy). If any item is performed at least once, it is coded as 'yes'; if not displayed, it is coded 'no'.

The Four-Habits Model (10–12)

Four sequential, inter-related patterns of behaviour form a family of attitudes and skills. The four habits are: invest in the beginning; elicit the patient's perspective; demonstrate empathy; and invest in the end. These authors highlight how the habits are inter-related. If the clinician does not elicit all of the patient's concerns and assess their importance at the beginning, empathy may be misplaced, diagnoses based on erroneous hypotheses or patient concerns left unresolved. Investing up front in the patient's issues while planning the visit ensures due attention to the patient's needs and the impact of the illness on their life-style. Such a person-centred approach depends on empathic exchanges. The closure is also crucial in establishing the diagnosis and buy-in to the management plan. The Four-Habits Coding Scheme is reliable, valid, and assesses 23 behaviours described in the model. This is an evaluative coding system that requires coders to consider several factors in giving each of the 23 behaviours a performance code.

Strengths and limitations

These models have been extremely valuable in implementing and assessing communication skills training programs. Each provides a set (ranging from thee to six) of components, further defined by more specific communication skills or behaviours. Each also has an accompanying assessment tool. These models suit primary care consultations, wherein a patient's problem needs to be diagnosed, understood and then managed. They are ideal for teaching in medical schools.

However, for healthcare professionals working in oncology settings, these models have limitations. They represent a generic approach to the first consultation, but not continuing care. For instance, a typical cancer patient at a comprehensive cancer centre may come to a first visit already knowing their diagnosis. The focus is not on eliciting information and trying to make a diagnosis. Instead, these visits often have complicated discussions about treatment options and can include difficult conversations about prognosis and end-of-life care. The models presented above may be too simplistic and abstract for these types of applied cancer consultations. Mindful of this, we undertook a further review of the communication skills training literature in search of an approach better suited to the highly specialized fields of cancer and palliative care.

Review of communication skills training research literature

In 2002, Cegala and Broz published a systematic review of 26 communication intervention studies from 1990 for practicing physicians and trainees in graduate medical education (13). They concluded there is good evidence that communication training is effective in improving skills. However, Cegala and Broz raised several concerns. First, they pointed out that very little information is usually provided about which skills were actually taught. Without such detail, it is impossible to judge (14) if correct outcome assessments were used. Second, where the skills being taught were named, there were several occasions of misalignment between the intervention's objectives (e.g. promoting patient-centred interviewing) and the assessment tool. Third, they asserted that 'little effort has been made to provide an over-arching framework for organizing communication skills' (13, p.1005). Since this review, 18 further studies have been published that would fit the criteria of Cegala and Broz. For the most part, Cegala and Broz's critiques hold true for this recently published literature; however, we did find several good examples of alignment between the stated objectives and the assessment (14).

In addition to Cegala and Broz's critiques, we carry an additional concern about the literature in general. The term 'communication skill' is used inconsistently across studies and is often ambiguous within studies. Terms such as: 'task' (9), 'element' (15), 'approach and technique' (16), 'strategy' (17), 'step' and 'component' (18) are found commonly. In some cases, these words are used interchangeably without explanation (15, 17). We found only one textbook definition of communication skills: 'the numerous acts that health workers express in caring for their patients' (19). Others, while offering no explicit definition, list skills of varying abstractness such as 'effective care', 'question style', and 'making eye contact' (19). Additionally, differing degrees of complexity are present in clinical encounters, ranging from 'greet and obtain patient name' to 'set consultation agenda' to 'determine and acknowledge patient's ideas' (20).

Because the peer-reviewed literature does not give explicit detail about curricula, we turned to copies of unpublished curricular material from training programmes throughout the world. We contacted recognized experts in the field and asked to review their material. Again the use of 'skills' remained unclear and needed to be extracted from the exemplars provided. For instance, a 'breaking bad news' workshop contained a step called 'encourage patients to express feelings', followed by an exemplar dialogue for this particular step (21, 22). We have broken this example down to highlight the skills necessary to convey the example (see Table 3.1). The left column contains the published 'steps', while the right column identifies the communication skills involved in this dialogue. The approach of providing examples of dialogue without naming the actual skill involved in this communication is not optimal, particularly in the context of teaching specific communication skills. Clearly identifying skills makes teaching and assessment more precise.

Development of the Comskil model

Our review highlighted the need for a model that:

◆ addressed communication challenges in illness settings characterized by continuous and ongoing care;

◆ made the skills necessary to meet these communication challenges explicit and unambiguous, and

◆ provided a direct linkage between the teaching curriculum and assessment.

Below we describe the development of the Comskil model.

Theoretical foundations of the Comskil model

Physician–patient communication is interpersonal communication in a particular context. Thus, as interpersonal communication scholars have developed a body of theory to aid in the understanding of this process, we have drawn on this work to inform our conceptual model. Two theories help explain how people formulate their communication:

◆ goals, plans, and action (GPA) theories; and

◆ sociolinguistic theory.

Table 3.1 Example from a breaking bad news module (21, 22)

Exemplar	Communication skill
'This is obviously bad news and it is understandable that you are very upset about it.'	Legitimizing
'Many patients feel upset or even angry when they receive this kind of news.'	Normalizing
'However, it is important not to jump to any conclusions. Although you have (disease) it is far too early to say what will happen to you.'	Offering hope.

Communication theorists provide a clear ordering of the components of interpersonal communication in GPA theories (23). These theories distinguish between communication elements that vary in abstractness. Originating in fields of communication and psychology (24, 25), the premise is that people rely on goals and plans (26) to guide their communication. Goals have been defined as the 'future states of affairs that individuals desire to attain or maintain' (27, p.68). Plans are more concrete than goals—they are mental representations of actions needed to achieve a goal (28). Plans vary in complexity and specificity. Actions are even more concrete, as they are the enacting of the behaviour that is planned.

As a second theoretical foundation, sociolinguistic theory clarifies communication styles. Two basic orientations are the position-centred and person-centred approaches. The position-centred communicator relies on a restricted code of communication, following the rules and norms of the predicament. The person-centred communicator adapts his or her communication in response to the perspectives, feelings, and intentions of others (23). Using a person-centred approach is one characteristic of what Epstein calls being a 'mindful practitioner' (29). We have endorsed a person-centred approach in our Comskil model. In other words, we recognize, as do GPA theories, that there is more than one way to meet a particular communication goal. The Comskil model offers potential strategies and skills that individuals can use, while adapting them to a variety of challenging situations (e.g. breaking bad news, discussing prognosis or treatment options) and allowing them to be congruent with each clinician's own interpersonal communication style. In using this theory, we concur with Kurtz and colleagues, who note that 'communication training should increase rather than reduce flexibility by providing an expanded repertoire of skills that physicians can adeptly and intentionally choose to use as they require' (20, p.45).

In order to address the difficulties inherent in earlier programmes of communication skills training, we have adapted the GPA and sociolinguistic theoretical frameworks as the basis of an innovative approach within which each component is defined, explicit, and unambiguous. This approach also enables more accurate and specific assessment to be made about how well trainees learn these skills, thus addressing an important limitation in the current literature.

Defining the core components of the Comskil model

In order to make the teaching of communication skills more explicit and to aid in the evaluation of the outcome of training, we conceive of five communication components in the typical consultation:

◆ goals;

◆ strategies;

◆ skills;

◆ process tasks; and

◆ cognitive appraisals.

In this section, we define these terms and describe how the components are integrated (14).

Communication goals

A communication goal is defined as the desired outcome of the consultation or portion of the consultation. For example, the communication goal of our breaking bad news module (30) is: 'To convey threatening information in a way which promotes understanding, recall, and a sense of ongoing support'. As GPA theories explain, this definition of a goal focuses on the desired state that the individual is attempting to attain. The communication goal is achieved through the use of communication strategies, skills, process tasks, and cognitive appraisals.

Communication strategies

Communication strategies are defined as a priori plans that direct communication behaviour toward the successful realization of a communication goal. The cumulative use of several strategies in a sequence facilitates goal achievement. For example, 'Respond empathically to emotion' and 'Provide information in a way that it will be understood' are both strategies that may help to achieve the communication goal for breaking bad news. As with the plans in GPA theories, strategies are more concrete than goals. Furthermore, a strategy can be accomplished in more than one way. In our curriculum, we recommend strategies that are useful to achieving a particular goal.

Communication skills

A communication skill is defined as a discrete mode (or unit of speech) by which a physician can further the clinical dialogue, and thus achieve fulfillment of a strategy. Unlike the definitions both implicit and explicit in the literature of communication skills, this definition describes the communication skill as verbal, concrete, teachable, and observable. Skills are similar to the notion of actions in GPA theories; they are the least abstract elements of the hierarchy. In addition, a variety of communication skills may be utilized in the attainment of any particular strategy. For example, the strategy of 'Respond empathically to emotion' could be accomplished through choice of skills like acknowledgment, validation, normalization, or praising patient's efforts. The strategy of 'Provide information in a way that it will be understood' could be accomplished through previewing information, summarizing information, and/or checking patient understanding. Communication skills exist and are expressed in certain contexts. As we have explored both the literature and various teaching modules (22, 31–33), we have compiled a list of 26 discrete communication skills (see Table 3.2). We have organized these skills into six higher-order categories to assist both teaching and assessment and to aid learners' understanding and recall. These are:

1. Establishing the consultation framework.

2. Information organization skills.

3. Checking skills.

4. Questioning skills.

5. Empathic communication skills.

6. Shared decision-making skills.

Process tasks

Process tasks are defined as sets of dialogues or non-verbal behaviours that create an environment for effective communication. These are similar to skills as they are concrete, while goals and strategies are abstract. Together with skills, process tasks help an individual enact a strategy as a means to meet a goal. Process tasks require thoughtful consideration and can range on a continuum from basic to more complex. Examples of basic process tasks include:

- introducing self to patient;
- providing a private space in which to break bad news; and
- ensuring that the doctor is at eye level.

Examples of more complex process tasks include:

- avoiding premature reassurance;
- paying attention to information framing (words or numbers); and
- using a randomization story to help explain a randomized clinical trial.

Table 3.2 Communication skills in six categories with descriptions and examples

Skill	Description	Examples
Checking skills		
Check patient understanding	Ask the patient about his or her understanding of previously conveyed information or the current situation. Optimally, understanding will be checked on more than one occasion and patients will be asked to reframe in their own words the information conveyed.	'Tell me what you know about your diagnosis.' 'Why don't you tell me what you understand about what I've said so far?'
Check patient medical knowledge	Ask the patient about his or her understanding of the medical words used.	'So, we have been talking about nodal status and I said they were positive. What does that mean to you?'
Check patient preference-information	Ask the patient about the amount and type of information desired. This needs to be done on more than one occasion. It is an iterative process—patients' information needs may vary throughout the consultation and across the course of the illness.	'Some people like to have lots of information about their illness and some people only want a little bit of information. How much would you like me to give you today?' 'Do you want me to give you information in numbers or words about the likely time frame?'
Shared decision-making skills		
Introduce joint decision-making	Offer joint decision-making and say why it is important.	'There are several options for treatment and we can decide together which is the most acceptable treatment for you. I think it is very important that you are comfortable with the final decision.'
Check patient preference—decision-making	Ask the patient about his or her preferred role in decision-making. This needs to be done on more than one occasion. It is an iterative process—patients' preferred roles may change throughout the consultation and across the course of the illness.	'It is important for me to know how you like to make decisions. Would you prefer for me to make the decision, for us to make the decision together or would you like to make the decision yourself or with your family?'
Reinforce joint decision-making	If joint decision-making has been introduced, review the concept at a later point in the illness or consultation (unless the patient has opted out of joint decision-making).	'Remember, I'm happy to talk with you about all the options and we can make this decision together.'
Make partnership statements	Convey alliance with the patient.	'Let's work together to figure out how to solve this problem.' 'Let's figure out together when we should start your chemo.'
Offer decision delay	Reinforce time to make treatment decision if applicable. If used, reassure patient that this delay will not affect treatment efficacy.	'We do have some time to make a decision. We know from previous studies that it does not make a difference if you wait up to six weeks after surgery before starting this type of treatment.'

(continued)

Table 3.2 (continued) Communication Skills in Six Categories with Descriptions and Examples

Skill	Description	Examples
Establishing the consultation framework		
Declare agenda items	State what you would like to accomplish in the consultation.	'Today, I would like to discuss with you the various treatment options available.'
Invite patient agenda items	Ask patient what items he or she would like to discuss today.	'Before we get started, I would like to hear what you are hoping to get out of our visit today?'
Negotiate agenda	Ask patient to help you prioritize agenda items.	'There may be more on your list than we have time to cover today. Which items do you prioritize as most important?'
Questioning skills		
Invite patient questions	Make it clear to the patient that you are willing to answer questions and address concerns.	'Do you have anything you want to discuss or do you want to ask me any questions? It is important that we cover the issues that are important to you.' 'If you think of things at home you would like to ask me, just write them down and bring them next time, ok?'
Endorse question asking	Express to the patient the importance of asking questions; provide a rationale for asking questions (i.e., that patients can gain salient information).	'Questions are a really good way for you to get the information that you need, or to get me to say things more clearly. I will try and answer any questions that you have. So feel free to stop me if you need me to answer something.'
Clarify	Ask a question to try to better understand what a patient is saying.	'When you asked about side-effects of the medication, was there a particular side effect to which you were referring?'
Restate	State in your own words what you think the patient is saying.	'It sounds like you have some questions about the treatment.' 'So, if I understand correctly, you are frustrated with what the nurse said to you?'
Make a 'take stock' statement	Pause in the dialogue to review the prior discussion. Seeking the patient's permission to move on.	'Now, so far we have talked about the standard treatments that are available. There is another possible choice that we could make about your treatment. That is a clinical trial which looks at different ways of giving chemotherapy. I know you have had a lot to take in today, but would you like to discuss it or leave it until another time?'

Table 3.2 (continued) Communication Skills in Six Categories with Descriptions and Examples

Skill	Description	Examples
Empathic communication skills		
Acknowledge	Make a statement that indicates recognition of the patient's emotion or experience.	'It sounds like this has been a tough time for you.' 'You do seem like you are feeling less anxious.'
Normalize	Make a comparative statement that expresses that a particular emotional response is not out of the ordinary.	'It's not uncommon to feel this way at a time like this.'
Legitimize	Make a statement expressing that a patient's emotional response to an event or an experience is appropriate and reasonable.	'It's understandable that you have been feeling anxious.' 'Yeah, it is hard to keep focused at work when you are going through treatment. It would be perfectly reasonable to take some leave from work during the next cycle of chemo.'
Encourage expression of feelings	Express to the patient that you would like to know how he or she is feeling.	'It's important to me to understand how you are dealing with all of this emotionally.'
Praise patient efforts	Make a statement that validates a patient's attempts to cope with treatment or side-effects, to make life-style changes, or to be adherent to treatment regime.	'You're doing really well with the nicotine patches.' 'It sounds like you have been taking good care of yourself through the treatment process.'
Express a willingness to help	Make a specific offer of help or a general statement about being available for future help.	'If you'd like, I could explain this to your daughter when she comes in with you next time?' 'Please let me know what I can do to help.'
Information organization skills		
Preview information	Give an overview of the main points that you are about to cover.	'First, I'd like to talk to you about the standard treatment. After we've discussed those options, I'd like to talk to you about a clinical trial on offer.'
Summarize	Recap the main details conveyed. As with checking behaviours, this should occur at various points during the consultation where appropriate.	'So, look I'll just summarize. You'll have three cycles of treatment initially and then we will repeat the scans.'
Review next steps	Go over with the patient the next things that the patient will do (e.g. make a follow-up appointment).	'I just want to go over the next steps that we've discussed to make sure we are on the same page.'

Cognitive appraisals

During consultations, doctors observe and then internally process patients' verbal and non-verbal behaviour. This process of reflection allows the clinician to formulate a hypothesis about the unstated or inexplicit needs and agendas the patient may have. This appraisal drives the selection of communication strategies. These cognitive appraisals are critical to the effective communication process, as some patient issues are not clearly articulated through conventional discourse. Patients may have needs or agendas that, if not uncovered, may impede the trajectory of the consultation. Bringing these to light is a complex communication challenge that is achieved through making cognitive appraisals that lead to selection of communication strategies, and thus the utilization of communication skills. Although clinicians are constantly making cognitive appraisals throughout each interaction, our model focuses on two specific types of cognitive appraisals: patient cues and barriers. We have chosen to include these in our training because, if they are not addressed, the physician–patient relationship may be impaired.

Patient cues

Patient cues are indirect behaviours or statements used to prompt doctors for informational or emotional support. For example, a patient may have a desire for particular information, yet lack confidence in asking direct questions. Consequently, in order to have the information need met, the patient may use an information cue such as 'I really don't know much about the different treatments' (34). As this is not a direct request for information, the doctor would have to make a cognitive appraisal of the patient's need for information. This is an iterative process, leading to an appropriate response to the patient cue through strategy and skill usage. Similarly, patients may cue their doctor for emotional support. An example of an emotional cue would be: 'I get so upset sometimes I can't stop crying' (34).

Patient barriers

Patient barriers are undisclosed perceptions of the patient that may impede effective communication. An example of a patient barrier may be particular fears about the prospect of chemotherapy, based on their previous knowledge and misconceptions of the side-effects. This undisclosed patient perception will impede an effective decision-making process and may be expressed by the patient's hesitancy to discuss treatment, use of blocking behaviours, or expression of anxiety in the discussion. Again, this is an iterative process and the use of strategies and skills will assist the clinician to uncover and resolve the hidden barrier (32).

Integrating the core communication components

Clearly, our definitions of communication goals, strategies, skills, process tasks, and cognitive appraisals are related to one another. We envision this connection in the Fig. 3.1.

The communication strategy is a higher-order category and is accomplished through the use of communication skills and/or process tasks. Communication skills differ from strategies and process tasks as they provide a building block for complex communication tasks. As noted by Kurtz, Silverman, and Draper, core skills are fundamental: 'Once core skills are mastered, specific communication issues are much more readily tackled' (20, p.38). As can be seen by the bi-directional arrows in Fig. 3.1, the components influence each other in a dynamic process to achieve the communication goal. In order to make the relationships between these components clear, we have developed comprehensive modular blueprints that provide the essential communication components for each of our applied modules, taught using the model described here. We have included as an example the modular blueprint for a breaking bad news module (see Table 3.3).

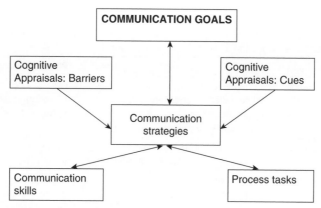

Fig. 3.1 Integrating core communication concepts.

Evaluation

In order to collect objective skill uptake data, we recommend video-recording two actual patient consultations (one new and one follow-up visit) before and after each learner has participated in training. To collect self-report data, at the conclusion of each of the individual communication training modules, learners can also complete evaluations eliciting their views about the value of the training provided.

Coding of strategies, skills, and process tasks

We have operationalized the computerized Comskil coding scheme to measure use of the strategies, skills, and process tasks described in this model. These are described in a coding manual that provides coding rules and multiple examples of each of the component parts. Coders are trained to use the manual to identify the presence of strategies, skills, or process tasks while viewing consultation video-recordings. A software program has been developed to provide a computerized environment, where it is possible to view the video-recording and simultaneously code for the presence of skills. These frequency data are then transferred to an SPSS database to allow for pre- and post-training statistical comparisons. In addition, the length of each consultation is recorded. The particular strength of this method is that we are able to ensure that the skills taught are directly matched to those measured as part of the evaluation process. This coding system is applied to these recordings to assess participants' baseline skills and post-training uptake. Inter-rater reliability for this coding has been good at kappa = 0.76. As we move forward with our coding, we plan to formally ensure that coders are blinded to whether the recordings are pre- or post-training. Inter-rater reliability needs repeated reassessment to sustain the quality of appraisal.

Conclusion

The Comskil model of communication skills training is a flexible, conceptual framework that can be adapted to meet the education requirements in a variety of healthcare contexts including: primary care, chronic disease, oncology, and other specialties. The model provides discrete and unambiguous definitions and hierarchy of communication strategies, skills, and process tasks enabling a systematic assessment process that is carefully matched to the curriculum.

In the next section of this Handbook, use will be made of this model to illustrate more fully how it can be applied in a curriculum developed for oncology and palliative care.

Table 3.3 Modular blueprint—breaking bad news

(*Goal:* To convey threatening information in a way that promotes understanding, recall, and support for the patient's emotional response and a sense of ongoing support.)

Strategies	Skills	Process tasks
Establish the consultation framework.	Declare your agenda items. Invite patient agenda items. Negotiate agenda. Check shared agreement about illness.	Greet patient appropriately. Make introductions. Ensure patient is clothed. Sit at eye-level.
Tailor the consultation to the patient's needs.	Check patient understanding. Check patient preference-information.	Avoid interruptions. Invite appropriate third party.
Provide information in a way that it will be understood.	Preview information. Invite patient questions. Check patient understanding.	Avoid jargon. Address all questions. Draw diagrams. Categorize.
Provide information in a way that it will be recalled.	Summarize.	Write information down. Repeat.
Respond empathically to emotion.	Encourage expression of feelings. Acknowledge. Normalize. Legitimize. Ask open questions.	Maintain eye contact. Allow time to integrate. Offer tissues. Provide hope and reassurance.
Check readiness to discuss management options.	Check patient preference—decision making. Preview information.	Provide literature.
Close the consultation.	Check patient understanding. Invite patient questions. Endorse question asking. Reinforce joint decision-making. Summarize. Review next steps.	Offer to talk to relatives. Offer follow-up phone calls or consultation.

References

1. Keller VF, Caroll JG (1994). A new model for physician–patient communication. *Patient Educ Couns* **35**, 121–40.

2. Kemp-White M, Goldstein MG (1999). Unpublished clinician patient communication global rating scale (CPCGRS): Bayer Institute for Healthcare Coder's Manual. West Haven, CT.

3. Cole SA, Bird J (2000). *The Medical Interview: the Three Function Approach.* Mosby Inc, St Louis, Missouri.

4. Novack DH, Dube C, Goldstein MG (1992). Teaching medical interviewing. A basic course on interviewing and the physician–patient relationship. *Arch Intern Med* **152**, 1814–20.

5. Makoul G (2001). Bayer-Fetzer conference on physician–patient communication in medical education. Essential elements of communication in medical encounters: the Kalamazoo consensus statement. *Acad Med* **76**, 390–3.

6. Kurtz SM, Silverman JD (1996). The Calgary–Cambridge Referenced Observation Guides: an aid to defining curriculum and organising teaching in communication training programmes. *Med Educ* **30**, 83–9.

7. ACGME (2006). Interpersonal and communication skills assessment approaches. In: **http://www. acgme.org/outcome/assess/IandC_Index.asp**, ed. A*CGME Outcome Project*: Accreditation Council of Graduate Medical Education, Chicago, IL.

8. Stewart M, Belle Brown J, McWhinney IR, *et al.* (1995). *Patient-centred Medicine: Transforming the Clinical Method.* Sage, Thousand Oaks, CA.

9. Makoul G (2001). The SEGUE Framework for teaching and assessing communication skills. *Patient Educ Couns* **45**, 23–34.

10. Frankel RM, Stein T (1999). Getting the most out of the clinical encounter: the four habits model. *The Permanente Journal* **3**, 79–88.

11. Krupat E, Frankel RM, Stein T, *et al.* (2006). The Four Habits Coding Scheme: validation of an instrument to assess clinician's communication behaviour. *Patient Educ Couns* **62**, 38–45.

12. Stein T, Frankel RM, Krupat E (2005). Enhancing communication skills in a large healthcare organization: a longitudinal case study. *Patient Educ Couns* **58**, 4–12.

13. Cegala DJ, Lenzmeier Broz S (2002). Physician communication skills training; a review of the theoretical backgrounds, objectives and skills. *Med Educ* **36**, 1004–16.

14. Brown RF, Bylund CL (2008). Communication skills training: describing a new conceptual model. *Acad Med* **83**, 37–44.

15. Makoul G (2001). Essential elements of communication in medical encounters: the Kalamazoo consensus statement. *Acad Med* **76**, 390–3.

16. Roter DL, Hall, JA (1992). *Doctors Talking with Patients, Patients Talking with Doctors: Improving Communication in Medical Visits.* Greenwood, Westport, CT.

17. Razavi D, Merckaert I, Marchal S, *et al.* (2003). How to optimize physicians' communication skills in cancer care: results of a randomized study assessing the usefulness of posttraining consolidation workshops. *J Clin Oncol* **21**, 3141–9.

18. Baile WF, Kudelka AP, Beale EA, *et al.* (1999). Communication skills training in oncology. Description and preliminary outcomes of workshops in breaking bad news and managing patient reactions to illness. *Cancer* **86**, 887–97.

19. Fielding R (1995). *Clinical Communication Skills.* Hong Kong University Press, Hong Kong.

20. Kurtz S, Silverman J, Draper J (1998). *Teaching and Learning Communication Skills in Medicine.* Radcliffe Medical Press Ltd, Abingdon.

21. Girgis A (1997). Overview of consensus guidelines on breaking bad news. In: **http://www.nbcc.org.au/ bestpractice/commskills/modules.html**, ed. NHMRC National Breast Cancer Centre, Sydney, NSW.

22. Girgis A, Smith J (1998). *Communication Skills Training Program.* Manual. University of Newcastle, Newcastle, NSW.

23. Miller K (2002). *Communication Theories: Perspectives, Processes, and Contexts.* McGraw–Hill, Boston, MA.

24. Austin JT, Vancouver JB (1996). Goal constructs in psychology: structure, process and content. *Psychol Bull* **120**, 338–75.

25. Clark RA, Delia JG (1979). 'Topoi' and rhetorical competence. *Q J Speech* **65**, 187–206.

26. Kellerman K (1992). Communication: inherently strategic and primarily automatic. *Commun Monogr* **61**, 210–35.

27. Wilson SR, Morgan WM (2006). Goals–plans–action theories: theories of goals, plans and planning processes in families. In: Braithwaite DO, Baxter LA, eds. *Engaging Theories in Family Communication: Multiple Perspectives*, p.68. Sage Publications, Thousand Oaks, CA.

28. Berger CR (1997). *Planning Strategic Interaction: Attaining Goals Through Communicative Action.* Lawrence Erlbaum, Mahwah NJ.

29. Epstein RM (1999). Mindful practice. *JAMA* **282**(9), 833–9.

30. Bylund C, Brown RF, Gueguen J, *et al.* (2006). *Breaking Bad News.* Monograph. Memorial Sloan–Kettering Cancer Center, New York, NY.

31. Back AL, Arnold RM, Tulsky JA, *et al.* (2003). Teaching communication skills to medical oncology fellows. *J Clin Oncol* **21**, 2433–6.

32. Brown RF, Butow PN, Butt DG, *et al.* (2004). Developing ethical strategies to assist oncologists in seeking informed consent to cancer clinical trials. *Soc Sci Med* **58**, 379–90.

33. Girgis A, Sanson-Fisher RW (1995). Breaking bad news: consensus guidelines for medical practitioners. *J Clin Oncol* **13**, 2449–56.

34. Butow PN, Brown RF, Cogar S, *et al.* (2002). Oncologists reactions to cancer patients verbal cues. *Psychooncology* **11**, 47–58.

Chapter 4

Shared treatment decision-making and the use of decision-aids

Cathy Charles and Amiram Gafni

Introduction

Over the past fifteen years or so, shared decision-making, a specific approach to making decisions in the medical encounter, has received considerable conceptual and practical attention among physicians, social scientists, and ethicists (1–10). In addition, governments and professional associations in different countries are developing patient charters/bills of rights to promote responsiveness to, and involvement of, patients in treatment decision-making (4, 11). The reasons for this widespread interest in shared decision-making are varied and have evolved over time (4). Most importantly, this interest derives from changes in ethical and legal notions of patient rights and is reflected in the language we now use to convey these: for example, patient rights of informed choice in treatment decision-making, rather than the more limited concept of informed consent (1, 4). The former is a stronger message, encompassing broader principles of patient autonomy, control, patient challenge to physician authority, and patient participation in treatment decision-making.

Definition

Despite the widespread interest in promoting shared treatment decision-making, there does not seem to be as yet a universally accepted consensus on the meaning of this concept. Many authors have attempted to define shared treatment decision-making (1–10). There has been some overlap in the dimensions identified as key characteristics of this model. Two recent articles, one by Makoul and Clayman (7) and another by Moumjid and colleagues (10) reviewed the most commonly cited definitions in the literature. Both found that the definition by Charles and colleagues (1, 4) was the most commonly cited and we will use this definition here. The particular clinical context that this definition pertains to is one of potentially life-threatening illness, such as cancer, where there are important decisions to be made at key points in the disease process, and several treatment options exist, with different possible outcomes and substantial uncertainty (1, 4).

Charles and colleagues (1) initially defined shared treatment decision-making as having four key characteristics:

- that at least two participants—physician and patient—be involved;
- that both parties share information;
- that both parties take steps to build a consensus about the preferred decision; and
- that an agreement is reached on the decision to implement.

In a subsequent follow-up paper (4), Charles and colleagues expanded on this model by explicitly identifying different analytic steps in the treatment decision-making process and identifying and comparing how, in implementation, these steps differ depending on whether the approach adopted to decision-making is paternalistic, shared, informed, or lies somewhere in-between. The authors also pointed out the dynamic nature of the treatment decision-making process by recognizing that the approach adopted at the outset of a medical encounter may change as the interaction evolves.

In Table 4.1, the different analytic steps that define the treatment decision-making process are presented: information exchange, deliberation or discussion of treatment options and preferences, and deciding on the treatment to implement. The three most prominent approaches to treatment decision-making are also presented in this table and compared in terms of how the different analytic steps are implemented in each model. The table also makes clear that the prominent models, as depicted in Table 4.1, are 'ideal or pure' types and that, in reality, actual decision-making approaches may well lie somewhere in-between. The framework does not assume that there is a right or wrong approach to arriving at a decision. Rather, it attempts to highlight the distinctive characteristics of each of the prominent models, which are described in more detail below.

Paternalistic model of treatment decision-making

In the purest form of the paternalistic model, information flow is one-way—from physician to patient—and is limited to medical information about the disease and its treatment, which physicians are legally required to inform the patient about. The physician alone, or in consultation with colleagues, decides on the treatment to implement and the patient passively acquiesces to professional authority by agreeing to the physician's choice of treatment. An assumption underlying this approach, which has increasingly been challenged in recent years, is that physicians will make the best treatment decision for their patients and can do so without eliciting from the latter information about their cultural beliefs, personal preferences for different treatment outcomes, and values that might influence the meaning that patients attribute to their illness and ways of coping with it. Many authors have argued that, in the past, this was the dominant approach to treatment decision-making in the medical encounter (12–14).

Informed model of treatment decision-making

At the other end of the spectrum lies the informed model of treatment decision-making (4). Here the patient is the sole decision-maker and the physician's role is to communicate to the patient all

Table 4.1 Comparison of treatment decision-making approaches

Analytic Stages	Paternalistic	Shared	Informed
Information exchange			
Flow	One-way (largely)	Two-way	One-way (largely)
Direction	Doctor > patient	Doctor > < Patient	Doctor > patient
Type	Medical	Medical and personal	Medical
Minimum	Legal requirement	Anything relevant for DM	Anything relevant for DM
Deliberation	Doctor alone or with other doctors	Doctor and patient (and potential others)	Patient (plus potential others)
Who decides on treatment to implement?	Doctor	Doctor and patient	Patient

relevant treatment options and their risks and benefits. The amount and type of information communicated includes, at a minimum, all relevant information on the above issues to enable the patient to make an informed choice. Communication of such information is one way—from physician to patient. In its pure type, this decision-making process involves a division of labour, whereby the physician communicates information to the patient and the latter adds her preferences in order to make the decision that is right for her. This model is thought to enhance patient control and autonomy over the decision-making process.

Some believe that the 'physician as a perfect agent' to her patient is an example of a paternalistic approach, where the choice of treatment that the physician makes for the patient will be the same as the choice that the patient would have made herself (an informed model). Note that in such a case, the treatment chosen by the patient in the informed decision-making process and by the physician, if she is a perfect agent, will be the same. While this is true in theory, Gafni and colleagues (15) have argued that this is not likely to happen in practice. They describe the 'physician as perfect agent' model as one where the patient delegates authority to her physician to make medical decisions and the challenge is to encourage the physician to find out the patient's preferences. In the informed model, the patient retains the authority to make medical decisions and the challenge is to encourage the physician to transfer knowledge about treatment options to the patient in a clear and non-biased way. Gafni and colleagues argue that for several reasons it is simpler for physicians to transfer technical knowledge to the patient than it is for patients to transfer their preferences to physicians. Because of this difference in the feasibility of implementation, while each of these approaches in the abstract would be expected to yield a similar result (i.e. the same decision), this is unlikely to be true in reality.

Shared model of treatment decision-making

The pure-type shared decision-making model lies between the other two above (4). The essential characteristic of this model is its interactional nature, in that the physician and patient share all stages of the decision-making process simultaneously. There is a two-way exchange of information. The physician communicates to the patient evidence-based information about the various relevant treatment options (including no treatment) and their risks and benefits, elicits information from the patient about her values, life-style and preferences, and, in the typical case, provides a treatment recommendation, taking into account both of the above sets of factors, plus the physician's own values about what is the best treatment for this particular patient. The patient communicates what she knows about her disease, and the risks and benefits of various treatment options she has heard about, as well as her values, life circumstances, and preferences that may influence which treatment she thinks would be best for her. Both parties agree on the decision to implement. This model assumes that the physician and patient each have a legitimate investment in the treatment decision. Hence, both declare treatment preferences and their rationale for these, while trying to build consensus on the most appropriate treatment to implement. If a consensus cannot be reached, shared decision-making will not occur.

Clinical contexts for partnership relationships

The above discussion has focused on what shared decision-making is, i.e. the defining characteristics of this model of decision-making in the context of other prominent models and in the context of acute care, such as cancer care. Even within a single disease, e.g. cancer, the decision-making context can vary substantially in terms of the nature, manifestations, and progress of the disease, as well as available treatment options, depending on the particular disease site and disease stage. Some form of shared decision-making may be appropriate in all these situations.

Increasingly, shared decision-making is also seen as appropriate for clinical contexts other than acute care, such as primary care (8) and chronic care (9), in a modified form and tailored to fit the specific clinical characteristics of that context.

Whether shared decision-making will actually occur in any given encounter depends on patient and physician preferences for different treatment decision-making models and the extent to which barriers and facilitators exist in a given care setting to facilitate or inhibit use of this approach (16–18). A number of studies undertaken in different countries have found that patient preferences for involvement in treatment decision-making vary (11, 19–23). There is no one model that fits everyone. For this reason, it is important to assess not simply the extent to which shared decision-making occurs, but also the match between what model the patient wants to use with her physician and what she receives.

The relationship between physician and patient is not symmetrical. The physician typically has more power by virtue of his greater knowledge, expertise, and professional authority, and the fact that he is not sick; yet it is the patient who bears the consequences of implementing the treatment decision. For these reasons, we feel that the onus is on the physician to ascertain the patient's preferences for the role she wants to play in decision-making and to facilitate patient involvement in decision-making as much as she wants.

It is increasingly argued that shared or informed treatment decision-making models are better than more paternalistic approaches, and should be universally promoted. Such statements are normative in nature, involving value judgments. If the underlying goal of this type of promotion is to allow patients to make decisions in a way that is consistent with their preferences, then we think that patients should be allowed to choose their preferred model of decision-making, including the option of choosing a paternalistic approach, if that is what they want.

It is not always clear from the literature whether shared decision-making is being promoted because it is seen as a positive end in itself or rather as a means to achieve other ends. Shared decision-making has been proposed, for example, as a means to increase patient autonomy and control in decision-making, to improve patient satisfaction, to enhance patient compliance with decisions made, to increase the extent to which decisions made are consistent with patient values, and to reduce healthcare costs (24). Many hoped-for patient outcomes are thus 'loaded on to' the concept of patient involvement in treatment decision-making, a concept that, when implemented in the clinical context, is expected to achieve multiple goals (24). As we will see in the next section, this expectation is also true of various forms of treatment decision-aids designed to help promote shared decision-making in the medical encounter.

Treatment decision-aids as a means to implement shared decision-making

Goals and assumptions

Like the concept of shared decision-making, treatment decision-aids have been defined in different ways with different emphases, depending on the author. Here we use the definition by O'Connor and colleagues (2007):

> Patient decision aids are interventions designed to help people make specific, deliberative choices among options (including the status quo) by providing information on the options and outcomes (e.g. benefits, harms) in sufficient detail that an individual could judge their value implicitly.

(25, p.554)

Two key components are inherent in this definition: first, that decision aids are designed to transfer technical information on available treatments and their potential benefits and risks to the patient; and, second, that such information is a necessary prerequisite for creating an informed patient, who is thereby enabled to participate in making a treatment decision that fits with her values. These two components are commonly cited in definitions of decisions aids. In addition, such aids are thought to be of benefit in establishing rapport between physicians and patients and in providing a structure that would encourage input from both parties in the treatment decision-making process (24).

In the cancer field, in particular, the number of decision aids developed over the last fifteen years has proliferated for several reasons (14). First, studies have shown that, without the use of such aids, the transfer of technical information on treatment options from physicians to cancer patients was often problematic, while, at the same time, the introduction of new cancer treatments has increased the number of options available. Second, many treatments offer varying mixes of potential benefits and side-effects, whose subjective values vary from patient to patient. For this reason, cancer patients are now encouraged to make these preferences known in the encounter, so that the decision made will reflect not only evidence on effective treatment but also patient preferences for different outcomes.

There are many forms of decision aids, most of which present information visually to patients on treatment options and the potential risks and benefits associated with each (24). Decision-aid formats include brochures, pamphlets, decision boards, interactive videos, and audio-taped workbooks, among others. The intent of these aids is to make the treatment options and their respective consequences clear to the patient, who can then make the choice that is right for her, given her own values and preferences. Decision aids may also include some form of values clarification exercise intended to help the patient clarify her preferences for various treatment outcomes and the kinds of trade-offs she is willing to make between risks and benefits associated with each, to arrive at her preferred decision (26).

Decision aids incorporate a number of assumptions that may or may not be made clear to the patient at the time of their use. For example, the developers of decision aids determine which treatment options to include for the patient to consider, as well as which risks and benefits (outcomes), the specific method (e.g. trade-off) that patients are to use to process the information presented, and the theoretical foundations of the method specified for making the treatment decision, e.g. expected utility theory (24). As long as both the physician and patient are aware of these assumptions, explicitly buy into them, and agree that the method presented is the best way to make treatment decisions, there is no problem. However, the extent to which physicians are aware of these assumptions and communicate them to patients, and the extent to which patients understand and accept these, are unknown and thus cast doubt on the validity of such exercises (24). Some forms of decision aids are designed for patients to go through on their own at home. In these contexts, outside the medical encounter, opportunities for assessing patient understanding of the assumptions, and the decision theory underlying different types of decision aids, may be even more problematic.

In addition, values clarification exercises specify the types of preferences patients are to consider and the process to use in incorporating these into decision-making. (26–27). A key issue with this type of exercise is that it may distort or be inconsistent with the way the patient usually makes decisions. In this case, the exercise itself becomes an intervention, imposing on the patient a different way of processing information, rather than allowing her to clarify and articulate her values in her own way, which is typically the stated goal of the exercise (24). In other words, the values clarification exercise has the potential to impede rather than help the patient choose a treatment in a way that is consistent with her own preferences.

Also underlying decision aids are cultural beliefs that frame their development and use. For example, decision aids are firmly embedded in a biological model of illness, an evidence-based medicine paradigm, medical concepts of risk, ethical precepts of informed choice, and a defined approach to decision-making (28). These common features of decision aids are not surprising given the Western medicine-oriented clinical and research contexts in which they have been developed. However, an interesting question for future research is the extent to which such aids are perceived as useful by patients from different cultural groups, whose beliefs about health and illness and the factors influencing these, as well as legitimate pathways to, and types of, healthcare may differ from those that underlie current decision aids (28).

Evaluation criteria and outcomes

The proliferation of decision aids has resulted in growing concern and interest among researchers to identify standardized methods to be used in their development, criteria to be used to evaluate decision aids, and measurements to apply these criteria in undertaking systematic reviews comparing outcomes from different studies. To this end, the International Patient Decision Aid Standards Collaboration (IPDAS) was formed to establish an internationally approved set of criteria to determine the quality of decision aids (29). The group consisted of more than 100 researchers, practitioners, and patients from 14 countries. The Collaboration published their criteria, developed through a consensus process, in 2006 (30). The criteria address three domains of quality: the clinical content, the development process, and the effectiveness of decision aids.

Using a similar format to that used in the Evidence-Based Medicine (EBM) users' guides (31), the criteria are presented as a series of questions (25) such as: does the decision aid provide information about treatment options in sufficient detail for decision-making (clinical content), use up to date scientific information that is cited in a reference section or technical document (the development process), and ensure that decision-making is informed and values-based (effectiveness)? Under each question is a list of items, which the evaluator is to mark as either present or absent from the tool (30). These questions provide a framework for both the development and evaluation of decision aids as a means to facilitate patient involvement in treatment decision-making. However, a major limitation of this framework is the absence of any criteria to judge the quality of the conceptual theory and assumptions underlying a given tool's development (i.e. the validity of the framework developed). Also, it remains to be seen whether all of the items addressed in the framework, some of which are fairly subjective, can be operationalized and measured in clear and consistent ways (24).

In recent years, a small number of systematic reviews have been undertaken to assess the impact of decision aids on different outcomes. Some of these reviews focus on decision aids in general, while others focus on cancer-related decision aids in particular. In addition, the Cochrane Collaboration keeps a computerized library of all decision aids that have been developed internationally, and updates these on a periodic basis (27).

A key issue in conducting evaluation studies and systematic reviews of decision aids is the determination of important outcomes to measure as indicators of effectiveness. In the early days of development, the focus was on measuring a small number of outcomes, reflecting the more limited goals of the decision aids developed. The most important of these outcomes was the extent to which decision aids increased patient acquisition of knowledge about treatment options and their benefits and risks, and how satisfied patients were with the decision-making process compared to a control group receiving 'usual care'.

Over time, the number and type of outcomes that decision aids have been posited to positively affect has increased considerably. In addition to knowledge acquisition and satisfaction, for example, decision aids have been studied for their effect on patient involvement in the decision-making process; the decision made; decisional burden, conflict, and regret; anxiety, depression, health status, and quality of life. In addition, the financial impact of changes in patients' treatment choices (either to more or less expensive treatments) after using some form of decision aid has been studied (24).

One question that arises from reading this list of outcomes is whether all of these were actually identified up-front as explicit goals of decision aids and whether the mechanisms through which they were hypothesized to have an effect were well thought through. Some studies simply state the outcomes to be measured without any reference to goals, but what is measured may not be what ought to be measured as important outcomes. The latter depends entirely on the goals set for the intervention in the first place. Whether decision aids can reasonably be expected to affect all the outcome measures listed above is a question worthy of further consideration (24, 32).

According to the IPDAS, the effectiveness of a decision aid should be assessed by the extent to which it improves the proportion of patients who choose and/or receive healthcare interventions that are consistent with their individual values (29). However, no measure currently exists that can fully capture all dimensions of this outcome (33). For example, to determine whether a choice made with a decision aid is consistent with a patient's values, you first need to know what those values are. But as we have shown elsewhere (24), measuring patient values is not an easy task, and using a values clarification exercise is likely to change, rather than accurately depict, the way that patients usually think about their preferences.

The outcomes measured in systematic reviews tend to be much smaller in number than the above list and reflect the most common outcomes measured across studies. Evidence from three recent systematic reviews, two published in 2007 (25, 33) and one published in 2008 (14), have yielded fairly similar results. Two of these reviews focused on decision aids used to support decision-making in the prevention, screening, and treatment of cancer care (14, 33), while the third included decision aids from different clinical contexts (25). All of the reviews focused on results of RCTs.

It is difficult to accurately and comprehensively summarize the results of the above systematic reviews, and the reader is encouraged to read each review paper in order to appreciate the range of methodological issues; for example, the types, number, and sample sizes of studies included, the comparability of the decision aids and clinical contexts of use, and the methods used to undertake the systematic reviews, including statistical analyses and the interpretation of results. However, a few comments can be made here. First, in both cancer-related reviews, decision aids were found to be consistently effective in increasing knowledge of treatment options compared to usual care for screening and treatment decisions (14, 33). The effect of decision aids on other outcomes is less clear.

O'Brien and colleagues (14) report that for cancer-screening decisions, use of decision aids had a variable impact on intentions to seek screening or on actual screening behaviour. Most studies showed no impact on the above outcomes, but a few did show an impact in the desired direction, with some increasing screening intentions or behaviour, for example, in colorectal screening, and others showing a decrease in these outcomes, for example, in prostrate screening. Measures of decisional conflict and the impact of the patient's role in treatment decision-making showed similar mixed results. In five screening studies (seven comparisons) in which general anxiety or cancer worry was measured, there were no significant differences between the group receiving the decision aid and the control group in four studies. However, when the results from three studies with sufficient data were pooled, the decision-aid group had significantly less anxiety than the group receiving usual care (14).

In terms of treatment decisions, O'Brien and colleagues (14) report that decision aids increased knowledge acquisition of treatment options, but did not show any statistically significant impacts in lowering patient anxiety or decisional conflict. Patients receiving decision aids tended to play a more active role in decision-making. Satisfaction with decision-making was increased in three of the four studies in which it was measured. The effect of decision aids on the decision made was variable across studies (14).

The above findings are essentially similar to those published by Neuman and colleagues (33) regarding the effects of decision aids in the cancer-care context. Again, a positive effect on knowledge acquisition is the most consistent beneficial effect found across studies, with some improvements too in patient involvement in treatment decision-making. But, as Neuman and colleagues (33) conclude: 'the efficacy of decision aids in facilitating other outcomes is less clear'. O'Connor and colleagues (25), in their systematic review of decision aids in different clinical contexts (not just cancer), also found that decision aids improved knowledge acquisition among recipients, compared to patients receiving usual care. Decision aids, in addition, increased patients' feeling informed and 'clear about values' compared to patients receiving usual care, although the meaning of this latter phrase is somewhat ambiguous (25).

Undertaking systematic reviews, especially those in which the results of different studies are pooled, is fraught with methodological challenges, since there are so many factors potentially influencing outcomes that can vary across studies. In addition, there does not yet appear to be consensus on what outcome measures are the most important to evaluate, or even consensus on the goals of decision aids. It may well be that our expectations of what decision aids should and can accomplish are too diffuse, and that the original intent of decision aids, to improve knowledge acquisition so that patients are better enabled to participate in treatment decision-making in different clinical contexts, is a sufficiently important goal, in and of itself, to merit promotion of such tools. This is also the area where decision aids appear to be most effective.

Conclusion

Shared decision-making between physicians and patients is often advocated as the 'best' approach to treatment decision-making in the clinical encounter. In reality, what is defined as 'best' can vary depending on whose perspective is being solicited and the criteria by which 'best' is judged. One rationale that is often cited for the promotion of shared decision-making is the achievement of greater patient autonomy and control in decision-making. But if this is the primary goal, then an informed model, where the patient has full control over decision-making, would seem to be better able to meet this objective. We think that the merit of a shared approach, or variant thereof, is that it incorporates physician transfer of key information on treatment options and their benefits and risks to the patient, and enables the latter to share in decision-making as much as she wants, rather than defining an ideal standard of participation that is thought to be best for everyone. The 'best' model is not some abstract and de-contextualized blueprint but rather a much more fluid, contextualized approach that fits with the patient's preferences and experiential comfort level with different approaches to decision-making.

We have seen from the above discussion of decision aids that they were originally designed as a means of implementing shared decision-making, by facilitating information transfer from physician to patient, thereby enabling more informed patient choice. Increasingly, decision aids are expected to positively affect a wide variety of additional outcomes, even though the rationale for these expectations and the mechanisms by which decision aids are to achieve these outcomes are rarely presented. Given the evidence of variability in the success of decisions aids to yield positive results in these areas, and the overwhelmingly consistent evidence of positive effects of decision aids on patient knowledge acquisition, we wonder whether expectations of what such aids should and can achieve have been overly optimistic. Perhaps we need to focus research attention more on developing decision aids for different clinical and cultural contexts, with the more limited goal of increasing patient knowledge of treatment options and their outcomes (what we know such aids are good at already), rather than attempting to search for an ever-expanding number of outcome measures that decision aids might possibly affect, but which were never included as up-front goals in the design of these instruments.

Finally, early decision aids were developed to be used in the context of the physician–patient relationship (34). Such aids were often thought to be of benefit in establishing rapport between physicians and patients, and in providing a structure that would encourage input from both parties in the process of treatment decision-making. One of the more interesting trends in the use of these tools has been an increase in the number of non-physicians who are now administering decision aids to patients, and the use of various take-home versions of such aids. To the extent that this trend continues, decision aids will, increasingly, be taken out of the context of the physician–patient encounter. An interesting question is whether this trend reflects an underlying assumption that anyone can administer such tools, with or without prior training, and that patient engagement in this process with the physician is not that important. In this case, decision aids may well become more of a stand alone and standardized intervention, more appropriate to an informed model of treatment decision-making, rather than a tool to encourage discussion and consensus building on the treatment to implement (i.e. shared decision-making) between physician and patient in the clinical encounter.

References

1. Charles C, Gafni A, Whelan T (1997). Shared decision-making in the medical encounter: what does it mean? (Or it takes at least two to tango). *Soc Sci Med* **44,** 681–92.

2. Guadagnoli E, Ward P (1998). Patient participation in decision-making. *Soc Sci Med* **47,** 329–39.

3. Charles C, Whelan T, Gafni A (1999). What do we mean by partnership in making decisions about treatment? *BMJ* **319,** 780–2.

4. Charles C, Gafni A, Whelan T (1999). Decision-making in the physician-patient encounter: revisiting the shared treatment decision-making model. *Soc Sci Med* **49,** 651–61.

5. Gwyn R, Elwyn G (1999). When is a shared decision not (quite) a shared decision? Negotiating preferences in a general practice encounter. *Soc Sci Med* **49,** 437–47.

6. Whitney SN (2003). A new model of medical decisions: exploring the limits of shared decision-making. *Med Decis Making* **23,** 275–80.

7. Makoul G, Clayman ML (2006). An integrative model of shared decision-making in medical encounters. *Patient Educ Couns* **60,** 301–12.

8. Murray E, Charles C, Gafni A (2006). Shared decision-making in primary care: tailoring the Charles *et al.* model to fit the context of general practice. *Patient Educ Couns* **62,** 205–11.

9. Montori V, Gafni A, Charles C (2006). A shared treatment decision-making approach between patients with chronic conditions and their clinicians: the case of diabetes. *Health Expect* **9,** 25–36.

10. Moumjid N, Gafni A, Brémond A, et al (2007). Shared decision-making in the medical encounter: are we all talking about the same thing? *Med Decis Making* **27,** 539–46.

11. Gattellari M, Butow P, Tattersall M (2001). Sharing decisions in cancer care. *Soc Sci Med* **52,** 1865–78.

12. Brock DW, Wartman SA (1990). When competent patients make irrational choices. *N Engl J Med* **322,** 1595–9.

13. Rose G (1990). Reflections on the changing times. *Br Med J* **301,** 683–7.

14. O'Brien MA. Whelan TJ, Villasis-Keever M et al. (2009). Are cancer-related decision aids effective? A systematic review and meta-analysis. *J Clin Oncol* **27,** 974–85.

15. Gafni A, Charles C, Whelan T (1998). The physician–patient encounter: the physician as a perfect agent for the patient *versus* the informed treatment decision-making model. *Soc Sci Med* **47,** 347–54.

16. Charles CA, Gafni A, Whelan T (2004). Self-reported use of shared decision-making among breast cancer specialists and perceived barriers and facilitators to implementing this approach. *Health Expect* **7**, 338–48.

17. Ford A, Schofield T, Hope T (2002). Barriers to the evidence-based patient choice (EBPC) consultation. *Patient Educ Couns* **47**, 179–85.

18. Holmes-Rovner M, Valade D, Orlowski C, *et al.* (2000). Implementing shared decision-making in routine practice: barriers and opportunities. *Health Expect* **3**, 182–91.

19. Charles C, Whelan T, Gafni A, *et al.* (1998). Doing nothing is no choice: lay constructions of treatment decision-making among women with early-stage breast cancer. *Sociol Health Illn* **20**, 71–95.

20. Salkeld G, Solomon M, Butow P (2004). A matter of trust—patient's views on decision-making in colorectal cancer. *Health Expect* **7**, 104–14.

21. Davey HM, Lim J, Butow P, *et al.* (2004). Women's preferences for and views on decision-making for diagnostic tests. *Soc Sci Med* **58**, 1699–1707.

22. Belcher VN, Fried TR, Agostini JV, *et al.* (2006). Views of older adults on patient participation in medication-related decision-making. *J Gen Intern Med* **21**, 298–303.

23. Nguyen F, Moumjid N, Charles C, *et al.* (2008). Shared treatment decision-making in the medical encounter: attitudes of physicians and their patients in breast cancer care. Unpublished document available from lead author of this chapter.

24. Charles C, Gafni A, Whelan T, *et al.* (2005). Treatment decision-aids: conceptual issues and future directions. *Health Expect* **8**, 114–25.

25. O'Connor AM, Stacey D, Barry MJ, *et al.* (2007). Do patient decision aids meet effectiveness criteria of the international patient decision aid standards collaboration? A systematic review and meta-analysis. *Med Decis Making* **27**, 554–74.

26. O'Connor A, Wells G, Tugwell P, *et al.* (1999). The effect of an explicit values clarification exercise in a woman's decision aid regarding postmenopausal hormone therapy. *Health Expect* **2**, 21–32.

27. O'Connor A, Stacy D, Entwistle V, *et al.* (2003). Decision aids for people facing health treatment or screening decisions. *The Cochrane Database of Systematic Reviews. The Cochrane Library.* Oxford: Cochrane Collaboration **1**, 1–213.

28. Charles C, Gafni A, Whelan T, *et al.* (2006). Cultural influences on the physician-patient encounter: the case of shared treatment decision-making. *Patient Educ Couns* **63**, 262–7.

29. O'Connor A, Llewellyn-Thomas H, Stacey D (2005). IPDAS (International Patient Decision Aid Standards) collaboration background document. **http://ipdas.ohri.ca/resources.html**

30. Elwyn G, O'Connor A, Stacey D, *et al.* (2006). Developing a quality criteria framework for patient decision aids: online international Delphi consensus process. *Br Med J* **333**, 417–9.

31. The Evidence-Based Medicine Working Group, Guyatt G and Rennie D (eds.) (2002). *Users' guides to the medical literature: a manual for evidence-based clinical practice.* AMA press, New York.

32. Nelson WL, Han Paul K, Fagerlin A, *et al.* (2007). Rethinking the objectives of decision aids: a call for conceptual clarity. *Med Dec Mak* **27**, 609–618.

33. Neuman HB, Charlson ME, Temple LK (2007). Is there a role for decision aids in cancer-related decisions? *Crit Rev Oncol Hematol* **62**, 240–50.

34. Levine MN, Gafni A, Markham B, *et al.* (1992). A bedside decision instrument to elicit a patient's preference concerning adjuvant chemotherapy for breast cancer. *Ann Intern Med* **117**, 53–8.

Chapter 5

The ethics of communication in cancer and palliative care

Laura A Siminoff

Introduction

There are two approaches to cancer communication and ethics. First, ethics in cancer communication can refer to the *ethical implications* of cancer communication. Second, it can refer to the *ethics of* cancer communication research, which entails the obligations of researchers working in this field of research. Cancer communication research is especially salient as cancer patients and practitioners have been one of the major laboratories for research in, and application of, bioethical theory. The majority of this chapter will focus on the importance and role of cancer communication research on our knowledge and understanding of bioethics and lastly the special ethical obligations of communication researchers.

Overview of ethical theories

Principlism

Bioethics as a field is based in moral reasoning. The major theoretical framework is 'Principlism' in which four basic principles of bioethics—beneficence, non-malfeasance, justice, and autonomy—are applied to the decisions made about healthcare, whether therapeutic or preventive. This approach is generally referred to as 'normative' ethics, in that it considers which rules or principles have merit. It is beyond the scope of this chapter to argue whether this is the best approach to moral reasoning; rather, it is the one most commonly applied within the field of bioethics.

Autonomy is a form of personal liberty where the individual is the agent determining his or her own course of action (1). Analogous to this is the concept of respect for autonomy in which others acknowledge that persons are ends in themselves and should not be treated as a means. The assumption is that the individual has the capacity to act intentionally, with understanding, and without controlling influences that would hamper the individual acting as a free and voluntary agent (1).

The principle of non-malfeasance is best drawn from the maxim, 'above all, do no harm.' This principle affirms the need for medical competence as the minimum standard for providing patient care. This principle is frequently combined with that of beneficence, referring to a duty to act in the interest of another, e.g. a physician's duty to help a patient when able. Thus, healthcare providers must not only refrain from harming patients, but are also obligated to aid them (1).

The principle of justice has probably received the least attention from bioethicists and policy-makers. Justice in healthcare is usually defined as a form of fairness, and implies the fair distribution of goods and services in society. The question of distributive justice (2) acknowledges that some goods and services are in short supply. In healthcare, where lack of supply can result in disability and death (for instance, in the case of distributing organs for transplantation or allocating drugs in short supply to treat cancer), there must be an equitable distribution system. How that distribution system should be structured in healthcare, and the criteria for distribution, vary greatly worldwide.

Casuistry

'Casuistry' is an alternative approach to moral reasoning. Casuistry is a case-based method of moral reasoning that does not rely on basic principles to guide decisions. Casuistry asserts that moral knowledge develops incrementally through analysis of specific cases through moral triangulation. An analogy is the development of English Common Law (3). A distinct advantage of casuistry is its rejection of the trend toward reductionism and the individualism of principlist-based ethics. It also lends itself to greater inclusivity of varying cultural perspectives and values, but can be criticized on the grounds that it is too 'relativist' and situationally dependent.

Virtue ethics

Another framework guiding the thinking of bioethicists is 'virtue' theory in which the character of the person, with their 'internal goods' or values, is seen to guide the behaviour and integrity of the clinician (1). Virtue ethics is a valuable addition to approaching moral conflicts, especially when principles are in conflict. In addition, virtue ethics can be seen as taking a more holistic, flexible, and relational approach to healthcare ethics (4). Compassion, practical wisdom, sincerity, trustworthiness, honesty, conscientiousness, and competence are some of the key virtues guiding medical practice. Medical education increasingly promotes recognition of these values that guide the principle of beneficence, yet recognize the relational nature of the encounter and form a motivating force for effective communication (4, 5).

Doctrine of informed consent

The concept of informed consent derives from the basic principles of beneficence, non-malfeasance, autonomy, and justice. The most important principle is respect for autonomy, which provides the basis for the practice of 'informed consent' in the healthcare provider–patient interactions regarding healthcare decisions. Ideally, informed consent is the process through which patients are fully informed about their health (diagnosis) and healthcare options (treatment choices), such that it enables them to participate in making decisions about their healthcare. There are five essential elements of informed consent:

(1) discussion about the rationale for the procedure;

(2) communicating the potential benefits of the procedure;

(3) understanding the risks involved;

(4) explanation of any treatment alternatives available; and

(5) assuring the decision of the subject is voluntary (6).

Informed consent by definition implies communication in both oral and written forms. Informed consent has at least two goals: to promote individual autonomy and to promote rational decision-making (7). The main mechanism of informed consent is communication, and the quality of the communication will determine the quality or 'trueness' of the consent.

Perhaps one of the most difficult issues, and most germane to health communication, is coercion. Coercion is defined as the imposition of another's will by means of a serious threat or even an irresistible offer or as influence by means of rational argument (8). The ability to differentiate persuasion from coercion, or even manipulation, can be difficult. Persuasion can appear controlling, as it may be used to elicit a desired decision, e.g. a patient chooses to participate in a clinical trial, but it is not defined as coercion if the decision is the result of appeal to reason (4, 6). Thus, medical research, especially interventional research, must carefully consider whether the techniques used to obtain informed consent are persuasive or coercive.

Finally, research on informed consent has examined how much information is needed for adequate consent. To date, most approaches to informed consent take a legalistic, rather than an empirical, approach to this question. Standard texts (1, 7) all identify three standards.

- There is a 'reasonable physician standard' that asks, 'What would a typical physician say about this intervention?'. This standard allows the physician to determine what information is appropriate to disclose. Most research has shown that the typical physician tells the patient very little, making this a standard of dubious value.

- The 'reasonable patient standard' asks, 'What would the average patient need to know in order to make an informed decision?'. This standard focuses on considering what a patient would need to know in order to understand the choices he or she is presented.

- Finally, there is a 'subjective standard' that asks, 'What would a specific patient need to know and understand in order to make an informed decision?'. This standard requires tailoring information to each patient.

None of these standards truly answer the question of how much information patients need to make informed decisions, and they evade altogether the question of how information should be delivered. Communication research can help answer these questions.

Communication and consent

Communication is the seminal activity to attain informed decision-making. Proper communication about the patient's illness and treatment options, including clinical trials, is necessary in order to respect patient autonomy and to ensure that participation is voluntary. The ways physicians must present patients with information during the informed consent process is two-fold: first, they need to provide all information to the patient as mandated by legal requirements; and, second, they must introduce and explain the information in an unbiased fashion, to ensure that patients can make an informed, voluntary choice (9).

Studies have shown that most physicians and researchers do not communicate all the domains of legal informed consent to patients. For example, a study by Sankar (10), examining the informed consent process for phase 1 clinical trials, found that compensation for injury was never discussed orally, and that confidentiality and the right to withdraw were discussed in only 6% of consent sessions. While most consent information is also covered in the consent form, the forms tend to have high reading levels, are difficult to follow, use technical or medical jargon, and may minimize risks and exaggerate potential benefits.

Sankar (10) also found that communication problems existed in the way investigators framed the information in their discussions with patients (leaving out or emphasizing certain information), discussed benefits that were unlikely, did not clearly discriminate between research and treatment, and mixed the unproven with the known (e.g. by making something seem effective, while also saying that the research is still needed). Other studies have found that this ambiguous, unclear presentation of information is not uncommon during the informed consent process, which underscores the importance of information being communicated clearly and effectively to patients in order for them to make their own informed, autonomous decisions (11, 12). It also underscores that clinicians continue to have their own difficulties understanding and incorporating the concept of equipoise (belief it is unknown whether or not one arm of a trial is better than the other) into their belief system. While some physicians have a good understanding of this concept and find it useful in conceptualizing clinical trials both for themselves and their patients (13), other physicians do not appear to understand the concept and report describing the experimental arm of a trial in such a way as to make it seem new, distinctive, or revolutionary to the patient, rather than explaining that it is not yet known if one arm of the study is better than the other (14).

Conversely, comprehensible, unambiguous communication between physicians and patients can aid the informed consent process. Research has shown that there are ways of communicating information that patients perceive as more understandable and personally tailored than others, which can reduce confusion in informed consent and decision-making. One study (15) reported that participants were better able to understand, and found it easier to make a decision, when chemotherapy-risk information was presented in a more personal manner and with a concise, positive framing, than when the same information was presented in a manner that was negative, impersonal, persuasive, ambiguous, or wordy and therefore confusing. Thus, communication must be clear, unbiased, and effective in order to aid in the decision-making process.

Intersection of cancer communication, decision-making, and consent

Cancer patients face several challenges when making decisions. The diagnosis of cancer can be very frightening because of the stigma attached to the disease, and the fear of disfigurement and death it evokes. Until recently, cancer was viewed as an inexorable disease that can affect anyone at any time. Despite the advances in prevention, early detection, and treatment, the public still ranks cancer as the illness of which they are most afraid. Second, with recent advances in cancer treatment has come the challenge of choice between multiple treatment options. However, this also makes the decision-making process more difficult for cancer patients because they must weigh the risks and benefits of each treatment (16). In addition, more responsibility is now being placed on patients for their own care, and patients are, therefore, making decisions that they may not be prepared or qualified to make (16). One proposed remedy to this situation is the use of decision aids. These tools were introduced in the 1980s and are designed to provide objective information to patients about various treatment options. Decision aids can assist in decision-making by helping patients make treatment choices that are consistent with their own values, increasing patient knowledge about risks and benefits, and allowing patients to participate in the decision-making process (17).

The use of decision aids also raises ethical questions. For example, Nelson and colleagues suggest that the structure of decision aids may actually interfere with patients' own decision-making strategies (18). When people scrutinize their decisions too closely or too much, they may actually be less likely to focus on information relevant to the situation at hand. Some data suggest that people are more satisfied with their decisions when they make them intuitively, rather than analytically. When considering decisions more rationally, individuals are at risk of weighing different aspects of the problem in a biased fashion, whereas when making decisions using less conscious thought, individuals can form more global impressions of their decisions. Therefore, decision aids may potentially distort patients' usual decision-making processes. Moreover, if patients do not have strong and stable values, decision aids cannot help them reach the decision that is most consistent with their values; rather, patients may construct temporary values while using the decision aid, and thus are susceptible to forming values based on the way the information is portrayed (18). Therefore, based on how information is framed, decision aids could actually persuade patients to make certain decisions rather than others. When the decision to enrol in a clinical trial is one possible result of the use of a decision aid, researchers must be especially careful. In order to be ethical, decision aids and interventions in communication research in general must focus on helping patients make informed decisions, not just helping patients see how particular decisions, such as the decision to enrol in a trial, may fit in with their value system. Finally, more basic research is needed to know what types of information are most valuable and influential to medical decision-making. These data could help to guide the design of better decision aids.

The decision to participate in a research study is a unique kind of decision in healthcare. Most decisions faced by patients are regarding what types of treatments will be the most likely to aid their medical problems or help maintain a high quality of life while ill. Informed participation in a clinical trial generally means that subjects must understand the diagnosis, the relationship between the illness and their future health and functioning, and the benefits of standard therapy options. They need to also obtain some understanding of how treatment received within the context of a clinical trial differs from standard care. Other exigencies are time constraints and dealing with medical uncertainty. For example, decisions may appear to need to be made quickly. Even when there is no medical reason to make the decision quickly, patients often feel pressured to do so by their fears for their health or by their physicians. It is well understood that simply handing a patient a written consent form does not constitute adequate consent. The information needs to be communicated in a meaningful way, so that the patient is prepared to participate in the decision-making process. However, clinical trials aim to test new medications or medical regimens that may be helpful to society and other patients in the future, rather than directly helping the patients actually participating in the study. Many patients still agree to participate in clinical trials with the belief that they may be getting 'better' treatment than they would receive from standard treatment or that the purpose of the trial is to provide them with better treatment. This misunderstanding has been termed the 'therapeutic misconception' (12). Health communication research can contribute to understanding phenomena such as these and contribute to ways to overcome these difficulties.

In order for communication between clinicians and patients to be effective, four essential topics must be addressed:

(1) the rationale for the procedure;

(2) the risks involved;

(3) the potential benefits of the procedure; and

(4) available treatment alternatives.

However, even these four basic topics are not always discussed (19). Although physicians are now providing patients with much more information than they did just thirty years ago (12–14), many physicians are still hesitant to disclose all relevant information to their patients. Some feel that full disclosure is burdensome to patients, causing unnecessary and excessive anxiety (15, 16). Thus, physicians struggle with deciding what information to convey to patients and what information will be helpful, as opposed to (what they perceive to be) harmful or overwhelming, for patients.

Physicians may also be unclear about what they should or should not communicate to patients. Until 10 years ago, there were gag clauses that could prevent physicians from discussing treatment options that insurance companies would not cover. Similarly, Health Maintenance Organizations would prohibit referral to medical specialists if they were not included in the insurance company's group of providers (20). Although these restrictive clauses have since been prohibited, some still believe that in order to maximize efficiency, physicians should not discuss options in which the benefit to the patient does not outweigh the cost of the therapy. Withholding information and options in this manner threatens the concept of informed consent.

While most patients desire to receive information about their diagnosis and possible treatment options, they vary much more on the extent to which they would like to participate in the decision-making process. Moreover, it must be recognized that while the majority of patients prefer a reasonable amount of detailed information, others do not. Matching studies, which examine the extent to which a patient's level of desire for information is met and the effect on patient outcomes, have somewhat mixed findings; however, the likelihood of positive outcomes (such as more satisfaction or less depression) is increased if treatment interventions are tailored to provide patients with the amount or method of providing information that they desire (21). For example, one study examined the amount of information patients wanted about the surgery they were to undergo (22). Patients who wanted more information received a problem-focused coping intervention, while patients who wanted less information received an emotion-focused coping intervention. Those who received the coping intervention that matched their information preference were better adjusted during surgery, more satisfied, and experienced less pain than patients whose preferences were discordant with the intervention they received (22). These studies demonstrate the importance of tailoring information preferences to each individual, as meeting patients' desire for information and decision-making can have a beneficial effect on patient outcomes. Health communication research can help develop mechanisms for intelligently tailoring information for individual patients.

Other ethically challenging communication predicaments

Many physicians are uncomfortable discussing poor prognoses with their patients, particularly when discussing a terminal prognosis. While physicians will answer patient questions truthfully when asked, they are often less likely to volunteer information about poor prognoses. A common rationale for this practice is to not deprive the patient with late-stage disease of hope. In addition, there is a fear that these patients are already psychologically fragile and explicit discussions of prognosis will damage an already delicate psyche. Moreover, many physicians are concerned as to how accurate their prognosis really is, whether or not patients understand probabilities and if these discussions hurt the doctor–patient relationship (23–25). However, if patients are not provided with sufficient information, or misinterpret the vague or optimistically-framed information provided by the physician, patients and their families frequently continue to hope for, or expect, a miracle. Some seek out futile care and endure advanced treatments for what may be small, if any, benefits, and some patients could undergo chemotherapy for a survival benefit of just one week (26).

Communication between patients and their family members at the end-of-life also raises certain ethical dilemmas. When patients are incapacitated, surrogates are often called upon to make medical decisions for patients. There is a presumption that these surrogates will carry out the patients' wishes. However, it is not uncommon for a patient's preferences for end-of-life care to be unknown to family members. This may be due to the patient's failure or inability to convey their preferences to family members before loss of capacity, or the absence of written advance directives. Often surrogates project their own preferences onto patients; that is, surrogates are more likely to predict that patients would want the same end-of-life treatments that the surrogates themselves would want, rather than what the patients would actually prefer (27). Even if surrogates do know patient preferences based on previous conversations, surrogates may not base their decisions for patient care on these preferences, but instead base the decision on their own beliefs about quality of life, possibility of change or recovery, or family burden (28–30). Therefore, clinicians need to be aware that the use of surrogates as decision-makers for patients is an imperfect ethical instrument.

Integration of ethics into communication research

Communication research has been a vital tool for providing observational data that have informed ethicists and policy makers about consent practices. The advisory committee formed by President Clinton in 1994 uncovered serious ethical violations in a series of radiation studies performed by the government approximately fifty years ago (31). This commission found that many consent forms did not properly address risks and may have over-emphasized benefits (31). Some patients believed it was a treatment option that was better than standard therapy, while others thought they had no choice. Consent forms were too complicated for many to read and understand—using technical language, small fonts, lengthy and technical descriptions, and requiring a high reading level. People involved in the radiation studies were hurt physically but also emotionally because they were deceived (32). Today, people are still confused about the difference between research and medical care.

Threats to effective communication occur not only when physicians withhold information from patients, but also when physicians and patients fail to communicate and comprehend each individual's preferences and goals. In their seminal work on communication in medical consultations, Byrne and Long (33) noted that lack of effective communication between doctor and patient was a result of several characteristics of how the physician conducted the consultation. Doctors had difficulty discussing issues besides symptoms and treatment (for instance, the psychosocial impact of the illness or family difficulties). They assumed patients would fit into certain categories and did not make accommodations if patients deviated from the presumed pattern. They seemed relatively unaware of the dynamics between the two inter-actants (i.e. the 'how' as opposed to the 'what' of the conversation), and asked questions in a stereotyped manner, rather than adapting to each patient. Through their analysis of hundreds of audiotapes, Byrne and Long discovered that when physicians and patients were not aware of each other's goals, both end up less satisfied with the outcome of the consultation (33). Byrne and Long wrote, 'There also appeared to be a clear degree of interactional confusion because many of the statements or questions made by the doctor bear no relationship to the apparent responses made by the patient and vice versa' (33, p.63).

Persuasion

There is a fine line between persuasion and coercion when obtaining informed consent. Many who participated in the radiation experiments said that initially they had declined to consent. Because there is no record of precisely what was said, it is unclear whether it was persuasion or coercion that caused their change of mind (33). Some reported they felt pressured by researchers to agree to participate. One definition of coercion is the use of manipulation or the threat of harm (be it physical or financial) to influence the decision. In contrast, persuasion is the use of techniques or reasonable incentives to change an individual's way of thinking (1). However, excessive threat or manipulation may not be necessary for patients to feel coerced into making certain decisions. Thus, Allmark and Mason (34) acknowledged that recruiting desperate participants to trials was not ethical because their decisions were essentially coerced. If participants believe that the trial is their only hope, and they cannot receive treatment without participating, it makes the decision less than voluntary and interferes with patient autonomy. In this example, patients may believe that they will suffer negative consequences if they do not consent, and that the incentive of survival or better quality of life fall outside of the realm of the 'reasonable' incentives used in persuasion. People feel coerced even when no direct communication occurs that could influence their opinion. Organ donation research highlights how individuals can feel coercion and loss of autonomy. If one person is found to be a good match, the potential recipient and related family members make assumptions that this individual will want to donate, creating a potential sense of pressure (35). Clearly, not only the words but also the predicament make people feel they are being coerced, rather than offered persuasive information and still able to make their own decision.

Shared decision-making

Patients vary in the extent to which they want to participate in the decision-making process about their care. There is a range of desire for information but, in general, studies show that about 92% want information about their illness and treatment options. Patients vary more in their wish to participate in treatment decisions (36). Before the 1980s, a paternalistic approach dominated and patients accepted the physician's recommendation. In this model, the flow of information passed unidirectionally from physician to patient, rather than both contributing to the discussion (37). The focus was medical in orientation, with the physician providing sufficient information to meet legal requirements for informed consent, but rarely full disclosure.

Charles *et al.* (37) identified four main assumptions making physicians dominant in decision-making:

(1) a single treatment was usually 'best';

(2) physicians would recommend this superior treatment;

(3) physicians were considered well-trained and educated; and

(4) physicians were motivated out of concern for their patient.

Patients therefore tended to allow, and indeed prefer, their doctor to make the choice. Parsons incorporated similar ideas into his concept of the 'sick role' (38). He posited from a sociological standpoint that a sick person is exempt from having to fulfill normal responsibilities, but that being sick is undesirable, and the ill individual is obliged to take steps to get better (38). According to this concept of the sick role, the relationship between physician and patient is inherently asymmetrical. While some individuals, particularly those who are older, less educated, and have a more severe illness still prefer the paternalistic style of decision-making (39), the development of a wider range of treatment options has led most patients to now prefer to participate in the decision-making process, to at least some degree.

At the other end of the spectrum is the fully informed model. This is more consumer-oriented as patients learn about their illness and treatment options so that they can make their autonomous choice. The content of the consultation focuses more on medical and other relevant information that informs patients about all treatment options, with their risks and benefits. This model assumes that patients will make the best decision for themselves, so that the deliberation is undertaken by the patient.

Falling in between these two extremes is the model of shared decision-making. There are four characteristics of the shared model:

(1) joint participation in decision-making;

(2) physician and patient exchange information about both medical (e.g. diagnosis and treatment options) and personal (e.g. impact of possible risks on patient's life topics);

(3) both express treatment preferences; and

(4) both eventually settle on what type of treatment will be implemented (16).

The physician and patient (and possibly the patient's family) discuss options and come to a treatment decision together. One specific paradigm of shared decision-making, the communication model of shared decision-making (CMSDM), puts emphasis on the transactional process that occurs between the physician and patient when communicating to come to a decision about cancer treatment (16). This model is based on four assumptions:

(1) the physician and patient (as well as any others participating in decision-making, such as spouses) work as a system and communicate with one another;

(2) both verbal and non-verbal messages are exchanged;

(3) physicians introduce patients to the consultation process and set the communication climate; and

(4) patients must convey their preferences regarding the extent to which they will participate in the decision-making process.

There are three influential factors involved in the interactional process between the physician and the patient. The first factor is patient–physician communication antecedents. Each individual has background characteristics that affect communication, namely, sociodemographic characteristics, personality traits (i.e. argumentative or docile), and communication competence (i.e. knowing what to communicate and how to do so). The second factor is the communication climate, which influences what happens during the consultation and takes the emotional, cognitive, and decisional preferences of each individual into account. The communication climate is affected by the patient's and physician's information and decision-making preferences, the severity of disease (i.e. patients tend to be more passive when illness is more severe), each inter-actant's emotional state, and the role expectations of each person. The third factor is the treatment decision in which the physician and patient, having hopefully established a relationship characterized by trust, jointly contribute to making a treatment decision.

Future directions

Communication research is the major vehicle for understanding the ethics of cancer communication, especially informed consent to treatment and to participation in clinical trials. Health communication researchers are deeply involved in attempting to develop 'better' ways for clinical communication to unfold and to help with treatment decision-making. The ethical obligations of communication researchers need to be sensitive concerning whose values are being upheld or promoted, and how we use effective models of communication persuasively but not coercively.

References

1. Beauchamp T, Childress J (2004). *Principle of Medical Ethics*, 6th edn. New York: Oxford University Press.
2. Rawls J (1971). *A Theory of Justice*. Harvard University Press, Boston.
3. Arras JD (1991). Getting down to cases: te revival of casuistry in bioethics. *The Journal of Medicine and Philosophy* **16**, 29–51.
4. Benner P (1997). A dialogue between virtue ethics and care ethics. *Theoretical Medicine* **18**(1–2), 47–61.
5. Randall F, Downie R (1996). *Palliative Care Ethics*. Oxford: Oxford University Press.
6. Siminoff LA (2003). Toward improving the informed consent process in research with humans. *IRB: Ethics & Human Research* **25**(5), S1–S3.
7. Lidz CW, Meisel A, Zerubavel E, *et al.* (1984). *Informed Consent: a Study of Decisionmaking in Psychiatry*. New York: Oxford University Press.
8. Faden RR, Beauchamp TL (1986). *A History and Theory of Informed Consent*. New York: Oxford University Press.
9. Siminoff LA (1992). Improving communication with cancer patients. *Oncology* **6**(10), 83–87.

10. Sankar P (2004). Communication and miscommunication in informed consent to research. *Medical Anthropology Quarterly* **18**(4), 429–446.

11. Applebaum PS (2002). Clarifying the ethics of clinical research: a path toward avoidigin the therapeutic misconception. *American Journal of Bioethics* **2**(2), 22–23.

12. Applebaum PS, Roth LH, Lidz CW (1982). The therapeutic misconception: informed consent in psychiatric research. *International Journal of Law and Psychiatry* **5**, 319–329.

13. Garcia J, Elbourne D, Snowdon C (2004). Equipoise: a case study of the views of clinicians involved in two neonatal trials. *Clinical trials* **1**(2), 170–178.

14. Ziebland S, Featherstone K, Snowdon C, *et al.* (2007). Does it matter if clinicians recruiting for a trial don't understand what the trial is really about? Qualitative study of surgeons' experiences of participation in a pragmatic multi-centre RCT. *Trials* **8**, 4.

15. Studts JL, Abell TD, Roetzer LM, *et al.* (2005). Preferences for different methods of communicating information regarding adjuvant chemotherapy for breast cancer. *Psychooncology* **14**(8), 647–660.

16. Siminoff LA, Step MM (2005). A communication model of shared decision making. Accounting for cancer treatment decisions. *Health Psychology* **24**(4 Suppl), S99–S105.

17. Weinstein JN, Clay K, Morgan TS (2007). Informed patient choice: patient-centered valuing of surgical risks and benefits. *Health Affairs* **26**(3), 726–730.

18. Nelson WL, Han PKJ, Fagerlin A, *et al.* (2007). Rethinking the objectives of decision aids: a call for conceptual clarity. *Medical Decision Making* **27**(5), 609–618.

19. Finucane TE, Beamer BA, Roca RP, *et al.* (1993). Establishing advance medical directives with demented patients: a pilot study. *The Journal of Clinical Ethics* **4**(1), 51–54.

20. Faden RR (1997). Managed care and informed consent. *Kennedy Institute of Ethics Journal* **7**(4), 377–379.

21. Kiesler DJ, Auerbach SM (2006). Optimal matches of patient preferences for information, decision-making and interpersonal behaviour: evidence, models and interventions. *Patient Education and Counseling* **61**(3), 319–341.

22. Martelli MF, Auerbach SM, Alexander J, *et al.* (1987). Stress management in the healthcare setting: matching interventions with patient coping styles. *Journal of Consulting and Clinical Psychology* **55**(2), 201–207.

23. Christakis NA (1999). Prognostication and bioethics. *Daedalus* **128**(4), 197–214.

24. Glare P, Virik K, Jones M, *et al.* (2003). A systematic review of physicians' survival predictions in terminally ill cancer patients. *BMJ* **327**(7408), 195–198.

25. Gordon EJ, Daugherty CK (2003). 'Hitting you over the head': oncologists' disclosure of prognosis to advanced cancer patients. *Bioethics* **17**(2), 142–168.

26. Matsuyama R, Reddy S, Smith TJ (2006). Why do patients choose chemotherapy near the end of life? A review of the perspective of those facing death from cancer. *Journal of Clinical Oncology* **24**(21), 3490–3496.

27. Fagerlin A, Ditto PH, Danks JH, *et al.* (2001). Projection in surrogate decisions about life-sustaining medical treatments. *Health Psychology* 2001;**20**(3), 166–75.

28. Arnold RM, Kellum J (2003). Moral justifications for surrogate decision making in the intensive care unit: implications and limitations. *Critical Care Medicine* **31**(5 Suppl.), S347–S353.

29. Rothchild E (1994). Family dynamics in end-of-life treatment decisions. *General Hospital Psychiatry* **16**(4), 251–8.

30. Vig EK, Taylor JS, Starks H, *et al.* (2006). Beyond substituted judgment: How surrogates navigate end-of-life decision-making. *Journal of The American Geriatrics Society* **54**(11), 1688–93.

31. Kass NE, Sugarman J (1996). Are research subjects adequately protected? A review and discussion of studies conducted by the advisory committee on human radiation experiments. *Kennedy Institute of Ethics Journal* **16**(3), 271–282.

32. Faden RR (1996). Chair's perspective on the work of the advisory committee on human radiation experiment. *Kennedy Institute of Ethics Journal* **6**(3), 215–221.

33. Byrne PS, Long BEL (1976). *Doctors Talking to Patients*. London: HMSO.

34. Allmark P, Mason S (2006). Should desperate volunteers be included in randomised controlled trials? *Journal of Medical Ethics* **32**, 548–553.

35. Olbrisch ME, Benedict SM, Haller DL, *et al.* (2001). Psychosocial assessment of living organ donors: clinical and ethical considerations. *Progress in Transplantation* **11**(1), 40–49.

36. Benbassat C, Jochanan E, Pipel Y, *et al.* (1998). Patients preferences for participation in clinical decision making: a review of published surveys. *Behavioural Medicine* **24**(2), 81–88.

37. Charles C, Gafni A, Whelan T (1999). Decision-making in the physician-patient encounter: revisiting the shared treatment decision-making model. *Social Science & Medicine* **49**, 651–661.

38. Parsons T (1975). The sick role and the role of the physician reconsidered. *The Milbank Memorial Fund Quarterly Health and Society* **53**(3), 257–278.

39. Auerbach SM (2001). Should patients have control over their own healthcare?: empirical evidence and research issues. *Annals of Behavioural Medicine* **22**(3), 246–259.

Chapter 6

Gender, power, and non-verbal communication

Marianne Schmid Mast, Christina Klöckner, and Judith A Hall

Introduction

Both non-verbal communication and gender play an important role in the clinical encounter. They not only affect the impact of the diagnosis, but also patient outcomes such as satisfaction and appointment-keeping. Dominance or power asymmetries in the provider–patient interaction have been assumed to affect the relationship, but have rarely been studied. Our goals in this chapter are:

(1) to give an overview of the empirical findings pertaining to non-verbal communication, gender, and power within the patient–clinician interaction;

(2) show how gender, non-verbal communication, and power are intertwined; and

(3) offer guidance about communication skills training to help physicians and improve outcomes for cancer patients.

Non-verbal communication

Definition

Non-verbal behaviour can be defined as 'communication effected by means other than words' (1, p.5). The distinction between verbal and non-verbal communication is not, however, clear-cut. Sign language, for instance, is 'non-verbal' behaviour through its use of gestures, but also 'verbal' in that each gesture has distinct linguistic meanings and there is an established grammar. Most non-verbal communication does not have such complex properties and, indeed, there is often ambiguity about how non-verbal cues should be interpreted. Examples of non-verbal behaviours include facial expressions conveying emotions, eye gaze, gestures, posture, touching, tone of voice and speech modulation and duration (2).

Whether verbal or non-verbal behaviour matters more as a source of information depends on the situation (3). In the case of an ambiguous verbal message or one of doubtful honesty, non-verbal cues provide key understanding. They become especially salient when they contradict the words being spoken or when the context is highly emotional. Non-verbal cues serve not just the expression of emotions but also signal attention, reflect physical symptoms like pain, convey attitudes about friendliness or dominance, and reveal personality characteristics such as shyness or extraversion.

Non-verbal communication in the medical encounter

In studying communication, researchers have paid relatively more attention to the verbal than the non-verbal. As a consequence, a number of different coding tools exist for the analysis of verbal content. Some of the most frequently used are: the Process Analysis System (4), the Verbal Response Mode (5), and the Roter Interaction Analysis System (RIAS) (6).

In the provider–patient relationship, emotions play a central role (7). Non-verbal behaviour is an important aspect to investigate because of its connection to emotions and interpersonal attitudes (7). Some of the verbal coding tools include ratings of non-verbal communication, like the global rating of provider dominance in the RIAS (6). With interest in non-verbal behaviours growing, non-verbal cue-coding schemes emerged. Gallagher and colleagues (8, 9) developed the Relational Communication Scale for Observational measurement (RCS-O), consisting of 34 items measuring intimacy, composure, formality, and dominance. Items such as 'The physician was willing to listen to the patient' are typically rated on non-verbal behaviours. Other studies use direct measures of non-verbal behaviour (e.g. how long the provider looked or how many times they smiled at the patient) and interpret their meaning based on knowledge about the correlates of certain non-verbal behaviours (10). However, because one and the same non-verbal behaviour can mean different things depending on context, the interpretation remains somewhat speculative.

Interplay between provider and patient non-verbal communication

The provider's non-verbal behaviour is not independent of the patient's, but dynamically interactive with it. Street and Buller (11) video-taped 38 patients and their 10 providers from a family practice clinic to analyse non-verbal behaviour. The more the provider gazed away from the patient, the more the patient looked away from the provider. Body orientation of clinician towards patient showed the same pattern. The authors concluded that when non-verbal behaviours are affiliative, the provider and patient show correspondence in their respective behaviours. This finding is in line with research reporting an association between feeling at ease in the medical encounter and ratings of interactional synchrony, including simultaneous movements, tempo similarity, and posture mirroring (12). In contrast, when behaviours are associated with power and dominance (e.g. speaking time), the provider and the patient show asymmetrical or complementary behaviour (11). The more the clinician talks, the less a patient talks. Reciprocity for affiliative and complementarity for dominance-related behaviours occur also outside the clinical setting in dyadic peer interactions (13).

Effect of a clinician's non-verbal communication on patients

The clinician's non-verbal behaviour can definitely have an impact on patients. Thus, the distancing behaviour of physical therapists, such as absence of smiling and looking away from the patient, was related to decreases in patients' physical and cognitive functioning (14). Also, surgeons with a more dominant tone of voice were more likely to have been sued for medical malpractice than surgeons with a less dominant tone (15). Moreover, non-verbal behaviour can help to make possible more accurate diagnosis. Bensing, Kerssens, and van der Pasch (16) found that provider-gazing at the patient was related to more successfully recognizing psychological distress.

Much of the research on the effects of non-verbal communication has investigated patient satisfaction as an outcome. More patient satisfaction is associated with reduced time spent by the provider reading the medical chart and more leaning forward, nodding, gesturing, gazing, and closer interpersonal distance (17). Griffith and colleagues (18) showed that patient satisfaction was higher when clinicians smiled a lot, increased eye contact, leaned forward, used an expressive tone of voice and face, and gestured more.

Depending on context, one and the same non-verbal behaviour can mean different things. As a consequence of this context dependency, there is no precise dictionary of non-verbal behaviour and our understanding of what specific non-verbal cues signify remains scattered, at best. Factors that can change the meaning of a non-verbal cue include gender, age, and severity of disease (19).

Provider non-verbal decoding skills

To reach a diagnosis and form an impression about a patient, the astute clinician observes the patient's non-verbal behaviour. Research addressing non-verbal decoding skills reveals that people can be very accurate when forming opinions about others. Correct judgments are invariably made about traits such as dominance or intelligence (20, 21), the nature of a social relationship, which of two individuals is the supervisor of the other (20, 21), what the intentions or motives of people are (22, 23) and what they feel or think (26–28).

Similarly, how well a physician can appraise the patient, or in other words, how well he or she can read the patient's non-verbal behaviour, impacts substantially their overall relationship. In one study, medical students were on average poorer at reading others' non-verbal cues compared to other students (24). However, medical students who indicated a preference for primary care specialization had better non-verbal decoding skills than both of the aforementioned groups. Research also shows that providers who are good at correctly interpreting their patient's non-verbal cues have more satisfied patients (25) who are more likely to return for their next appointment (26). A pronounced ability to understand patients' non-verbal cues is advantageous for clinicians, because their patients are more satisfied and more willing to return for further appointments.

For cancer patients, the healthcare provider's ability to decode non-verbal cues is particularly important because of the frequency of psychological distress (27). Often, symptoms of distress are not detected and go untreated, with the potential for deterioration in a patient's well-being (27, 28). Given that affect is expressed non-verbally, the correct assessment of a patient's demeanour and non-verbal cues becomes crucial to the provision of responsive care.

Gender

Female and male providers communicate differently (29) and these differences affect patient outcomes, in particular patient satisfaction. Moreover, depending on the provider's gender, patients communicate differently (30). Thus both the gender of the clinician and the patient affect communication in the medical setting.

Differences in communication styles of male and female providers

In comparison to men, women in general differ in their communication style: they self-disclose more (31) and use a greater relationship-oriented style (2), with more smiling, more gazing at the other, less physical distance, and increased emotional expressiveness. Women also tend to adjust their status to equal their partner's, whereas men underscore status differences (32). In like manner, female clinicians differ from their male counterparts. On the one hand, Roter and colleagues' (29) meta-analysis revealed that both providers share the same amount and quality of medical information, as well as social conversation (medically irrelevant information), with their patients. However, female providers talked more about the psychosocial impact of a diagnosis or treatment and used more partnership building (e.g. soliciting expectations from, and including, the patient in decision-making processes).

Moreover, female clinicians used more positive communication (e.g. encouragement), emotionally focused talk (e.g. emotional probes, empathy), and supportive behaviours such as smiling and nodding (29). Last, but not least, consultations with female providers were on average two minutes longer than with male providers.

All in all, when clinicians are women, they talk more about the effects of an impediment on the patient, communicate in a more egalitarian manner, and like their patients more (33). These conclusions are valid for general practitioners, but may differ across other medical specializations.

For gynaecologists, for instance, these results are reversed: male gynaecologists create a more emotional interaction and their consultations last longer than female gynaecologists (29).

Patients communicate differently with male and female providers

The gender of the provider affects how patients communicate. One explanation is that, outside of the medical consultation, people react differently to women and men. Women are looked at and smiled at more, and are given more confidential information than men (2, 31). Another explanation is that, because female and male providers communicate differently (29), this directly affects the communication style of patients (11).

In a meta-analysis, Hall and Roter (30) showed that patients of female doctors talked more and conveyed more biomedical and psychosocial information than did patients of male physicians. Patients communicate more positively (e.g. reach agreement) with a female clinician and use more partnership-building statements. Interestingly, patients talk about emotions to the same extent with female and male providers.

In sum, female clinicians appear to have a diagnostic advantage because patients convey more medical information, despite the fact that providers do not differ in how much medical data they convey in return. As we shall see, patients are more assertive and dominant with women; they feel more empowered.

Effect of patient gender

Women seek medical advice more often than men and become more active in the medical encounter (34, 35). Thus, they ask more questions and show more interest than male patients (36). Moreover, the behaviour of the provider changes in response to the patient's gender. Female patients are treated more empathically (37, 38), asked more about their opinion and feelings, and may receive more information (39). This is most likely the result of asking more questions (34). Importantly, clinicians use a calmer and less dominant voice when speaking to a woman (37, 38). In sum, providers communicate with female patients in a more emotional and partnership-oriented way.

Gender composition of the dyad

Because both patient and provider gender affect medical communication, studies that consider both aspects simultaneously prove helpful in extricating the role of gender (19, 45–47). One noteworthy finding is that when the clinician and patient are the same gender, providers show more interest and prefer discussing personal matters (40). Comparison of all-male with all-female dyads reveals further differences. For all-female dyads, the patient and provider talk for fairly equivalent periods, whereas in male dyads, the provider speaks much more (37). Because speaking time is one indicator of dominance, (41) we conclude that an all-female interaction is more egalitarian, an all-male dyad more hierarchical. In a study including Western-European general practitioners, the woman-to-woman interaction was most likely to follow the biopsychosocial model in showing concern for the patient, her situation and treating her as a partner in decision-making (47).

In the case of behaviours that interrupt a conversation, patient satisfaction is reduced in all-male, and increased in all-female, consultations (37). Interruptions are experienced as a sign of dominance within the more hierarchically oriented male structure (42). In contrast, interruptions in all-female groups are welcomed and understood as mutual participation, with encouragement to go on talking, hence a sign of interest (43).

Consultations between a female clinician and male patient are the most problematic—the younger the provider and older the patient, the less satisfied the patient is (19, 37). When female providers interact with men, they can develop a potentially ambiguous style in that, although they smile more and use less jargon, they convey dominance and less friendliness through their voices (37). Female clinicians appear less at ease with male patients. In their turn, male patients tend towards a more dominant and bored vocal expression, and they share less biomedical information with a female doctor (44). This raises the question of role conflicts. The stereotypical view of a physician or surgeon is male (45). We will shed light on the effects of gender role expectations in the next section.

Role expectations

Patient satisfaction has a positive effect on outcomes and is an important indicator of the quality of the clinical interaction. From the patients' perspective, male and female patients are equally satisfied with their providers (36, 46). On average, patients are not more or less satisfied with female or male providers (19). This finding is surprising, given ample research showing that patients are more satisfied with a patient-centred orientation, characterized by putting oneself in the shoes of the patient, exploring feelings, responding empathically, and promoting a sense of partnership (55–57). Female clinicians are more likely to exhibit exactly this communication style (29, 40, 47). Here we have a paradox! Patients seek a specific communication style, but are not more satisfied with female providers who demonstrate this. One explanation for this astonishing finding could be the gender role expectations that patients carry.

Patients arrive at a consultation expecting different communication styles from male and female clinicians. Schmid Mast and colleagues (48) found that patient satisfaction correlated with stereotypically female behaviours (e.g. more gazing, less interpersonal distance, softer voice) from women providers. Correspondingly, satisfaction was high when male clinicians adhered to stereotypically male behaviours (e.g. more interpersonal distance, greater expansiveness, louder voice). In the same vein, participants—especially female patients—who were confronted with an emotional communication style in a female provider were more satisfied than when meeting a non-emotional style (49). This effect only emerged for female doctors' relational style. In sum, patients harbour specific expectations about how a provider should behave, based on gender. Particularly for female providers, patient satisfaction depends on the congruence of the provider's communication style with existing gender-role expectations.

Dominance and power

The clinician–patient relationship is hierarchical, with the provider having more power, defined as 'access to scarce resources', than the patient (50). In general, doctors have more medical knowledge, thus more clinical competence than patients. Furthermore, help-seeking is fundamentally a position of powerlessness. Discomfort, pain, or anxiety about the prognosis or treatment might accompany the patient and contribute to his or her loss of power. In many cases, the provider has higher status in terms of social standing and earning capacity. Nevertheless, there will be differences in how dominantly any clinician behaves towards his or her patient; these affect outcomes, such as satisfaction. Schmid Mast *et al.* (51) found that patients spoke less, provided less medical information, and agreed more when interacting with 'high-dominance' compared to 'low-dominance' providers. The clinician who adopts a dominant style might, therefore, be at a disadvantage because the diagnosis is largely based on provision of the medical history. Moreover, provider dominance has correlated with reduced patient satisfaction (52).

Distribution of power in the provider–patient relationship

How much power or influence the clinician and patient have, respectively, during the medical encounter varies. Different models to explain the distribution of power have been proposed (53, 54). Roter and Hall (54) distinguish between a provider with high or low power interacting with a patient with high or low power, resulting in four different patterns.

◆ A 'high-power' provider linked with a 'low-power' patient is termed a paternalistic relationship, in which the clinician sets the goals and agenda for the visit, makes the decisions, and takes control. The patient's actual values and treatment preferences are bypassed, while the clinician acts as a guardian. This traditional form of the doctor–patient relationship is based on a biomedical paradigm of healthcare (55).

◆ The reverse of this pattern is called consumerist. The patient sets the goals and agenda, and takes on the role of a consumer seeking a specific service. The provider becomes the source of information but the patient makes all the decisions.

◆ When provider and patient have both relatively high power and value this balance, the relationship is called mutual. In this pattern, both are involved in decision-making about treatment, negotiate the goals and agenda for the visit, and the patient's values are respected. The role of the provider becomes one of advisor. This is the interaction advocated by the 'relationship-centred care' approach (56).

◆ Finally, in the default relationship, both patient and provider exercise 'low-power' and, therefore, remain relatively uninvolved. Neither of them wants to take responsibility for setting any goals or agenda, so that the patient's values and the provider's role remain vague.

This classification is a useful framework for studying communication between a clinician and patient. Either can show a more or less dominant stance. In the next section, we will discuss which non-verbal cues are related to dominance.

Non-verbal signs of dominance

Hall and colleagues (10) investigated which non-verbal behaviours are related to the perception of dominance, as well as those that dominant persons exhibit. Their meta-analysis showed that many different cues are assumed to be markers of dominance, whereas, in reality, the non-verbal cues indicating actual dominance (personality dominance or high status) are few and far between. People are perceived as dominant when they use less interpersonal distance, gaze at another more and smile less, use more gesture and self-touch, use a louder or deeper voice, interrupt more, speak faster and without pause, and so on. On the other hand, truly dominant people do approach others more closely, have louder voices, and interrupt more frequently. Note that many of the behaviours thought to reflect dominance were inconsistently related to actual dominance.

To investigate which non-verbal cues are perceived as dominant in providers, we presented short video-clips of 11 clinical consultations to observers who were asked to step into the shoes of the patient and judge how dominant each clinician was (57). Behaviours perceived as being dominant included: speaking more; looking at, smiling and nodding less; frowning and gesturing more; talking while doing something else; body orientation toward the patient. People use the same non-verbal indicators to judge dominance in clinicians as they do in other social settings.

In oncology, three different styles of breaking bad news (patient-centred, disease-centred, and emotion-centred) were assessed for dominance (58). The disease-centred approach was perceived as significantly more dominant than the patient- or the emotion-centred styles. When the oncologist was disease-centred, bad news was conveyed bluntly, with a focus on facts and not on the patient's reactions.

Gender and dominance

Within society, women behave less dominantly and are less likely to embrace hierarchies, be competitive, take on leadership positions, or emerge as group leaders than men (69). Although the sexes do not differ in how effectively they lead teams (59), their leadership style is different (32). Women are more democratic or participative, while men are rather autocratic and directive as leaders. In general, women exert influence more gently (e.g. offer advice), whereas men tend to be forceful and explicit (60).

Women in social positions of considerable power, who behave in a rather dominant or directive way, can be evaluated negatively because their behaviour does not correspond to gender-role expectations (61, 62). Healthcare providers are reacted to similarly. Female clinicians are perceived in a negative light if they adopt gender-incongruent behaviours. Burgoon *et al.* showed that variations in aggressive communication (non-aggressive, moderately aggressive, and aggressive) affected patients differently depending on the clinician's gender (63). Patient satisfaction decreased with greater aggressiveness in female providers, whereas satisfaction was less affected by male aggression.

There appears to be a greater expectation that female clinicians adhere to gender-specific norms. Because providers differ naturally in how they communicate (29), communication skills training should focus less on 'drilling' a particular communication style but rather encourage clinicians to be authentic individually. By authentic, we mean that if female physicians communicate in a certain way and male physicians in another, this should be accepted because patients make due allowance for gender. Nevertheless, avoiding a dominant communication style seems beneficial for all providers.

Significance in the cancer setting

The importance of communication in cancer care has been well documented (64). Care delivery may be different from standard medical settings in the length of relationships, nature of the treatment decisions, and complexity of medical data. The emotional dimension is omnipresent, given the fear related to diagnosis, treatment, recurrence, or threat of death. One vital element is establishing an interpersonal relationship characterized by support and empathy (64, 65). Indeed, research suggests that positive provider behaviour (e.g. support, empathy) is related to better cancer patient outcomes (e.g. quality of life, reduced anxiety) (66). For instance, Fogarty *et al.* (67) suggested that more provider compassion (touching the patient's hand, expressing reassurance, and support) would reduce patient anxiety. Moreover, in palliative care, emotional support is of the utmost importance: accompaniment, empathy, touch, and comfort (68, 69).

Given that researchers concur about the paramount importance of emotional connectedness in cancer care, the lack of research addressing which behaviours are associated with better patient outcomes is astonishing. Given the evidence supporting the importance of positive non-verbal communication (e.g. gazing, smiling, nodding) in standard clinical interactions, one can speculate that the relationship is even stronger in cancer care. Moreover, because the patient is regarded as a partner in decision-making (64), the negative impact of dominant communication might even be more pronounced and thus particularly to be avoided.

The role that gender plays in communication in oncology has been insufficiently explored. If the empathic and emotional aspect of communication is so important and female providers are more likely to offer this, cancer patients may prefer their clinicians to be women. However, as with patient satisfaction, although patients in general prefer the communication style that is more likely exhibited by women, patients are not dissatisfied with male, when compared to female, providers. Unless we have empirical evidence, the question posed above cannot be answered in a conclusive way.

Conclusion

As in standard provider–patient dyads, the gender composition might play an important role for adequate communication in cancer care. Moreover, it is very likely that, depending on the type of cancer, there might be preferences for one gender or the other. Women with breast cancer, for instance, might prefer a female provider, whereas men with prostate cancer might have a preference for a male provider.

It becomes clear, with respect to cancer care, that more research on the impact of non-verbal communication and the contribution of gender is needed.

References

1. Knapp ML, Hall JA. *Nonverbal communication in human interaction*, 5th edition. Fort Worth: Thomson Learning; 2002.
2. Hall JA. *Nonverbal sex differences: Communication accuracy and expressive style*. Baltimore, MD: Johns Hopkins University Press; 1984.
3. Hall JA, Schmid Mast M. Sources of accuracy in the empathic accuracy paradigm. *Emotion* 2007; **7**: 438–446.
4. Bales RF. *Interaction process analysis: a method for the study of small groups*. Cambridge, MA: Addison-Wesley; 1950.
5. Stiles WB. *Describing talk: a taxonomy of verbal response modes*. Newbury Park, CA: Sage; 1992.
6. Roter DL, Larson S. The Roter interaction analysis system (RIAS): utility and flexibility for analysis of medical interactions. *Patient Education and Counseling* 2002; **46**: 243–251.
7. Roter DL, Frankel RM, Hall JA, *et al.* The expression of emotion through nonverbal behaviour in medical visits. *Journal of General Internal Medicine* 2005; **21**: 28–34.
8. Gallagher TJ, Hartung PJ, Gerzina H, *et al.* Further analysis of a doctor-patient nonverbal communication instrument. *Patient Education and Counseling* 2005; **57**: 262–271.
9. Gallagher TJ, Hartung PJ, Gregory SW. Assessment of a measure of relational communication for doctor patient interactions. *Patient Education and Counceling* 2001; **45**: 211–218.
10. Hall JA, Coats EJ, Smith LeBeau L. Nonverbal behaviour and the vertical dimension of social relations: a meta-analysis. *Psychological Bulletin* 2005; **131**: 898–924.
11. Street RL, Buller DB. Nonverbal response patterns in physician-patient interactions: A functional analysis. *Journal of Nonverbal Behaviour* 1987; **11**: 234–253.
12. Koss T, Rosenthal R. Interactional synchrony, positivity and patient satisfaction in the physician-patient relationship. *Medical Care* 1997; **35**: 1158–1163.
13. Tiedens LZ, Fragale AR. Power moves: complementarity in dominant and submissive nonverbal behaviour. *Journal of Psychology and Social Psychology* 2003; **84**: 558–568.
14. Ambady N, Koo J, Rosenthal R, *et al.* Physical therapists' nonverbal communication predicts geriatric patients' health outcomes. *Psychology and Aging* 2002; **17**: 443–452.
15. Ambady N, LaPlante D, Nguyen T, *et al.* Surgeons' tone of voice: a clue to malpractice history. *Surgery* 2002; **132**: 5–9.
16. Bensing JM, Kerssens JJ, van der Pasch M. Patient-directed gaze as a tool for discovering and handling psychosocial problem in general practice. *Journal of Nonverbal Behaviour* 2005; **19**: 223–242.

17. Hall JA, Harrigan JA, Rosenthal R. Nonverbal behaviour in clinician-patient interaction. *Applied & Preventive Psychology* 1995; **4**: 21–37.

18. Griffith CH, Wilson JF, Langer S, *et al.* House staff nonverbal communication skills and standardized patient satisfaction. *Journal of General Internal Medicine* 2003; **18**: 170–174.

19. Hall JA, Irish JT, Roter DL, *et al.* Satisfaction, gender, and communication in medical visits. *Medical Care* 1994; **32**: 1216–1231.

20. Barnes ML, Sternberg RJ. Social intelligence and decoding of nonverbal cues. *Intelligence* 1989; **13**: 263–287.

21. Schmid Mast M, Hall JA, Murphy NA, *et al.* Judging assertiveness in female and male targets. *Facta Universitatis* 2003; **2**: 731–743.

22. Malone BE, DePaulo BM. Measuring sensitivity to deception. In: Hall JA, Bernieri FJ, eds. *Interpersonal sensitivity: Theory and measurement.* Mahwah, NJ: Lawrence Erlbaum Associates; 2001, pp.103–124.

23. Rosenthal R, ed. *Skill in nonverbal communication: individual differences.* Cambridge, MA: Oelgeschlager, Gunn, & Hain; 1979.

24. Giannini AJ, Giannini JD. Measurement of nonverbal receptive abilities in medical students. *Perceptual and Motor Skills* 2000; **90**: 1145–1150.

25. DiMatteo MR, Taranta A, Friedman HS, *et al.* Predicting patient satisfaction from physicians' nonverbal communication skills. *Medical Care* 1980; **18**: 376–387.

26. DiMatteo MR, Hays RD, Prince LM. Relationship of physicians' nonverbal communication skills to patient satisfaction, appointment noncompliance, and physician workload. *Health Psychology* 1986; **5**: 581–594.

27. Ryan H, Schonfield P, Cockburn J, *et al.* How to recognize and manage psychological distress in cancer patients. *European Journal of Cancer Care* 2005; **14**: 7–15.

28. Fallowfield L, Ratcliffe D, Jenkins V, *et al.* Psychiatric morbidity and its recognition by doctors in patients with cancer. *British Journal of Cancer* 2001; **84**: 1011–1015.

29. Roter DL, Hall JA, Aoki Y. Physician gender effects in medical communication: a meta-analytic review. *Journal of the American Medical Association* 2002; **288**: 756–764.

30. Hall JA, Roter DL. Do patients talk differently to male and female physicians? A meta-analytic review. *Patient Education and Counseling* 2002; **48**: 217–224.

31. Dindia K, Allen M. Sex differences in self-disclosure: a meta-analysis. *Psychological Bulletin* 1992; **112**: 106–124.

32. Eagly AH, Johnson BT. Gender and leadership style: a meta-analysis. *Psychological Bulletin* 1990; **108**: 233–256.

33. Hall JA, Epstein MA, DeCiantis ML, *et al.* Physicians' liking for their patients: more evidence for the role of affect in medical care. *Health Psychology* 1993; **12**: 140–146.

34. Wallen J, Waitzkin H, Stoeckle JD. Physician stereotypes about female health and illness: a study of patient's sex and the informative process during medical interviews. *Women & Health* 1979; **4**: 135–146.

35. Gabbard-Alley AS. Health communication and gender: a review and critique. *Health Communication* 1995; **7**: 35–54.

36. Hall JA, Roter DL. Patient gender and communication with physicians: results of a community-based study. *Women's Health* 1995; **1**: 77–95.

37. Hall JA, Irish JT, Roter DL, *et al.* Gender in medical encounters: an analysis of physician and patient communication in a primary care setting. *Health Psychology* 1994; **13**: 384–392.

38. Hooper EM, Comstock MS, Goodwin JM, *et al.* Patient characteristics that influence physician behaviour. *Medical Care* 1982; **20**: 630–638.

39. Stewart M. Patient characteristics which are related to the doctor-patient interaction. *Family Practice* 1983; **1**: 30–36.

40. Zaharias G, Piterman L, Liddell M. Doctors and patients: gender interaction in the consultation. *Academic Medicine* 2004; **79**: 148–155.

41. Schmid Mast M. Dominance as expressed and inferred through speaking time: a meta-analysis. *Human Communication Research* 2002; **28**: 420–450.

42. Ng S, H., Brooke M, Dunne M. Interruption and influence in discussion groups. *Journal of Language and Social Psychology* 1995; **14**: 369–381.

43. Aries EJ. *Men and women in interaction: reconsidering the differences.* New York: Oxford University Press; 1996.

44. van den Brink-Muinen A, van Dulmen S, Messerli-Rohrbach V, *et al.* Do gender-dyads have different communication patterns? A comparative study in Western-European general practices. *Patient Education and Counseling* 2002; **48**: 253–264.

45. Lenton AP, Blair IV, Hastie R. Illusions of gender: stereotypes evoke false memories. *Journal of Experimental Social Psychology* 2001; **37**: 3–14.

46. Hall JA, Dornan MC. Patient sociodemographic characteristics as predictors of satisfaction with medical care: a meta-analysis. *Social Science and Medicine* 1990; **30**: 811–818.

47. Roter DL, Hall JA. Physician gender and patient-centred communication: a critical review of empirical research. *Annual Review of Public Health* 2004; **25**: 497–519.

48. Schmid Mast M, Hall JA, Klöckner C, *et al.* Physician gender affects how physician non-verbal behaviour is related to patient satisfaction. *Patient Education and Counseling* 2007; **68**: 16–22.

49. Schmid Mast M, Hall JA, Roter DL. Disentangling physician gender and communication style effects on patient satisfaction and behaviour in a virtual medical visit. *Patient Education and Counseling* 2007; **3**: 1–28.

50. Schmid Mast M. Dominance and gender in the physician-patient interaction. *Journal of Men's Health and Gender* 2004; **1**: 354–358.

51. Schmid Mast M, Hall JA, Roter DL. Caring and dominance affect participants' perceptions and behaviours during a virtual medical visit. *Journal of General Internal Medicine* 2007; **23**: 523–527.

52. Buller MK, Buller DB. Physicians' communication style and patient satisfaction. *Journal of Health and Social Behaviour* 1987; **28**: 375–388.

53. Emanuel EJ, Emanuel LL. Four models of the physician–patient relationship. *Journal of the American Medical Association* 1992; **267**: 2221–2226.

54. Roter DL, Hall JA. *Doctors talking with patients/patients talking with doctors: improving communication in medical visits.* Westport, CT: Praeger; 2006.

55. Engel GL. The need for a new medical model: a challenge for biomedicine. *Science* 1977; **196**: 129–136.

56. Beach MC, Inui T. Relationship-centered care: a constructive reframing. *Journal of General Internal Medicine* 2006; **21**: 3–8.

57. Schmid Mast M, Hall JA, Klöckner C. Which physician non-verbal cues do patients perceive as dominant? Unpublished manuscript 2007, available from first author on request.

58. Schmid Mast M, Kindlimann A, Langewitz W. Patients' perception of bad news: how you put it really makes a difference. *Patient Education and Counseling* 2005; **58**: 244–251.

59. Eagly AH, Karau SJ, Makhijani MG. Gender and the effectiveness of leaders: a meta-analysis. *Psychological Bulletin* 1995; **117**: 125–145.

60. Bjorkqvist K, Lagerspetz KMJ, Kaukiainen A. Do girls manipulate and boys fight? Developmental trends in regard to direct and indirect aggression. *Aggressive Behaviour* 1992; **18**: 117–127.

61. Eagly AH, Karau SJ. Role congruity theory of prejudice toward female leaders. *Psychological Review* 2002; **109**: 573–598.

62. Eagly AH, Makhijani MG, Klonsky BG. Gender and the evaluation of leaders: a meta-analysis. *Psychological Bulletin* 1992; **111**: 3–22.

63. Burgoon M, Birk TS, Hall JR. Compliance and satisfaction with physician-patient communication: an expectancy theory interpretation of gender differences. *Human Communication Research* 1991; **18**: 177–208.

64. Arora NK. Interacting with cancer patients: the significance of physicians' communication behaviour. *Social Science and Medicine* 2003; **57**: 791–806.

65. Finset A, Smedstad LM, Ogar B. Physician–patient interaction and coping with cancer: the doctor as informer or supporter? *Journal of Cancer Education* 1997; **12**: 174–178.

66. Baile W, Aaron J. Patient–physician communication in oncology: past, present, and future. *Current Opinion in Oncology* 2005; **17**: 331–335.

67. Fogarty LA, Curbow BA, Wingard JR, *et al.* Can 40 seconds of compassion reduce patient anxiety? *Journal of Clinical Oncology* 1999; **17**: 371–379.

68. Kruijver IP, Kerkstra A, Bensing JM, *et al.* Nurse-patient communication in cancer care: a review of the literature. *Cancer Nursing* 2000; **23**: 20–31.

69. Yates P, Hart G, Clinton M, *et al.* Exploring empathy as a variable in the evaluation of professional development programs for palliative care nurses. *Cancer Nursing* 1998; **21**: 402–410.

Chapter 7

Medical student training in communication skills

Joshua Hauser and Gregory Makoul

Introduction

Communication is increasingly understood to be a fundamental clinical skill. It is critical to effective diagnosis and management, as well as connecting with patients on a cognitive and emotional level. In addition, communication skills themselves have been linked with patient outcomes, including satisfaction, adherence, and decreased malpractice incidence (1–3). In addition, poor communication skills in a Canadian medical licensing exam have recently been found to be predictive of complaints to medical licensing authorities (4).

Communication skills are a basic competency advocated by the Accreditation Council on Graduate Medical Education (ACGME) (5), American Board of Medical Specialties (ABMS) (6), Joint Commission (7), and Liaison Committee on Medical Education (LCME) (8). For instance, ACGME has mandated that 'interpersonal and communication skills that result in effective information exchange and teaming with patients, their families and other health care professionals are a core area of competency for all physicians' (9).

For medical students, communication skills training generally begins in the pre-clinical years and extends into the clinical years, where increasing levels of sophistication and more *in vivo* experiences can be taught. In this chapter, we review general approaches to teaching communication skills in medical school and then consider several specific aspects to communication skills in oncology and palliative care for medical students.

Approaches to teaching and assessment in medical school

Approaches to communication teaching and assessment in medical school include: small-group teaching and role play, interviews with real patients, and interviews with simulated patients.

Small-group teaching and role play

Small-group teaching and role play allows students to have the opportunity to learn, practice, and receive feedback on communication skills. They are able to do this in a safe environment without the anxiety of being with actual patients.

Role-play techniques have been used in settings ranging from palliative care to cross-cultural training to human sexuality (10). In role plays, a specific case is developed and key roles are assigned to students (e.g. patient, oncologist, family member) and students enact a communication task such as breaking bad news. It is generally preferable to prepare a case scenario ahead of time, as opposed to asking for a case. This gives the facilitator more control and allows for more familiarity. Developing cases from the group of students can be done, but is more time-consuming; there is also a risk that students might not have examples of cases. Role plays require some structure and careful facilitation, but they also need to be flexible enough to allow spontaneity.

Some of the key components of role plays include that they be based on a scenario, but not scripted, have a focused objective (i.e. 'discuss a new biopsy that shows breast cancer' as opposed to 'talk to this patient'), and that they be appropriately debriefed. In general, debriefing a role play should proceed from the role players to a more open discussion with the audience of other learners.

There are multiple ways to facilitate role plays, including a 'fishbowl' technique and multiple, parallel role plays. In the fishbowl method, a case is presented to a whole group of students, two or three people are assigned roles, and the role play is run in front of the whole group. The role play is then debriefed and discussed as a group. In the method of multiple, parallel role plays, a case is presented to the whole group of students and then role plays are done in groups of two or three. The role play is then debriefed as a whole group.

Some of the challenges of role plays include that they can feel too artificial to students and that they can elicit anxiety in the role players. They are, by definition, a re-creation of an event and so may feel artificial; acknowledging that up-front—and being clear that the goal is to try to feel what it is like to be in a patient's, family member's, or physician's role—can help to alleviate this. The anxiety that accompanies role plays is usually linked to:

(1) the possibility that the student may have had a similar experience in his or her (or a family member's) life; and

(2) more general 'performance anxiety'.

To alleviate the former, it is critical for the facilitator to recognize this possibility and allow students to excuse themselves from the situation if it is similar to one of their own personal experiences. While doing this, the facilitator needs to assure the student that he or she need not reveal this experience. To alleviate the latter, it can be helpful for the facilitator to emphasize that the role play is not about the realism or un-realism or quality of the performance, but about giving students the opportunity to try a new role.

Role play can also be combined with more innovative approaches: as one example, investigators have used role play combined with exercises designed to engage medical students on an emotional level, and have shown positive outcomes in self-reported communication behaviours with seriously ill patients (12).

In our palliative care teaching, we use role plays to discuss challenging topics, such as revealing a new diagnosis of cancer, discussing prognosis, or introducing the topic of hospice care with a patient and family. As these are difficult topics, many students benefit from the ability to practice and get feedback from colleagues before seeing actual patients.

Simulated patients

Simulation techniques, such as standardized patients, have been used for many years for teaching communication skills to medical students. They have been used to teach in areas as diverse as breaking bad news, genetics, pain, and overall clinical reasoning skills (13–16). They can also be trained to portray patients' family members, a role that is especially important in palliative and intensive care unit medicine (17). When simulated patients are incorporated into teaching, they serve as 'patient instructors' (PIs) who may change their general demeanor and/or the personal details of the role they are playing. For instance, with different students, a PI might portray patients with different types of relationships, coping styles, life-styles, work situations, family dynamics, and so forth. In contrast, when involved in assessments, simulated patients function as 'standardized patients' (SPs). The term 'standardized' means just that: truly standardized patients are trained to enact the same patient role—with the same demeanor and same information—during each student encounter. They are, in essence, the test. Accordingly, they are also trained to use consistent criteria for evaluating each student.

When working with standardized patients, students can receive feedback from the standardized patient, self-evaluation, and evaluation from a preceptor. Encounters with standardized patients can also be video-taped to allow for review and self or preceptor assessment (18). This triangulation approach increases the validity of the evaluation. In addition to actual standardized patients, at least one centre has experimented recently with virtual standard patients, where students interact with a standardized patient by computer (19). At least one investigator has examined the relationship between medical students' competence with standardized patients and their competence with actual patients; findings indicate a moderately strong relationship (20).

The advantages of simulated patients include opportunities to get direct feedback, to implement multiple observation points, and to practice both basic and advance skills in a safe environment. Potential disadvantages include cost, the need for support staff, and the challenge of sustaining authenticity.

The SEGUE framework for teaching and assessing communication skills

A key need for students is a conceptual framework with which to approach patients. This needs to be flexible enough to adapt to many situations and specific enough to give guidance. One example is the SEGUE framework. In this framework, five basic steps include: Set the stage, Elicit information, Give information, Understand the patient's perspective, and End the encounter. Within each of these steps are specific communication tasks that comprise effective encounters (see Appendix 7.1).

While the SEGUE framework benefits from parallels with the more traditional content of a medical history, it has the advantage of emphasizing a more general approach to communication tasks that can be adapted to multiple medical contexts. This approach has been used for more than 15 years for communication skills training and has been adopted widely in undergraduate medical education in the United States and in Canada. The SEGUE framework is a validated approach to teaching and assessing communication skills for medical students (21).

Using the SEGUE framework in oncology and palliative care

A palliative care assessment emphasizes not only symptoms, but also goals of care, whole-patient assessment, and understanding of patients and families in the context of their illness. For patients who are in palliative care, the recognition that suffering may be multidimensional and may include aspects of physical, emotional, spiritual, and existential pain is a fundamental observation first made by Cicely Saunders (22, 23). As a framework that focuses on setting the stage, eliciting and giving information, and understanding the patient perspective, the SEGUE framework is an important tool in palliative care, where different frames of reference (e.g. patient, family, medical team) are often heightened.

What is unique about palliative care as a context for communication?

Although the cancer and palliative care settings share many aspects with general medical encounters, there are noteworthy differences of emphasis. Each of these might make some of the communication tasks more challenging for students and practitioners alike.

1. *Role of the physician.* Palliative care physicians are often, but not always, consultants to patients and their families, and consequently do not have a long-term relationship, with shared expectations and knowledge of the patient and family. In terms of communication skills, this makes eliciting information and assessing their understanding of their current illness all the more crucial.

2. *More serious illness and less serious illness.* Although patients are referred to palliative and hospice care for a number of different reasons, the predominant one is a life-threatening or life-limiting illness. This clearly distinguishes palliative care from more general primary care. At the same time, patients in palliative care also have multiple co-morbid illnesses requiring management. Communication necessitates a focus on the primary reason that the patient is referred for palliative care alongside co-morbid illnesses.

3. *Multidisciplinary team members.* Oncology and palliative care emphasize interdisciplinary teamwork. In this regard, understanding the roles, strengths and limitations of different team members is vital.

4. *End of the road.* Many patients or families perceive that a hospice is where you go to die. 'Throwing in the towel' or 'giving up' is a common expression that we hear from patients and their families. The crucial strategy here is not to defend the hospice as 'not giving up' but to try to understand where this feeling comes from and how to cope with that feeling.

5. *Involvement of families.* Palliative care views the family as vital to the care of patients. This is for practical reasons—patients may be unable to communicate, may be reliant on family members to give medications, and so on—and philosophical reasons. At the same time, there are data that show that family members of seriously ill patients are at increased risk for morbidity, mortality, and financial hardship (24, 25). The communication skill that is important here is to help students expand from the traditional doctor–patient paradigm to one that incorporates third parties, as discussed in Chapter 14.

Advanced communication skills for medical students

If basic communication skills include opening and closing an interview, performing a history of present illness, past medical history, and social history, cancer care presents many predicaments that require use of the category of advanced skills. While training for these skills begins in medical school, they are likely to continue to develop during residency and beyond, and become increasingly efficient. Although we focus on cancer in this book, these advanced skills can serve those caring for a broad group of patients. In the remainder of this chapter, we explore several domains of these advanced communication skills and consider the implications for medical student communication training.

We believe that each of these areas can be taught to medical students in small groups with role play and standardized patients. Medical students in the course of clinical exposure can also see these types of interactions and reflect upon them with preceptors. Advanced medical students, with adequate support, preparation, and with physicians in the room, might also have the chance to 'take the lead' on some of these areas as well.

Breaking bad news

Breaking bad news is a fundamental and teachable set of skills, one that medical students and residents clearly feel they need. Practitioners such as Baile and Buckman have developed a widely-adhered to approach, abbreviated by the acronym SPIKES (see Chapter 9). SPIKES stands for: setting, preparation, invitation, knowledge, empathy, summary/plan. SPIKES has been subject to clinical trials and shown to be effective (27, 28). SPIKES has much in common with SEGUE, but is tailored specifically to disclosing bad news.

Basic communication principles are reinforced in SPIKES, such as providing privacy, minimizing interruptions, checking what the patient understands about his or her illness, asking about the level of detail that a patient wants concerning information, then giving information clearly and simply, and encouraging questions. Empathic skills include developing comfort with silence, recognizing the emotions that the patient might be feeling, and validating these. Phrases such as 'This must be sad news to hear' or 'You seem very distressed by the news' are useful ways for this.

SPIKES is a guideline for any segment of a clinical interview in which new and difficult information needs to be revealed. As with any guideline, it need not be adhered to rigidly, but represents touch points for the clinician to be aware of. A key example of this is the idea of 'empathy' as a step. Clearly, expressions of empathy (whether verbal or non-verbal) need to be present at all stages of a medical encounter. For medical students, it is necessary to help them move from treating models, such as SEGUE or SPIKES as scripts, to using them as a flexible framework for an interaction.

Prognosis/uncertainty

Prognosis remains a challenging topic for students and trainees at all levels. There is growing literature concerning physicians' discomfort with providing prognostic information, coupled with patients' and families' desire to receive this (29, 30). There is a relative neglect of prognosis in medical textbooks (31) and improvements in prognostic scales used in palliative care (32–34). Despite our improved knowledge of how to prognosticate, the act of prognosticating, and the secondary act of communicating prognosis, are continued challenges.

Medical students can be taught to estimate prognosis using clinical rules and scales. By definition, these cannot predict with certainty for any given patient, but can give an idea of prognosis for populations of patients. From a communication perspective, two extremes are best avoided: first, giving a specific number ('you have 6 months') and second, saying 'I don't know' and leaving it at that. While it is literally true that one doesn't know exactly what the future will bring, saying 'I don't know' neglects the knowledge and expertise that we do have, and does not allow the patient and family to plan. (See Chapter 10 for a detailed discussion of how to discuss prognosis.)

When teaching medical students about prognosis, we favour a model that is similar to breaking bad news: first, asking what patients already know and what level of detail they would like to have; second, presenting our prognostic estimate using ranges of time, words, and diagrams, while also acknowledging our uncertainty. This serves to give patients and families a general idea without being inappropriately definitive or inappropriately vague.

Conflict management

Conflict has been considered a challenge in multiple oncology situations, especially around futility decisions. One basic paradigm holds that many cases of medical futility arise from a conflict of understanding, values, or goals between two or more parties (patient, family, and healthcare professionals) (35). More generally, investigators have begun to identify the high prevalence of family conflict that may be exacerbated by having a family member with a life-threatening illness (36).

Given this paradigm, the idea of focusing communication skills around conflict management has merit. Skills such as facilitation, negotiation, and understanding multiple perspectives, are examples of this. At least one investigator has developed curricular materials specifically in conflict management for medical students (37) and found positive outcomes in terms of their confidence to negotiate confliction situations. In addition to conflict within families, there may be conflicts between healthcare professionals, and between families and healthcare professionals (such as in situations of futility) (38).

Goals of care/introducing palliative care

As hospice services continue to expand, the communication task of transitioning patients and families to palliative care is called for. There are data associating the hospice with attitudes of 'giving up' or 'not being appropriately treated' (39, 40). The balance of maintaining hope in the face of life-threatening illness is a core skill in this regard (41). Commentators suggest using some of the effective strategies from breaking bad news (42).

More specifically, the types of questions that medical students can consider asking revolve around goals of care: 'What are you hoping for?' or 'What are you expecting to happen?' are the most open-ended way of doing this. Sometimes when asked these questions, a patient may talk spontaneously about dying or acknowledge the value of good symptom control.

When such an open-ended approach is unfruitful, a second level of questions tries to frame the situation a little more specifically: 'We are concerned that things have worsened and treating with chemotherapy may do more harm than good. I imagine that you might have thought about this too.' This can be followed up with: 'Given that this is the case, what are the things that would be most important for you now?'. For some patients, endorsement of the palliative approach could be undertaken thus, 'In these situations, we often find that a focus on symptoms and quality of life and support for you and your family is most helpful'.

It is less important what the specific words are than to preserve the overall approach of beginning with an open-ended elicitation of the patient's perspective on their illness, but not being afraid to make a more focused inquiry that acknowledges the need for palliative care.

Family meetings

Conducting family meetings is a core competency, which is increasingly recognized as a set of skills needed throughout medical practice (see Chapter 15). As a field, palliative care has focused on the fundamental belief that the patient and the family together are the unit of care. Although the patient is the one with the illness, he or she is accompanied by a family in most circumstances. Although definitions of families vary, the one that we and others have found most flexible and applicable is considering a family to be anyone who is important to a patient, whether related by blood or marriage or neither. This definition is a broad one and accommodates friends and significant others of many types. While it is outside the topic of this chapter to explore the varieties of family types and dynamics, a couple of basic points are critical to consider:

◆ *Families bring multiple perspectives.* Because of their varied educational and professional backgrounds, family members have differing perspectives on medical decisions, goals, and preferences.

◆ *Families may have conflicts.* In addition to different opinions about any illness, families often have a history of long-term disagreements or conflicts, which may be accentuated with the stress of illness. Families have styles of negotiating, coping, and reaching consensus. While they may need time and space to work through decisions, they may also be looking for help along the way. The strategy of acknowledging multiple perspectives ('We often see families having different points of view about things') and recognizing that there might be conflict ('There are some families that not only have different perspectives but also have disagreements') are important to keep in mind.

Although families have varied contacts with healthcare professionals, one common setting is a family meeting. Here, a team of practitioners gather to discuss a patient's condition, treatment, goals, and next steps. Like any meeting, having a clear agenda, strong leadership, and defined roles are critical. There are three stages of a family meeting: preparatory (about who will attend, lead, and guide the agenda); the meeting itself; and a post-meeting phase, where the plan is carried out. Family meetings need to have room for emotions, conflict, and difficult decisions. When they are well-structured and facilitated, there is more room for the difficult topics and decisions. Investigators have shown efficacy in teaching these types of communication skills to medical and social work students (43). In another intervention, investigators developed a standardized family meeting as a teaching tool for medical students in the ICU. When video-tapes of actual family meetings were compared, those who received the standardized meeting scored higher in tasks of: introduction; gathering information; imparting information; and setting goals and expectations (44).

Palliative care training programmes such as the Education in Palliative and End-of-Life Care (**www.epec.net/EPEC/webpages/index.cfm**), End of Life/Palliative Education Resource Center (**www.eperc.mcw.edu**), and Harvard's Program in Palliative Care Education and Practice (**www.hms.harvard.edu/cdi/pallcare/pcep.htm**) have workshops on the conducting of family meetings.

Communication and teamwork in palliative care

In the setting of cancer and palliative care, interdisciplinary teamwork and communication are crucial. Care by interdisciplinary teams has shown mixed outcomes for patients in both geriatrics and palliative care. In geriatrics, functional decline and mental health measures have been shown to improve, while survival did not change (45). In palliative care, the most consistent outcome findings have been around family satisfaction with care. In a smaller numbers of studies, symptom management improved and costs decreased (46, 47).

Not unusually, patients have multiple professional caregivers in palliative care, including medical students, residents, fellows/registrars, and attending physicians. On the nursing side, hospitalized patients receive care from multiple staff nurses and nurse's assistants. In a typical hospital-based palliative care programme, patients typically have 4–8 physicians, 2–4 staff nurses, 2 nurse's assistants, and 1–2 social workers across a week-long hospitalization. Given this diversity, the communication between professional caregivers is a crucial skill. In addition to systemic interventions that support such communication (e.g. daily interdisciplinary team meetings), it is important to attend to basic interpersonal and communication skills.

At least one study has shown difficulties in communicating between medical students and nurses (48). Thus, medical students need awareness of the different roles that professionals can have in interdisciplinary care. Strategies for efficient and focused communication include making sure nurses, social workers, and other team members are included in critical care decisions, eliciting the perspectives of all team members, and active listening during multidisciplinary team meetings (see Chapter 21).

Conclusion

In theory, all medical students receive training in basic communication skills; some are exposed to advanced communication skills training as well. In any case, residency programmes are expected to further develop and assess communication skills to suit each discipline. In this chapter, we provided an overview of communication skills education for medical students as a foundation for subsequent chapters that will develop a curriculum for oncology and palliative care. In this manner, we hope that a continuum of training can be established, which steadily matures the skills of young clinicians as they embrace increasingly sophisticated clinical tasks and predicaments. Building excellence in communication is at the core of establishing a healing profession.

Appendix 7.1 SEGUE checklist

The SEGUE Framework   Patient: _____   Physician of Student: _____

Set the stage

		Yes	No
1.	Greet patient appropriately		
2.	Establish reason for visit _____		
3.	Outline agenda for visit (e.g. 'anything else?', issues, sequence)		
4.	Make a personal connection during visit (e.g. go beyond medical issues at hand)		
→5.	Maintain patient's privacy (e.g. close door)		

Elicit information

		n/a	Yes	No
6.	Elicit patient's view of health problem and/or progress			
7.	Explore physical/physiological factors			
8.	Explore psychosocial/emotional factors (e.g. living situation, family relations, stress)			
9.	Discuss antecedent treatments (e.g. self-care, last visit, other medical care)			
10.	Discuss how health problem affects patient's life (e.g. quality-of-life)			
11.	Discuss life-style issues/prevention strategies (e.g. health risks)			
→12.	Avoid directive/leading questions			
→13.	Give patient opportunity/time to talk (e.g. don't interrupt)			
→14.	Listen. Give patient undivided attention (e.g. face patient, verbal acknowledgement, non-verbal feedback)			
→15.	Check/clarify information (e.g. recap, ask 'how much')			

Give information

		n/a	Yes	No
16.	Explain rationale for diagnostic procedures (e.g. exam, tests)			
17.	Teach patient about his/her own body and situation (e.g. provide feedback from exam/tests, explain rationale)			
18.	Encourage patient to ask questions/check understanding			
→19.	Adapt to patient's level of understanding (e.g. avoid/explain jargon)			

Understand the patient's perspective

		n/a	Yes	No
20.	Acknowledge patient's accomplishments/progress/challenges			
21.	Acknowledge waiting time			
→22.	Express caring, concern, empathy			
→23.	Maintain a respectful tone			

End the encounter

		Yes	No
24.	Ask if there is anything else patient would like to discuss		
25.	Review next steps with patient		

If suggested a new or modified treatment/prevention plan:

		n/a	Yes	No
26.	Discuss patient's expectation/goal for treatment/prevention			
27.	Involve patient in deciding upon a plan (e.g. options, rationale, values, preferences, concerns)			
28.	Explain likely benefits of the option(s) discussed			
29.	Explain likely side-effects and risks of the option(s) discussed			
30.	Provide complete instructions for plan			
31.	Discuss patient's ability to follow plan			
32.	Discuss importance of patient's role in treatment/prevention			

Comments:

Items without an arrow focus on *content*; mark 'Yes' if done *at least one time* during the encounter.

Items with an arrow (→) focus on *process* and should be maintained throughout the encounter; mark 'No' if at least one relevant instance when not done (e.g. just one use of jargon).

© 1993/2008 Gregory Thomas Makoul, PhD—makoul@northwestern.edu—All Rights Reserved. The SEGUE Framework may be used for educational/non-commercial purposes without permission.

References

1. Stewart M, Brown JB, Boon H, *et al.* (1999). Evidence on patient–doctor communication. *Cancer Prev Control* **3**, 25–30.
2. Cegala DJ, Marinelli T, Post D (2000). The effects of patient communication skills training on compliance. *Arch Fam Med* **9**, 57–64.
3. Levinson W, Roter DL, Mullooly JP, *et al.* (1997). Physician–patient communication. The relationship with malpractice claims among primary care physicians and surgeons. *JAMA* **277**, 553–9.
4. Tamblyn R, Abrahamowicz M, Dauphinee D, *et al.* (2007). Physician scores on a national clinical skills examination as predictors of complaints to medical regulatory authorities. *JAMA* **298**, 993–1001.
5. Batalden P, Leach D, Swing S, *et al.* (2002). General competencies and accreditation in graduate medical education. *Health Affairs* **21**, 103–11.
6. Horowitz SD (2000). Evaluation of clinical competencies: basic certification, subspecialty certification, and recertification. *Am J Phys Med Rehab* **79**, 478–80.
7. Applicable Joint Commission Standards. **http://www.jointcommission.org/NewsRoom/PressKits/ Behaviours+that+Undermine+a+Culture+of+Safety/app_stds.htm.** Accessed 15 September 2008.

8. http://www.lcme.org/functions2007jun.pdf. Accessed 15 September 2008.

9. http://www.acgme.org/outcome/comp/GeneralCompetenciesStandards21307.pdf. Accessed 15 September 2008.

10. Steinert Y (1993). Twelve tips for using role-plays in clinical teaching. *Med Teacher* **15**, 283–91.

11. Nestel D, Tierney T (2007). Role-play for medical students learning about communication: Guidelines for maximising benefits. *BMC Med Educ* **7**, 3.

12. Torke AM, Quest TE, Kinlaw K, *et al.* (2004). A workshop to teach medical students communication skills and clinical knowledge about end-of-life care. *J Gen Intern Med* **19**, 540–4.

13. McGovern MM, Johnston M, Brown K, *et al.* (2006). Use of standardized patients in, undergraduate medical genetics education. *Teaching Learn Med* **18**, 203–7.

14. Windish DM, Price EG, Clever SL, *et al.* (2005). Teaching medical students the important connection between communication and clinical reasoning. *J Gen Intern Med* **20**, 1108–13.

15. Wakefield A, Cooke S, Boggis C (2003). Learning together: use of simulated patients with nursing and medical students for breaking bad news. *Int J Pall Nurs* **9**, 32–8.

16. Mavis BE, Ogle KS, Lovell KL, *et al.* (2002). Medical students as standardized patients to assess interviewing skills for pain evaluation. *Med Educ* **36**, 135–40.

17. Lorin S, Rho L, Wisnivesky JP, *et al.* (2006). Improving medical student intensive care unit communication skills: a novel educational initiative using standardized family members. *Crit Care Med* **34**, 2386–91.

18. Zick A, Granieri M, Makoul G (2007). First-year medical students' assessment of their own communication skills: a video-based, open-ended approach. *Patient Educ Couns* **68**, 161–6.

19. Stevens A, Hernandez J, Johnsen K, *et al.* (2006). The use of virtual patients to teach medical students history taking and communication skills. *Am J Surg* **191**, 806–11.

20. Colliver JA, Swartz MH, Robbs RS, *et al.* (1999). Relationship between clinical competence and interpersonal and communication skills in standardized-patient assessment. *Acad Med* **74**, 271–4.

21. Makoul G (2001). The SEGUE Framework for teaching and assessing communication skills. *Patient Educ Couns* **45**, 23–34.

22. Saunders C (1983). *Beyond All Pain: a Companion for the Suffering and Bereaved.* SPCK Publishing, London.

23. Saunders C, Baines M (1983). *Living with Dying: the Management of Terminal Disease.* Oxford University Press, Oxford.

24. Christakis NA, Allison PD (2006). Mortality after the hospitalization of a spouse. *N Engl J Med* **354**, 719.

25. Schulz R, Beach SR (1999). Caregiving as a risk factor for mortality: the Caregiver Health Effects Study. *JAMA* **282**, 2215–9.

26. Makoul G (1998). Medical student and resident perspectives on delivering bad news. *Acad Med* **73**, S35–S37.

27. Buckman R (1992). *How To Break Bad News: a Guide for Health Care Professionals.* Johns Hopkins University Press, Baltimore, MD.

28. Baile WF, Buckman R, Lenzi R, *et al.* (2000). SPIKES—a six- step protocol for delivering bad news: application to the patient with cancer. *Oncologist* **5**, 302–11.

29. Christakis N (1999). *Death Foretold.* University of Chicago Press, Chicago, IL.

30. Butow P, Dowsett S, Hagerty R, *et al.* (2002). Communicating prognosis to patients with metastatic disease: what do they really want to know? *Support Care Cancer* **10**, 161–8.

31. Christakis NA (1997). The ellipsis of prognosis in modern medical thought. *Soc Sci Med* **44**, 301–15.

32. Glare PA, Eychmueller S, McMahon P (2004). Diagnostic accuracy of the palliative prognostic score in hospitalized patients with advanced cancer *J Clin Oncol* **22**, 4823–8.

33. Morita T, Tsunoda J, Inoue S, *et al.* (2001). Improved accuracy of physicians' survival prediction for terminally ill cancer patients using the Palliative Prognostic Index. *Palliat Med* **15**, 419–24.

34. Lamont EB, Christakis NA (2003). Complexities in prognostication in advanced cancer: 'To help them live their lives the way they want to.' *JAMA* **290**, 98–104.

35. Goold SD, Williams B, Arnold RM (2000). Conflicts regarding decisions to limit treatment, a differential diagnosis. *JAMA* **283**, 909–14.

36. Kramer BJ, Boelk A, Auer C (2006). Family conflict at the end-of-life: lessons learned in a model program for vulnerable older adults. *J Pall Med* **9**, 791–801.

37. Ang M (2002). Advanced communication skills: conflict management and persuasion. *Acad Med* **77**, 1166.

38. Back AL, Arnold RM (2005). Dealing with conflict in caring for the seriously ill: 'It was just out of the question.' *JAMA* **293**, 1374–81.

39. Daugherty CK, Steensma DP (2002). Overcoming obstacles to hospice care: an ethical examination of inertia and inaction. *J Clin Oncol* **20**, 2752–5.

40. Friedman BT, Harwood MK, Shields M (2002). Barriers and enablers to hospice referrals: an expert overview. *J Pall Med* **5**, 73–84.

41. Delvecchio Good MJ, Good BJ, Schaffer C, *et al.* (1990). American oncology and the discourse on hope. *Cult Med Psychiat* **14**, 59–79.

42. Casarett DJ, Quill TE (2007). 'I'm not ready for hospice': strategies for timely and effective hospice discussions. *Ann Int Med* **146**, 443–9.

43. Fineberg IC (2005). Preparing professionals for family conferences in palliative care: evaluation results of an interdisciplinary approach. *J Pall Med* **8**, 857–66.

44. Lorin S, Rho L, Wisnivesky JP, *et al.* (2006). Improving medical student intensive care unit communication skills: a novel educational initiative using standardized family members. *Crit Care Med* **34**, 2386–91.

45. Cohen, HJ, Feussner, JR, Weinberger, M., *et al.* (2006) A controlled trial of inpatient and outpatient geriatric evaluation and management. *New England J Medicine* **346**, 905–12.

46. Hearn J, Higginson IJ (1998). Do specialist palliative care teams improve outcomes for cancer patients? A systematic literature review. *Pall Med* **12**, 317–32.

47. Zimmermann C, Riechelmann R, Krzyzanowska M, *et al.* (2008). Effectiveness of specialized palliative care: a systematic review. *JAMA* **299**, 1698–709.

48. Nadolski GJ, Bell MA, Brewer BB, *et al.* (2006). Evaluating the quality of interaction between medical students and nurses in a large teaching hospital. *BMC Med Educ* **6**, 23.

Chapter 8

Enhancing cancer patients' participation in medical consultations

Donald J Cegala and Dana Eisenberg

Introduction

Over the last thirty years of research in primary care settings, considerable attention has been given to physician communication skills, but comparatively little to patient communication skills (1). This trend is also true for research involving specialist physicians and cancer patients. Our goal in this chapter is to examine interventions designed to enhance cancer patients' communication with physicians.

There is ample research in primary care supporting the value of enhanced patient participation (2). Thus, it is reasonable to ask if cancer patients might also benefit from taking a more active role in medical consultations. While there is variance in research findings, the majority of cancer patients prefer at least a collaborative role in consultations, which requires a good degree of participation (e.g. asking questions, expressing preferences and opinions). Thus, most cancer patients will be open to, and can benefit from, communication skills training.

Cegala (3) discussed implications of patient communication skills interventions for cancer patients, but did not review studies that tested the effects of such interventions. Recently, Parker *et al.* (4) picked up where Cegala left off and reviewed interventions to enhance cancer patients' participation in consultations. In an effort to avoid duplicating this review by Parker and colleagues, we focus primarily on two issues. We direct most attention to the communication skills addressed in interventions and, secondly, the extent to which interventions include specific guidance or instruction in communication skills. We believe these issues are central to an accurate assessment of the current literature and provide especially fruitful directions for future research.

Research on patient communication skills interventions

We do not provide an exhaustive review of the literature into cancer patient communication skills interventions. Given our stated focus, we excluded several studies reviewed by Parker *et al.* (4), which were not centrally concerned with communication skills (e.g. studies examining the effects of audio-taping consultations on patient recall or satisfaction). Additionally, we experienced some difficulty in developing search terms that appeared to capture relevant research (e.g. even including key terms from titles of captured studies sometimes did not result in searches that included those studies). Ultimately, we conducted searches from 1994 to the present on all authors previously identified, in an effort to uncover any subsequent research, which resulted in one additional study. While we cannot claim to have located every study of communication skills interventions for cancer patients, we believe the corpus of studies in our review is likely to be representative of the current literature.

Twelve studies met our basic inclusion criterion, which was an intervention with at least minimal attention to one or more communication skills. Essential information for each study is summarized in Table 8.1.

Nature of the studies

There are less than 30 studies of patient communication skills interventions in primary care. On balance, the amount of research activity devoted to cancer patients' communication skills is what might be expected. Of positive note, all but two studies are randomized control designs. As is typical of research on physician–patient communication, the sample sizes of participants varies from rather small to quite substantial. Also, there is variance in the medical status of the samples. Some focus on patients with a single cancer, while others cover multiple cancers.

Another commonality with research into physician–patient communication in general is that the 12 studies vary considerably in the number of physicians included, or the actual number is either unspecified or unclear. Only three studies include as many as eight or nine physicians, while the remaining studies that specify a number include less than five physicians. Given the variability of physicians' personal communication style and the inherent interactivity between each physician's style and the patient's, inclusion of so few physicians questions the generalizability of some studies. Such methodological concerns could be addressed by using designs and methods of analysis that block on physicians (e.g. nesting patients within physicians). But, none of the studies including two or more physicians reported any such design or analysis. Consequently, it is difficult to tell to what extent observed results are due to differences in physicians' communication style. Future research should correct these design and methods of analysis issues.

Training patients to ask questions

Turning to one of our main foci, it is clear from Table 8.1 that most studies examined a single communication skill, namely question-asking. In some respects this is not surprising, indeed perhaps expected. Most of the patient studies in primary care also focus on question-asking, although some include other skills as well. Much of the literature on physician–patient communication from the 1970s through the 1990s suggested that patients, especially older or less educated ones, tended to ask few, if any, questions during consultations. Thus, it is reasonable that researchers focus on question-asking in patient interventions.

Clearly, asking questions is an important component of participation and should be included in patient interventions. However, other communication skills are also important and probably should not be ignored. For example, expressing preferences, opinions, and disagreements are centrally important to patients engaging in a collaborative partnership with physicians, as would be the case when patients adopt an active (i.e. consumer type) role. Such communication skills are essential to discussing the benefits and risks of various treatment options, and selecting what best meets the needs and values of the patient. While treatment selection may be of relevance to just about any medical consultation, it is often at the very centre of consultations with cancer patients. Consider, for instance, the complex and uncertain set of issues about the treatment of patients with localized prostate cancer, which may be further complicated by conflicting views from different disciplines. Under such circumstances, patients need more than the ability to ask questions, for they must also know how to express what is important to them in relation to the various treatment options. This entails talking about one's values, life-style preferences, and opinions. Only one of the 12 studies summarized in Table 8.1 included any attention to expressing concerns (see 26).

Table 8.1 Summary of essential information from corpus studies of patient communication training interventions

Source[a]	Design[b]	Patient sample[c]	Number of physicians[d]	Communication skill(s)	Intervention type	Dependent measure(s)[e]	Outcome(s)[f]
(19)	RC	$N_c = 71$ $N_i = 71$ MC	1	Question-asking	Low	SR & D	NS in # of Qs overall I>C # of prognosis Qs NS for satisfaction, psychological adjustment, recall
(20)	RC	$N_c = 30$ $N_i = 30$ Newly diagnosed prostate cancer patients	2	Question-asking, combined with treatment information	Moderate	SR	I>C in reported active participation in treatment decision making NS for anxiety, depression
(21)	RC	$N_c = 20$ $N_{i1} = 20$ $N_{i2} = 20$ MC	2	Question-asking	High	SR & D	NS for # of Qs overall among three arms, but when I groups are combined I>C I>C for # of Qs about tests NS for anxiety, satisfaction, psychological adjustment
(22)	RC	$N_c = 244$ $N_i = 206$ MC	?	Unclear	Low	SR	NS on global health status, emotional functioning, cognitive functioning, satisfaction with communication or participation in own care
(23)	RC	$N_c = 158$ $N_{i1} = 79$ $N_{i2} = 81$ MC	9	Question-asking	Low	SR & D	NS in # of Qs between I groups, so combined Combined I>C in # of Qs about prognosis Physicians gave more diagnostic information to I than C NS on satisfaction

(continued)

Table 8.1 (continued) Summary of essential information from corpus studies of patient communication training interventions

Source[a]	Design[b]	Patient sample[c]	Number of physicians[d]	Communication skill(s)	Intervention type	Dependent measure(s)[e]	Outcome(s)[f]
(24)	RC	$N_c = 250$ $N_i = 251$ MC	?	Question-asking	Low	SR	NS on QoL, patients' understanding, remembering, asking about worries (all 6 months post-appointment)
(25)	RC	$N_c = 367$ $N_i = 367$ Breast cancer Patients 4–10 years post-diagnosis	?	Unspecified guidance in topics for discussion and involvement preference	Moderate	SR	I participants were three times more likely to report assuming a more passive role than initially intended NS on satisfaction
(26)	NRC	$N_c = 52$ $N_i = 42$	9	Question-asking Expressing Concerns	Moderate	SR	NS on self-reported reduction in communication barriers and patient satisfaction I>C on physicians' satisfaction with consultation
(27)	RC	$N_c = 30$ $N_i = 30$ Breast cancer patients for initial visit	?	Question-asking	Low	SR & D	NS on # of Qs overall I>C on # of diagnosis Qs I>C on helpfulness of prompt sheet in communicating with physician NS on satisfaction, speaking duration
(28)	SG/NC	23 palliative care patients	?	Question-asking	Low	SR	Decrease in anxiety scores (16/19 patients) 22/23 patients said booklet was helpful
(29)	RC	$N_c = 35$ $N_i = 30$ MC	8	Asking-questions Verifying Information Expressing Opinions	High	SR & D	I>C in declaring preferences and perspectives NS in # of Qs NS in information or involvement preferences, decisional conflict, satisfaction, or depression

(30)	RC	$N_c = 84$	4	Question-asking	Low	SR & D	I>C on overall # of Qs
		$N_i = 80$					I>C in # of prognosis Qs
		MC					I>C on challenges (NS on 9 other behaviours)
							NS on satisfaction with consultation or treatment decision-making, anxiety, or depression

[a]Numbers in refer to reference numbers.

[b]RC = randomized control; NRC = non-randomized control; SG/NC = single group, no control.

[c]N_c = control group N; N_i = intervention group N; MC = multiple cancers.

[d]? = unspecified number.

[e]SR = self-report; D = discourse (e.g. number of questions asked).

[f]NS = non significant; Qs = questions; C = control group; I = intervention group. Statistically significant difference is indicated by the symbol > to mean greater than.

Emotional expression

Another important component of patient participation is the expression of affect or emotion, particularly negative emotion. Cancer patients are typically under a great deal of stress and worry. Articulation of their fears and other concerns is as important to effective physician–patient communication as reporting new symptoms and an accurate medical history. While it could be assumed that the expression of emotion 'comes naturally', such may not be the case for many patients, especially when interacting with oncologists. Interestingly, the literature on the experience of cancer is overwhelmingly attentive to the resultant emotions, but none of the interventions in Table 8.1 gave attention to the identification and articulation of patients' emotions.

Information provision

A communication skill that is often not included in patient interventions, or definitions of patient participation, is information provision. Yet, most physicians agree that effective information provision is indeed an important patient communication skill. For example, 70–80% of diagnoses in primary care are based on the patients' reported medical history (5, 6). The clarity and completeness of patients' reports of symptoms, co-occurrences, applied remedies, and the like, are very important to effective physician–patient communication, and have significant implications for patients' health outcomes. Patients' information provision is no less important in a cancer environment. For instance, breast cancer patients undergoing chemotherapy often experience pain, fatigue, and/or depression. These effects occur at different stages of treatment and whether or not they are experienced, and to what extent, vary greatly. Physicians are able to ameliorate such discomfort, but only if patients effectively convey their experiences.

In summary, we believe that virtually all of the communication skills interventions in oncology have been too narrowly focused on information seeking. Additionally, most attention has been directed to asking questions, with little to information verifying skills. In only one study (30) was a distinction made between seeking new information and verifying one's understanding of the information already conveyed. However, this distinction was apparently made only at the analysis stage in probing categories of obtained data. It is less clear if this distinction was illustrated or otherwise addressed in the intervention. Future research should expand information seeking skills and include other skills important to patient participation.

Classification of intervention intensity

Regarding our second main focus, under 'Intervention type' in Table 8.1, we classified each intervention as low, moderate, or high in intensity. The following definitions were used to make these coding decisions.

- *Low intensity.* Patients are merely given a written prompt sheet or orally encouraged to participate in the medical interview (e.g. ask questions). No additional guidance or training is provided.

- *Moderate intensity.* Patients are given a written prompt sheet or shown a video, which is then discussed with a health educator (HE). Discussion with the HE may include aiding the patient in formulating questions, reporting concerns or symptoms, articulating preferences in information and/or involvement in decision-making. The attention to specific skills or guidelines varies from vague encouragement (e.g. ask questions) to greater assistance, like helping patients to identify and discuss topics of concern.

- *High intensity.* Patients are given explicit material (e.g. printed booklet, video) and engaged by a HE, but they are also presented with material (e.g. definitions, explanations, illustrations, rationales) about relevant communication skills. Additionally, patients are provided with models of the skills (e.g. printed examples of questions, videos of patients expressing preferences) and/or the opportunity to practice communication skills (e.g. role-playing exercises) with feedback.

These definitions are based on our familiarity with a variety of communication skills interventions reported in the literature (for reviews, see 1, 7, 8). Perhaps immediately evident is that most (58.3%) of the studies reported in Table 8.1 employed a low-intensity intervention. As the definition indicates, such interventions do not involve any sort of instruction or training, but instead merely suggest to patients that they might note items of interest (e.g. a printed list of questions they may want to ask).

An examination of the Outcome(s) column in Table 8.1 indicates that these low-intensity interventions have, at best, mixed results. For example, one study (22) found no significant differences between control and intervention groups, while five of the studies reported partial support (i.e. at least one result was statistically significant). One study (28) found two positive results, although no statistical analysis was reported and this study used a single group, no control design.

Three studies (25%) were identified as including a moderate intensity intervention. One (25) reported no significant difference between control and intervention groups for one variable and a significantly negative result (i.e. opposite of what was expected) for the other variable. The The Davison and Degner study (20) found one significant result, but it was for self-reported participation in decision-making, rather than being directly observed. The third study (26) also reported mixed results. Two points might be noted: first, the significant result was based on physicians' perceptions of patients' communication, indicating that physicians were more satisfied with intervention patients' communication than that of controls. This is in contrast to patients' perceptions, which were not significant. Second, the intervention could be coded as 'moderate plus' intensity, as it included attention to question-asking and expressing concerns, and patients role played these skills with the HE. Unfortunately, there is no report of how many patients actually took part in role play, nor were data analysed with respect to those who did and did not engage in role play.

Only two (16.6%) studies were coded as including a high-intensity intervention. These also report mixed results. One study (21) found no significant difference in the number of questions asked among the three arms of the design. However, upon combining the two intervention groups and comparing their result to the controls, significant differences emerged for the total number of questions asked and also the number asked about tests. No significant differences were found for self-reported anxiety, satisfaction, or psychological adjustment. The second study (29) reported significant differences between the intervention and control groups on patients' declaration of preferences and perspectives, but there was no difference in the number of questions asked. There were also no significant differences in self-reported information or involvement preferences, decisional conflict, satisfaction, or depression.

In summary, an initial examination of the outcome of studies in Table 8.1 suggests that the interventions produced mixed support, regardless of their intensity. Such an observation may lead some to call for more research, while others could conclude that the effort to develop these interventions is not in balance with observed patient benefits. Our position is that more research is indeed needed on cancer patient communication skills interventions, but that future research should be improved methodologically. There is not adequate space to examine the details of each study in Table 8.1, consequently, we have identified the important issues that, in varying degrees, cut across the studies comprising the corpus, and that provide an organizing scheme for improving future research.

Recommendations for future research

One issue is the need to include multiple skills in interventions, rather than only focusing on question-asking or another single skill. Researchers should examine the work on patient participation (9), shared decision-making (10), and reviews of patient communication skills interventions (1, 7, 8, 11) for ideas about important communication skills to consider in developing interventions for cancer patients. Additional direction may be found in the details of each targeted cancer (12). We discuss this below.

Training for patients with homogeneous types of cancer

Several studies included samples of patients with heterogeneous cancers. This is problematic because the needs of patients vary with the type of cancer. Additionally, some studies included mixed stages of cancers (e.g. 30). Others (e.g. 25) were homogeneous for the cancer, but the time from initial diagnosis varied significantly (in the Davison & Degner case, 4 to 10 years). Despite these differences, the apparent assumption of researchers was that a single intervention was sufficient for meeting all patients' communication needs (note that retrospectively, Davison and Degner recognized sample differences as a potential problem). This 'one-size-fits-all' approach is probably not valid in many applications, especially in oncology. Researchers should not only include multiple communication skills in their interventions, but also carefully examine the particulars of each cancer and adjust the relative emphasis placed on skills to accommodate these.

Overall, we believe that expanding the scope and appropriateness of patient-based communication interventions will produce results that show clear benefits. However, as discussed below, researchers must align their assessment procedures with each intervention's particular set of skills to ensure adequate evaluation of effectiveness.

Assessment procedures

Turning to the issue of assessment, one half of the studies in Table 8.1 assessed both self-reported and discourse data. Audio-recordings of physician–patient interviews are needed to assess the latter. Then transcripts are prepared[1] and content-coded for discourse units of interest. Assessing patients' self-reports of their communication is less labour-intensive than coding actual discourse, and research has shown that patients' (and physicians') perceptions of their communication do correlate with what is actually said (13–15).

Nevertheless, we argue that assessment of actual discourse is essential to measure how much an intervention impacts patients' communication style as intended. For example, consider a researcher using a low-intensity intervention and assessing only patients' self-reported question-asking. Without measuring the actual number of questions patients asked, there is little confidence in assessing the intervention's efficacy because there is no way of knowing how many questions patients actually asked. Yet, only half of the corpus studies assessed patients' discourse. Given this, an examination of the discourse-based outcomes in Table 8.1 shows that:

(1) of the low-intensity intervention studies, 57% (4 of 7) had at least one significant result;

(2) no moderate-intensity studies included discourse assessment; and

(3) 100% (2 of 2) of the high-intensity intervention studies had at least one significant result.

---

[1] Some discourse-coding schemes are applied directly to audio-taped discourse. However, we recommend that transcripts be prepared to facilitate reliability in unitizing the portions of discourse that are to be content-coded into various categories.

This pattern is consistent with literature reviews that conclude that high-intensity interventions are more effective in modifying patients' communication (8, 16–18). Overall, we recommend that both patients' and physicians' discourse be assessed and that interventions strive to achieve a high intensity.

Some previous observations made by Cegala and Lenzmeier Broz (17) are relevant to both discourse and self-report assessment in future research. They noted that several studies of physician communication skills training had a mismatch between the skills addressed in the intervention and the dependent variables used to test the intervention's effectiveness. Consequently, in several studies the efficacy of the intervention was not supported by results.

We observed a similar mismatching problem in several of the studies in Table 8.1, particularly with respect to self-report outcomes. There was an inadequate or unspecified connection made between the specific skills taught in the intervention (e.g. sample questions) and the outcome measure, often assessed at a more global level (e.g. depression, satisfaction). No study included an intervention that addressed patients' emotions specifically, yet several used a measure of self-reported anxiety to assess differences between the intervention and controls. Why, for example, would asking more questions necessarily lead to reduced anxiety? Indeed, asking more questions about one's cancer may increase anxiety, depending on the questions asked and the information obtained. Similarly, several studies included measures of patient satisfaction to assess intervention and control differences, but typically it was unclear or unspecified as to how the intervention (e.g. a list of possible questions) was conceptually linked to the measure of satisfaction.

Given these conceptual and operational mismatches, it is not surprising that nearly all of the studies in Table 8.1 report at least one non-significant difference for a self-report measure and, in many instances, the results of all of the self-report measures are non-significant. The potential for mismatching is not limited to self-report measures. Several studies assessed discourse (e.g. 19, 21, 23, 27, 29, 30) and coded multiple, discrete categories (e.g. questions about various topics such as diagnosis, tests, prognosis), but the connection between these categories of questions and the specifics of the intervention was mostly unclear. For instance, if patients were to check and ask questions of interest from a list, then there would be considerable variance among the topics chosen, thus increasing the chances of mismatching between the intervention and the frequency of various questions asked. Thus, it would not be surprising to find no significant differences between intervention and control groups in the frequencies of particular questions asked.

Our main point in addressing this matter of intervention and assessment mismatching is to offer another reason to question the lack of striking outcome for many of the corpus's interventions. More appropriate matching of intervention components with assessment variables could result in more positive outcomes. Future research should take special care in selecting its method of assessment of effectiveness.

Educational information

Our final concern is with the interplay of information about one's disease and the communication skills used to talk about it. This interplay is particularly important in complex illnesses like cancer, where a minimum baseline of information is often needed to recognize what one's information needs are and which questions to ask. This issue is especially relevant when studies focus on question-asking. Communication skills training for cancer patients must be integrated with educational information about each cancer. While some studies examined here did include information about cancer, many others did not. The failure to include disease-relevant information (at least as an option for patients who need it) is especially problematic for low-intensity interventions, where patients are merely handed material (e.g. a list of questions) for use during consultations. Future research should examine this interplay between cancer education and communication skills, particularly with respect to patients' baseline knowledge about their cancer. When patients vary greatly in this, the intervention should integrate educational information or provide separate educational material to the patients who need it.

Conclusion

We recommend caution in evaluating the outcome of recent research into cancer patient communication skills interventions. While the results overall are not particularly encouraging, our review has identified several methodological improvements. More comprehensive interventions are needed that include training in multiple communication skills. Another important recommendation is to avoid interventions that only minimally attend to communication. The more successful ones specify key skills and illustrate how they are beneficial with modelling and guided practice components. Along with these major recommendations, we have discussed patient sampling, the value of gathering and coding participants' discourse, and the importance of matching evaluation procedures with the specifics of each intervention. Attention to these matters will improve the quality of research into communication skills training of cancer patients, and as such, will both improve physician–patient communication and bring benefits to cancer patients.

References

1. Cegala DJ, Lenzmeier Broz S (2003). Provider and patient communication skills training. In: Thompson TL, Miller K, Parrott R, eds. *Handbook of Health Communication*, pp.95–119. Lawrence Erlbaum, Mahwah, NJ.

2. Griffin SJ, Kinmonth AL, Veltman MW, *et al.* (2004). Effect on health-related outcomes of interventions to alter the interaction between patients and practitioners: a systematic review of trials. *Ann Fam Med* **2**, 595–608.

3. Cegala DJ (2003). Patient communication skills training: a review with implications for cancer patients. *Patient Educ Couns* **50**, 91–4.

4. Parker PA, Davison BJ, Tishelman C, *et al.* (2005). What do we know about facilitating patient communication in the cancer care setting? *Psychooncology* **14**, 848–58.

5. Frederikson LG (1995). Exploring information-exchange in consultation: The patients' view of performance and outcomes. *Patient Educ Couns* **25**, 237–46.

6. Peterson MC, Holbrook JH, Von Hales D, *et al.* (1992). Contributions of the history, physical examination, and laboratory investigation in making medical diagnoses. *West J Med* **156**, 163–5.

7. Haywood K, Marshall S, Fitzpatrick R (2006). Patient participation in the consultation process: a structured review of intervention strategies. *Patient Educ Couns* **63**, 12–23.

8. Rao JK, Anderson LA, Inui TS, *et al.* (2007). Communication interventions make a difference in conversations between physicians and patients: a systematic review of the evidence. *Med Care* **45**, 340–9.

9. Cegala DJ, Street RL, Jr., Clinch CR (2007). The impact of patient participation on physicians' information provision during a primary care medical interview. *Health Communic* **21**, 177–85.

10. Makoul G, Clayman ML (2005). An integrative model of shared decision making in medical encounters. *Patient Educ Couns* **60**, 301–12.

11. Cegala DJ (2006). Emerging trends and future directions in patient communication skills training. *Health Communic* **20**, 123–9.

12. Cegala DJ (2007). Patient participation, health information, and communication skills training: Implications for cancer patients. In: O'Hair D, Kreps GL, Sparks L, eds. *The Handbook of Communication and Cancer Care.* Pp.383-94. Hampton Press, Cresskill, NJ.

13. Cegala DJ, Gade C, Lenzmeier Broz S, *et al.* (2004). Physicians' and patients' perceptions of patients' communication competence in a primary care medical interview. *Health Communic* **16**, 289–304.

14. Elstein AS, Chapman GB, Knight SJ (2005). Patients' values and clinical substituted judgments: the case of localized prostate cancer. *Health Psychol* **24**(4 Suppl), S85–S92.

15. Street RL, Jr (1992). Analyzing communication in medical consultations: do behavioral measures correspond to patients' perceptions? *Med Care* **30**, 976–88.

16. Anderson LA, Sharpe PA (1991). Improving patient and provider communication: A synthesis and review of communication interventions. *Patient Educ Couns* **17**, 99–134.

17. Cegala DJ, Lenzmeier Broz S (2002). Physician communication skills training: A review of theoretical backgrounds, objectives, and skills. *Med Educ* **36**, 1–13.

18. Epstein AM, Street RL, Jr (2007). *Patient-Centered Communication in Cancer Care: Promoting Healing and Reducing Suffering.* NIH Publication No. 07-6225. National Cancer Institute, Bethesda, MD

19. Butow PN, Dunn SM, Tattersall MH, *et al.* (1994). Patient participation in the cancer consultation: Evaluation of a question prompt sheet. *Ann Oncol* **5**, 199–204.

20. Davison BJ, Degner LF (1997). Empowerment of men newly diagnosed with prostate cancer. *Cancer Nurs* **20**, 187–96.

21. Brown R, Butow PN, Boyer MJ, *et al.* (1999). Promoting patient participation in the cancer consultation: evaluation of a prompt sheet and coaching in question-asking. *Br J Cancer* **80**, 242–8.

22. Drury M, Yudkin P, Harcourt J, *et al.* (2000). Patients with cancer holding their own records: a randomised controlled trial. *Br J Gen Pract* **50**, 105–10.

23. Brown RF, Butow PN, Dunn SM, *et al.* (2001). Promoting patient participation and shortening cancer consultations: a randomised trial. *Br J Cancer* **85**, 1273–9.

24. Williams JG, Cheung WY, Chetwynd N, *et al.* (2001). Pragmatic randomised trial to evaluate the use of patient held records for the continuing care of patients with cancer. *Qual Health Care* **10**, 159–65.

25. Davison BJ, Degner LF (2002). Feasibility of using a computer-assisted intervention to enhance the way women with breast cancer communicate with their physicians. *Cancer Nurs* **25**, 417–24.

26. Sepucha KR, Belkora JK, Mutchnick S, *et al.* (2002). Consultation planning to help breast cancer patients prepare for medical consultations: effect on communication and satisfaction for patients and physicians. *J Clin Oncol* **20**, 2695–700.

27. Bruera E, Sweeney C, Willey J, *et al.* (2003). Breast cancer patient perception of the helpfulness of a prompt sheet versus a general information sheet during outpatient consultation: a randomized, controlled trial. *J Pain Symp Manage* **25**, 412–9.

28. Clayton J, Butow P, Tattersall M, *et al.* (2003). Asking questions can help: Development and preliminary evaluation of a question prompt list for palliative care patients. *Br J Cancer* **89**, 2069–77.

29. Brown RF, Butow PN, Sharrock MA, *et al.* (2004). Education and role modelling for clinical decisions with female cancer patients. *Health Expect* **7**, 303–16.

30. Butow P, Devine R, Boyer M, *et al.* (2004). Cancer consultation preparation package: Changing patients but not physicians is not enough. *J Clin Oncol* **22**, 4401–9.

Section B

A core curriculum for communication skills training for oncology and palliative care

Section editor: David W Kissane

In this section, we offer a basic curriculum for teaching communication skills that has been developed from the literature on communication skills training in oncology and palliative care. This modular approach is structured to follow the life-cycle of illness from diagnosis to survivorship or death. Experts offer consensus guidelines based on the best available research evidence to guide clinicians to communicate optimally. While this curriculum breaks the encounter up into teachable modules, in the real world, clinicians would combine appropriate components to respond to each patient and their relatives.

Chapter 9

Breaking bad news

Walter F Baile and Patricia A Parker

Introduction

The importance of the topic of 'breaking bad news' is underscored by a recent Medline search, which revealed close to 500 articles published on this subject in the past ten years, and by the fact that the cancer clinician is likely to give bad news many thousands of times during the course of his or her career (1). Paradoxically, however, despite the argument for its importance, very few training programmes in oncology thoroughly cover the topic and provide adequate learning experiences for trainees. Only a minority of oncologists have formal training in breaking bad news and other key communication skills (2, 3).

The goal of this chapter is to review the concept of breaking bad news, highlighting salient points and controversies in the literature and making training recommendations. It will consider a definition of bad news, why the topic is so important, the challenges to clinicians in breaking bad news, protocols for giving bad news, research on bad news disclosure and directions for the future.

Definition of 'bad news'

Bad news in the oncology context has been defined in many different ways. One common definition is 'any news that seriously and adversely affects the patient's view of her future' (4). In other words, the 'badness' of the news is the gap between the patient's expectations of the future and the medical reality. It cannot be determined a priori, but is dependent on an individual's subjective evaluation (5). This is a key point because it distinguishes bad news from other types of more emotionally neutral information about cancer, such as information about chemotherapy. It also cautions the practitioner that what he/she might think is good news to one patient ('I'm glad this tumor can definitely be removed') might be perceived as troubling to another ('Oh my god... I just can't handle another surgery'). Thus, it is essential to discover the recipient's expectations and understanding of their medical situation as part of the discussion.

Breaking bad news is a complex communication task and involves a verbal component (giving the news), as well as recognizing and responding to patients' emotions, involving the patient in decision-making, and finding ways to frame 'hope' and provide support (2). Ideally, bad news disclosure is a dynamic interaction between the clinician and patient in which information is not only transmitted to the patient, but the patient's reactions provide cues to the clinician regarding how the information has been received (2, 6, 7) and what concerns the patient may have (8).

Why skills in breaking bad news are important

Breaking bad news is a key aspect of communicating with cancer patients

Over the course of a 40-year career in caring for cancer patients and families, an oncologist may give bad news many thousands of times (9). As the cancer trajectory lengthens and patients survive longer but are not necessarily cured of their disease, patients experience multiple cycles of disease remission, surveillance and recurrence. Thus, patients may experience bad news at several points during the course of the illness, including initial diagnosis, recurrence, disease progression and transitioning to palliative care, as well as end-of-life discussions. Bad news not only includes medical setbacks but also events that could be life-changing, such as the occurrence of irreversible side-effects of cancer (e.g. peripheral neuropathy) or the discussion of resuscitation. Including these events acknowledges the fact that protocols for giving bad news are widely applicable (10). Box 9.1 lists key events along the cancer trajectory that are likely to involve bad news discussions. Furthermore, as genetic testing becomes more available, patients are told about additional risks for many common malignancies (11).

Box 9.1 Cancer events warranting 'bad news' discussions and key communication challenges at these points on the cancer trajectory

- **The cancer diagnosis**. Most patients want as much information as is available on treatment. Patients may not hear the information conveyed because of an emotional response to their diagnosis. In some countries, the diagnosis is withheld because of culture, family and other issues.

- **Prognosis of the illness**. Discussing prognosis can be tricky and a major concern of clinicians is not to destroy hope. Checking with the patient may provide information as to what information the patient wants about the likelihood of success of treatment.

- **Prescription of harsh treatments**. Patients may have preconceived ideas about treatments or side-effects. Others may underplay potential side-effects. Asking them what they know and expect can help clarify misconceptions.

- **Disease recurrence**. Patients may want less detailed information than at the time of diagnosis. Demoralization is a common psychological response.

- **Unexpected or severe side-effects**. Even when patients are cured, side-effects may diminish quality of life. Patients may feel angry or cheated when their disease is cured but they are left with disabilities.

- **Treatment failure**. Discussing the possibility of cancer treatments not working while 'hoping for the best' may be a useful strategy to use when first- and second-line treatments fail.

- **End of anti-cancer treatment/DNR**. Transitioning patients to palliative care is one of the most difficult tasks for cancer clinicians. The doctor's own emotions, lack of communication skills and fear of destroying patient hope are significant barriers to overcome in not unnecessarily continuing anti-cancer therapy.

- **Discussion of discontinuation of ventilation**. Goal-setting with families early on in an ICU stay can reduce unrealistic expectations and shorten ICU stay when the prognosis is grim. Family meetings are an important way of accomplishing this.

- **Sudden unexpected death**. The physician should be prepared to handle very strong emotions in the patient and family and often him/herself.

- **Genetic test results**. It helps to be familiar with current protocols for disclosure since this is a highly specialized discussion.

Giving bad news sensitively is a prime concern of patients, who can be traumatized when bad news is given bluntly or matter-of-factly (12). Giving bad news is the 'gateway' to many important aspects of patient care, such as discussing a treatment plan, shared decision-making, obtaining informed consent and involving the family in the patient's care. If bad news is given poorly, it can increase patients' distress and suffering, resulting in dissatisfaction with medical care (13, 14). Poor communication has also been found to be associated with medical malpractice suits (15, 16).

Patients have a right to information about their health status

In Western societies, ethical guidelines and the lack of available cancer treatments have influenced bad news disclosure since the 1950s. At one time, the principle of beneficence took precedence over that of autonomy, and physicians made the decision as to how much and what kind of information to give patients. Many patients were not told about their cancer due to the fear that it would send them into a deep depression (17). Since the 1970s, as better treatments became available, the principle of autonomy has prevailed to allow patients to make important healthcare decisions. Today, patients in Western cultures are uniformly told about their diagnosis, although worldwide only about 50% of cancer patients receive full disclosure. However, despite international trends towards truth-telling, and growing ethical and legal requirements for informed consent, partial and non-disclosure still takes place in many areas of the world (18). This is more common where medical paternalism predominates, where families play a major role in decision-making and where cultural beliefs influence non-disclosure (19).

Safeguards have been implemented to protect individuals from medical experimentation against their will. After World War II, the Nuremberg trials established that the physician's judgment that a treatment would help a patient (beneficence) was insufficient to protect individuals from abuse. Every patient needs to consent before receiving a medical procedure (20). This agreement has established principles for codes of ethics and rules for informed consent, both for treatments and clinical trials. However, controversies still exist over application of these standards. These include whether or not a doctor's claim of therapeutic exception (that bad news will harm a patient) is valid, whether these codes cover discussion of prognosis or the probability of a specific treatment working, and the complex interactions when families seek to have the information disclosed to them first. However, the overarching position of many patients is that decisions made about them should not be made without them (21).

Patients wish to receive as much information as possible about their health

Studies across a variety of cancer populations have shown that patients desire information about their cancer status (22, 23). This is true even in countries where traditionally bad news (especially that with a dire prognosis) has been withheld from patients. Jenkins and colleagues, for example, found that 98% of patients wanted to know their diagnosis and 87% wanted all possible information, both good and bad (22). Not all patients, however, desire complete information. Thus, an important first step may be to ask patients about their information preferences.

A few recent studies have asked patients about their perspective on how they would like to be given bad news. Parker and colleagues asked 351 patients with varied cancers at different stages about their communication preferences when given bad news about diagnosis or recurrence (24). The highest rated concerns included: the doctor being up to date with the latest research, informing the patients about the best treatment options, taking time to answer all questions, being honest about the disease severity, using simple language, giving the news directly and giving full attention to the patient. Differences were noted in patients' preferences based on gender, age and level of education, underlying the importance of tailoring the discussion to each individual. Cancer type did not predict patients' preferences. Through elicitation of each patient's perspective, many incorrect beliefs can be clarified beneficially (24).

Patients can be traumatized by the way that bad news is given

When patients receive bad news, they may be shocked or demoralized. Rates of post-traumatic stress disorder are up to 19% among cancer survivors (25). Women who experienced less emotional support are at significantly increased risk for partial PTSD (26). These psychological states are worsened by the bad news being given abruptly or insensitively (12). On the other hand, physicians are a vital source of support for patients who are receiving bad news (24).

The stigma of cancer

There continues to be stigma surrounding a cancer diagnosis. In 2007, the American Institute of Cancer Research found that half of America believed that it was impossible to prevent cancer. Moreover, one-third feared it more than any other catastrophe. More than half still believed that stress caused cancer (27).

These health beliefs are analogous to the primitive fears of children of the dark or a 'boogeyman'—a monster popularized by folklore. The boogeyman metaphor denotes something that is feared irrationally (28). The concept is portrayed in titles like 'Beating the boogeyman. A cancer patient's diary' (29). Here Sikes writes, '…emotions associated with this disease do not easily lend themselves to logic. Because cancer is still mysterious, insidious and life-threatening, it calls forth feelings that few other diseases can inspire. That is enough to rupture any protective membrane of intellectualization' (29, p.28). Another metaphorical image of cancer came from John Dean, President Nixon's White House counsel, who, in describing the seriousness of the Watergate problem, stated, 'we have a cancer…within, close to the Presidency, that's growing. It's growing daily. It's compounding, it grows geometrically because it compounds itself' (30).

The diagnosis is an essential prelude to treatment planning

Giving bad news is an imperative to 'patient-centred' care. In many Western countries, there are administrative sanctions associated with non-disclosure, including malpractice suits and censure (31–33). Patients cannot be given treatments against their will. Without disclosure, the criteria for informed consent or shared decision-making cannot be fulfilled.

Disclosure can promote psychosocial adjustment

Although honest disclosure can have a negative emotional impact in the short term, most patients adjust well over time. Gratitude and peace of mind, positive attitudes, reduced anxiety and better adaptation are some of the benefits arising from sharing the truth. Relief from uncertainty can also be therapeutic (33). An increased understanding of illness promotes a sense of order within the context of chaos theory (34). Bad news should be delivered tactfully, honestly and in a supportive fashion. Not being told the severity of their condition, or being denied the opportunity to express their worries and concerns, may limit understanding and even lead some to believe that nothing can be done to help them (9, 35). Transmission of bad news bluntly or too quickly can exacerbate distress. Being told 'there is nothing more we can do' tends to engender feelings of abandonment (35). In a survey of 497 cancer patients, significant predictors of patient satisfaction included perceiving the physician as personally interested, being able to understand the information, being informed in a private setting (doctor's office) and having more time to discuss the situation (36). Although the majority wishes to receive complete and accurate information, many still feel the news is forced upon them. This could be protected against by allowing the patient to declare their preferences for how much they want to hear ('Are you the type of person who wants to know all the details about your condition?').

Current practices in disclosing bad news

There are significant geographic and cultural differences in the information given to cancer patients about their diagnosis and prognosis. In the United States and other parts of North America, attitudes toward disclosure about cancer have evolved considerably. Prior to the 1970s, most physicians did not inform their patients of the diagnosis (37). The discussion of diagnosis matured during the 1960s and 1970s. By 1979, 97% of physicians indicated in a survey that they disclosed the diagnosis of cancer (17). Improved treatment modalities, changing societal attitudes and legislation enforcing the patient's right to informed decision-making, drove physician–patient communication in a more open direction (38, 39). Consequently, today in many Western countries, there is total open disclosure of cancer. Physicians report various types of bad news discussions in a typical month: amid an average of 36 discussions, they had 12.8 about a new cancer diagnosis, 7.6 about recurrent disease and 7.4 about treatment failure (40). Conversations about prognosis and disease progression are now occurring more frequently (23). If actively encouraged to ask questions, prognosis is the one area in which patients' desire information and actually increase their question asking (41, 42). Prognostic information was rated as most important by women with early-stage breast cancer, who wanted to know the probability of cure, disease stage, chance of curative treatment, and 10-year survival figures comparing receipt and non-receipt of adjuvant therapy (43). However, patients vary in their desire for prognostic information. Those with more advanced cancer may be more ambivalent (44).

Cultural influences on disclosure

In non-Western cultures, and some European countries, the diagnosis of cancer is often revealed to the family first (45). There are a number of reasons for non-communication of the cancer diagnosis—treatment may not be available, may be too expensive or the physician may feel that the patient will not understand. By far and away the main argument for not telling the patient is one of non-malfeasance, the concept that it would do irreparable harm to the patient (18). The counter to this argument is that most patients want to know and already suspect, so that telling the family without a discussion with the patient violates the patient's autonomy. Lack of enforcement of medical laws plays a part, since in the United States, where the big change in doctors revealing the diagnosis came after the threat of malpractice suits (18). In other cultures, patients may prefer that the family be told first. However, when families insist that the news not be given to the patient, an ethical and care dilemma is created for the doctor, who enters into a conspiracy of misinformation, which can undermine trust and the therapeutic alliance, not to mention thwart the notion of informed consent and shared decision-making. In such circumstances, the contemporary 'patient-centred' model of practice is voided.

Patients in Italy, China and Japan (38), Spain (46), Tanzania (47), Korea and Mexico (39) believe in a culturally determined value inherent in non-disclosure of diagnosis and terminal prognosis (38, 40, 46). In this family-centred model of decision-making, autonomy is seen as isolating (38, 46). Patients from an Egyptian background believe that dignity, identity and security are conferred by belonging to a family; illness is managed by the family (48). Navajo patients are another example who feels that order and harmony are disrupted by receiving negative information (38). Giving patients an unfavourable diagnosis and prognosis is seen as a curse (46). Sometimes, the negative stigma associated with the word 'cancer' is so strong that its use is perceived as rude, disrespectful and even causal. In Taiwan, families believe that patients can be happier without knowing the truth (49). For Ethiopian refugees, the tradition is to tell the family first and not give bad news at night to prevent disturbed sleep (46). Awareness of the power of non-verbal communication and the impact of words like 'cancer' is helpful. Phrases like 'malignant tumour' or 'growth' can be less inflammatory and better accepted (46), as is approaching threatening topics indirectly. While sensitivity to culture is crucial, it is difficult to tease apart the various ethnic, family, economic and related issues from the stigma of giving bad news.

Barriers to bad news disclosure

Bad news disclosure is made difficult by several factors. Giving bad news has not been conceptualized as an acquirable skill, but seen rather as an innate ability that doctors should have. Additionally, oncologists have rarely been trained in techniques for giving bad news, with only about 5% of oncology training programmes historically teaching communication skills (40, 50). Certification exams have not demanded proficiency in communication skills and there has been a lack of qualified teachers among oncology faculty. Additionally, when physicians have to tell that treatment has not worked, they can experience negative emotions, such as anxiety, or fear being blamed (51, 52). They may react to the patient's emotions by offering false hope, premature reassurance or they may omit salient information (4, 53). Moreover, patients may process information through a repertoire of coping styles including denial and 'blunting' (54). They may avoid asking questions, be overly optimistic about the outcome and distort information to put it in a better light.

Giving bad news evokes strong emotions in both the deliverer and the recipient

Physicians may experience anticipatory anxiety when preparing to give the news, subject to the type of news and the physician's perceptions about their ability to convey it effectively (4). Ptacek and Eberhardt describe a dynamic model of the delivery process, which suggests that physicians may be more stressed prior to, and during, delivery, whereas the height of patient stress is after the news has been given (53). Patients' blood pressure and heart rate become elevated while receiving bad news (55). In a simulated physician–patient scenario of breaking bad news, natural killer cell function increased in medical students (56). However, oncologists do not typically see themselves as a source of support for the patient, whereas patients often mention the oncologist as one of their most important sources of support. Patients assess a supportive style as highly desirable in their clinicians. Supportive processes include expressions of concern, provision of comfort, if the patient is distressed, and encouragement to talk about feelings (24).

Communicating with dying patients readily generates anxiety, sadness and frustration in clinicians, combined with the historic tendency of Western medicine to focus on cure (51). Physicians strive to achieve a delicate balance between providing honest information sensitively and not discouraging hope (57). Consistent with the assumption that one needs hope to battle cancer, physicians fear that the revelation of a grim prognosis may dash hope and take away patients' will to survive. Physicians avoid putting odds on longevity, recurrence and cure, since they do not know how each individual patient will fare (38). Patients may not measure hope solely in terms of cure, but their hope may represent achieving goals, having family and clinician support, and receiving the best treatment available (58).

Concerns about destroying hope

Clinicians fear that hearing bad news will destroy a patient's hope (58, 59). Discussions about poor prognosis or transitioning to palliative care may especially reduce hope. Protective features to preserve hope include the physician being up-to-date on all treatment options and stating that he/she will not abandon the patient (58, 59).

Guidelines for giving bad news

Learning to give bad news is a complex task, which involves major communication skills such as establishing rapport, obtaining information from the patient, providing information in understandable language without jargon, responding to patient emotions and providing a treatment plan to guide the patient through cancer therapy (60). Insight into how drastically bad news may alter a person's perception of their reality is helpful. Thus the dictum 'ask, before you tell' becomes relevant. If an individual is prepared for bad news, their reaction will be different to a person who is oblivious to the danger. Secondly, awareness of what type of crisis the news will precipitate will also help the clinician to prepare.

Historically, the majority of physicians had not formed a consistent plan when they broke bad news (61). At an annual meeting of the American Society of Clinical Oncology, 22% of clinicians reported that they did not have a consistent approach to breaking bad news, while 51.9% used several techniques or tactics, but not an overall plan. Determining what patients believe to be important helps refine guidelines to create evidence-based recommendations for this task (2). Several general guidelines for delivering bad news were developed over the past two decades (2, 4, 24, 62, 63). Much of this has been based on experience or expert opinion, with little empirical foundation. Girgis and Sampson-Fisher described the published literature from 1973 to 1993: only 23% of authors reported descriptive data on breaking bad news, and almost two-thirds were opinions, reviews, letters, case reports or non-data-based descriptive studies (61).

Many common elements emerge from these approaches recommended for giving bad news. The news should be broken in an appropriate setting (quiet place, with uninterrupted time), assessing the patient's understanding of their illness, providing information the patient wants, allowing the patient to express their emotions and responding empathically, before summarizing the information provided and coming up with a plan for the next step(s).

Both the structure and content of the consultation influence the patient's ability to remember what has been said in several ways:

(1) patients usually recall facts provided at the start of a consultation more readily than those given later;

(2) topics deemed most relevant and important to the patient (which might not be those considered most pertinent to the doctor) are recalled most accurately;

(3) the greater the number of statements made by a doctor, the smaller the mean percentage recalled by the patient; and

(4) items that patients do manage to recall do not decay over time as do other memories (9).

One protocol for disclosing bad news is represented by SPIKES (2), a six-step approach shown in Table 9.1. The schema of strategies is short, easily understandable and leads to specific skills that can be practised. Moreover, it can be applied to most breaking bad new situations including diagnosis, recurrence, transition to palliative care and even error disclosure. Its reflective style helps the physician deal with his/her own distress as the 'messenger of bad news'. It incorporates many of the historical recommendations for giving bad news.

When threatened, individuals mobilize different types of coping responses including denial, reframing the threat as a challenge or mobilizing family support. For most people, the diagnosis of cancer is an immediate threat and elicits strong emotional reactions. These can include shock, helplessness, fear of dying, uncertainty, loss of control/vulnerability and lowered self-esteem.

Table 9.1 Strategies to discuss bad news using the SPIKES protocol

Strategies using the SPIKES anagram	Key skills and tasks	Examples of the clinician's comments
1. **Set up** the interview.	Use a private space with uninterrupted time; seated; tissues available; consider who should be there. Review the agenda with the aim of building rapport and settling the patient into the process.	'We're here today to discuss the results of your pathology.' 'Before we turn to the results, do you have any issues or concerns that you'd like to put on our agenda?'
2. Review the patient's **Perception** of the illness.	Check understanding. Determine information gaps and expectations. Correct misunderstanding and define your current role and goal.	'I'd like to make sure you understand the reasons for the tests.' 'Do you remember that we sent the tissue from your operation to the pathologist for examination?' 'Most patients have some ideas about what's causing their symptoms. What do you suspect?'
3. Get an **Invitation** from the patient to deliver the news.	Determine what type and how much information the patient wants. Acknowledge that information needs change over time.	'Are you the type of person who wants every bit of detail, or do you prefer an overview of what we found?'
4. Give the patient **Knowledge** and information.	Forecast what will come. Share the information in chunks, avoiding jargon. Draw diagrams and write down details. Check understanding.	'I'm afraid I've got some bad news for you.' 'The pathology shows that the cancer has spread through the wall of the bowel into a nearby lymph gland.'
5. Respond to the patient's **Emotions**.	Explore emotions. Acknowledge empathically. Validate the emotions. Promote a sense of support.	'I can see how upsetting this is for you.' 'Can you tell me what you are feeling right now?' 'It is very common for patients to feel this way.'
6. **Summarize** the treatment plan and review all that has been communicated.	Discuss future treatment options. Check understanding and future needs. Review next steps.	'We have good treatments using chemotherapy and radiation for your situation. I can tell you about these in due course.' 'Can you summarize for me what you've learnt so that I can see how much you've been able to take in.'

The clinician needs to recognize the patient's response to be able to empathize appropriately with them. When discussing diagnoses and treatment options with patients from different cultures, consider the balance between frank discussion and respect for their cultural values (64).

Teaching breaking bad news

Guidelines provide a useful roadmap for key steps or issues to focus on in giving bad news. However, as with any other skill development, giving bad news is best learned through practice. One training model is described in the programme 'Oncotalk' (see Chapter 54), where oncology fellows were given a didactic lesson in how to give bad news and then afforded practice with standardized patients (65). Each fellow was given the opportunity to practice across a spectrum of giving bad news, including discussing abnormal laboratory findings, disclosing the diagnosis of cancer, discussing disease recurrence, transitioning to palliative care and end-of-life conversations, including how to say goodbye to patients. Compared with standardized patient assessments (SPA) before the workshops, post-workshop SPAs showed that participants acquired significantly more skills in breaking bad news (65).

Conclusion

Communicating in ways that address patients' information needs and provide emotional support increases the likelihood of trust, hope, respect and a willingness to partner with the doctor to achieve the best possible outcome. As is the reality with research about prescribing morphine, there has been little study of the efficacy of methods of giving bad news on patient outcomes. Nonetheless, communication skills training has been shown to produce significant patient outcomes, as described in Chapter 59 in this book. Most recommendations about the delivery of bad news are based on 'best practices' and derive from patient preferences for receiving information.

Communication skills training has been shown to be effective in enhancing oncologists' skills and competencies in giving bad news. Alas, to date, very few oncology training programmes have created experiential learning opportunities for fellows to build skills in breaking bad news (50). Nothing less than a commitment on the part of oncology programmes to regard training in improving communication to be as equally important as other skills associated with care provision will propel this forward. Multiple opportunities exist to teach skills in clinics, hospital inpatient rounds, seminars and case-based conferences. A major barrier to training is a narrow biomedical approach, often characteristic of academic cancer centres, where a focus on research is to the exclusion of preparing well-rounded trainees (66, 67). The addition of core competency requirements in communication skills is a bright light for an improved future.

References

1. Fallowfield L, Lipkin M, Hall A (1998). Teaching senior oncologists communication skills: results from phase I of a comprehensive longitudinal program in the United Kingdom. *J Clin Oncol* **16(5)**, 1961–8.
2. Baile W, Buckman R, Lenzi R, *et al.* (2000). SPIKES A six-step protocol for delivery bad news: Application to the patient with cancer. *The Oncologist* **5**, 302–11.
3. Sullivan AM, Lakoma MD, Block SD (2003). The status of medical education in end-of-life care: a national report. *J Gen Intern Med* **18(9)**, 685–95.
4. Buckman R (1984). Breaking bad news: why is it still so difficult? *Br Med J (Clin Res Ed)* **288**, 1597–9.
5. Fallowfield L, Jenkins V (2004). Communicating sad, bad, and difficult news in medicine. *Lancet* **363(9405)**, 312–9.

6. Lee SJ, Back AL, Block SD, *et al.* (2002). Enhancing physician–patient communication. *Hematology (Am Soc Hematol Educ Program)* **1**, 464–83.

7. Ptacek J, Fries, EA, Eberhardt, TL, *et al.* (1999). Breaking bad news to patients: physicians' perceptions of the process. *Support Care Cancer* **7**, 113–20.

8. Maguire P (1999). Improving communication with cancer patients. *Eur J Cancer* **35**, 1415–22.

9. Fallowfield L, Jenkins V (1999). Effective communication skills are the key to good cancer care. *Eur J Cancer* **35**, 1592–7.

10. von Gunten CF, Ferris FD, Emanuel LL (2000). The patient-physician relationship. Ensuring competency in end-of-life care: communication and relational skills. *Jama* **284(23)**, 3051–7.

11. Forrest K, Simpson SA, Wilson BJ, *et al.* (2003). To tell or not to tell: barriers and facilitators in family communication about genetic risk. *Clin Genet* **64(4)**, 317–26.

12. Bedell SE, Graboys TB, Bedell E, *et al.* (2004). Words that harm, words that heal. *Arch Intern Med* **164(13)**, 1365–8.

13. Cherny NI, Coyle N, Foley KM (1994). Suffering in the advanced cancer patient: a definition and taxonomy. *Journal of Palliative Care* **10(2)**, 57–70.

14. Ong L, Visser M, Lammes F, *et al.* (2000). Doctor-patient communication and cancer patients' quality of life and satisfaction. *Patient Educ Couns* **41**, 145–56.

15. Levinson W, Roter DL, Mullooly JP, *et al.* (1997). Physician–patient communication. The relationship with malpractice claims among primary care physicians and surgeons *Jama* **277(7)**, 553–9.

16. Beckman HB, Markakis KM, Suchman AL, *et al.* (1994). The doctor-patient relationship and malpractice. Lessons from plaintiff depositions *Archives of Internal Medicine* **154(12)**, 1365–70.

17. Novack DH, Plumer R, Smith RL, *et al.* (1979). Changes in physicians' attitudes toward telling the cancer patient. *Jama* **241(9)**, 897–900.

18. Surbone A (2006). Telling the truth to patients with cancer: what is the truth? *Lancet Oncol* **7(11)**, 944–50.

19. Surbone A (2008). Cultural aspects of communication in cancer care. *Support Care Cancer* **16(3)**, 235–40.

20. Shuster E (1998). The Nuremberg Code: Hippocratic ethics and human rights. *Lancet* **351(9107)**, 974–7.

21. McIntyre P (2008). Not trials about us without us! Patient advocates demand a seat at the table. *Cancer World* **22**, 16–20.

22. Jenkins V, Fallowfield L, Saul J (2001). Information needs of patients with cancer: results from a large study in UK cancer centres. *Br J Cancer* **84(1)**, 48–51.

23. Degner LF, Kristjanson LJ, Bowman D, *et al.* (1997). Information needs and decisional preferences in women with breast cancer. *Jama* **277(18)**, 1485–92.

24. Parker PA, Baile WF, de Moor C, *et al.* (2001). Breaking bad news about cancer: patients' preferences for communication. *J Clin Oncol* **19(7)**, 2049–56.

25. Vachon M (2006). Psychosocial distress and coping after cancer treatment. How clinicians can assess distress and which interventions are appropriate–what we know and what we don't. *Am J Nurs* **106(3 Suppl)**, 26–31.

26. Ronson A (2004). Psychiatric disorders in oncology: recent therapeutic advances and new conceptual frameworks. *Curr Opin Oncol* **16(4)**, 318–23.

27. American Institute for Cancer Research Facts and Fears Survey/ AICR (2007) [updated 2007; cited July 1, 2008]; Available from: **www.aicr.org**

28. Wikipedia. Boogeyman. [cited July 1, 2008]; Available from: **http://en.wikipedia.org/wiki/Boogeyman**

29. Sikes S (1984). Beating the boogeyman. A cancer patient's diary. *Bull Menninger Clin* **48(4)**, 293–317.

30. Watergate Trial Conversation Transcript (1971–77). *Records of the Watergate Special Prosecution Force* 1362, Conversation #668.8.

31. Goldberg RJ (1984). Disclosure of information to adult cancer patients: issues and update. *J Clin Oncol* **2(8)**, 948–55.

32. Annas GJ (1994). Informed consent, cancer, and truth in prognosis. *N Engl J Med* **330(3)**, 223–5.

33. Girgis A, Sanson-Fisher RW (1998). Breaking bad news 1: Current best advice for clinicians *Behav Med* **24(2)**, 53–9.

34. Mishel MH (1990). Reconceptualization of the uncertainty in illness theory. *Image J Nurs Sch* **22(4)**, 256–62.

35. Friedrichsen MJ, Strang PM, Carlsson ME (2002). Cancer patients' interpretations of verbal expressions when given information about ending cancer treatment. *Palliat Med* **16(4)**, 323–30.

36. Loge JH, Kaasa S, Hytten K (1997). Disclosing the cancer diagnosis: the patients' experiences. *Eur J Cancer* **33(6)**, 878–82.

37. Oken D (1961). What to tell cancer patients. A study of medical attitudes. *Jama* **175**, 1120–8.

38. Gordon EJ, Daugherty CK (2003). 'Hitting you over the head': oncologists' disclosure of prognosis to advanced cancer patients. *Bioethics* **17(2)**, 142–68.

39. Arber A, Gallagher A (2003). Breaking bad news revisited: the push for negotiated disclosure and changing practice implications. *Int J Palliat Nurs* **9(4)**, 166–72.

40. Baile WF, Lenzi R, Parker PA, *et al.* (2002). Oncologists' attitudes toward and practices in giving bad news: an exploratory study. *J Clin Oncol* **20(8)**, 2189–96.

41. Hagerty RG, Butow PN, Ellis PM, *et al.* (2005). Communicating with realism and hope: incurable cancer patients' views on the disclosure of prognosis. *J Clin Oncol* **23(6)**, 1278–88.

42. Butow PN, Dowsett S, Hagerty R, *et al.* (2002). Communicating prognosis to patients with metastatic disease: what do they really want to know? *Support Care Cancer* **10(2)**, 161–8.

43. Lobb EA, Butow PN, Kenny DT, *et al.* (1999). Communicating prognosis in early breast cancer: do women understand the language used? *Med J Aust* **171(6)**, 290–4.

44. Helft PR (2005). Necessary collusion: prognostic communication with advanced cancer patients. *J Clin Oncol* **23(13)**, 3146–50.

45. Mystakidou K, Parpa E, Tsilila E, *et al.* (2004). Cancer information disclosure in different cultural contexts. *Support Care Cancer* **12(3)**, 147–54.

46. Mitchell JL (1998). Cross-cultural issues in the disclosure of cancer. *Cancer Pract* **6(3)**, 153–60.

47. Harris SR, Templeton E (2001). Who's listening? Experiences of women with breast cancer in communicating with physicians. *Breast J* **7**, 444–9.

48. Butow P, Maclean M, Dunn S, *et al.* (1997). The dynamics of change: Cancer patients' preferences for information, involvement, and support. *Annals of Oncology* **8**, 857–63.

49. Hu WY, Chuang RB, Chen CY (2002). Solving family-related barriers to truthfulness in cases of terminal cancer in Taiwan. A professional perspective. *Cancer Nurs* **25**, 486–92.

50. Hoffman M, Ferri J, Sison C, *et al.* (2004). Teaching communication skills: an AACE survey of oncology training programs. *J Cancer Educ* **19(4)**, 220–4.

51. Wallace JA (2006). Emotional responses of oncologists when disclosing prognostic information to patients with terminal disease: Results of qualitative data from a mailed survey to ASCO members. *J Clin Oncol* **24(18S)**, 8520.

52. Buckman R (2002). Communications and emotions. *Bmj* **325(7366)**, 672.

53. Ptacek JT, Eberhardt TL (1996). Breaking bad news. A review of the literature. *Jama* **276(6)**, 496–502.

54. Miller S (1987). Monitoring and blunting: validation of a questionnaire to assess styles of information under threat. *Journal of Personality and Social Psychology* **52**, 345–53.

55. Biondi M (2006). The implications of neurosciences in communication and doctor-patient relationship. 8th World Congress of Psycho-Oncology. Wiley: Ferrara-Venice, Italy.

56. Cohen L, Baile WF, Henninger E, *et al.* (2003). Physiological and psychological effects of delivering medical news using a simulated physician–patient scenario. *J Behav Med* **26(5)**, 459–71.

57. Ellis PM, Tattersall MH (1999). How should doctors communicate the diagnosis of cancer to patients? *Ann Med* **31**(**5**), 336–41.

58. Sardell AN, Trierweiler SJ (1993). Disclosing the cancer diagnosis: procedures that influence patient hopefulness. *Cancer* **72**(**11**), 3355–65.

59. Links M, Kramer J (1994). Breaking bad news: realistic versus unrealistic hopes. *Support Care Cancer* **2**(**2**), 91–3.

60. Back AL, Arnold RM, Baile WF, *et al.* (2005). Approaching difficult communication tasks in oncology. *CA Cancer J Clin* **55**(**3**), 164–77.

61. Girgis A, Sanson-Fisher RW (1995). Breaking bad news: consensus guidelines for medical practitioners. *J Clin Oncol* **13**(**9**), 2449–56.

62. Fallowfield L, Jenkins V, Farewell V, *et al.* (2002). Efficacy of a Cancer Research UK communication skills training model for oncologists: a randomised controlled trial. *Lancet* **359**(**9307**), 650–6.

63. Blanchard C, Labrecque, MS, Ruckdeschel, JC, *et al.* (1988). Information and decision-making preferences of hospitalized adult cancer patients. *Soc Sci Med* **27**, 1139–45.

64. Hern HEJ, Koenig BA, Moore LJ, *et al.* (1998). The difference that culture can make in end-of-life decisionmaking. *Camb Q Healthc Ethics* **7**, 27–40.

65. Back AL, Arnold RM, Baile WF, *et al.* (2007). Efficacy of communication skills training for giving bad news and discussing transitions to palliative care. *Arch Intern Med* **167**(**5**), 453–60.

66. Greer S (2003). Healing the mind/body split: bringing the patient back into oncology. *Integr Cancer Ther* **2**(**1**), 5–12.

67. Gadacz TR (2003). A changing culture in interpersonal and communication skills. *Am Surg* **69**(**6**), 453–8.

Chapter 10

Discussing prognosis and communicating risk

Phyllis N Butow, Martin HN Tattersall, and Martin Stockler

Introduction

'Prognosis' and 'risk' in the context of healthcare are terms usually used to refer to the chances of a health state occurring, including the development of an illness or disability, symptoms of the illness, benefits and side-effects of treatment, and the likelihood of, or likely time to, death.

Estimating how long people diagnosed with cancer have to live, and the likely outcomes of various treatment options, is not easy. Communicating these concepts to patients in a way that is both clear and supportive is even harder. Over the past thousand years, there has been an ongoing philosophical dialogue concerning whether information harms or benefits patients. Many health professionals are uncertain how much risk information to give and in what format.

There is a vast literature on communicating the risk of developing illness (including cancer) at both a population and individual level, which is beyond the scope of the current chapter. Our purpose in this chapter is to help health professionals better communicate prognosis and risk to people who have cancer. The discussion below presents evidence regarding the legal, patients' and doctors' views on these issues, patients' understanding of prognosis and the impact of discussing prognosis on patient outcomes. Finally, summary guidelines are provided for the health professional, and strategies for training in this communication challenge are included.

Background and evidence from the literature

The legal position

There has been a shift towards greater provision of medical information about cancer over the past twenty years in the Western world. This has been for many reasons, including better treatments and improved outcomes, reduced stigmatization of cancer, the development of the medical consumer movement and increased medico-legal concerns.

The legal view pertaining to information provision is that the patient has a basic human right of self-determination. This is protected by the written constitutions of many countries, in which the standard of disclosure focuses on the informational needs of the *reasonable patient*, in the particular patient's position (1). This approach may, however, fail to protect those whose fears, religious or cultural beliefs and information needs lie outside the mainstream of society.

In addition to the law, many health councils have published guidelines, which, while not legally binding, may be consulted in disciplinary or civil proceedings. These attempt to take a more flexible approach to information provision; however, in attempting flexibility, they are often anything but clear. For example, the relevant document produced by the National Health and Medical Research Council (NHMRC) of Australia states that information provided to patients should cover such aspects as known severe risks of treatment, even when occurrence is rare, the degree of uncertainty of any diagnosis or therapeutic outcome and any significant long-term physical, emotional, mental, social, sexual or other outcome that may be associated with a proposed intervention. However, the information should be 'appropriate to the patient's circumstances, personality, expectations, fears, beliefs, values and cultural background' and may be influenced by 'current accepted medical practice' (2). This leaves considerable latitude on the part of the doctor.

What do patients want?

The literature shows that a clear majority of cancer patients in Westernized countries, at all stages of the disease trajectory, prefer detailed information about their disease and prognosis, and that this information is given in a direct and honest manner (3–24). Two recent systematic reviews, encompassing over 100 studies, concluded that most patients want specific information about their risks and prognosis, including the chances of cure, the extent of disease spread, their life-expectancy (e.g. the chances of living one year or five years), best and worst case scenarios, the possible effects of cancer on their life and possible side-effects of treatment (3, 4).

However, a small minority (2–10%) consistently report a preference for not knowing their prognosis and for never discussing it (5), while in palliative care, a larger proportion may prefer not to discuss their likely survival time (11). Palliative patients have highlighted the conflict between wanting to know and fearing bad news (11). Many patients would like the physician to check with them first to see if they want prognostic information (3).

Patients also have strong views on the format for receiving prognostic information (3). For example, Kaplowitz et al. found that 80% of 352 patients in their study wanted a qualitative prognosis but only 50% wanted a quantitative estimate (22). Another study found that patients preferred written prognostic information in positively framed language (e.g. survival probabilities as opposed to chances of mortality) (6). More metastatic patients surveyed in Australia preferred words (47%) or percentages (42%) to graphical presentations (21%), which they described as 'too cold, clinical and confronting' and difficult to understand (5).

There is, however, diversity in preferences. For instance, more educated patients prefer graphical presentations, probably because they find them easier to process and understand (5). Patients of Anglo-Saxon background are more likely to prefer words when being given survival statistics, while those without good English understand numbers more easily. Furthermore, patients' views change. In a study of 80 patients followed over a 3–6-month period, patients who had deteriorated by their follow-up visit were significantly more likely to shift towards wanting less information (14).

Clearly, information preferences need to be re-negotiated over time. In prognostic discussion towards the end of life, patient and caregiver information needs tend to diverge as the illness progresses, with caregivers needing more and patients wanting less (3). Caregivers may desire more information as the patient gets sicker, to enable them to prepare mentally and to feel confident that they can provide appropriate physical care and emotional support.

Who wants what?

Several studies have identified predictors of prognostic information preferences. In early-stage cancer, younger, female and rural patients, those with a better prognosis and those who were less anxious were more likely to want full disclosure of prognosis (10). Anxious patients were more likely to prefer the physician to tell a loved one the prognosis (10), and to avoid discussions about death (22). Patients who were being treated more intensively were more likely to want to know information about treatment side-effects and the chances of cure (15), perhaps to assist them in making an informed choice about an arduous treatment.

In the advanced cancer setting, patients whose prognosis is better are more likely to want to discuss prognosis at the first consultation (5). Depressed patients are also open to a discussion of prognosis, including the worst news (shortest time to live without treatment) (5). Patients without children are more willing to discuss death and dying earlier than those with children, perhaps because they can face these issues more readily. Additionally, those with strong religious faith are more likely to want to discuss prognosis (25).

Cultural expectations differ considerably. In some communities, it is believed that the doctor should not disclose prognosis to the patient or involve them in decision-making. These cultures prefer the family to have a high level of involvement and, in some cases, the family is informed first so that the patient is either told gradually or not at all (26, 27). However, even within ethnic groups that are perceived by outsiders to be strongly unified, there may be variations in their expectations. Doctors need to avoid stereotypes when discussing diagnosis and prognosis (28).

Overall, assumptions cannot be made about individuals' information needs based on their demographic characteristics or cultural background. Both patients and caregivers indicate that doctors should clarify individual information needs and tailor information provision accordingly (3, 4). Each person's needs will vary at different time points throughout an illness.

Patients' understanding of prognostic information

In most studies of patient's understanding, wide discrepancies exist between doctor prognostication and patient understanding. Cancer patients frequently misunderstand much of what they are told (29, 30), incorrectly state the extent of disease and the goal of treatment (29), and overestimate their prognosis (31–34). Both patient optimism and poor health professional communication appear to contribute to this misunderstanding (29).

Doctors' views regarding prognostic discussions

Medical views about discussing prognosis have been influenced by the struggle between different ethical principles: beneficence (acting for the good of others), paternalism (the doctor takes responsibility for the patient's presumed best interests) and autonomy (the patient's integrity and right to self-determination are respected). Reticence to provide information to patients is often derived from the paternalistic model, which assumes that sickness makes the patient vulnerable, and, therefore, places responsibility for deciding what constitutes benefit or harm firmly upon the doctor. Providing information that portrays a gloomy prognosis or offering choice in treatments may cause psychological distress in some patients, albeit temporarily; therefore, it is advisable to 'first, do no harm' and withhold information. Doctors endorsing this philosophy argue vehemently that the modern practice of full disclosure is cruel and insensitive, contrary to patients' best interests (35, 36) and disruptive to the benefits arising from denial and hope (37, 38).

Those arguing from the principle of autonomy adopt a different stance. Now in the ascendance within the Western world, this group argues that patients have a right to control what is done to their body, to be provided with full information and to make their own decisions. These ideas have been embodied in the principles of informed consent and shared decision-making. The process of informed consent ensures an ethical dialogue about treatment options between doctor and patient. The risks and benefits of all treatments (including prognosis with and without treatment) are discussed, the level of patient understanding is checked and then the patient is asked for their preferred option (39). Within this model, information about prognosis is essential to informed decision-making and integral to any medical discussion.

In practice, most doctors argue for a combination of these positions, suggesting that the way information is given is as important as the content; honest disclosure is only effective when given compassionately and sensitively (7). The need for optimism and hope to be sustained in the process of honestly delivering bad news and information about a limited life-expectancy is an ideal sought by all (7, 40). However, a delicate balance exists between fostering realistic hope and creating false expectations of longevity (41).

How do doctors and patients discuss prognosis?

While most doctors in Western countries now tell their patients the diagnosis of cancer (42), information about prognosis is less commonly presented. Only 27% of 187 people with breast cancer or melanoma reported any discussion of prognosis at the time of their diagnosis (16). In another study, 10 medical and radiation oncologists were asked what they had told 244 patients by their second treatment session. The oncologists reported informing 72% about their chances of cure (29). Patients with a good prognosis were significantly more likely to have been given this information.

Studies in which consultations were audio-taped and audited also indicate that many patients are not told their prognosis, particularly if it is poor. In one study, patients commencing adjuvant therapy received some information about their prognosis, both with and without treatment, but the data presented were most likely to be risk of relapse (70%) rather than survival rates (30%) (43). In the advanced cancer setting, prognosis is discussed less frequently (34, 44–46). If a prognostic discussion has occurred, it is more likely between the doctor and someone other than the patient (46). There is often a lack of clarity in what is provided (44). Estimates of anticipated survival are often not given (46). Both doctors and patients tend to avoid discussing prognosis by focusing on the treatment plan. While patients can be well-informed about the aim of their treatment and the incurable status of their disease, few understand the expected survival (47).

Clearly, prognosis is a difficult area for both patients and doctors to broach, and becomes more difficult, the worse the news to be delivered. Doctors face particular difficulties when discussing life-expectancy with patients with a 'poor' prognosis. Such information raises immediate issues for the patient when the life-expectancy is short. Health professionals and patients may fall into a 'conspiracy of silence', where both are too frightened to raise the issue of prognosis (44).

Communication of risk and prognosis by the multidisciplinary team

The management of persons with cancer is increasingly conducted within a multidisciplinary team. Inevitably there is the potential for inconsistent information to be presented to the patient by different members of the team, with resulting confusion. There is a paucity of research on information flow within the multidisciplinary team, but the patient's general practitioner is rarely informed of what prognostic information has been communicated (48). It is usually absent from the patient's medical record.

Outcomes of discussing prognosis and risk

Increased question-asking and discussion of prognosis does not increase anxiety, but rather leads to greater patient satisfaction, lower anxiety and depression, and less likelihood of using alternative therapies (32, 49). Variations in the communication of risk do influence decision-making about medical treatments. For example, people are more likely to choose riskier treatment options if information is worded positively (chances of surviving) rather than negatively (chances of dying) (50). Similarly, treatments offering long-term benefits are more likely chosen when a longer discussion has taken place, suggesting that additional explanation does assist understanding (51). Discussion about prognosis takes on special importance during treatment decision-making. Here clear, balanced presentation of facts is imperative, with sufficient time and explanation to assist patients to understand and adjust to the facts being presented.

Suggestions for discussing prognosis

Determining what and how people want to know

Since people vary in whether they want to know their prognosis, and how they want to hear it, it is important to directly negotiate the approach to this discussion. Experts in the field recommend an individualized disclosure that takes into account the patient's intellectual capacity, coping style and preferences for involvement (16). Stepwise disclosure is a process wherein specific prognostic data are only offered after patients first understand the nature of the information and then indicate their interest in receiving it. This process may take several consultations. Box 10.1 depicts a short negotiation between a doctor and patient on this topic.

Patients will often raise prognosis themselves, not necessarily in a straightforward manner. For example, they may comment that they are thinking of travelling overseas in about 6 months, and then wait for a response from the health professional. This may be a request for information

---

Box 10.1 Discussion between patient and doctor about prognosis

Dr: Most patients in your situation do very well, but in a small proportion the cancer will come back. Having chemotherapy reduces the chances of the cancer coming back. Unfortunately we don't know up-front who will do well and who won't. Therefore, we have to give chemotherapy to everyone to achieve that reduction in risk. So we would normally recommend chemotherapy to someone like you.

Now, are you the sort of person who likes numbers? Some people like to know what their risk is in numbers, other people don't like that degree of preciseness.

Pt: Well, will it make a difference to the treatment I get?

Dr: It won't change my recommendation, but this is a trade-off between reducing risk and putting up with the side-effects of chemotherapy for a few months. You may feel differently to me about that trade-off.

Pt: Oh, I see. Well yes, I would like to know what we are dealing with here.

Dr: OK. About 3 in 10 people in your situation would have their cancer come back without treatment. If they have treatment, only 2 in 10 will have the cancer come back. How do you feel about that? Was it what you expected?

Pt: Well, actually, I guess I was hoping for better odds than that. Even a 2/10 chance still sounds awfully high to me. Is there nothing else we can do to reduce that risk down further?

Dr: Not that we know of today, but there is always research going on trying to improve outcomes for people, so other treatments may become available in the future. I'm sorry I can't offer you better odds. But remember, a 2 in 10 chance of the cancer coming back also means you have an 8/10 chance of everything going well.

Pt: Thanks I appreciate that. It does sound a bit better that way!

Dr: Please feel free to ask me questions about this, or anything else about your cancer and the treatment, at any time. If you feel you would like some support, because you are worrying a lot about the cancer coming back, we can arrange for you to see our social worker or psychologist who are great to talk to.

about whether they will still be alive in 6 months. Exploration of what the question really means is helpful. For example, the doctor might say: 'So this is what you are thinking about. Do you want me to help you with that decision? Do you want advice on how well you are likely to be in 6 months, and whether you are likely to be able to travel?'.

One method proven to facilitate prognostic communication is a question prompt-list provided before the first or subsequent consultations (see Chapter 29). Question prompt-lists endorse question-asking and contain lists of questions in categories that patients can ask, if and when they wish. The questions are devised by asking patients, carers and health professionals in focus groups what questions they asked, were asked, should ask or wish they had asked. Question prompt-lists increase question-asking in oncology and palliative care settings, particularly about prognosis (52-54).

Accurately conveying prognosis and uncertainty

Any estimate of survival should always be accompanied by a clear explanation of the inherent uncertainty in forecasting. Assuming the health professional has all the data required to calculate prognosis (often not the case!), median survival and the interquartile range are probably the best statistics to convey prognosis (54). Best and worst case scenarios can also be given, using the 10th and 90th percentiles. Thus the recommended answer to the question, 'How long have I got?' might be something like:

> This is a hard question. The typical person with your kind and stage of cancer lives about 12 months. This means that half the people live longer than 12 months and half live shorter than 12 months. If we had 100 people exactly like you, then we'd expect that the 10 who did worst might only live a few (2) months, but the 10 who did best might still be around in a few (3–4) years, and that most (about half) would live somewhere between 6 months and 2 years.

Formats for presenting prognosis

Prognosis can be presented in a variety of formats, including, words, numbers and graphs (see Figs 10.1 and 10.2). Most people find numbers and 100-person diagrams the easiest to understand (55), although some find the latter confronting (6). Pie charts and survival graphs are harder to take in, and some find them too clinical and cold when discussing their own life (6). The bar graphs generated by adjuvant-online for breast, colon and lung cancers (**www.adjuvantonline.com**) appear to be well-understood by patients.

The way prognosis is discussed is just as important as what is said about it. Stop often and check that people have understood what has been said, invite questions, explore whether the information was as they expected, what this means to them in the context of their lives (e.g. its impact on holiday, home and work plans) and how they are coping with the news. If they are upset, the oncology team's support and reassurance that they will be working with them to maximize their chances and quality of life will be very important. Write down important messages for them to take home (9, 56).

Maintaining hope

Most doctors and patients emphasize the importance of maintaining hope when discussing prognosis. Communication strategies found to increase patient hope (5, 57–60) include:

- ◆ Talking about psychosocial issues and providing emotional support.
- ◆ Answering questions and providing information honestly and openly.
- ◆ Offering the most up-to-date treatment and demonstrating expertise.
- ◆ Discussing outliers.

Words: **You have a good chance of being alive in five years time. Most people in your situation are alive five years after they are diagnosed and some people live much longer than that.**

Numbers: **You have a fifty-fifty chance of being alive in five years. In other words, half of the people with your sort of cancer are alive five years on. This means that half the people like you live more than five years and half live less than five years. About 10 per cent, or 1 in 10, live for less than one year, but another 10 per cent live for 15 years or more.**

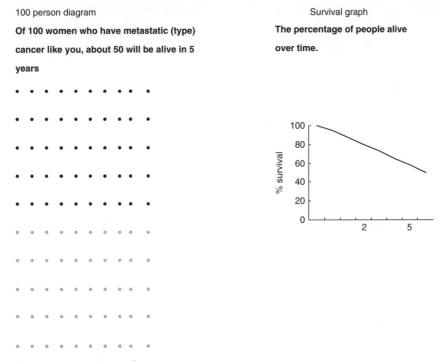

100 person diagram

Of 100 women who have metastatic (type) cancer like you, about 50 will be alive in 5 years

Survival graph

The percentage of people alive over time.

Fig. 10.1 Ways to present prognosis.

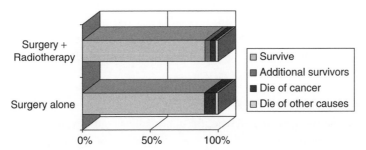

Fig. 10.2 A bar graph is useful for communicating relative prognosis with and without therapy.

- ◆ Focusing on positive and achievable goals.
- ◆ Couching the patient's prognosis in terms of reaching goals or 'landmarks', or overcoming 'hurdles'.
- ◆ Normalizing preparations for death, as something that everyone needs to do. Reassuring the patient that discussing death does not make it an inevitable event.

Summarizing, recording and communicating to others

Documentation in letters to referring doctors about what has been said to patients in oncologist consultations is important so that the potential for multiple and differing estimates being conveyed to patients is reduced (48).

Guidelines

The Australian National Breast Cancer Centre has produced a set of evidence-based guidelines for clinicians on communicating prognosis. Consensus-based guidelines for discussing prognosis and end-of-life issues have also been recently published in Australia (61). Recommended steps for discussing prognosis, based on these guidelines, are shown in Box 10.2.

Box 10.2 Recommended steps for discussing prognosis with people with cancer[a]

Prior to discussing prognosis:

- ◆ Ensure that the discussion will take place in privacy.
- ◆ Ensure, as much as possible, that there will be no interruptions (e.g. switch off mobile phones and pagers; inform staff).
- ◆ Check if the patient would like to have a friend or relative present.
- ◆ Check if the patient would like another medical person present (if applicable).

Negotiating the agenda:

- ◆ Ask first if the person wants to be given information about prognosis (e.g. 'I can tell you what happens to most people in your situation. Would you like me to do that?') and explore what he or she currently understands and expects.
- ◆ Explore and negotiate with the patient the type (e.g. staging details; the chances of being cured; short- and long-term side-effects of treatment; survival estimates) and format (e.g. words, numbers, graphs) of prognostic information desired and adhere to these preferences.

Aspects of prognosis to discuss:

Adhere to the person's stated preference for information about prognosis. If/when desired, the following can be provided:

- ◆ Staging details and their implications for prognosis.
- ◆ Chances of being cured or that cancer will never return.

Recommended steps for discussing prognosis with people with cancer *(continued)*

- Likely benefits and risks of treatment.
- Chances of the cancer shortening the individual's life compared to other life events, e.g. heart disease.
- Average and longest survival times, emphasizing a range rather than a single time point.

How to discuss prognosis:

- Adopt an honest and straightforward, yet sensitive approach.
- Encourage a collaborative relationship with the patient (e.g. provide opportunity to ask questions).
- Use the most up-to-date information and, if desired, explain its source. Explain how this may be revised by additional information. Suggest a time-frame for when additional prognostic information is likely to be available.
- Preface any statement of prognostic estimates with the limitations of prognostic formulations. Explain that you can't predict how the person, as an individual, will respond to the illness and its treatment.
- If giving a time-frame, emphasize a range and not specific endpoints.
- Use mixed framing, i.e. give the chances of cure first, then chances of relapse.
- Present information in a variety of ways (e.g. words, graphs, statistics).
- Present absolute risks with and without treatment.
- Broaden discussion of the prognosis to include effect of the cancer on the individual's life-style.
- Emphasize hope-giving aspects of the information, e.g. extraordinary survivors.
- Repeat negotiation of information preferences and needs over time.
- When explaining relative risk reduction, provide several examples of the calculations.
- Only use statistical terminology (e.g. median, hazard risk ratio) if a person is familiar with these concepts.

Concluding the discussion:

- Summarize main points of the consultation and reassess the person's understanding.
- Emphasize hope-giving aspects of the information.
- Check the patient's emotional reaction to the information and offer support or referral, if needed.
- Indicate your availability for contact to address any questions or concerns and arrange a further appointment to review the situation within a stated time period.

[a]Adapted with permission from National Breast Cancer Centre Australia guidelines for discussing prognosis (2).

Box 10.3 Role-play scenario for discussing prognosis

Mary Green, aged 57, has early-stage breast cancer. Mary has had a lumpectomy. The axillary dissection showed three positive lymph nodes. Mary is married, with three adult children, two of whom are married with children of their own. Mary is a home-maker; her husband is a dentist. Mary wants a lot of information. She has searched the internet and has found a range of numbers concerning her chance of cure. She wants to know facts and figures, and what this means for her as an individual. She will not be fobbed off with words or reassurance.

Surgeons: Mary is meeting you for the post-surgical consultation.

Oncologists: Mary is meeting you to discuss radiotherapy or chemotherapy. The surgeon has told her that she has an excellent chance of cure.

Nurses: Mary tells you that the surgeon said she is most certainly cured, while the oncologist told her she has a 50% chance that the cancer will return, and she is now confused and upset.

Social workers/psychologists: Mary says she cannot make a decision about whether or not to have chemotherapy. She cannot make sense of the figures she has been given, and what they mean for her as an individual.

Learning to discuss prognosis

Role-play practice of how to discuss prognosis is invaluable to try out and develop new skills. The scenario illustrating a breast cancer patient with possible variations for different health professionals is provided in Box 10.3.

Conclusion

The discussion of prognosis and risk is revisited frequently in cancer care, needs to be tailored to the needs of each individual and considered in every treatment plan. Adept communication of prognosis contributes greatly to supportive care provision.

References

1. Giesen D (1993). Legal accountability for the provision of medical care: a comparative view. *Journal of the Royal Society of Medicine* **86**, 648–52.
2. National Health and Medical Research Council (2004). *General guidelines for medical practitioners on providing information to patients*. National Health and Medical Research Council, Commonwealth of Australia, Australian Government Publishing Service, Canberra.
3. Hancock K, Clayton JM, Parker SM, *et al.* (2007). Discrepant perceptions about end-of-life communication: a systematic review. *J Pain Symptom Manage* **34**, 190–200.
4. Hagerty RG, Butow PN, Ellis PM, *et al.* (2005).Communicating prognosis in cancer care: a systematic review of the literature. *Ann Oncol* **16**, 1005–53.
5. Hagerty RG, Butow PN, Ellis PA, *et al.* (2004). Cancer patient preferences for communication of prognosis in the metastatic setting. *J Clin Oncol* **22**, 1721–30.
6. Davey HM, Butow PN, Armstrong BK (2003). Patient preferences for written prognostic information. *Br J Cancer* **89**, 1450–56.

7. Butow PN, Dowsett S, Hagerty RG, *et al.* (2002). Communicating prognosis to patients with metastatic disease: what do they really want to know? *Support Care Cancer* **10**, 161–8.

8. Schofield PE, Beeney LJ, Thompson JF, *et al.* (2001). Hearing the bad news of a cancer diagnosis: the Australian melanoma patient's perspective. *Ann Oncol* **12**, 365–71.

9. Lobb EA, Kenny DT, Butow PN, *et al.* (2001). Women's preferences for discussion of prognosis in early breast cancer. *Health Expectations* **4**, 48–57.

10. Marwit SJ, Datson SL (2002). Disclosure preferences about terminal illness: an examination of decision-related factors. *Death Studies* **26**, 1–20.

11. Kutner JS, Steiner JF, Corbett KK, *et al.* (1999). Information needs in terminal illness. *Soc Sci Med* **48**, 1341–52.

12. Ravdin PM, Siminoff LA, Harvey JA (1998). Survey of breast cancer patients concerning their knowledge and expectations of adjuvant therapy. *J Clin Oncol* **16**, 515–21.

13. Greisinger AJ, Lorimor RJ, Aday LA, *et al.* (1997). Terminally ill cancer patients: their most important concerns. *Cancer Practice* **5**, 147–54.

14. Butow PN, McLean M, Dunn S, *et al.* (1997). The dynamics of change: Cancer patients' preferences for information, involvement and support. *Ann Oncol* **8**, 857–63.

15. Meredith C, Symonds P, Webster L, *et al.* (1996). Information needs of cancer patients in west Scotland: cross sectional survey of patients' views. *BMJ* **313**, 724–26.

16. Butow PN, Kazemi J, Beeney LJ, *et al.*M (1996). When the diagnosis is cancer: Patient communication experiences and preferences. *Cancer* **77**, 2630–7.

17. Derdiarian AK (1986). Informational needs of recently diagnosed cancer patients. *Nurs Res* **35**, 276–81.

18. Degner LF, Kristjanson LJ, Bowman D, *et al.* (1997). Information needs and decisional preferences in women with breast cancer. *JAMA* **277**, 1485–92.

19. Merriman L, Perez DJ, McGee R, *et al.* (1997). Receiving a diagnosis of cancer: the perceptions of patients. *New Zealand Med J* **110**, 297–8.

20. Eidinger RN, Schapira DV (1984). Cancer patients' insight into their treatment, prognosis and unconventional therapies. *Cancer* **53**, 2736–40.

21. Lobb EA, Butow PN, Kenny DT, *et al.* (1999). Communicating prognosis in early breast cancer: do women understand the language used? *Med J Aust* **171**, 290–4.

22. Kaplowitz SA, Campo S, Chui WT (2002). Cancer patients' desire for communication of prognosis information. *Health Commun* **14**, 221–41.

23. Fried TR, Bradley EH, O'Leary J (2003). Prognosis communication in serious illness: perceptions of older patients, caregivers, and clinicians. *J Amer Ger Soc* **51**, 1398–403.

24. Sapir R, Catane R, Kaufman B, *et al.* (2000). Cancer patient expectations of and communication with oncologists and oncology nurses: the experience of an integrated oncology and palliative care service. *Support Care Cancer* **8**, 458–63.

25. Steinhauser KE, Christakis NA, Clipp EC, *et al.* (2000). Factors considered important at the end of life by patients, family, physicians, and other care providers. *JAMA* **284**, 2476–82.

26. Goldstein D, Thewes B, Butow PN (2002). Communicating in a multicultural society II: Greek community attitudes towards cancer in Australia. *Int Med J* **32**, 289–96.

27. Iconomou G, Viha A, Koutras A, *et al.* (2002). Information needs and awareness of diagnosis in patients with cancer receiving chemotherapy: a report from Greece. *Pall Med* **16**, 315–21.

28. Moore R, Butow P (2005). Culture and Oncology: Impact of Context Effects. In: Spiegel D, ed. *Cancer, Communication and Culture*. Kluwer Academic/ Plenum Publishers, New York.

29. Gattellari M, Butow PN, Tattersall MH, *et al.* (1999). Misunderstanding in cancer patients: why shoot the messenger? *Ann Oncol* **10**, 39–46.

30. Mackillop WJ, Stewart WE, Ginsburg AD, *et al.* (1988). Cancer patients' perceptions of their disease and its treatment. *Br J Can* **50**, 355- 59.

31. Weeks JC, Cook EF, O'Day SJ, *et al.* (1998). Relationship between cancer patients' predictions of prognosis and their treatment preferences. *JAMA* **279**, 1709–14.

32. Chochinov HM, Tataryn DJ, Wilson KG, *et al.* (2000). Prognostic awareness and the terminally ill. *Psychosom* **41**, 500–4.

33. Siminoff LA, Fetting JH (1991). Factors affecting treatment decisions for a life-threatening illness: The case of medical treatment of breast cancer. *Soc Sci Med* **32**, 813–8.

34. Chan A, Woodruff R (1997). Communicating with patients with advanced cancer. *J Pall Care* **13**, 29–33.

35. McIntosh J (1976). Patients' awareness and desire for information about diagnosed but undisclosed malignant disease. *Lancet*, 300–3.

36. Editorial (1995). Your baby is in a trial. *Lancet* **345**, 805–6.

37. Tobias JS, Souhami RL (1993). Fully informed consent can be needlessly cruel. *BMJ* **307**, 1199–201.

38. Druss RG, Douglas CJ (1988). Adaptive responses to illness and disability: health denial. *Gen Hosp Psychiat* **10**, 163–8.

39. Levine RY (1986). *Ethics and Regulation of Clinical Research*, 2nd edn. Verland Schwarzenburg, Baltimore.

40. Hagerty RG, Butow PN, Ellis PM, *et al.* (2005). Communicating with realism and hope: Incurable cancer patients' views on the disclosure of prognosis. *J Clin Oncol* **23**, 1278–88.

41. Clayton JM, Butow PN, Arnold RM, *et al.* (2005). Fostering coping and nurturing hope when discussing the future with terminally ill cancer patients and their caregivers. *Cancer* **103**, 1965–75.

42. Charlton RC (1992). Breaking bad news. *Med J Aust* **157**, 615–21.

43. Leighl N, Gattellari M, Butow P, *et al.* (2001). Discussing adjuvant cancer therapy. *J Clin Oncol* **19**, 1768–78.

44. The AM, Hak T, Koeter G, *et al.* (2001). Collusion in doctor-patient communication about imminent death: an ethnographic study. *West J Med* **174**, 247–53.

45. Kim MK, Alvi A (1999). Breaking the bad news of cancer: the patient's perspective. *Laryngoscope* **109**, 1064–7.

46. Bradley EH, Hallemeier AG, Fried TR, *et al.* (2001). Documentation of discussions about prognosis with terminally ill patients. *Am J Med* **111**, 218–23.

47. Gattellari M, Voigt KJ, Butow PN, *et al.* (2002). When the treatment goal is not cure: are cancer patients equipped to make informed decisions? *J Clin Oncol* **20**, 503–13.

48. McConnell D, Butow PN, Tattersall MHN (1999). Improving the letters we write: An exploration of doctor-doctor communication in cancer care. *Br J Cancer* **80**, 427–37.

49. Pruyn JF, Rijckman RM, van Brunschot CJ, *et al.* (1985). Cancer patients' personality characteristics, physician-patient communication and adoption of the Moerman diet. *Soc Sci Med* **20**, 841–7.

50. O'Connor AM (1989). Effects of framing and level of probability on patients' preferences for cancer chemotherapy. *J Clin Epidemiol* **42**, 119–26.

51. Mazur DJ, Jickam DH (1994). The effect of physicians' explanations on patients' treatment preferences. *Med Decis Making* **14**, 255–8.

52. Brown RF, Butow PN, Dunn SM, *et al.* (2001). Promoting patient participation and shortening cancer consultations: a randomised trial. *Br J Cancer* **85**, 1273–9.

53. Clayton JM, Butow PN, Tattersall MHN, *et al.* (2007). Randomized controlled trial of a prompt list to help advanced cancer patients and their caregivers to ask questions about prognosis and end-of-life care. *J Clin Oncol.* **25**, 715–23.

54. Stockler MR, Tattersall MHN, Boyer MJ, *et al.* (2006). Disarming the guarded prognosis: a cohort study of predicted and actual survival in newly referred people with incurable cancer. *Br J Cancer* **94**, 208–12.

55. Feldman-Stewart D, Kocovski N, McConnell BA, *et al.* (2000). Perception of quantitative information for treatment decisions. *Med Decis Making*, **20**, 228–38.

56. Parker PA, Baile WF, de Moor C, *et al.* (2001). Breaking bad news about cancer: patients' preferences for communication. *J Clin Oncol* **19**, 2049–56.

57. Koopmeiners L, Post-White J, Gutknecht S, *et al.* (1997). How healthcare professionals contribute to hope in patients with cancer. *Oncol Nurs Forum* **24**, 1507–13.

58. Ptacek JT, Ptacek JJ (2001). Patients' perceptions of receiving bad news about cancer. *J Clin Oncol* **19**, 4160–4.

59. Peteet JR, Abrams HE, Ross DM, *et al.* (1991). Presenting a diagnosis of cancer: patients' views. *J Fam Practice* **32**, 577–81.

60. Sardell AN, Trierweiler SJ (1993). Disclosing the cancer diagnosis. Procedures that influence patient hopefulness. *Cancer* **72**, 3355–65.

61. Clayton JM, Hancock KM, Butow PN, *et al.* (2007). Clinical practice guidelines for communicating prognosis and end-of-life issues with adults in the advanced stages of a life-limiting illness, and their caregivers. *Med J Aust* **186(12 Suppl)**, S77, S79, S83–108.

Chapter 11

Communication training to achieve shared treatment decisions

David W Kissane

Introduction

Many decisions in oncology and palliative care involve difficult choices about a range of potential benefits alongside burdens. As the treatment of cancer becomes increasingly complex, accurate information provision and its effective delivery to the patient and their family is crucial. Moreover, as the ethos of care provision shifts from a paternalistic model to a climate where patient autonomy is greatly respected, the actual process of communication to achieve treatment decisions comes more to the fore. In this chapter, the focus is on the pragmatics of communication skills training to achieve the goal of a shared treatment decision. A patient-centred approach to care provision is central as a theoretical underpinning to this approach (1).

In the first section of this book, Charles and Gafni (Chapter 4) laid the foundation for this chapter in considering the nature of a shared treatment decision. Based on a two-way exchange of information and identification of preferences about the treatments involved, this model respects the investment of both parties in the treatment choice and works towards the achievement of consensus. Patient variation in the extent to which they want to make this choice individually, with their family and with the help of their clinician, is built into the negotiation, as is also the clinician's willingness to eventually deliver the selected treatment. The inherent process is both asymmetrical and dynamically evolving, as information is mutually shared and preferences explored. Nonetheless, the goal of optimizing satisfaction with the choice, through a process of iteratively increasing common understanding, identifies communication as central to a successful outcome.

In the next section of this book, Tattersall (Chapter 29) presents a clinician's perspective on shared decision-making with an up-to-date review of recent research. Much of this starts to examine how information is framed, with multiple modalities being used to enrich the presentation and completeness of message delivery. The future will be enriched through these developments. Here, I hone in on the typical sequence that unfolds in a clinical dialogue, which aims to develop decisions about the management of any condition. I only briefly touch on the background literature, as it is well covered elsewhere in this book. Instead, I illustrate a method of communication skills training that makes explicit what is taught (2) and include role-play scenarios that can be helpful in such training exercises.

A participatory model of management choices

Clinicians and patients bring differing values and preferences to each clinical predicament that necessitates a treatment choice. Slevin and colleagues presented a hypothetical treatment scenario to (a) cancer patients prior to receiving chemotherapy, (b) cancer doctors and nurses, and (c) the general public, to determine levels of risks and benefits that would be acceptable before commencing treatment (3). Cancer patients accept higher risks of potential side-effects and reduced likelihood of benefit than do others in the community. In taking such values into the equation, shared decision-making provides a method to optimally reach consensus for the benefit of all.

In a prospective study in the United Kingdom, women with early-stage breast cancer who perceived they were offered a choice between lumpectomy and mastectomy had significantly improved psychological outcomes (4). In addition, there were no differences in outcome between women whose tumour characteristics allowed a real treatment choice and those that precluded this (5). Being offered genuine participation in the decision-making process is what counts here.

In another prospective evaluation of outcomes from achievement of desired roles in the decision-making process, patients who were not as involved in the process as they desired fared more poorly in that they carried higher unmet needs for specific information and assurance, were less satisfied with the consultation, and were more anxious (6). Least satisfied were those who reported that the decision had been made by physician alone or themselves alone. Furthermore, those who participated less than desired experienced negative psychological outcomes that were not evident in those achieving what they desired. Thus, while tailoring the treatment-decision approach to patient needs may be optimal, offering more participation in the decision produces demonstrably better outcomes than offering less.

Culture is a further dimension adding complexity to the clinical encounter. Promoting participation of the patient from a culturally diverse background ensures that their health beliefs about illness are incorporated into the process of decision-making (7). Not only does this enhance trust between patient and clinician, but it ensures that each understands the other's explanatory model of illness, a process that promotes eventual adherence to the management plan. In addition to culture, the evidence-base informing clinical practice is a vital ingredient that guides the process of information provision in shared decision-making (8). Arranging material from research studies and framing this in a manner conducive to integration by the patient is a prerequisite to the interactive process.

A structured approach to shared treatment decisions

In the clinical setting, consultations that are focused on developing a management plan often follow ones that have generated investigations aimed at confirming the diagnosis or extent of disease. A commonly used format for these consultations has been developed from clinical wisdom, but matured by the evidence-base supporting shared treatment decisions (9). This can be laid out as a sequence of strategies to achieve the communication goal, which in turn are supported by both process tasks and communication skills to complete each strategy (see Table 11.1).

The objective of a shared decision-making consultation is to make sure that the patient achieves a fully informed treatment choice based upon a comprehensive understanding of:

(1) the disease or clinical predicament and the available treatment options to deal with this;

(2) the benefits and risks of each treatment choice; and

(3) the capacity to appreciate the significance of each outcome for the life-style and values of the person, so that the choice can be weighed up and selected to optimally suit the person.

Having established the consultation framework, which is dependent on reaching agreement about the agenda for this conversation, a sense of partnership is initially developed through an exploration of the patient's preferences for receipt of information and involvement in decision-making. Younger patients tend to want greater detail and more personal autonomy in their

Table 11.1 Shared decision making about treatment options – The goal is to ensure the patient makes a fully informed decision based upon (1) a thorough understanding of the clinical condition and its available treatment options; (2) a dialogue about the implications of treatment on the patient's life, and (3) the capacity to integrate the key aspects of the information into the decision-making process. This objective is best achieved within a partnership between the clinician and patient.

Communication strategies	Process tasks	Communication skills
1. Establish the consultation framework.	Greet patient appropriately. Make introductions of third parties. Ensure patient is clothed. Sit at eye-level.	Declare your agenda items. Invite patient's agenda items. Negotiate agenda.
2. Establish the physician–patient team.	Introduce the approach to shared decision-making, offering choices to the patient and the goal of reaching a mutual understanding of which is preferred.	Check patient preferences for information and decision-making style. Endorse question-asking. Make partnership statements.
3. Develop an accurate, shared understanding of the patient's situation: (a) disease features; (b) prognosis without treatment; (c) psychosocial needs and concerns; (d) other factors influencing the treatment decision.	Begin with patient's understanding, Include any third party's understanding when others are present. Correct misunderstandings.	Check patient understanding. Clarify. Invite patient concerns.
4. Present established treatment options.	Categorize into chunks. Present treatment benefits. Present treatment side effects and potential inconveniences. Present the source and strength of evidence for each treatment. Avoid jargon. Draw diagrams.	Preview the information. Summarize the information. Check patient understanding. Endorse question asking. Offer decision delay.
5. Discuss patient's values and lifestyle factors that may impact on the standard treatment decision.	Consider the impact of treatment on employment, lifestyle and relationships. Explore patient views and feelings about treatment options. Avoid interruptions or blocking.	Ask open questions. Clarify. Empathically acknowledge, validate or normalize emotional responses. Reinforce value of joint decision-making. Make a partnership statement.
6. Present a clear statement of the recommended treatment option and invite patient choice.	It is generally helpful for the clinician to state their treatment recommendation clearly. Work towards consensus and confidence with the treatment choice.	Summarize. Ask open questions. Offer decision delay.
7. Close the consultation.	Arrange for signing of consent forms as needed. Arrange for any additional consultations or referrals. Create plan for next steps.	Affirm value of the discussion. Bid goodbye.

treatment choices, while older patients may seek greater physician involvement in the process (10). There can be no better way than to ask a patient directly how much detail they like in the descriptions of treatment approaches—a simple overview, moderate attention to major benefits and side-effects, or considerable detail about all potential risks and benefits (11).

In like manner, asking the patient about their preferred role in making decisions proves to be useful in engaging them in the process (12). Do they generally like to make their own decision about what happens to their body, or are they guided by the views of their physician and family? In an effort to make explicit the process of shared decision-making, the clinician might helpfully comment about the modern trend towards shared decision-making in medical practice. A partnership statement is useful here, such as, 'Let us try during this discussion to understand together the benefits and risks of treatments for your condition'. Table 11.2 illustrates some of the comments that clinicians make to achieve each strategy in this clinical encounter.

It is wise to clarify the patient's, and any third party's, understanding of the illness, the seriousness of its threat or prognosis, and what they expect the treatment will need to be. This approach ensures that everyone is on the same page before commencing the discussion. Establishing pre-existing concerns empowers the clinician to address them as the conversation unfolds, while any misunderstandings can be corrected early.

Offering a preview of the range of options proves helpful first, with data being categorized into portions large enough to digest readily. Be clear about the benefits of each treatment option alongside its risks and side-effects. Categorize outcomes into early, long-term and late effects. Present the source and strength of evidence for each treatment modality as a means to optimize knowledge and the rationale behind each treatment choice. Draw diagrams, whenever possible, to illustrate a surgical technique or outcome from a treatment approach. Thus, 100-person diagrams are very useful ways of promoting understanding about the benefits of adjuvant chemotherapy. List of side-effects and take-home literature about a treatment method will usually be appreciated.

At this stage of the dialogue, clarification of any potential impact on life-style, employment, relationships, or family life is worthwhile. Consider personal issues like any effect on sexual functioning or fertility. Invite questions and empathize with any emerging emotional responses to what is being discussed. Reinforce the value of joint decision-making and offer a partnership statement as a reminder of the collaborative nature of the process.

The recent ascendance of patient autonomy does not mean that physicians should be passive about recommending their preferred mode of treatment for each patient. Their insight is governed by their training and experience; their clear treatment recommendation helps guide uncertain and anxious patients (13). In working towards a consensus (14), clinicians retain a responsibility to avoid endorsement of futile treatments and to provide a strong rationale for what they recommend. Offering a decision delay can helpfully provide time for more deliberative persons.

Patient scenarios to guide role-play exercises

- ◆ Breast cancer. A 38-year-old, divorced actor and mother of one is about to see you with a diagnosis of ductal carcinoma-in-situ, with unclear margins following a recent initial lumpectomy. Radiation therapy, mastectomy with implant, or mastectomy with free flap reconstruction are potential treatment options. Her new partner, accompanying her, is a corporate lawyer and life-style factors will likely impact upon her treatment choice.

- ◆ Prostate cancer. A 58-year-old physician comes to you for a second opinion about treatment of his recently diagnosed prostate cancer. After a serial rise in his prostate specific antigen titres, biopsy has revealed a moderately undifferentiated carcinoma with a Gleason score of 7.

Table 11.2 Exemplary statements made by clinicians to achieve the desired communication strategies in shared treatment decision-making

Communication strategies	Exemplary comments by clinicians
1. Establish the consultation framework.	'We're here today to talk about the treatment options for your cancer.' 'Before we begin, are there particular agenda items that you want to ensure we cover today? Making me aware of these will help me to cover them at the appropriate time in our conversation.'
2. Establish the physician–patient team.	'People differ in the amount of information they like to receive from their doctor. Help me to understand whether you are the sort of person who only likes to hear overviews, or sufficient detail to inform your choice, or all possible information about the issue.' 'People also differ in their decision-making style. Some are very independent and make the decision completely on their own, some consult in a shared manner with their physician, family and friends; others want to follow precisely what their doctor recommends. Do you know which style suits you best?' 'Well, let us now work together to understand your treatment options and consider which choice may be best for you.'
3. Develop an accurate, shared understanding of the patient's situation: (a) disease features, (b) prognosis without treatment; (c) psychosocial needs and concerns; (d) other factors influencing the treatment decision.	'Let me check on what sense you've been making of this diagnosis? What was it called? How serious do you perceive this illness to be?' 'What have you discovered already about your treatment options?' 'Have you known other family members or friends to receive treatment for this illness?' To a relative, 'Are there any issues or concerns that you think will influence X's decision about this treatment?'
4. Present established treatment options.	'Let me first of all summarize each of the three treatments that are possible for you. Then we'll discuss each in turn.' 'Are there questions that you want to ask?' 'Let me clarify what you've understood about each of these treatment options. Can you summarize the key points for me please?' 'Remember that you don't have to reach a final choice about your treatment today. It will be fine to think it over, talk more with your family, and let me know when you feel confident about your choice.'
5. Discuss patient's values and life-style factors that may impact on the standard treatment decision.	'Let me check if you carry any concerns about the impact of this treatment on your employment, lifestyle, fertility or sexuality?' 'Help me to understand if a treatment preference is emerging for you and why?'
6. Present a clear statement of the recommended treatment option and invite patient choice.	'Now that you understand the range of treatment options, I want to make sure that you understand what I recommend for you. If you were my father/wife, I'd …' 'Are you in a position to make a treatment choice today, or would you prefer to think about it for a few days?'
7. Close the consultation.	'Let me tell you what the next steps are. You'll need to sign an informed consent form, see our booking officer and get an appointment to see the anaesthetist.' 'If further queries come up for you, please don't hesitate to give me a call.'

MRI imaging suggests localized disease. He has expressed interest in brachytherapy, but wonders what the Da Vinci Robotic approach to radical prostatectomy surgery may have to offer him. His wife from his third marriage will accompany him.

◆ Rectal cancer. A 62-year-old, married stockbroker has been referred with a quite low-lying rectal cancer. One surgeon has offered him an abdominoperineal resection with a permanent stoma, but he has heard about the development of neorectal pouches. He declares that he has become confused about the side-effects of these different approaches and wants to discuss the potential benefits versus risks of each treatment option. His wife suffers from chronic anxiety and is known to be a very fussy woman.

◆ Lung cancer. This 55-year-old woman has suffered from chronic obstructive pulmonary disease and emphysema, consequent upon many years of smoking. Her biopsy was recently positive for non-small cell lung cancer in her right upper lobe, but her respiratory reserve makes uncertain her suitability for attempting lung resection. She wants to discuss both surgical and non-surgical approaches to management and comes to you as an oncologist to learn about recent advances in the chemotherapeutic treatment of lung cancer.

Guide to training actors for decision-making role-plays

The actor can be directed to play a well-educated, confident, and somewhat narcissistic individual, who likes always to make his/her own choices or, alternatively, an uncertain and timid person, who worries constantly and is unsure about what is best to choose. Irrespective of the role selected by the facilitator, the actor should strive to ask questions about the potential advantages and disadvantages of each treatment option, and consider the impact of these on their workplace, relational and family life. The actor will value the opinion of the clinician, seek the views of any accompanying third party, ask about reliable websites for further consideration, and indicate that they like to learn a lot about the disease and its possible treatment. The worth of a second opinion should be queried routinely.

Conclusion

The framing of information messages is becoming a sophisticated science, but the process of dialogue in the clinical decision-making encounter must of necessity transverse a series of sequenced steps. Time is a necessary ingredient to assure integration of knowledge and its application to the needs of each individual. The greater use of decision aids and question prompt-sheets in the future will deepen each patient's understanding and satisfaction with these interactions. Person-centred care leads to individualized treatment planning, with wide variations in any patient's and family's level of interest and assertiveness in the process. The adaptiveness of the clinician to each patient's needs is vital. The strategies, skills, and process tasks presented here offer a blueprint that has broad applicability for cancer care and is also readily modifiable to the specifics of complex decision-making processes.

References

1. Epstein RM, Street RL Jr (2007). *Patient-Centered Communication in Cancer Care: Promoting Healing and Reducing Suffering.* National Cancer Institute, NIH Publication No. 07–6225, Bethesda, MD.

2. Brown RF, Bylund CL (2008). Communication skills training: describing a new conceptual model. *Acad Med* **83**, 37–44.

3. Slevin M, Stubbs L, Plant H, *et al.* (1990). Attitudes to chemotherapy: comparing views of patients with cancer with those of doctors, nurses and the general public. *BMJ* **300**, 1458–60.

4. Fallowfield L, Hall A, Macguire GP, *et al.* (1994). Psychological effects of being offered choice of surgery for breast cancer. *BMJ* **309** (6952), 448.

5. Fallowfield L, Hall A, Macguire GP, *et al.* (1994). A question of choice; Results of a prospective 3 year follow up study of women with breast cancer. *Breast* **3**, 202–8.

6. Gattellari M, Butow PN, Tattersall MH (2001). Sharing decisions in cancer care. *Soc Sci Med* **52**, 1865–78.

7. Charles C, Gafni A, Whelan T, *et al.* (2006). Cultural influences on the physician-patient encounter: the case of shared decision-making. *Patient Educ Couns* **63**, 262–7.

8. Ford S, Schofield T, Hope T (2003). What are the ingredients for a successful evidence-based patient choice consultation? A qualitative study. *Soc Sci Med* **56**, 589–602.

9. Brown RF, Bylund CL, Gueguen J, *et al.* (2005). *Shared Decision Making*. Communication Skills Training and Research Laboratory, Memorial Sloan-Kettering Cancer Center, New York, NY.

10. Coulter A, Jenkinson C (2005). European patients' views on the responsiveness of health systems and healthcare providers. *Eur J Public Health* **15**, 355–60.

11. Finney-Rutten LJ, Arora NK, Bakos AD, *et al.* (2005). Information needs and sources of information among cancer patients: a systematic review of research (1980–2003). *Patient Educ Couns* **57**, 250–61.

12. Bradley JG, Zia MJ, Hamilton N (1996). Patients preferences for control in medical decision making: A scenario based approach. *Fam Med* **28**, 496–501.

13. Brown RF, Butow PN, Butt DG, *et al.* (2004). Developing ethical strategies to assist oncologists in seeking informed consent to cancer clinical trials. *Soc Sci Med* **58**, 379–90.

14. Montgomery A, Fahey T (2001). How do patients' treatment preferences compare with those of clinicians? *Qual Health Care* **10** Suppl 1, i39-i43.

Chapter 12

Responding to difficult emotions

Jennifer Philip and David W Kissane

Introduction

Clinicians must be prepared to allow the expression of a variety of emotions in cancer care. There are times during the illness when emotional responses may be anticipated, such as when a patient is first diagnosed with cancer, when a recurrence occurs or when the disease is progressing despite anti-cancer treatments. There will be other times when the physician is unaware of the particular stimulus for distress. A seemingly benign discussion can result in an unexpected response. Additional sources of vulnerability do occur in the lives of patients, not directly related to the cancer care. To be supportive, physicians must be skilled in the delivery of empathic responses. We contend that these are teachable skills.

The assessments of physicians and their responses will vary according to the acuity or chronicity of the emotions expressed. We will divide this chapter accordingly. We take the angry patient as one example of an emotionally difficult encounter and offer a model as to how the clinician can respond. This approach can be applied to a range of other challenging interactions.

Acute emotional distress

The implications of a cancer diagnosis, its treatment and prognosis ensure that emotions will inevitably be expressed. For many patients, these reactions are private or confined to home and family (1). Indeed, it is surprising that physicians are witness to relatively few intense emotional outbursts in view of the losses and existential threats that occur.

Patients exhibit a range of emotions post-diagnosis including, but not limited to, mood changes such as worry, sadness, anger and frustration; existential concerns like fear of recurrence and living with uncertainty; concerns about body image, sexuality, changing roles, employment and finances; and relational issues including the family's emotional response (2–4). The prevalence of anxiety in cancer patients is between 25 and 48% (5–7), with acute stress disorder present in almost one-third of patients after diagnosis (8, 9). Meanwhile, in advanced cancer, depression affects between 5 and 28% of patients (9).

While the form of expression of emotions may vary, there are some commonalities in the approaches taken by physicians that patients find helpful. These are outlined in Box 12.1. Physicians will be discomforted by extreme emotions, but quiet acknowledgement of the discomfort to oneself may be sufficient to remain aware of the patients' needs and take care not to use avoidant behaviours or strategies. Some examples of the latter behaviours are given in Box 12.2.

'Difficult emotions'

Not infrequently, there will be consultations where the patient's particular acute emotional expressions make communication more difficult. The so-termed 'difficult patient' may be one who is extremely distressed, demanding, unable to make decisions or angry (10). In cancer care,

Box 12.1 Responses of the physician to the emotional distress of patients

- Be prepared to 'be present' with the distress as one human being to another.
- Listen, ask open-ended questions and show care, compassion and interest.
- Allow time to understand the experience and gain insight into what may have prompted this response, particularly at this time.
- Take care not to use distancing techniques or strategies that indicate the emotional response is unwelcome. For example, do not focus only on physical questions when emotional cues are offered by the patient.
- Show empathy by acknowledging the emotional distress you see.
- Provide support: this may be from the clinician, but also recruited from the patient's own networks. Therefore, determine who the patient's usual supports are, and consider ways, with the patient's permission, to mobilize their supportive role.
- Follow-up: this should be formally organized.

these situations may also encompass 'difficult families', since family members can have a very active role in support and care provision. Hahn and colleagues suggest that one-sixth of all out-patient consultations are 'difficult' (11). The presence of co-morbid psychiatric conditions increases the likelihood of this: depression and alcohol create a three-fold increase, anxiety disorders a seven-fold increase and somatoform disorders a twelve-fold increase (11).

The following discussion will use the difficult patient as a model to discuss strategies to respond to challenging encounters. This approach is one that will have applicability across a number of consultations, where communication is more difficult.

An approach to 'the difficult patient'

The construct of patients being considered 'difficult' should be treated with caution, as it suggests a punitive situation where the patient is not adopting the proper role or expected response. The problem may not lie with the patient, but instead in a breakdown of the clinician–patient

Box 12.2 Defensive behaviours to be avoided by physicians in cancer care

- Asking closed questions.
- Asking leading questions.
- Interrupting the patient, changing the subject, cutting him short.
- Giving premature reassurance or advice 'Don't worry, most people think that…'.
- Becoming irritable or angry.
- Concentrating on physical symptoms and ignoring psychological symptoms and cues.
- Talking to relatives rather than the patient.

relationship (12). More usefully, we suggest the clinician understand the difficulty as lying with the communication between the patient and physician. Within this framework, the challenges are more appropriately located in the space between those present in the encounter. It is within this space that a shared understanding and partnership may be formed, leading to a constructive clinical relationship. Equally, however, when there is misunderstanding or reluctance to engage, difficulties arise.

Such misunderstanding may result from different expectations. In clinical interactions, people bring their cultural understanding of the body. These explanatory models of illness will influence how they consider health, including how it is defined, and the means by which it is maintained or regained (13). Even within the same culture, there can be variation in the adherence to certain practices. And then, in addition to their formal cultural background, people bring other influences. The health professional will represent his or her discipline and will bring its language. Kagawa-Singer has produced a model of the cultural intersections that occur for the clinician. The physician's identity is derived from her native culture, gender, clinical specialty and the healthcare system within which she works (13). To this model should be added the physician's personal expectations and roles (14).

Misunderstandings arising from different expectations may be conferred by roles, beliefs, values, basic understandings of disease and well-being, culture and many other parameters in life, not all linked with the medical concerns at hand (15). Shimoji and Miyakawa have noted that '[i]n the gap, loophole, between the two epistemological systems [of the doctor and patient] is the space where clinical dialog is pursued at its deepest level' (16). The approach to negotiating this interpersonal space is common to each 'difficult' clinical encounter, with the same strategies being helpful in a number of situations. We use anger as an illustration.

Anger

The widespread influence of Elisabeth Kübler-Ross has led to anger being considered a normal emotional response to the diagnosis of a terminal illness (17). Certainly anger is highly prevalent in clinical care. In patients with cancer, anger is reported to be a feature in the clinical encounter in 9–18% (18–21) with some suggestion that it is becoming more prevalent (22, 23). Possible explanations include changing systems of clinical care that are less responsive to individual needs, greater confidence to question doctors' fallibility, a more acceptable response to threat that does not admit vulnerability, a normalization of aggression (24) and a recognition that the 'squeaky gate gets attention'. There may be wider social phenomena at play, such as an increasing set of expectations about healthcare that suggests there is fault in the event of poor physical outcomes (25).

For patients with cancer, there are many possible sources of anger. They are forced to deal with many potential and real losses, and the resulting anger may be stated directly or be expressed as another complaint, such as discontent at a perceived or real neglect, and sometimes abandonment (26). At times, physicians will feel that anger is being voiced despite appropriate care.

Anger can be expressed as a component of other symptoms, in particular, pain. Among suffering patients, Cohen *et al.* suggest that angry outbursts may be linked to episodes of increased pain (13, 27). In this study, anger resulted from an awareness of dying and was expressed more openly than complaints of pain.

Anger may be regarded as an opportunity for more creative channelling of energy (28). By encouraging emotional expression, health professionals assist with the emergence of these constructive emotional responses. Attempts to 'deal with' anger may occur at some personal cost to the health professionals involved. Such impact is little discussed, yet most physicians will readily recall a clinical encounter where they were the object of anger, and express discomfort despite the incident having occurred several years earlier.

Clinicians meeting anger may feel threatened, become defensive or, indeed, angry in response (29). These reactions are generally considered unhelpful as they are likely to result in an escalation of the patient's anger (26, 29, 30).

Longer term results from angry encounters have included absenteeism, substandard patient care and reduced job satisfaction in health professionals (31). Taylor *et al.* reported that among United Kingdom hospital physicians, 32% had psychiatric morbidity and 41% suffered from emotional exhaustion (32). Among those in cancer care, this stress and burnout was attributed, among other things, to dealing with distressed, angry and blaming relatives.

Response to anger

For the majority of patients expressing anger, due attention to their concerns, allowing them to feel heard and facilitating some shift in perspective, will result in a useful outcome for all concerned (26). This ideal outcome is nevertheless challenging to achieve and often dependent upon careful attention to a sequence of strategies that help ameliorate the distress. A practical approach to this is summarized in Box 12.3.

Step 1. Preparation

It is useful to be forewarned if a patient is angry so that some personal preparation can be made before the encounter, especially if the clinician concerned is the focus of the anger. If the patient is in a hospital ward, move the conversation from a shared room or corridor to a quiet room, showing a willingness to provide uninterrupted attention. By ensuring everyone is seated, a sense of 'making time' is created and, simultaneously, any power inequalities conferred by height differences are reduced.

Step 2. Listen

The angry patient needs to be heard and understood. Ventilation alone, however, is unlikely to lead to improved interpersonal communication in the clinical encounter (26). Instead, the

---

Box 12.3 Sequence of strategies for the difficult communication encounter

1. Preparation. Be clear about clinical details and investigation results prior to meeting the patient. Make time.

2. Listen. Using open-ended questions, allow the narrative to unfold. Develop a shared understanding of the experience, and develop shared goals from this point.

3. Offer an empathic acknowledgment of the emotions expressed.

4. Provide symptom relief.

5. Involve experienced clinicians.

6. If anger persists, reconsider your approach. Important role for senior staff to guide this approach and model appropriate behaviour.

7. Consider limit-setting to the expression of emotion, where behaviours present danger or disruption to care.

8. Support of the team.

9. Consider a second opinion or the involvement of an independent broker.

approach must attempt to establish a shared understanding of the patient's experience and emotion, and may ultimately involve encouragement to direct the energy as constructively as possible (26, 29).

A practical way of facilitating these psychotherapeutic tasks is to invite the angry patient or family member to tell her story. 'I can see you are angry. I wonder if you could tell me what has been happening. Perhaps you could take me back to the beginning of this.' The patient's story should be allowed to unfold. The clinician must take care to avoid interruptions or defensiveness, and, in the first instance, should not attempt to correct misunderstandings. Instead, the story should be heard in its entirety. Throughout this narrative, there will be opportunities for clarification and reflection on occasions of triumph and disappointment. Questions that may facilitate the recounting of grievances and allow insights into the patient's experience are listed in Box 12.4.

As the narrative nears the present, the doctor and patient reach a common understanding of what happened, which creates a connection within the consultation. This should be followed by an exploration of the patient's understanding of the present predicament and then, after careful clinical assessment, with the physician's understanding of the reality. Differences of perception should be examined and, if possible, a common position reached. Finally, some goals of care need to be negotiated and agreed upon. When taking this approach, it is almost always possible to agree to some common goals. Though anger may still be present, this usually allows the patient and family to direct the energy of anger into another avenue.

Step 3. Offer empathic acknowledgment

While hearing the story, simple strategies such as repeating phrases or stating, as appropriate, 'that must have been very upsetting' may be useful. Such phrases used in the context of empathetic listening serve not only to acknowledge the distress, but also to rename the anger as an alternative emotion. These psychotherapeutic strategies may be encapsulated as: allowing the patient to recount grievances; working towards a shared understanding of the patient's emotion and experience; and showing empathy (10).

If anger is justified, then validation of its expression frequently results in its amelioration. Even if anger is seemingly incomprehensible, its non-judgemental acknowledgement can be helpful for many patients. 'I can see you are very angry and upset by this.' Unhelpful responses, including indifference, lack of empathy, rushing consultations, blocking questions with premature reassurance and failure to conduct a deeper enquiry, may all result in anger escalating. Clinicians need self-awareness about defensive behaviours that could be adopted in the face of anger, so that they can elect to adopt more constructive behaviours. This will lead to improved patient outcomes in the longer term.

Box 12.4 Questions to prompt the patient narrative

- Help me to understand what has been happening.
- Tell me what you thought went wrong, and the events leading up to this.
- What do you think caused the problem?
- Can you take me back to when all this began. When was this, and what was the first thing you noticed?

The narrative approach described in this section is effective for many and frequently results in improvement of the patient–physician relationship. This approach does, however, require a significant commitment of time. A busy outpatient clinic allows little time and scant remuneration for these tasks. By contrast, in palliative care, there is a legitimacy given to the time taken to explore these issues and experience suggests the time is well spent (33). Anger is recognized as a symptom requiring exploration, expression and understanding (28). For palliative care workers, the expression of anger is viewed as an opportunity to facilitate the emergence of alternative and more creative emotional responses to the illness. When anger is transformed into more mature emotions, relationships are enriched and the clinical team satisfied. Patients and families often ascribe great value to the fact that the doctor has taken the time to listen and this, in itself, can assist to dissipate anger.

Step 4. Provide symptom relief

The approach to anger should also include careful attention to, and relief of, symptoms that may be exacerbating the complexity of the emotional experience. The reduction of pain, for example, will allow the space for a distressed patient to consider alternative emotional responses.

Step 5. Involve experienced clinicians

The capacity of physicians to interact constructively with angry patients and families increases with experience. Patterns may be recognized and, without dismissing the events precipitating anger, appropriate responses follow. The skilled physician has an educational responsibility to model constructive responses to anger for junior staff.

On occasion, anger may persist unabated, despite intensive and conscientious efforts by the physician (26). For some, anger may persist because the initial grievances have not been adequately addressed, but for a few, anger may represent a lifelong pattern of response to a challenge or crisis. When anger is persistent, there are frequently unfortunate consequences for patient care. If the competence or effort of staff is continually questioned, confidence will be undermined. Staff may be reluctant to engage with the patient, thereby protecting themselves, but also reducing the opportunities for therapeutic relationships. Ultimately, care may become fragmented and adversarial positions between the patient (or family) and staff become fixed, further limiting the opportunities for discourse and negotiation. In such a challenging situation, staff should be supported but efforts must also be made to prevent intransigent positions being adopted.

Step 6. If anger persists, reconsider the approach

When anger persists despite the thoughtful efforts of experienced staff, then the approach should be reconsidered. In such a situation, the aims should change from attempting to resolve the anger to supporting the healthcare team. Firstly, early recognition of a patient or family who appear to be persistently angry is important. When anger is unabating, junior staff need guidance to cease making themselves vulnerable to the expression of such anger. Secondly, once recognized, senior staff should be actively involved. Junior staff should feel comfortable to defer complaints to their senior colleagues, who in turn must be willing to show leadership and model adaptive behaviours. Thirdly, team unity is critical and must be reinforced to staff, patients and families. This will both support staff and reduce the ambiguity of 'mixed messages', thus providing certainty to patients. On occasion, a single member of staff and a single member of the family concerned may be nominated as persons through which all communication occurs.

Step 7. Consider limit setting

On occasion, anger is so extreme that limits on behaviour and interactions are required. Staff have responsibilities to a number of patients, and they must be confident that they can conduct their duties in a safe, non-threatening (verbally and physically) environment. The use of limit-setting can be a constructive way of containing anxieties and best use of the time available. A family meeting may be helpful (see Chapter 15). Take care that senior staff are involved, more than one staff member is present and use the formality of the process to achieve containment. Senior staff should always be involved in the negotiation of such limits, and it may be helpful to involve non-clinical staff (such as the director of nursing). In this way, limits that initially appear unpalatable may be negotiated without compromising what remains of the therapeutic relationship.

Step 8. Support of the team

In the presence of resolute anger, support of the health professional team is critical. Actively inform all staff of the goals of care through regular meetings and through the development of a detailed care plan for the patient concerned. Involve all disciplines as appropriate, including medical, nursing, allied health, security and food services, since all may be subject to the anger expressed. Staff should actively facilitate the collegiate support of all within this team.

Step 9. Involve an independent broker

In the presence of continued dissatisfaction and questioning of competence, offer a second medical opinion. Another approach is the involvement of an outside independent broker. Such mediation may take the form of a clinical ethics consultation or a patient's representative or advocate. This independent opinion may be particularly helpful in an extreme situation, where seemingly intransigent positions between staff and the patient are set.

In effect, the model delineated here for anger is useful in its application to a number of difficult clinical encounters, including patients who are anxious, resentful, distressed or fearful. In each scenario, a response from the empathetic physician, which involves listening, hearing the illness narrative and, as necessary, involving senior clinicians, will contain distress.

Prolonged emotional distress

Suffering

The lay press might consider suffering as synonymous with pain, but in clinical care the two are not so easily equated. One person may feel pain but not be suffering. Another may suffer when they lose something central to their life, such as losing employment, yet they have no physical injury. Instead, a richer understanding of suffering stems from the notion that human beings exist with a sense of their wholeness, identity and embodiment. Suffering results when this integrity is threatened.

> Suffering is experienced by persons not merely by bodies, and it has its source in challenges that threaten the intactness of the person as a complex social and psychological entity.

> (34, p.639)

In this sense, suffering is understood as a dis-integration of the self. Suffering is not universal in terminal illness. Its causes are intensely personal. These cannot be predicted, so that we must enquire directly as to their nature (34). Cassell writes, 'Suffering is not only personal—that is, involving the person—it is also individual' (35, p.532). An approach to suffering, therefore, requires not only an understanding of pain and its relief, but also the nature of what it is to be human in all its complexity. It is difficult to characterize the suffering person, but adjectives that have been used include despairing, helpless, melancholic and demoralized. The patient may or may not have symptoms that are distressing.

If suffering is understood as a dis-integration, then the approach to assisting the person who is suffering should be aimed at re-integration. The use of open-ended questions, attentive listening and encouraging personal narratives may all assist some form of re-integration. The phrase 'tell me what you were like at the top of your game' (36) may be useful. Hearing each person's description of him or herself when they were at their best not only reminds them that they exist apart from the current illness, but it also recalls a time when they were fully integrated. For some, the evocation of that embodied self assists them towards re-establishing a relationship with that self, and allows them to move, in some way, towards re-integration. Aspects of this approach have been formally developed in an intervention for terminally ill patients termed Dignity Therapy (37). Such an approach not only helps patients redevelop a sense of meaning in their lives, but also assists their families during bereavement (37). Some phrases that may be useful when caring for a patient who is suffering are outlined in Box 12.5.

Demoralization

Demoralization may be understood as a particular reaction to threat experienced by patients with significant illness, which is characterized by anxiety and an inability to determine the way forward (38). This helplessness may progress to a more generalized hopelessness, where the patient feels a loss of direction and pointlessness to his or her life. If help is not forthcoming, the patient feels isolated and, if coupled with reduced self-esteem, a severe form of demoralization may result. This state of severe demoralization can be equivalent to the existential distress of suffering discussed previously.

The patient who is demoralized may be able to laugh and enjoy the moment, but is unable to anticipate the future with any pleasure, while the depressed patient cannot experience pleasure at any level. The demoralized patient does not know how to act or what to do, with a pervasive helplessness about their state, but for the patient with depression, even though the path to act may be evident, he or she has lost the motivation to pursue that course (38).

Once again the approach to the demoralized patient is not significantly different to other 'difficult' clinical encounters. Such an approach should include:

+ The relief of symptoms.
+ The use of open-ended questioning, empathic listening to encourage connectedness, valuing and relationships.

Box 12.5 Phrases that may be useful in the presence of someone suffering

+ Take me back to before this cancer started or to when you last felt really well in yourself. Tell me when this was, how you were, how you spent your time, your interests.
+ Now can you describe to me what first made you go to the doctor, and then…. How were you getting on then, how did the treatments go from your point of view?
+ You seem to be having a very difficult time at the moment.
+ Are you suffering? Can you help me understand what you are feeling and what is making you suffer?
+ Can you take me back to when you were 'at the top of your game', when you were feeling absolutely on song. When was that? What were you doing? Tell me about your life at that time.

◆ An exploration of life's meaning, including views on relationships, beliefs and roles. The patient should be encouraged to consider his or her life as a whole, including times when they were connected and integrated.

Conclusion

A number of emotions will be expressed in the journey with cancer. Some will occur at times when bad news is delivered; others will be unexpected and may take the physician by surprise. Skills that help acute distress include listening with empathy, using open-ended questions to allow gentle exploration of the related feelings, avoiding strategies that tend to distance patients and providing the information and appropriate reassurances to enable a person to recruit their own coping responses.

It is both surprising and humbling that most patients negotiate this journey with little or no significant assistance from their physician, but instead draw upon their personal resources and those of their immediate family and community.

The difficult clinical encounter is one characterized by essential differences between the patient and their clinician. This difference lies in the expectations of the participants, their beliefs, cultures, understanding of illness, approach and roles, and results in a mismatch in communication. Our model of negotiating this difference has utility across a number of different clinical scenarios and settings.

Finally, when emotional responses have become more chronic, a state of demoralization may result. Here the helplessness becomes overwhelming and, if help is not offered or proves ineffective, a state of existential distress may develop. When severe, this represents a form of suffering. The approach to care for such patients must include a careful and gentle exploration of the source of distress in the context of a caring clinical relationship. For some patients telling their story to a physician who is truly listening will be of great benefit. For others, an exploration and improved understanding of his or her beliefs, values and sense of meaning may allow some mobilization of personal resources to assist the intensely personal task of re-integration. The amelioration of suffering is personal and individual, and cannot be proscribed. But the care of a clinician who is willing to be open and to spend time in the space occupied by the suffering patient will enable some patients to emerge, even in some small way, from a state of suffering. In turn, there may be rich rewards, which flow to the clinician himself. Michael Kearney suggests that the physician who is prepared to accompany 'another as he journeys into the depths of his experience' (39) may himself be enriched. For,

> …the healing on offer may be there not just for the patient and his family but also for us as people who are physicians, and in some small way for western medicine itself.

(39, p.46).

References

1. Cowley L, Hayman B, Stanton M, *et al.* How women receiving adjuvant chemotherapy for breast cancer cope with their treatment: a risk management perspective. *J Advanced Nursing* 2000; **31**(2), 314–321.
2. Tish Knobf M. Psychosocial responses in breast cancer survivors. *Sem Oncol Nurs* 2007; **23**(1), 71–83.
3. Reddick BK, Nanda JP, Campbell L, *et al.* Examining the influence of coping with pain on depression, anxiety, and fatigue among women with breast cancer. *J Psychosoc Oncol* 2005; **23**(2–3), 137–157.
4. Anderson BL, Shapiro CL, Farrar WB, *et al.* Psychological responses to cancer recurrence. *Cancer* 2005; **104**(7), 1540–1547.

5. Derogatis LR, Morrow GR, Fetting J, *et al.* The prevalence of psychiatric disorders among cancer patients. *JAMA* 1983; **249**(6), 751–757.

6. Mehnert A, Koch U. Prevalence of acute and post-traumatic stress disorder and comorbid mental disorders in breast cancer patients during primary cancer care: a prospective study. *Psychooncology* 2007; **16**(3), 181–188.

7. Stark D, Kiely M, Smith A, *et al.* Anxiety disorders in cancer patients: their nature, associations, and relation to quality of life. *J Clin Oncology* 2002; **20**(14), 3137–3148.

8. Kangas M, Henry JL, Bryant RA. Correlates of acute stress disorder in cancer patients. *J Trauma Stress* 2007; **20**(3), 325–334.

9. Miovic M, Block S. Psychiatric disorders in advanced cancer. *Cancer* 2007; **110**(8), 1665–1676.

10. Bylund C, Gueguen J, Brown R, *et al.* 2006. *Responding to Patient Anger.* Communication Skills Training and Research Laboratory, Memorial Sloan-Kettering Cancer Center, New York.

11. Hahn SR, Kroenke K, Spitzer RL, *et al.* The difficult patient: prevalence, psychopathology, and functional impairment. *J Gen Int Med* 1996; **11**, 1–8.

12. Pearce C. The difficult patient. *Aust Fam Physician* 2002; **31**(2), 177–178.

13. Kagawa-Singer M, Kassim-Lakha S. A strategy to reduce cross-cultural miscommunication and increase the likelihood of improving health outcomes. *Acad Med* 2003; **78**(6), 577–87.

14. Komesaroff P. 1995. Introduction: postmodern ethics. In: Komesaroff P, editor. *Troubled Bodies*, pp.1–19, Melbourne University Press, Melbourne.

15. Komesaroff P. 1995. From bioethics to microethics; ethical debate and clinical medicine. In: Komesaroff P, editor. *Troubled Bodies*, pp.62–86, Melbourne University Press, Melbourne.

16. Shimoji A, Miyakawa T. Culture-bound syndrome and a culturally sensitive approach: From a view point of medical anthropology. *Psych Clin Neurosci* 2000; **54**, 461–466.

17. Kubler Ross E. 1969. *On Death and Dying.* Macmillan, New York.

18. Craig TJ, Abeloff MD. Psychiatric symptomatology among hospitalised cancer patients. *Am J Psychiatry* 1974; **131**, 1323–1327.

19. Farber JM, Weinerman BH, Kuypers JA. Psychosocial distress in oncology outpatients. *J Psychosoc Oncol* 1984; **2**, 109–118.

20. Kissane D, Bloch S, Burns WI, *et al.* Psychological morbidity in the families of patients with cancer. *Psychooncology* 1994; **3**, 47–56.

21. Stefanek ME, Derogatis LP, Shaw AI. Psychological distress among oncology outpatients. *Psychosomatics* 1987; **28**, 530–539.

22. Menckel E, Viitasara E. Threats and violence in Swedish care and welfare—magnitude of the problem and impact on municipal personnel. *Scand J Caring Sci* 2002; **16**(4), 376–385.

23. Richards B. From respect to rights to entitlement, blocked aspirations and suicidal behaviours. *Int J Circumpolar Health* 2004; **63**(Suppl 1), 19–24.

24. Fry AJ, O'Riordan D, Turner D, *et al.* Survey of aggressive incidents experienced by community mental health staff. *Int J Ment Health Nurs* 2002; **11**(2), 112–120.

25. White D. 1995. Divide and multiply: culture and politics in the new medical order. In: Komesaroff P, editor. *Troubled Bodies*, pp.20–37, Melbourne University Press, Melbourne.

26. Kissane D. Managing anger in palliative care. *Aust Fam Physician* 1994; **23**(7), 1257–1259.

27. Cohen M, Williams L, Knight P, *et al.* Symptom masquerade: understanding the meaning of symptoms. *Support Care Cancer* 2004; **12**(3), 184–190.

28. Philip J, Gold M, Schwarz M, *et al.* Anger in palliative care: a clinical approach. *Intern Med J* 2007; **37**, 49–55.

29. Cunningham W. The immediate and long-term impact on New Zealand doctors who receive patient complaints. *NZ Med J* 2004; **117**(1198), U972.

30. Houston R. The angry dying patient. *Primary Care Companion J Clin Psychiatry* 1999; **1**, 5–8.

31. Rowe MM, Sherlock H. Stress and verbal abuse in nursing. *J Nurs Manag* 2005; **13**(3), 242–248.

32. Taylor C, Graham J, Potts HWW, *et al.* Changes in mental health of UK hospital consultants since the mid-1990s. *The Lancet* 2005; **366**, 742–744.

33. Philip J. 2007. *Lowering One's Net Deeper and Deeper. An Exploration of the Cultural and Ethical Components in Palliative Care.* Monash University, Melbourne.

34. Cassell EJ. The nature of suffering and the goals of medicine. *N Eng J Med* 1982; **306**, 639–645.

35. Cassell EJ. Diagnosing suffering: a perspective. *Ann Int Med* 1999; **131**, 531–534.

36. Cassem E. 2002. *Patient Narratives in Palliative Care.* Lecture given at Center for Palliative Care, University of Melbourne, Melbourne,.

37. Chochinov H, Hack T, Hassard T, *et al.* Dignity therapy: a novel psychotherapeutic intervention for patients need the end of life. *J Clin Oncology* 2005; **23**(24), 5520–5525.

38. Clarke D, Kissane D. Demoralization: its phenomenology and importance. *Aust N Z J Psychiatry* 2002; **36**(6), 733–742.

39. Kearney M. Palliative medicine—just another specialty? *Palliat Med* 1992; **6**(1), 39–46.

Chapter 13

Denial and communication

Linda Sheahan and Simon Wein

And again his thoughts dwelt on his childhood, and again it was painful and he tried to banish them and fix his mind on something else.

Tolstoy, The Death of Ivan Ilyich

Introduction

Patients who appear not to acknowledge the diagnosis of an illness, or its gravity, are said to be 'in denial'. A patient's history readily illustrates this in Box 13.1.

Denial is a common reaction, especially when an illness is life-threatening. After being told of the diagnosis, approximately 20% of patients deny they have cancer; 26% partially suppress awareness of impending death, and 8% demonstrate complete denial (1, 2). In a recent meta-analysis, Vos and Haes suggested that the prevalence of denial of the cancer diagnosis ranged from 4 to 47% and denial of negative affect from 18 to 42% (3).

Although the term 'denial' is an accepted part of the medical vernacular, a review of the literature reveals that it is used in a variety of clinical circumstances, with varying definitions and little consensus. This explains the unwieldy ranges in Vos and Haes's meta-analysis (3). As with all of the body's defences—physiological, immunological, psychological—denial can become maladaptive.

This chapter will establish a pragmatic view of denial, explore how it functions within the clinician–patient relationship, and then demonstrate when intervention is appropriate and how that intervention is best undertaken. Specific attention will be given to the communication skills required for an effective clinical response to denial.

Definition

The term denial has not acquired a monolithic meaning—that is, there is no common agreement as to when and how to use the word. Psychoanalysts describe it as one of several cognitive defence mechanisms, which serve to protect a person against anxiety (4). A patient demonstrates denial by refusing (self-aware) or being unable (unaware) to acknowledge some painful aspect of reality or emotion that would ordinarily be apparent to self or others. The term psychotic denial is used when there is, in addition, gross impairment in reality testing (see Box 13.2).

Box 13.1 Denial leading to morbid consequences

TC was a 36-year-old man with recently diagnosed metastatic colorectal cancer. Clearly told it was incurable, he received palliative chemotherapy. TC was admitted to hospital for pain management and multiple medical complications related to progressive disease. He was cooperative with staff and treatment plans, but remained convinced that his disease was curable. The treating team sensed his reluctance to discuss prognosis, and subsequently avoided speaking directly about the cancer and his deterioration. His family and his 9-year-old son were not informed about the extent of his illness. TC wanted to go home. His mood deteriorated and the psycho-oncologist diagnosed depression with denial, complicated by collusion of the treating team. A family meeting, including the patient, discussed the overall goals of care, gradually achieving a realistic consensus.

Throughout the medical literature, the construct of denial is used to describe anything from illogical behaviour and non-compliance, to the patient's pretence to family that all is well, to non-integration of medical information into the patient's world view (3). To make matters more complicated, there is also denial as a specific clinical sign associated with neurological damage (5). This leads to confusion and uncertainty as to how to manage denial. The importance of defining denial, or at least setting functional parameters, is to enable management. The key to management of denial is thoughtful communication.

How should we define denial? The term 'denial' is applied to patients who, consciously or unconsciously, alleviate their anxiety (primarily directed at death or pain) by portraying a serious health situation as either exaggerated or non-existent (6). Why do people deny? One answer is that the human brain is designed to enable it to accommodate practically any trauma that it confronts. When an event is too difficult or painful to integrate immediately, denial is used as a coping mechanism, as a self-protective buffer (7). Sometimes this defence mechanism is adaptive, and sometimes maladaptive. The pathogenesis of how a protective defence-mechanism becomes maladaptive is unknown. An analogy might be drawn to the body's immune system, to diseases that fail to distinguish self from non-self. Furthermore, denial is dynamic—it comes

Box 13.2 Psychotic denial associated with late presentation of advanced cancer

JN was a 71-year-old retired oncology nurse, who presented to the emergency department with abdominal pain. She was found to have a large fungating chest wall lesion, consistent with advanced breast cancer. Investigations confirmed malignancy, with chest wall invasion and liver metastasis. On questioning, she insisted that she had extensive experience with cancer in her work, and that this was not cancer. She also claimed that the mass had been there for over 20 years, and was due to severe dermatitis. On being asked why she had not sought a medical opinion, she simply said that she thought it was nothing to worry about. On further questioning, JN admitted that it had changed slightly over the last few months. Gradually, after a number of consultations with the medical staff, she began to exhibit inconsistencies in her belief that it was dermatitis, and began to accept the possibility that it might be cancer.

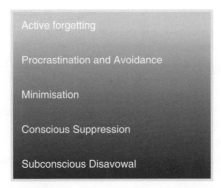

Fig. 13.1 Spectrum model of denial.

and goes 'at will', as needed. Factors that influence the presentation of denial include level of anxiety (primarily of death), the passage of time, professional relationships and stage of disease. The clinician's job is to assess whether denial is adaptive or not.

We propose conceptualizing denial as a spectrum (see Fig. 13.1). The key variables are:

(1) the degree to which the patient is aware of their denial; and

(2) how effectively the denial functions in striking a balance between subjective fear and the threat of illness.

Denial in the clinical environment

To help us understand the clinical application of denial, we will examine four clinical parameters:

(1) beneficial;

(2) detrimental;

(3) clinician's complicity; and

(4) familial and cultural.

Denial as beneficial

Denial functions as a form of self-protection. For example, it is the first step in the 'normal' stages of dying, as described by Kubler-Ross: denial, anger, bargaining, depression and acceptance (8). Longitudinal studies of breast cancer patients showed that those patients who denied the seriousness of a cancer diagnosis, experienced significantly less mood disturbance than those with 'acceptance' coping styles (9). Denial is negatively correlated with anxiety in adult cancer patients (3), and positively correlated with good adjustment in survivors of childhood cancers (1). Denial may also lead to patients experiencing fewer physical complaints, and it may have a positive effect on function (3).

Furthermore, the use of denial as a coping strategy may be predictive of a more favourable disease trajectory (10). In a 15-year prospective study of adjustment styles in breast cancer, Greer and colleagues followed a group of non-metastatic breast cancer patients at 5, 10 and 15 years after surgical intervention (11). They demonstrated that women who used fighting spirit or denial as coping strategies survived longer than those who reacted with stoic acceptance or helplessness (11). This finding has been corroborated in some follow-up studies (1), although not by others (12). The overall trend in meta-analysis suggests a positive relationship between denial and survival (10). Recent studies look more closely at minimization, as opposed to subconscious denial. Minimization techniques in patients with both metastatic melanoma and metastatic breast cancer have also been associated with longer survival (13, 14).

Then there is the question of denial in relation to hope. Druss and Douglas correlate healthy denial with optimism and resilience, where what is being denied is not the disease or infirmity itself, but rather the fearful implications and emotional impact (15). Patients may interpret what they are told about their condition according to the fear they experience or the hope they wish to maintain. In early studies of hospital patients interviewed with a diagnosed but undisclosed malignancy, 88% suspected they had cancer on admission, but 68% had no wish to augment that knowledge. Patients used denial paradoxically to maintain uncertainty and to support hope (16).

Denial as detrimental

However, denial can also be detrimental. In spite of the success of public screening for certain cancers, denial still contributes to late clinical presentation (17–19). Denial creates a barrier between clinician and patient, which can reduce effective communication. This in turn effects the patient's ability to make informed health choices and, in extreme cases, to poor compliance with treatment. Denial may prevent patients from preparing for death, both pragmatically and psychologically; and lead to complicated grief in the bereaved (9). It appears as an obstacle to open discussion of death, dying at home, stopping 'futile' treatments, advanced care planning and symptom control (20).

Clinician's complicity with denial

Traditionally, the term denial has been applied to patients; however, the clinician is not immune from denial as part of the therapeutic relationship (21). A physician may deny information to patient or family, thereby encouraging hope. Cousins states, 'In a sense the physician who treats a terminally ill patient is himself practicing a form of denial. He battles malignancy against heavy odds, employing his special knowledge and a wide array of methods and techniques' (6, p.211).

Denial by physicians may be employed as part of their defences against the difficult feelings evoked by their work, including any sense of mortal vulnerability. While these defences are protective, they can seriously hamper communication. This is characterized by emotional distancing,

---

Box 13.3 Denial as a pathway towards futile medical care

AH was a 19-year-old girl with metastatic osteosarcoma refractory to chemotherapy. AH and her family were from the Middle East and held strong religious beliefs that she would be cured, despite multiple discussions with her oncologist regarding the palliative nature of her treatment. They were adamant that every modality of treatment should be trialled since 'where there is life, there is hope'. Staff became increasingly concerned that the family were 'living in denial', which resulted in an almost daily discussion regarding prognosis and the futility of chemotherapy. AH then developed spinal cord compression. She and her family remained steadfast in their insistence on attempting further treatment, and her physician acquiesced by giving her a dose of 'emergency' chemotherapy in the early hours of the morning. There was no effect, and she died a couple of days later in hospital.

detachment, intellectualization, nihilism and even aggression. In turn, this may affect patient's adherence to treatment, pain control, information recall and overall satisfaction with care (22).

Family's complicity and cultural context

Some families use denial to cope with the patient's illness. Tacit agreement between family members to 'deny' illness can appear as 'mutual pretence awareness'. At times it can be distressing or detrimental for the patient, particularly when communication patterns are disturbed, leading to anxiety, isolation and suspicion. Cultural and religious variance has a significant impact on the use of denial as a psychological mechanism of coping (3, 24, 25). To what extent do we respect these variances, and 'allow' ongoing denial? Box 13.3 illustrates the potential for futile medical care to be administered through collusion with a family's process of denial. At its most extreme, futile care could lead to extended suffering and prolonged dying from advanced cancer in the intensive care unit.

A 'functional' or clinical definition

When should denial be broached? Only when it is causing self-harm? Or when it is judged that denial is blocking acceptance? What role do cultural or individual values play?

Clinicians need a functional definition of denial. Denial scales have been trialled in various studies without much success, but perhaps the most effective way to view denial is dimensionally, as displayed in Fig. 13.1. At one extreme is completely subconscious disavowal, and at the other, active forgetting. Elements of denial are evident within each of the labelled domains in this spectrum. Patients' level of denial may fluctuate and move from one domain to the other, depending on the patient's perceived—conscious or not—level of threat. However, only certain domains in certain circumstances require active intervention.

Role of self-awareness

Denial is often assumed to be by definition unconscious, in contradistinction to more 'healthy' coping mechanisms, such as minimization and avoidance, in which there may be some self-awareness. Nevertheless, elements of denial in minimization and avoidance are recognizable and these coping mechanisms should be integrated into the dimensional nature of denial. Active forgetting involves consciously setting aside or pushing into the background information that is too painful, as in the epigram from Tolstoy.

Role of context

The central question is whether denial is functioning in a beneficial or a maladaptive way. Adaptiveness is judged by how well a person can cope with the practicalities of the illness (and its implications) despite anxieties and fears. Thus, if the denial is accompanied by self-harm or neglect, it could reasonably be labelled as maladaptive and require healthcare intervention. The definition of 'self-harm' is relative and requires the prudent judgment of the healthcare team. Broad parameters include: non-compliance; unrealistic expectations by patient or family regarding goals of care; damage to relationships with family and loved ones (21); and inability to find 'closure'.

'Acceptance' is not always necessary. Patients may die without ever acknowledging the full extent of their illness or the imminence of death. In these cases, the priority is symptom control—physical, emotional and spiritual—notwithstanding denial. There is no rationale for intervening in cases of benign or adaptive denial by forcing acceptance upon patients, as this may only serve to increase distress and, indeed, may not be ethically prudent.

Summary

Denial is a response to fear, typically of death. The expression of denial depends on personality, coping styles, degree of self-awareness ('I'm not going to think about it any more') and the extent to which the patient can manoeuvre their illness-pathway through the healthcare system. It ranges on a spectrum from beneficial coping to maladaptive self-harm. The best approach is to develop a 'feel' for their coping style, support the patient and note the balance between fear and adaptation. Generally, a trusting relationship and good communication will be all that is required to allow the patient to open up and 'let go' of denial.

Communication with patients using denial

Although there are no empirical studies exploring the best way for a physician to challenge denial in their patient, physicians are not confident of their communication skills in dealing with denial (25). When 'breaching' the defence of denial, oftentimes an indirect approach is best. Given that denial functions as a response to a fear (of death), then by shoring up a person's self-esteem, dignity, morale and life's meaning, the fear will likely recede and denial will commensurately cease to have a function. The following recommendations are a compilation of findings based on case study reviews and expert opinion about communication in the face of denial (1, 9, 23, 26–30):

- Exclude neuropathology, misunderstanding or inadequate information.
- Determine whether denial is maladaptive or adaptive.
- Determine whether denial requires management.
- Explore emotional background to fears.
- Provide information tailored to the needs of the patient and clarify goals of care.
- Be aware of cultural and religious issues.
- Monitor the shifting sand of denial as the disease progresses.

These strategies, together with their related communication skills and process tasks, are outlined in Table 13.1.

Table 13.1 Strategies and communication skills to use in response to denial

Strategies	Skills	Process tasks	Model statements
1. Recognize the presence of denial, and exclude misunderstanding, neuropathology or misinformation.	Ask open questions. Check patient understanding.	Find out how much the patient knows about their disease. Correct any misunderstandings. Identify denial in self or team, and ensure it is not impacting on management; Gather collaborative history from family and supportive others.	'Could you describe for me in your own words what you have been told about your illness?' 'Just to ensure that I understand you correctly, you think...' 'Is it clear to you why you had treatment?' 'Have you asked any of the hospital staff for information regarding your treatment, and was the information they gave to you clear?'

Table 13.1 (continued) Strategies and communication skills to use in response to denial

Strategies	Skills	Process tasks	Model statements
2. Determine whether it is maladaptive or adaptive for the given circumstance.	Declare your agenda items (explore patient coping style and its effect). Determine and normalize past psychological coping style.	Determine if denial concurs with the patient's previous response to stress. Evaluate the effect of denial on treatment compliance. Determine if it is causing difficulties within the patient's support group/ family. Decide whether it is obstructing the patient's treatment.	'I would like to explore how you are coping with your illness. Would that be ok with you?' 'How have you coped with difficult things in the past?' 'How are you managing at home or at work?' 'What is difficult for you living with the illness?'
3. Provide information tailored to the needs of the patient.	Clarify. Acknowledge. Normalize.	Clarify the patient's preference for information and decision-making, including goals of care.	'Different patients request different levels of information from their clinician. Are you someone who likes to be given a lot of information and detail, or are you someone who prefers minimal information?' 'Have you talked to your family about this health problem?' 'Would you like me to arrange a family meeting?'
4. Explore emotional reactions and respond with empathy.	Ask open questions regarding emotional response and coping. Empathize. Validate. Acknowledge. Normalize. Simplify. Praise the patient's efforts. Express a willingness to help.	Ask about and acknowledge their emotional response. Demonstrate empathy for the difficulty they are having confronting the threatening aspect of their illness. Validate this difficulty. Divide the emotional issues into smaller more manageable packets.	'How are you feeling at this stage in your illness?' 'I can see that you are afraid/uncertain, and I know that must be extremely difficult for you.' 'Difficulty coping is normal and understandable.' 'If we can put names to our emotions, it is sometimes easier to deal with them. Let's try that for you and see if it is helpful?' 'If something I am saying makes you too uncomfortable, please let me know.'

(continued)

Table 13.1 (continued) Strategies and communication skills to use in response to denial

Strategies	Skills	Process tasks	Model statements
5. Where denial is maladaptive, identify and gently challenge inconsistencies in the patient's narrative; Maintain an open dialogue, particularly so that shifts in denial can be addressed, if required.	Clarify. Endorse question-asking. Summarize. Review next steps.	Ask the patient to identify their disease status and phases of management; Explore the factors which support a more realistic understanding of the situation. Confront ambivalence sensitively. Be wary of abrupt interventions that may precipitate overwhelming anxiety. Confrontation often requires repeated visits. Encourage optimism. Work with family and treating team re collusion. Involve psychosocial services if required.	'Could you explain to me why you think this lesion is severe dermatitis?' 'Is there a time, even just for a moment, when you consider that it might not be as simple as dermatitis?' 'Does the fact that it has changed over the last few months make you suspicious that it is not simply dermatitis?' 'How do you explain the recent changes?' 'It looks as though part of you prefers to believe that it is not serious, but another part of you is willing to consider that it is something more serious?'
6. Follow up and monitor denial in context as disease progresses	Reinforce joint decision steps.	Monitor for gradual adjustment to the stressor, and acceptance of next steps as context changes. Monitor adaptive denial for signs that it is becoming maladaptive.	'I understand that this is how you feel about your illness currently. I would like us to meet again in... just to check how things are going, and discuss things a little further.'

Conclusion

Denial can be a temporary, adaptive coping mechanism to help a person deal with a difficult and usually frightening new circumstance. Generally, it is best to support the patient's method of coping with their illness. Where denial is seen to function in a maladaptive way, however, it may be necessary to tackle and expose the denial, albeit with care and wisdom.

References

1. Greer S (1992). The management of denial in cancer patients. *Oncology* **6**, 33–6.
2. Hinton J (1994). Which patients with terminal cancer are admitted from home care? *Pall Med* **8**, 197–210.
3. Vos MS, De Haes JCJM (2007). Denial in cancer patients, an explorative review. *Psycho-Oncology* **16**, 12–25.
4. Straus DH, Spitzer RL, Muskin PR (1990). Maladaptive denial of physical illness: a proposal for DSM IV. *Am J Psychiat* **147**, 1168–72.

5. Ellis SJ, Small M (1993). Denial of illness in stroke. *Stroke* **24**, 757–9.

6. Cousins N (1982). Denial. *JAMA*, **248**, 210–2.

7. Ness DE, Ende J (1994). Denial in the medical interview. *JAMA* **272**, 1777–81.

8. Kubler-Ross E (1973). *On Death and Dying*. Routledge, New York.

9. Watson M, Greer S, Blake S, *et al.* (1984). Reaction to a diagnosis of breast cancer: Relationship between denial, delay and rates of psychological morbidity. *Cancer* **53**, 2008–12.

10. Garssen B (2003). Psychological factors and cancer development: evidence after 30 years of research, *Clin Psychol Review* **24**, 315–38.

11. Greer S, Morris T, Pettingale KW, *et al.* (1990). Psychological response to breast cancer and 15-year outcome. *Lancet* **335**, 49–50.

12. Petticrew M, Bell R, Hunter D (2002). Influence of psychological coping on survival and recurrence in people with cancer: systematic review. *BMJ* **325**, 1066–76.

13. Brown JE, Butow PN, Culjak G, *et al.* (2000). Psychosocial predictors: time to relapse and survival in patients with early stage melanoma. *Br J Cancer* **83**, 1448–53.

14. Butow PN, Coates AS, Dunn SM (1999). Psychosocial predictors of survival: metastatic breast cancer. *Ann Oncol* **11**, 469–74.

15. Druss RG, Douglas CJ (1988). Adaptive responses to illness and disability. *Gen Hosp Psychiat* **10**, 163–8.

16. McIntosh J (1976). Patients' awareness and desire for information about diagnosed but undisclosed malignant disease. *Lancet.* **2**(7980), 300–3.

17. Phelan M, Dobbs J, David AS (1992). 'I thought it would go away': patient denial in breast cancer. *J Royal Soc Med* **85**, 206–7.

18. Zervas IM, Augustine A, Fricchione GL (1993). Patient delay in cancer. *Gen Hosp Psychiat* **15**, 9–13.

19. Hackett TP, Cassem NH, Raker JW (1973). Patient delay in cancer. *N E J Med* **289**, 14–20.

20. Zimmermann C (2007). Death denial: obstacle of instrument for palliative care? An analysis of clinical literature. *Soc Health Illness* **29**, 297–314.

21. Helft PR (2005). Necessary collusion: Prognostic communication with advanced cancer patients. *J Clin Oncol* **23**, 3146–50.

22. Favre N, Despland JN, De Roten Y, *et al.* (2007). Psychodynamic aspects of communication skills training. *Support Cancer Care* **15**, 333–7.

23. Erbil P, Razavi D, Farvacques C, *et al.* (1996). Cancer patients psychological adjustment and perceptions of illness: cultural differences between Belgium and Turkey. *Support Cancer Care* **4**, 455–61.

24. Gall TL (2004). The role of religious coping in adjustment to prostate cancer. *Cancer Nursing* **27**, 454–61.

25. Travado L, Grassi L, Gil F, *et al.* (2005). Physician-patient communication among southern European cancer physicians: the influence of psychological orientation and burnout. *Psycho-oncology* **14**, 661–70.

26. Schofield PE, Butow PN, Thompson JF, *et al.* (2003). Psychological responses of patients receiving a diagnosis of cancer. *Ann Oncol* **14**, 48–56.

27. Maguire P, Faulkner A (1988). Communicate with cancer patients: 2 Handling uncertainty, collusion and denial. *BMJ* **297**, 205–7.

28. Maguire P, Pitceathly C (2003). Managing the difficult consultation. *Clin Med* **36**, 532–7.

29. Faulkner A (1998). ABC of palliative care: communication with patients, families, and other professionals. *BMJ* **316**, 130–2.

30. Hudson PL, Schofield P, Kelly B, *et al.* (2006). Responding to desire to die statements from patients with advanced disease: recommendations for health professionals. *Pall Med* **20**, 703–10.

Chapter 14

Communicating with relatives/ companions about cancer care

Terrance L Albrecht, Susan S Eggly, and John C Ruckdeschel

Introduction

The oncologist–patient interaction is frequently situated in a triadic relationship consisting of the physician, the patient, and a third party, usually at least one key family member or companion (1). The presence and involvement of a third party inevitably increases the challenge and complexity of information exchange in the clinical encounter. Research during the past three decades has demonstrated the important influence that relatives or companions can have on the clinician–patient interaction (2–4). Patients and their families/companions add extraordinary dynamics to the clinical interaction due to their knowledge, coping styles, willingness to challenge or question the physician, and prior experience interacting with oncologists and members of the medical team. The need for clinicians to garner their support is critical in order to provide the highest quality care to the patient.

In this chapter, we describe the importance of family/companions in cancer clinical interactions, their role in strategic communication goals, interaction strategies for achieving these goals, and implications for translating, implementing, and disseminating this information to the training of clinicians.

The importance and role of families or companions in clinical encounters

Family members and companions potentially influence most oncologist–patient relationships simply because they are more likely than not to be present during outpatient clinic visits (4, 5). Whether the role played by a family member/companion helps or hinders the partnership-building process between, and among, the parties in the encounter, will depend in part on the extent to which he/she shares the physician's and/or patient's views, expectations (2), and understanding regarding the disease, the diagnosis/prognosis, and/or treatment plan. Moreover, the relative/ companion may be in a great deal of distress themselves over the patient's condition and the caregiving demands they are facing (3), further exacerbating any anxieties, uncertainties, or contentiousness they may bring to the interaction.

Interestingly, results from at least one study show that oncologists generally perceive that the presence of a family member/companion has a positive effect on patient outcomes. Specifically, third parties serve to foster greater patient participation in the interaction, particularly in matters related to treatment decision-making (4). Still, oncologists' positive perceptions are distinct from the extent to which the interactions that they have with patients and family members/companions are observed to be actually 'patient-centred' (5). In other words, though physicians may report enhanced patient participation in decision-making, it may or may not be the case that systematic observation and analysis of these clinic visits would show them to be facilitative and participative, based on the types and range of behaviours exhibited by the family member/companion during the exchange.

For example, an observational study conducted by Eggly and colleagues (6) found that family/companions asked more questions of oncologists than cancer patients, but this was more likely to occur in interactions where oncologists were observed to be less conversationally dominant, and coders' ratings for oncologist–family/companion trust were relatively higher than for other interactions. Further, in addition to the physician's perceptions, whether the *patient* perceives the family member/companion as helpful is likely to be related to the type of role and activity level that the patient needs and wants the family member/companion to play (7).

In short, a family member/companion's pattern of behaviour (or sets of different behaviours) affects the dynamics of the interaction. Even in a single visit, the family member/companion may range from being facilitative and supportive to argumentative and controlling with the patient and the physician. He or she may also be assertive, contentious, submissive, silent, disinterested, fearful, optimistic, nervous, confused, and/or angry with either the physician or the patient. Such positive, negative, or neutral emotional displays, whether uniform or varied, affect the course of the information exchange and the quality of the discussion, and ultimately the nature of the patient–physician interaction.

Issues of family member/companion characteristics of race and age remain empirically important with an increasing number of studies examining these effects (8). In their observations of 235 video-recorded oncology interactions, Eggly and colleagues (9, 10) found that Black patients were significantly less likely be accompanied by a family member/companion to the oncology visit ($P < 0.001$); similar findings have been reported by others (11). Companions of Black lung cancer patients were found to be less involved in clinic interactions than companions of White patients and the oncologists were observed to be correspondingly somewhat less engaged and supportive (12).

Elderly patients are generally accompanied by a third party during medical interactions. Findings regarding the effects of family/companions on patient decision-making are inconsistent across types of medical encounters, with two studies showing that the presence of a family member may inhibit the cancer patient's involvement (11, 16) and two studies reporting family/companions as 'autonomy-enhancing' and non-distracting (17–18). Given the mixed results in the literature and the inherent differences in primary care versus acute/specialty care contexts, it is our choice to focus on conclusions drawn from research conducted in oncology medical settings.

Triadic communication in the cancer setting

Clinical communication occurs when oncologists, cancer patients, and their family/companions attend to each other and begin interpreting one another's verbal and non-verbal, explicit and implicit, obvious and subtle interactional behaviour (13). Like patients, family members may or may not have concerns, questions, and feelings of fear, uncertainty, optimism, and/or hope (14). In light of this emotion-laden interaction, communication can be considered relatively effective if shared understanding and shared perspectives enable all parties to engage in coordinated behaviour. Alternatively, communication may be ineffective if messages exchanged create mutual misunderstanding, confusion, and disturbance, leading to errors, mistakes, and uncoordinated behaviour.

The convergence model

The process of physician communication with families and companions is best captured in the convergence model of communication (15). Following Rogers and Kincaid (15), convergence is the extent to which physicians, patients, and family/companions create mutual understanding by communicating with one another. Communication that leads to convergence is the centerpiece of quality cancer care in clinical settings and plays an important role in improving patient outcomes, both large and small, affecting adherence to medical regimens (20, 22), clinical trial accrual (16), adjustment and functioning following a diagnosis (18), reactions to treatment (18), racial disparities in patterns of care (19, 20), and stress (21). As physicians, patients, and family/companions simultaneously transact and interpret messages during medical encounters, they may converge (share varying degrees of meaning regarding the content of information such as the diagnosis, medication, treatment procedures, prognosis), or not converge, resulting in mutual misunderstanding and possible disagreement concerning key aspects of a patient's disease and care. Whether physicians, patients, and family/companions communicate in ways that produce convergent or non-convergent meanings has likely consequences for the quality of cancer care.

Convergence (mutual understanding) between and among the patient, physician, and family member/companion (if present) is depicted in a Venn diagram (see Fig. 14.1) by overlapping portions of the circles. In our view, the overlapping (converging) segments may expand and/or contract throughout the discussion and even afterwards, depending on the shifting levels of mutual understanding and shared perspective that exists at any point in time among and between the parties.

Understanding and misunderstanding

Physicians, patients, and family/companions may agree or disagree about concerns discussed and they may understand or misunderstand (accurately or inaccurately perceive) each others' views. If they 'understand that they disagree' (understand that they have different views), they can address and attempt to resolve that disagreement. However, if they fail to recognize that they disagree, they will proceed as if in agreement. This situation is likely to result in subsequent misunderstandings (e.g. creating serious errors in administering medication, recognizing symptoms, understanding whether or not they are enrolled in a clinical trial).

Message functions

Messages may function in ways that provide both content (e.g. diagnosis, prognosis) and relationship information (e.g. social support, common ground, liking/disliking, etc.). As participants

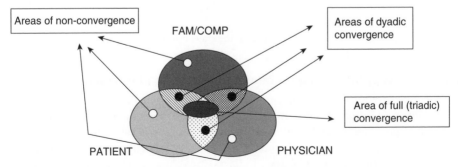

Fig. 14.1 Convergence/Non-Convergence Model of Physician-Patient-Family/Companion Communication (adapted from Rogers and Kincaid, 1981).

interact around content, they are also creating, exchanging, and interpreting messages about their relationship. Relational messages produced by physicians, patients, and family/companions can be explicit (e.g. I'm glad you have your family here with you; I'm glad you are my doctor; I think my sister is in good hands) or implicit, signalling a variety of feelings, such as alliance and affiliation (e.g. liking, agreement, connection, supportiveness), disinterest (e.g. boredom, disengagement), and/or negativity (e.g. disliking, distrust, disappointment).

Content and relational messages and meanings may be congruent, complementary, and mutually reinforcing, or they may be incongruent, discrepant, and mutually conflicting. When an oncologist describes treatment options in language that the patient and family member/companion comprehend, offers the patient and family member/companion his/her home phone number and e-mail address to discuss further questions, and does so in a friendly manner, these coherent, consistent behaviours likely convey messages of alliance, that 'we are facing this diagnosis and treatment situation together'. Conversely, when an oncologist abruptly interrupts the patient and/or the family member/companion and is obviously time-pressured, yet states, 'I am happy to answer any questions', this likely creates confusion, anxiety, as well as other negative patient and family reactions, such as distrust and frustration. The situation is compounded by the fact that cancer patients develop their own reactions as to how they perceive that their family members/companions were treated by their oncologists during the encounter and this has effects on how they feel about their doctor and their treatment decisions (16).

Strategies for achieving convergence and interaction goals with relatives or companions

Establishing shared understanding and reaching interaction goals requires skill on the part of the physician (3). Communication skills training is important for physicians, and results of controlled studies to assess behaviour-change are promising. Breast cancer physicians in Belgium, who were randomized to a training arm, were subsequently more open towards family members' needs and concerns, more empathic, and more likely to engage in 'educated guessing, alerting to reality, confronting, negotiating, and summarizing' types of skills (pp. ii210) (3). However, members of the same research group concluded in a later study that physicians still need training to detect the distress of relatives, particularly since they can be trained to detect patients' distress levels (22).

Skills for building convergence and the triadic relationship

Lang and colleagues (23) present some of the most useful and relevant general guidelines for enhancing physicians' communication with third parties. Several of their 'core' and 'advanced' skills are highly relevant to oncology interactions. Similarly, Casarett and Quill (24) describe a set of techniques for effective communication that also have relevance for cancer consultations and other acute care medical encounters. Several of the excellent strategies described by these authors inform the discussion below.

Harnessing support: engaging family/companions in interactions

Given that the visit is usually at least a triadic relationship, making personal introductions with each family member/companion at the beginning of the encounter is a good way to initiate the process of rapport-building and acknowledging their presence on behalf of the patient. Previewing the components of the visit (usually comprised of history-taking, a physical exam, tests to be scheduled and/or results to be reviewed, diagnostic issues, and treatment options) helps orient the patient and third party to the initial agenda. At this point, eliciting the concerns and expectations of each person is important for establishing consensus on the agenda (a precursor for creating convergence about the nature of the ensuing discussion). Strategies include, for example, asking whether each person has additional topics to address. If there are additional topics, suggesting when during the discussion those topics will be most relevant. Clarifying the issues to be addressed and when the focus will be on each specific person's concerns, helps reduce uncertainty at the beginning by creating a roadmap for the discussion, and reassures all parties that the physician will be responsive to their concerns at the appropriate time. In addition, if the physician acknowledges that he/she sees the family member/companion as an 'ally' and 'advocate', this can help reinforce, validate, and acknowledge the family member/companion as a participant in the patient's care. Gaining early consensus is a first step for creating convergence because it becomes a process of assessing and reinforcing an initial degree of common ground.

Family members and companions are not always physically present at the visit, yet they are still emotionally and psychologically present in the patient's mind. They may be absent for many reasons (e.g. employment, infirmity, childcare needs, distance/travel), yet they remain important to the patient's life and will most likely influence the patient's decision-making, particularly regarding treatment choices and subsequent adherence/compliance (13). Thus, if the patient comes to the visit alone, it is important for the physician to inquire whether there is another person that will be relied upon when any decisions are made and if the patient wants that person to be somehow involved in the discussion (e.g. remotely by speaker-phone or a later arranged call with the physician).

As a plan is being developed and once it is set (whether for diagnostic purposes, treatment, and/or post-treatment monitoring), it is essential for the physician to continue to check and validate each person's feelings and concerns about the plan and its anticipated challenges regarding implementation and possible outcomes. Once again, this checking should serve to reinforce convergence around important elements, mutual agreement and accuracy regarding the prescribed plan, the anticipated issues involved in implementation, and commitment to undertaking the necessary steps to put the plan in action.

Addressing challenges to convergence, relationships and alliances

Family members/companions, especially when physically present, may present challenges for physicians and patients alike. Perhaps the most frequent problem arises when family members/ companions dominate the discussion in disruptive ways. They may unduly control the floor (creating disproportionate and excessive talk time), interrupt others, talk over the patient, and finish others' sentences prematurely. The physician's communicative task in such circumstances involves offering verbal reinforcement, control, and curtailment. He/she should reinforce the family member/companion's presence and earnest need to help the patient, but then firmly redirect conversational turn-taking to others for equal time and help more reticent parties (e.g. the patient or others in the room) to express themselves.

Additional strategies to maintain convergence include avoiding the tendency to 'take sides' with a patient or family member/companion that may polarize parties or create defensiveness. If, indeed, any two or more parties share a view counter to another (e.g. the patient and family member/companion share a view counter to that of the physician), it is important for the physician to acknowledge that the difference in perspectives exists, and whether there might be room to explore ways that the differences might be bridged. Messages in the encounter will be experienced at a cognitive level (in terms of the information value) and at a relational level (in terms of the emotions and feelings associated with the situation and the relationships among those in the room). Inquiring about, and acknowledging, each person's reactions and feelings are important for supporting and validating each person during an emotionally charged and/or difficult segment of the discussion.

Finally, family members/companions can thwart convergence by exhibiting counterproductive resistance to the physician as he or she is providing information and/or recommendations. Such resistance can take several forms: denial, challenging the expertise of the physician, and dismissing the patient's perspective and feelings. Again, the physician's role is to:

(1) validate the family member/companion's right to their perspective and feelings;

(2) restate the information in clarifying terms, perhaps using examples or analogies; and

Table 14.1 Example strategies and model statements for communicating with cancer patients' families/companions[a]

Strategy	Model statement
Engaging family members/companions in interactions	
Personal introduction.	'I'm Dr…it is good to meet you; I'm glad you are here.'
Identify others important but not present.	'Are there other family members or people close to you that you want to be included, either at the next visit or by a phone call?'
Elicit concerns and expectations.	'Do you have particular questions or concerns that you would like us to discuss today?' 'Some things that the family members of other patients have expressed as concerns include…. Are these on your mind too?'
Check for accuracy.	'Am I correct that your question/concern about your wife's condition is …?'
Check for agreement.	'It seems that we agree that treatment X looks like it might be a good choice for us to consider…. Do you think so too?'
Validate convergence.	'It is helpful that together we understand and agree about the best treatment choices…let's talk now about what to do and how to get started.'
Reassure.	'It is good that you are here so we can talk openly about these things.' 'You have every reason to feel hopeful and reassured that you are doing everything possible to help your husband.' 'It is okay if you and [the patient] want more time to think about your options. I'll continue to care for him/her and be here for you no matter what you decide.'
Addressing Challenges to Convergence, Relationships and Alliances	
Managing resistance to experimental treatment options.	'It is certainly understandable to feel that this may be too risky, but let me assure you that we are offering this option because we think it is a good one and because we have already taken the risks into consideration. The primary risks are the side-effects that he/she may or may not experience—let's talk again about each one and what we can do in case any of them arise.'
Control conversational dominance.	'I understand how you feel about this; now I'd like to hear it in his/her words.'
Acknowledge family member/companion's response.	'It may be hard to understand the test results given that he doesn't seem to feel sick or have any symptoms.'
Addressing anger at medical recommendation.	'These treatments don't always work the way we hope and expect they will. We are all understandably upset when this happens.'

(3) offer some suggestions for coping with potentially difficult information. Examples of the latter include: 'I know this is a lot to take in at once, you might want to take some time to think this through and then we can talk again' or 'Getting another opinion may help and I will be happy to assist you in arranging that if you would like' or 'Not everyone sees this the same way—it can be frustrating, but keep in mind that this happens in many families and it might help you to talk with someone from our counselling service, who can work with you individually and together'.

These and other communication strategies and model statements for achieving convergence are presented in Table 14.1.

Conclusion

Unfortunately, there remains a dearth of empirical research examining the complex dynamics of physician–patient–family member/companion interactions in the cancer context. However, promising conceptual frameworks in clinical communication research are being used to drive observational investigations. These frameworks are assisting researchers in developing better descriptions and explanations for how and why functional and dysfunctional dynamics may arise in medical encounters. This work is shifting the basis for guidelines for training physicians. That is, guidelines that are largely evidence-based are gradually replacing guidelines that have been traditionally derived from anecdotal information and opinion (6).

In this chapter, we posit the convergence model of communication as a strong framework for creating shared meaning and understanding with family and companions, whether physically present at the visit or not. Specific strategies for achieving convergence and managing challenging communication behaviours are also reviewed here and fit well with many of the 'tried and true' guidelines already reported in the literature. Finally, we emphasize that the true value of the convergence model serves not only to direct research efforts, but also provides a useful mindset for physicians to adapt, as they think about interacting with family members and companions. This mindset provides a potentially rich platform for creatively and strategically planning and enacting their clinical goals in the context of providing patient-centred, quality care.

References

1. Blanchard CG, Albrecht TL, Ruckdeschel JC (2000). Patient-family communication with physicians. In: Baider L, Cooper CL, Kaplan De-Nour A, eds. *Cancer and the Family*, 2nd edn, pp.477–495. Wiley, London.
2. Gleason ME, Harper FW, Eggly S, *et al.* (2009). The influence of patient expectations regarding cure on patient treatment decisions. *Patient Educ Couns* **75**, 263–9.
3. Merckaert I, Libert Y, Delvaux N, *et al.* (2005). Breast cancer: communication with a breast cancer patient and a relative. *Ann Oncol* **16** (Suppl 2), ii209–12.
4. Shepherd HL, Tattersall MH, Butow PN (2008). Physician-identified factors affecting patient participation in reaching treatment decisions. *J Clin Oncol* **26**, 1724–31.
5. Epstein RM, Street RLJ (2007). Patient-centered communication in cancer care: promoting healing and reducing suffering. Report No.: 07–6225. National Cancer Institute, NIH Publication, Bethesda, MD.
6. Eggly S, Penner LA, Greene M, *et al.* (2006). Information seeking during 'bad news' oncology interactions: question asking by patients and their companions. *Soc Sci Med* **63**, 2974–85.
7. Ishikawa H, Roter DL, Yamazaki Y, *et al.* (2006). Patients' perceptions of visit companions' helpfulness during Japanese geriatric medical visits. *Patient Educ Couns* **61**, 80–6.
8. Roter DL (2003). Observations on methodological and measurement challenges in the assessment of communication during medical exchanges. *Patient Educ Couns* **50**, 17–21.

9. Eggly S, Harper FWK, Penner L, *et al.* (2008). Information seeking by patients and companions during cancer clinical interactions. In: International Psycho-Oncology Society (IPOS) 10th World Congress of Psycho-Oncology, Madrid, Spain.

10. Eggly S, Harper FWK, Penner L, *et al.* (2007). Question asking by black and white patients and companions during clinical trial offers. In: *Proceedings of the American Association for Cancer Research Science of Cancer Health Disparities in Racial/Ethnic Minorities and the Medically Underserved*, p.82. Atlanta, GA.

11. Gordon HS, Street Jr RL, Sharf BF, *et al.* (2006). Racial differences in doctors' information-giving and patients' participation. *Cancer* **107**, 1313–20.

12. Street RL, Gordon HS (2008). Companion participation in cancer consultations. *Psycho-Oncology*, **17**, 244–51.

13. Albrecht T, Eggly S, Cline R, *et al.* (2009). Clinical communication issues in cancer diagnosis and treatment. *J Health Communication*, **14**(Suppl 1), 47–56.

14. Ballard-Reisch DS, Letner JA (2003). Centering families in cancer communication research: acknowledging the impact of support, culture and process on client/provider communication in cancer management. *Patient Educ Couns* **50**, 61–6.

15. Rogers E, Kincaid DL (1981). *Communication Networks: A Paradigm for New Research*. Free Press, New York.

16. Albrecht TL, Eggly SS, Gleason MEJ, *et al.* (2008). The influence of clinical communcation on patients' decision-making about clinical trials. *J Clin Oncol* **26**, 26666–73.

17. Clayman ML, Roter D, Wissow LS, *et al.* (2005). Autonomy-related behaviours of patient companions and their effect on decision-making activity in geriatric primary care visits. *Soc Sci Med* **60**, 1583–91.

18. Cline RJ, Harper FW, Penner LA, *et al.* (2006). Parent communication and child pain and distress during painful pediatric cancer treatments. *Soc Sci Med* **63**, 883–98.

19. Penner LA, Eggly S, Harper FW, *et al.* (2007). Patient attributes and information about clinical trials. In: American Association of Cancer Researchers, *Science of Cancer Health Disparities in Racial/Ethnic Minorities and the Medically Underserved*. Atlanta, GA.

20. Dovidio JF, Penner LA, Albrecht TL, *et al.* (2008). Disparities and distrust: the implications of psychological processes for understanding racial disparities in health and health care. *Soc Sci Med*, **67**: 478–86.

21. Arora NK (2003). Interacting with cancer patients: the significance of physicians' communication behaviour. *Soc Sci Med* **57**, 791–806.

22. Merckaert I, Libert Y, Delvaux N, *et al.* (2008). Factors influencing physicians' detection of cancer patients' and relatives' distress: can a communication skills training program improve physicians' detection? *Psychooncology* **17**, 260–9.

23. Lang F, Marvel K, Sanders D, *et al.* (2002). Interviewing when family members are present. *Am Fam Physician* **65**, 1351–4.

24. Casarett D, Quill TJ (2007). 'I'm not ready for hospice': strategies for timely and effective hospice discussions. *Ann Int Med* **146**, 443–9.

Chapter 15

Conducting a family meeting

Nessa Coyle and David W Kissane

Introduction

Family meetings in oncology occur most commonly in four settings. The first is soon after diagnosis, when the patient and family are being oriented to the disease, potential treatment options and the system of care with available supports. The second is in the setting of an inpatient admission, when goals of care need to be re-defined and treatment options reviewed. The third is during palliative care, where the support of the family in planning ongoing care is essential to optimize such care. And the fourth is when there is conflict about the direction of care, sometimes in the setting of a patient without capacity, when the medical staff and the patient's healthcare agent disagree with goals of care and treatment. Family meetings are commonly held in paediatric oncology or genetic counselling settings. Some meetings are held 'impromptu'—the opportunity presents itself when staff and the family are available and the meeting is held.

Here we describe a model of conducting the basic, planned family meeting in the setting of a patient with advanced disease. The overall goals of such a meeting are:

(1) to educate about the illness and its management;

(2) to assess caregiver needs regarding the cancer illness;

(3) to understand wishes about end-of-life care and views about place of death;

(4) to address the pragmatics of advance directives and who are the decision-makers within the family;

(5) to discuss discharge planning issues; and

(6) to assess family coping and identify high-risk families or members so that appropriate referrals can be made.

The principles we outline for conducting a family meeting in palliative care apply broadly to meetings in other settings. The family meeting is often co-facilitated by an oncologist or physician and a social worker, psychiatrist or advance practice nurse. This co-facilitated approach is ideal to meet broader biopsychosocial goals and is dependent on mutual respect and collaboration.

Why a family meeting and who is the family?

The family is a crucial resource for patients living with cancer and facing life-threatening illness. Family members often serve as primary caregivers: they guide the provision of support for loved ones during their final days, actively participate in the decision-making processes and serve as liaisons and proxy informants to healthcare practitioners. The journey of illness is thus a shared one. Distress reverberates through the family, leading to recognition that members are second-line patients through a model of family-centred care (1). As a result, practitioners and researchers alike have taken an interest in understanding how the family accommodates the strain of serious illness, and in identifying ways to ensure optimal functioning. This attention to the family has been a striking development over the 50 years since Arthur Sutherland at Memorial Hospital in New York first described cancer in a family context, drawing attention to the intimate reciprocity of suffering (2).

As caregiving has been progressively transferred into the living room, the roles of the family carers have become more pronounced. The principle caregiver is the spouse in 70% of cases, children (daughters and daughters-in-law predominate) in 20%, and approximately 10% comprise friends or more distant relatives (2–4). The family is best defined as 'a fictive-kin', namely, whoever the patient says their family is. Hence, visiting relatives from overseas, best friends, same-sex partners, or neighbours of those without direct kin, could all be involved if they contribute to caregiving and support of the patient.

The resilient family

Resilience can be defined as a positive adaptation arising in a setting of significant adversity, so that the family is seen to strengthen its functioning to the benefit of its membership and community. Central family functions include: (a) cohesion, membership and family formation (e.g. the family maintains a sense of belonging, including personal and social identity for its members); (b) economic support (e.g. the family provides for basic needs of food, shelter and health resources); (c) nurturance, education and socialization (e.g. the family affirms social values, fosters productivity and compatibility with community norms); and (d) protection of vulnerable members (e.g. the family protects members who are young, ill or disabled) (5).

The adaptive family is able to re-organize its roles, rules and interaction patterns to ensure adequate care and protection of an ill member. Family assets empower growth and transformation via a style of functioning in which members communicate effectively, provide mutual support and resolve differences of opinion through flexibility and buoyancy (6). Resilience is a likely outcome for those families who believe that strength is derived from teamwork, adversity is a shared challenge to be overcome together, and whose optimism and spirituality deliver new meaning and transcend suffering (7, 8).

The family considered 'at risk'

Observational studies of families during palliative care and bereavement led Kissane and colleagues to develop a typology that defines families at risk of morbid outcomes during bereavement (9, 10). Poor family cohesion, communication and conflict resolution were determinative of this classification, which, in turn, was highly predictive of psychiatric disorder occurring during bereavement for the membership of these families. Dysfunctional families fell into two types: the first, fractured, argumentative and help-rejecting; the second, sullen, depressed yet help-accepting. An intermediate type between well-functioning and dysfunctional families had mid-range communication, restricted cohesion and also carried high rates of psychosocial morbidity among members.

When it is recognized that these families are at greater risk for morbid outcome during palliative care, a preventive model of family therapy commenced while the cancer patient is still alive has been shown, in a randomized control trial, to ameliorate the distress of bereavement for the survivors and support their overall adaptation (11). This may be an important approach as Higginson and colleagues recently conducted a meta-analysis of 26 studies of palliative and hospice care teams and contrasted a slightly positive effect size on patient symptom outcomes [26 studies, weighted mean 0.33, SE 0.12 (95% CI 0.10, 0.56)] with no proven benefit on caregiver and family outcomes [13 studies, weighted mean 0.17, SE 0.16 (95% CI 0.14, 0.48)]

(12). Palliative care as a discipline understands the need for family-centred care, but has struggled to find an effective model to accomplish this comprehensively.

How then do clinicians recognize those families in greatest need? While resilient families do well and are not in need of additional psychosocial resources, families with some limitation in their functioning as a group—reduced communication, limited teamwork and prominent conflict—are worthwhile referring for prophylactic family therapy in the palliative care setting (13). Sometimes a basic family meeting clarifies these relational characteristics and helps to have the family agree to accept help through referral for ongoing work together. Additionally, families where members are already distressed, having suffered cumulative stress, loss and tragedy, profit by early family therapy referral.

Range of family needs

Systematic reviews of interventions to support family caregivers (14, 15) have identified the following challenges to optimally informing caregivers about their role:

◆ conspiracies of silence about the prognosis;

◆ the timing and amount of information to be delivered;

◆ overcoming impaired concentration;

◆ avoidant responses;

◆ not wanting to bother; or

◆ outright rejection of the health provider's help.

Health systems, in their turn, need adequate staffing, skill training, educational materials and a model of delivering carer training to achieve the desired goal.

Clarity about the content of carer educational sessions is derived from nursing research into key roles and tasks undertaken by carers in the home as they assist a dying relative. These tasks include:

◆ symptom assessment and management;

◆ medication administration;

◆ help with ambulating, transferring the patient in and out of bed or dressing the patient;

◆ liaising with doctors;

◆ instrumental care activities like meal preparation or transportation; and

◆ coordinating visits from volunteers and friends to achieve respite for the carer (16–18).

Information provision stands out as the key unmet need in assisting the carers' preparation for these roles, thus helping to minimize their burnout and exhaustion (19–21).

Family education about caregiving is a fundamental service requirement that is applicable to families whose relative is at home, but also relevant to the family of an inpatient. A number of the latter families might be preparing for an eventual death at home. In addition to information about caregiving roles as described above, a number of other themes worthy of discussion with the family are listed in Box 15.1. Coverage of these has been shown to be immensely helpful to families (22).

Families with special needs include those with young children losing a key parent or when a single parent is dying and will leave children orphaned; families with elderly parents, while also burdened by physically handicapped or mentally ill offspring; and families that are isolated through migration or in some way disenfranchised from relatives and support. Listening to a family's story and assessment of its needs is a crucial clinical task.

Box 15.1 Themes often discussed in family meetings in the palliative care setting

1. The nature of the illness and its symptoms.

2. Prognosis and future predictions about the course of the illness.

3. Caregiving roles about symptom management, medications, nursing care.

4. Liaison with medical team.

5. The emotional demands of the role.

6. Importance of self-care and respite from caregiving.

7. What to expect as death approaches.

8. How to talk with the patient about death and dying.

9. The process of saying goodbye.

10. How to manage a death in the home.

11. The positive aspects of the caregiver's role.

12. Teamwork and sharing the role of caregiver.

13. When to seek help and how.

14. Support from volunteers and other community resources.

Communication principles in conducting a family meeting

Facilitators of a family meeting do well to join initially with each person present through a round of introductions that identify names, ages (if appropriate), occupations, place of residence and relationship to the ill person. Agendas and expectations of meeting together are also shared so that all concerns are placed initially on the table at the beginning of the conversation. The unifying or common focus of the meeting is, 'What is best for the patient?'. Linear questions tend to be used here as an exchange occurs between facilitator and individuals speaking about their personal point of view. Facilitators wisely avoid taking sides with individuals expressing contentious issues, lest loss of neutrality damages the ability to guide the family-as-a-whole to their preferred solution (23).

The use of circular questions is a communication skill through which the facilitator preserves this neutrality and promotes the family's search for a solution from among its members (24–26). Using such circularity, each member can be invited to express an opinion about the needs, functioning, health or interaction styles of other members of the family unit. Thus, 'Who talks to whom about the patient's illness?', 'Who provides transport, food, or material support?', 'Who is most stressed?', 'How will the family cope?'.

As facilitators embed a potential solution into the wording of a question, it becomes strategic in style as a communication skill. Thus, 'Is it possible that sharing feelings together will help you grow closer?'. Strategic questions can also harness a direction of change: 'What might help motivate your son to visit more often?'.

Other questions might raise a hypothesis that invites the family to reflect on a range of possible choices that it could adopt, such reflexive questions serving a catalytic function for the family. There is generally a better outcome for the family as a group when more problem-solving is done by the family, rather than the clinician.

Box 15.2 Communication skills used in family meeting facilitation

- *Circular questions.* Ask each family member to comment in turn on aspects of others to promote curiosity and reflection by the group as a whole. For example, 'How are your parents and sisters coping with Dad's illness? Who is most upset in your view?' (25, 26).

- *Reflexive questions.* Invite the family to reflect on possibilities, hypotheses and a range of outcomes to stimulate their internal efforts to improve family life. For example, 'What benefits might come from caring for Dad at home? In what ways might this be hard for you as a family group?' (25, 26).

- *Strategic questions.* Here a solution might be incorporated into the wording of the question to more directly guide the family toward an outcome that is considered preferable. For example, 'What change in Dad's symptoms would need to occur for you to realize that admission to an inpatient hospice bed is necessary?' (24).

- *Summary of family focused concerns.* The family's views are reflected back to highlight levels of tension or discordance in different member's opinions, while maintaining professional neutrality, yet inviting further problem solving by the family. For example, 'As a family, you recognize your father's desire to die at home, your mother's commitment to meet his wishes, and yet your concern that his confusion is becoming unmanageable and a burden to your mother. There is no easy answer here, as whichever solution you adopt will appear to demand more of each of you for a time.' (27).

A useful communication skill to promote movement towards consensus, or at least accommodation of differing views among the family, is for the facilitator to offer a summary that reflects the tension between two or more points of view aired by members (27). The goal is not to offer a solution, but to make explicit the advantages and disadvantages of the options, while leaving the choice blatantly as the familiy's. Further problem-solving with consensus-building or accommodation is then evoked from the family. In circumstances involving future treatment recommendations or avoidance of futile care, the clinician may wish to make a firm recommendation. Delaying delivery of this recommendation for a time, while searching for their point of view, may allow the family to reach that position readily and with greater acceptance than were the outcome imposed. Partnership statements that acknowledge shared deliberation also prove supportive.

The family meeting often falls into two distinct parts: a clinician-led part and a psychosocial-led part. The clinician-led part or first phase of the meeting discusses the medical illness, including the course of the disease, medical management along the way and future treatment options. These include palliative care, hospice care and site of care. The goal of this phase of the meeting is to educate, clarify and plan for the patient's future care. The psychosocial-led part focuses on coping issues and the emotional response to the illness, including its impact on the patient and the life of each family member. Families often express their feelings through narrative—stories of life before the diagnosis and through the lived experience of cancer.

During the process of this two-phase meeting, the family participants have the opportunity to learn exactly what is happening to their loved one and why. They may also come to understand in a different way the complexities and uncertainties of medical care. The healthcare team may deepen their understanding of who this patient and family are, their strengths and their vulnerabilities, and what the experience of cancer has been like for them. The importance of the family is acknowledged, the present situation and goals of care are clarified, problem-solving and counselling occur and role modelling takes place, demonstrating team work, mutual respect and open and honest communication.

The family meeting offers an opportunity to introduce the family to members of the interdisciplinary team, who will be helping to organize the patient's care. The family is brought into partnership in planning such care. They have the chance to express their fears and concerns, and be offered support. One objective is to harness their energy into joint meaningful action. Additionally, the team starts to get to know the patient and family as individuals and a social group. They learn what the family values, their style of communication and decision-making, which members carry significant levels of distress, and how the family can best benefit from the team. Problems that have remained un-addressed and festering can be brought to the surface with good potential for resolution.

Key process tasks in conducting family meetings

Process tasks are both plans and actions that are fundamental to achieve the communication goals of the family meeting. Several are important and considered here:

- **Set-up the meeting.** This involves identifying who are the important family members or significant individuals in the patient's life that need to be present.

  Who are the influential relatives and significant others that may bring wisdom and value to the session?

  Will the patient contribute usefully to the meeting and be important to include?

  Will there be any barriers to meeting?

  What clinical staff will be needed to address relevant medical, nursing, psychosocial and spiritual issues?

- **Co-facilitation.** Here it is important to clarify whether there are key medical agendas that differentiate from psychosocial needs. Should these be separated as distinct agendas for different phases of the meeting? Co-facilitators need to talk about their respective roles and the order of approach, before the meeting starts. Medical issues place a greater emphasis on education, planning and clarifying; psychosocial issues require more focus on listening, empathetic skills and fostering a sense of support. The tenor of these phases of the meeting can be distinctly different and hence the wisdom, as reviewed earlier, of structuring the session to complete one domain before moving to an exploration of the other.

- **Cultural sensitivity while avoiding collusion.** Ethnicity and family background impact directly on a family's approach to coping with illness. Clarification of the family's detailed understanding of the illness and its treatment, its progression and seriousness, their values and religious beliefs, and the appropriate goals of care for this stage of illness is necessary. In addition, points of consensus and dissonance need to be identified.

- **Understanding the family's strengths and vulnerabilities.** Family traditions, norms and values can be harnessed adaptively when they are recognized as strengths and balanced with the family's worries and concerns. Achieving understanding of the reality of their family life is vital to any pragmatic planning for their future.

- **Familiarity with resources that are available to the patient and family.** These include educational materials, DVD or website resources, other information sources, and community nursing and related support services.

◆ **Follow-up.** Explain details of where to go from here, what are the next steps and who will coordinate these with the patient and family. Is there an identified family member through whom ongoing communication can be channelled?

Typical sequence of strategies in conducting a family meeting in oncology

The concept of a sequence of strategies involves the *a priori* plans of an ordered method that experience teaches will generally facilitate the communication goals of the meeting. The sequence need not be rigidly applied, but can be adapted to the family's needs (see Box 15.3). Nevertheless, there is considerable logic to this sequence, as the patient's medical reality directly impacts upon the emotional consequences that follow.

After welcoming the family, an agenda is created by stating the goals of meeting together:

◆ to review where the patient is in his/her illness trajectory;

◆ to consider the family's needs in providing care; and

◆ to aim at optimizing the journey ahead.

The facilitators check for any other agenda the family might have, clarify the family's understanding of the gravity of the illness and explore their understanding of the current goals of care. Questions are then asked about any key symptoms that are of concern to the family and that need to be addressed. The family's views of what the future holds are clarified including, if appropriate, advance directives and whether the preferred place of death has been discussed. If the preference is for care to occur at home, who from the family will be the primary carer? If the preference is for care in an inpatient setting, who will support the patient? Once goals of care and methods for achieving these have been considered, the facilitators clarify how the family is doing emotionally. Are there any questions that have been left unanswered? Finally, the facilitators affirm the family's caring commitment to the patient and to each other, while also affirming the team's commitment to be there for them.

A blueprint summarizing the core communication components employed in this model of conducting a family meeting are outlined in Table 15.1. The communication skills listed in this

---

Box 15.3 Typical sequence of strategies for the conduct of a family meeting in oncology and palliative care

1. Planning and prior set-up to arrange the family meeting.

2. Welcome and orientation of the family to the goals of the family meeting.

3. Check each family member's understanding of the illness and its prognosis.

4. Check for consensus about the current goals of care.

5. Identify family concerns about the management of key symptoms and care needs.

6. Clarify the family's view of what the future holds.

7. Clarify how family members are coping and feeling emotionally.

8. Identify family strengths and affirm their level of commitment and mutual support for each other.

9. Close the family meeting by final review of agreed goals of care and consensus about future care plans.

Table 15.1 Core communication components in conducting a family meeting

Strategy	Skills	Process tasks
1. Planning and prior set-up to arrange the family meeting.	Clarify. Invite questions. Restate.	Consider who should attend and extend invitations; explain rationale and benefits; acknowledge challenges in attending. Will the patient be included? Who will facilitate? What disciplines will help? Co-facilitators? Plan seating, privacy, availability of tissues.
2. Welcome and orient to the goals of the family meeting.	Declare agenda items. Invite family agenda. Negotiate agenda. Ask open questions. Clarify. Restate.	Round of introductions and orientation. Include all present at the meeting. Normalize anxiety.
3. Check each family member's understanding of the illness and its prognosis.	Ask open questions. Ask circular questions. Check understanding. Acknowledge/legitimize.	Clarify name of the illness. Clarify seriousness of the illness. Clarify reasons for admission. Clarify each person's concerns. Normalize both concordance and divergence of views among family members. Respect culturally sensitive views. Acknowledge protective urges and any expressed desire to help.
4. Check for consensus about the current goals of care.	Ask open and circular questions. Clarify. Restate. Summarize.	Compare and contrast oncological, nursing, social, psychological and spiritual goals of care. Reality test sensitively where needed. Correct misunderstanding.
5. Identify family concerns about their management of key symptoms or care needs.	Ask open questions. Preview information. Check understanding. Clarify. Summarize. Make partnership statements.	Consider medication or treatment concerns? Any hygiene issues? Any concerns about walking, moving, transferring? Any concerns about nursing? Any concerns about assessing palliative care resources—extra help? Financial issues? Any need for respite? Any concern about a sense of helplessness? Promote problem-solving; Educate as appropriate.
6. Clarify the family's view of what the future holds.	Ask circular questions. Clarify. Restate. Summarize. Make partnership statements.	Are there advanced care directives? Health proxy appointed? Has the place of death been discussed? Consider cultural or religious concerns. If at home, who from the family will be providing care? If in the hospital, who will accompany? Help? Support? Educate as appropriate.

Table 15.1 (continued) Core communication components in conducting a family meeting

Strategy	Skills	Process tasks
7. Clarify how family members are coping and feeling emotionally.	Ask circular questions. Ask strategic or reflexive questions. Acknowledge, legitimize or normalize.	Review family functioning as a group, asking specifically about their communication, cohesion and conflict resolution. Identify any member considered to be 'at risk' or a concern to others. Discuss future care needs of family or individual when concerns exist. Avoid premature reassurance.
8. Identify family strengths and affirm their level of commitment and mutual support for each other.	Ask circular questions. Ask strategic and reflexive questions. Praise family efforts. Acknowledge, legitimize.	Review family traditions, spirituality, mottos, cultural norms.
9. Close the family meeting by final review of agreed goals of care and future plans.	Summarize. Invite questions. Acknowledge. Make partnership statements. Express willingness to help. Review steps.	Provide educational resources. Clarify future needs, funeral plans. Refer those 'at risk' to psychosocial services for further care. Consider feedback to patient if they were not present.

schema have been defined in detail in Chapter 3 of this book. Skills that are listed against each strategy are not intended to be used exhaustively, but selected as appropriate for the family at hand. The combination of skills and process tasks outlined here help in the accomplishment of each communication strategy. The family meeting follows the agreed agenda until themes are worked through and the communication goal is completed. A final step is documentation of what happened in the patient's chart.

Documentation of the family meeting

This is a necessary part of communication among care providers in any institution. The note is comprised of the following:

- who was present at the meeting, including the various disciplines of the healthcare providers and the relationship of the family members present to the patient;
- whether the patient was present and, if not, what was the reason;
- a brief medical and social history;
- a genogram that sketches out the genders, ages, names and relationships within the family;
- a process summary of the meeting with the various issues outlined and options discussed;
- the outcome of the meeting, including agreed goals of care;
- the follow-up plan; and
- whether the outcome of the meeting was shared with the patient if he/she was not able to be present.

Conclusion

Family meetings play an important role in comprehensive cancer care, especially in the setting of advanced disease and when palliative care is the primary focus. The importance of family is acknowledged and an environment of support is created therein. Information exchange often includes 'hard news'. The family's dynamics are assessed and the family is 'engaged' in the partnership of care provision. Both the goals of care and the next steps in management are suitably discussed. In addition, specific problems are defined, steps to resolve these are outlined, who is missing is identified, commitment is demonstrated, role modelling is illustrated about how to build consensus, and family problem-solving skills are promoted.

A resiliency focus guides the identification of family strengths alongside any concerns, empowering the members to work together to optimize their mutual support. Any distress created by the cancer journey is thus ameliorated, with the prospect of family harmony creating a peaceful environment for the ill family member. A model of shared family care and partnership with the medical team is promoted.

References

1. Rait D, Lederberg MS (1989). The family of the cancer patient, In: Holland JC, Rowland JH, eds. *Handbook of Psychooncology. Psychological Care of the Patient with Cancer*, pp.585–97. Oxford University Press, New York.

2. Sutherland AM (1956). Psychological impact of cancer and its therapy. *Med Clin North Am*, **40**, 705–20.

3. Given B, Given W (1989). Cancer nursing for the elderly. *Can Nurs* **12**, 71–7.

4. Ferrell BR, Ferrell BA, Rhiner M *et al.* (1991). Family factors influencing cancer pain management. *Postgrad Med J* **67 Suppl 2**:S64–9.

5. Patterson JM (2002). Understanding family resilience. *J Clin Psychol* **58**, 233–46.

6. Kissane DW (1994). Grief and the family. In: Bloch S, Hafner J, Harari E, *et al.* eds. *The Family in Clinical Psychiatry*, pp. 71–9. Oxford University Press, Oxford.

7. Walsh F (2002). Family resilience framework: innovative practice applications. *Fam Relations* **51**, 130–8.

8. Walsh F (2003). Family resilience: a framework for clinical practice. *Fam Proc* **41**, 1–18.

9. Kissane DW, Bloch S, Burns WI, *et al.* (1994). Perceptions of family functioning and cancer. *Psychooncology* **3**, 259–69.

10. Kissane DW, Bloch S, Dowe DL, *et al.* (1996). The Melbourne family grief study, 1: perceptions of family functioning in bereavement. *Am J Psychiatry* **153**, 650–8.

11. Kissane DW, McKenzie M, Bloch S, *et al.* (2006). Family focused grief therapy: a randomized controlled trial in palliative care and bereavement. *Am J Psychiatry* **163**, 1208–18.

12. Higginson IJ, Finlay IG, Goodwin DM, *et al.* (2003). Is there evidence that palliative care teams alter end-of-life experiences of patients and their caregivers? *J Pain Symptom Manage* **25(2)**:150–68.

13. Kissane DW, McKenzie M, McKenzie DP, *et al.* (2003). Psychosocial morbidity associated with patterns of family functioning in palliative care: baseline data for the Family Focused Grief Therapy controlled trial. *Palliat Med* **17**, 527–37.

14. Harding R, Higginson IJ (2003). What is the best way to help caregivers in cancer and palliative care? A systematic literature review of interventions and their effectiveness. *Palliat Med* **17**, 63–74.

15. Hudson PL, Aranda S, Kristjanson LJ (2004). Meeting the supportive needs of family caregivers in palliative care: challenges for health professionals. *J Palliat Med* **7**, 19–25.

16. Barg FK, Pasacreta JV, Robinson KD, *et al.* (1998). A description of a psycho-educational intervention for family caregivers of cancer patients. *J Fam Nurs*, **4**, 394–413.

17. Yang CT, Kirschling JM (1992). Exploration of factors related to direct care and outcomes of caregiving. Caregivers of terminally ill older persons. *Cancer Nurs* **15**, 173–81.

18. Aranda SK, Hayman-White K (2001). Home caregivers of the persons with advanced cancer: an Australian perspective. *Cancer Nurs* **24**, 300–7.

19. Kristjanson LJ, Leis A, Koop PM, *et al.* (1997). Family members' care expectations, care perceptions, and satisfaction with advanced cancer care: results of a multi-site pilot study. *J Palliat Care* **13**(4):5–13.

20. Milne D (1999). When cancer won't go away: the needs and experiences of family caregivers. Unpublished Master of Nursing Thesis. University of Melbourne, Melbourne.

21. Rose KE (1999). A qualitative analysis of the information needs of informal carers of terminally ill cancer patients. *J Clin Nurs* **8**, 81–8.

22. Hudson PS, Aranda S, McMurray N (2002). Intervention development for enhanced lay palliative caregiver support—the use of focus groups. *Eur J Cancer Care* **11**, 262–70.

23. Selvini MP, Boscolo L, Cecchin G *et al.* (1980). Hypothesizing–circularity–neutrality: three guidelines for the conductor of the session. *Fam Process* **19**(1):3–12.

24. Tomm K (1988). Interventive interviewing: part 111. Intending to ask lineal, circular, strategic, or reflexive questions? *Fam Process* **27**, 1–15.

25. Tomm K (1987). Interventive interviewing: part 1. Strategizing as a fourth guideline for the therapist. *Fam Process* **26**, 3–13.

26. Tomm K (1988). Interventive interviewing: part 11. Reflexive questioning as a means to enable self-healing. *Fam Process* **26**, 167–83.

27. Kissane DW, Bloch S. (2002) *Family Focused Grief Therapy: a Model of Family-Centred Care During Palliative Care and Bereavement*. Open University Press, Buckingham.

Chapter 16

Communication about coping as a survivor

Linda E Carlson and Barry D Bultz

Introduction

As medical cancer treatments become more and more successful, a growing cohort of cancer survivors is emerging. Maintaining effective communication with survivors poses a host of new challenges that have not received much attention in the literature to date. This chapter covers a number of areas relevant to enhancing communication with survivors including: various definitions of who is considered a cancer survivor; prevalence of survivors; key issues faced by cancer survivors; coping strategies, including the use of care plans and clinical practice guidelines; communication challenges with cancer survivors; models for survivorship care and details about communication techniques in the survivorship consultation. Our objective is to cover the issues that are important for ongoing care and communication with cancer patients who will go on to live post-treatment and require continuity of care for many years.

Definition of survivorship

The term 'survivor' has been adopted into the mainstream lexicon when referring to people who have been diagnosed with, and treated for, cancer; however, there is still some debate as to the meaning of the term. Historically, the survivorship movement began in the United States in 1986 with the formation of the National Coalition for Cancer Survivorship (NCCS). The NCCS, a grass-roots organization of people living with cancer, adopted a broad stance and defined 'survivor' as anyone who has been diagnosed with cancer. That is, one becomes a survivor at the time of diagnosis and remains so for the balance of life. Under the NCCS definition, caregivers and family members were also considered cancer survivors. The mainstream medical community, on the other hand, adopted a narrower definition of 'survivor' as someone who has lived for at least five years beyond their initial cancer diagnosis. A middle-ground definition defines someone as a survivor after the completion of active primary treatment, such as surgery, chemotherapy and radiation. However, the definition varies across professionals and agencies, so it is prudent to determine what operational definition of 'survivor' is being used in any given context. In this chapter, the moderate definition of a survivor, as someone who has completed active primary cancer treatment, is the definition being applied.

In a widely cited paper published by an oncologist, who himself contracted cancer, Mullan (1) described three distinct 'seasons' of survival:

1. Acute survival begins at the time of diagnosis and is dominated by the process of diagnostic tests and treatment. Fear and anxiety are the most persistent psychological features during this phase.

2. Extended survival is the period of remission, when rigorous treatments are completed and the patient enters a period of surveillance. There may also be lingering physical limitations caused by aggressive treatments during the acute phase, which may affect a person's ability to function in the home, community and workplace. Psychologically, this period is dominated by fears of recurrence.

3. Permanent survival is roughly equated with 'cure' and is characterized by longer term consequences of the cancer experience, including problems with employment or insurance.

Welch-McCaffrey and colleagues (2) describe several potential cancer survival trajectories within this characterization:

◆ Live cancer-free for many years and die of something else.

◆ Live long cancer-free, but die rapidly of late recurrence.

◆ Live cancer-free (first cancer), but develop a second primary cancer.

◆ Live with intermittent periods of active disease.

◆ Live with persistent disease.

◆ Live after expected death.

Hence, there are many types of 'cancer survivors', who may be dealing with an array of different concerns and issues, depending on which of these scenarios best describes their experience. One version of the cancer care trajectory (Fig. 16.1) depicts survivorship care as occurring at the juncture between the completion of active treatment and any return of disease. Survivorship care, as shown in the diagram, can follow any number of trajectories, interacting with other stages of care throughout the cancer journey. Regardless of the recurrence of cancer, survivorship care may last the duration of one's life.

Prevalence of cancer survivors

Advances in the use of effective biomedical screening for cancer, and improvements in treatment, have contributed to the ever-increasing significance of survivorship as part of the patient experience.

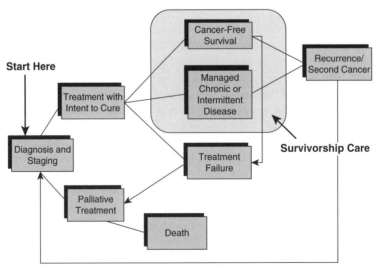

Fig. 16.1 Cancer care trajectory (from the report Implementing Cancer Survivorship Care Planning; 9).

The number of cancer survivors (diagnosed and currently alive) in the United States has risen from approximately 3 million in 1971 to over 11 million in the year 2004 (3); and, in 2007, the number of cancer survivors was estimated closer to 12 million. The largest group of survivors were diagnosed with breast (23%), followed by prostate (19%), colorectal (10%), gynaecological (9%), haematological (8%) and urinary tract (7%) cancers (3). The most notable difference between incidence and survivorship figures is in lung cancers, which account for greater than 15% of the incidence of overall cancer, but account for only 3% of survivors (3). This inconsistency is a testament to the continued poor prognosis for lung cancer.

In terms of age, 50% of all cancer survivors are over 70 years of age, with another 22% in their 60s and 16% in their 50s (3). Hence, only 14% of all cancer survivors are under the age of 50 years. This demographic must be borne in mind when considering all aspects of survivorship care. In terms of longer term survival, approximately two-thirds of all cancer patients diagnosed in 2007 will be alive five years later. For children diagnosed with cancer, the 10-year survival is 75% (3). Taking into account the ageing Baby Boomer demographic, prevalence rates for cancer survivors are predicted to double between the years of 2000 and 2050 (4). Hence, there is a growing cohort of largely elderly cancer survivors requiring, and indeed demanding, specific care programmes that meet their unique needs.

Until recently, there had been quite a paucity of research into cancer survivorship. However, with the formation of the Office of Cancer Survivorship (OCS) in the United States in 1996, there has been an increased awareness. Survivorship has become an important political issue in the United States, due in part to the high level of grass-roots activism. This politicization of cancer has resulted in the creation of a number of comprehensive reports, which summarize the research and can serve as excellent references for obtaining an overall picture of the state of the science in survivorship research and care (5–8).

Arguably the most important of these government reports came in 2006 when the Committee on Cancer Survivorship: Improving Care and Quality of Life released *From Cancer Patient to Cancer Survivor: Lost in Transition* (4). This report focuses on the phase of survivorship that follows primary treatment and lasts until cancer recurrence or end-of-life. Many detailed recommendations for survivorship care are provided, in addition to documenting the various issues facing survivors of all ages and types of cancer. This was followed by a 2-day workshop in which experts from the National Cancer Policy Forum discussed issues arising from the *Lost in Transition* report. Their resultant report summarized the discussions that took place and recommendations that followed (9).

Key issues for survivors

The survivorship experience may touch individuals at every level of their existence, from the existential to the very practical. Inevitably, survivorship also touches family and friends. However, the survivorship experience is a dynamic and subjective one. Survivorship issues may vary considerably between survivors of different types of cancer and even within cancer type, requiring different treatment and supportive care regimens.

One theme that arises across survivors is resiliency. Indeed, many people do quite well in the face of this terrifying disease, returning to adequate or good health-related quality of life (10). However, there are many lingering biopsychosocial effects with which survivors often have to contend. Researchers distinguish between 'late effects' and 'long-term effects' of cancer treatment. Late effects are defined as unrecognized toxicities that are absent or subclinical at the end of therapy, but which manifest later with the unmasking of injury; for example, during later developmental processes, due to the failure of compensatory mechanisms over the passage of time, or organ senescence (11). Long-term effects refer to any side-effect or complication of treatment for which patients must compensate. They are also known as persistent effects and usually begin during treatment and continue beyond the end of treatment. Late effects, in contrast, appear months to years after the completion of treatment.

Long-term and late effects can span domains including: physical and medical issues (e.g. second cancers, cardiac dysfunction, pain, lymphoedema, sexual impairment, infertility); psychological functioning (e.g. depression, anxiety, uncertainty, isolation, altered body image, cognitive impairments); social functioning (e.g. changes in interpersonal relationships, concerns regarding health or life insurance, return to work, return to school, financial burden); and existential and spiritual issues (e.g. sense of purpose or meaning, appreciation of life). Figure 16.2 illustrates the wide range of life areas that are affected by cancer survivorship. In this model, based on Ferrell's model of Quality of Life (12), the larger categories include physical, psychological, social and spiritual well-being.

Cancer survivors are also at higher risk for secondary cancers; about 8% of current cancer survivors have reported second malignancies, three-quarters of which were in different sites than the original primary cancer (13). In terms of disability, almost 60% of survivors—a number more than twice as high as in the general population—reported one or more functional problems, such as difficulties with self-care, completing household activities or driving (14). Reasons for these and other late effects are varied, but many of the common treatments for cancer have their own long-term consequences. Some of the potential effects of surgery, radiation therapy, chemotherapy and hormonal therapy are summarized in Table 16.1.

Keeping in mind both the psychological and medical late and long-term effects of cancer and its many treatments, cancer survivors need follow-up well beyond the period of acute treatment. This care should be specific to the type of cancer and treatment regimen. Although there are many similarities across types of cancer, there are also many issues that are quite specific (22).

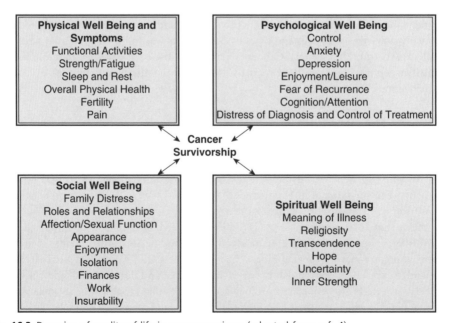

Fig. 16.2 Domains of quality of life in cancer survivors (adapted from ref. 4).

Table 16.1 Possible late effects of cancer treatments

Organ system/ tissue	Radiation therapy effects	Chemotherapy/ Hormonal therapy effects	Type of Surgery	Surgery effects
All tissues	Second cancers	Second cancers	Any procedure	Pain, cosmetic, wound healing
Nervous system	Thinking, learning, memory problems; bleeding into brain; structural changes	Thinking, learning, memory problems; paralysis; seizure; numbness; tingling; hearing loss	Brain, spinal cord	Impaired cognition, motor function, sensory function, vision, language
Dental/oral	Dental cavities; dry mouth	Temporomandibular joint necrosis	Head and neck	Problems talking, swallowing, breathing; cosmetic
Lymphatic	Lymphoedema	—	Lymph node removal	Lymphoedema; retrograde ejaculation in testicular cancer
Bone and soft tissue	Atrophy; fibrosis; bone death	Bone death and destruction; risk of fractures	Amputation	Functional changes; disability; accelerated arthritis in other joints; pain (phantom/ neuropathic)
Pulmonary	Lung scarring; decreased lung function	Lung scarring; inflammation	Lung resection	Difficulty breathing; fatigue; weakness
Immune system	Impaired immune function; immune suppression	Impaired immune function; immune suppression	Splenectomy	Impaired immune function; risk of infection, hernia
Gastrointestinal	Malabsorption	Mobility disorders	Abdominal	Possible intestinal obstruction; hernia; altered bowel function
Hepatic	Abnormal liver function; liver failure	Abnormal liver function; cirrhosis; liver failure	Ostomy	Bowel obstruction; constipation; nausea; vomiting; loss of appetite; fatigue
Renal	Hypertension; impaired kidney function	Impaired kidney function; delayed-onset renal failure	Pelvic	Sexual dysfunction: incontinence; hernia
Genitourinary	Bladder scarring, small bladder capacity; bowel bleeding/ulceration	Haemorrhagic cystitis	Prostatectomy	Urinary incontinence; sexual dysfunction
Endocrine	Low thyroid function; sterility	Diabetes; sterility in men and women	Oophorectomy	Premature menopause and infertility
			Orchiectomy	Infertility; testosterone deficiency
Ophthalmologic	Cataracts, dry eyes, visual impairment	Cataracts	Ocular enucleation	Blindness

Table 16.1 (continued) Possible late effects of cancer treatments

Organ system/ tissue	Radiation therapy effects	Chemotherapy/ Hormonal therapy effects	Type of Surgery	Surgery effects
Cardiovascular	Scarring, inflammation of the heart; coronary artery disease	Inflammation of the heart; congestive heart failure		
Haematologic	Low blood counts; myelodysplastic syndrome and acute leukaemia	Myelodysplastic syndrome and acute leukaemia		

Adapted from *Lost in Transition* (4)

Coping strategies for survivors

Treatment summaries and care plans

Given the breadth of potential issues, survivorship care needs a team of caregivers and mechanisms for communication between these providers and survivors. The President's Cancer Panel, in its 2004–05 Report, recommended that each patient and their primary care provider be given a treatment summary following discharge (7). This should document all treatment received and include a number of elements of a follow-up care plan (see Box 16.1). The care plan includes not only continued surveillance for late effects and potential cancer recurrence, but also psychosocial elements, including relationship issues, sexuality, fertility, parenting and social support, as well as legal and financial issues.

Another important aspect of the care plans are recommendations regarding health behaviours that will enhance overall health and decrease the likelihood of contracting further cancers or chronic diseases. An excellent paper by Jones and Whanefried (15) was included as an appendix to the survivorship care-planning report (9). Areas comprehensively reviewed included weight management, nutrition and diet, exercise, smoking cessation, alcohol consumption, sunscreen use, complementary and alternative therapies, prevention of osteoporosis, and immunizations. Current life-style guidelines are summarized in Box 16.2.

Clinical practice guidelines

Many clinical practice guidelines (CPGs) exist for the treatment of different forms of cancer; for example, in the National Academy of Sciences Institute of Medicine (IOM) Report, 24 sets of CPGs for breast cancer were identified (4). These CPGs were evaluated in terms of their coverage of the following survivorship domains:

1. Surveillance for recurrent disease.

2. Monitoring/prevention of second primary cancer.

3. Management of late sequelae of disease.

4. Management of late complications of treatment.

Box 16.1 Survivorship care plan

Upon discharge from cancer treatment, including treatment of recurrences, every patient should be given a **record of all care received and important disease characteristics**. This should include, at a minimum:

1. Diagnostic tests performed and results.

2. Tumour characteristics (e.g. site(s), stage and grade, hormone receptor status, marker information).

3. Dates of treatment initiation and completion.

4. Surgery, chemotherapy, radiotherapy, transplant, hormonal therapy, or gene or other therapies provided, including agents used, treatment regimen, total dosage, identifying number and title of clinical trials (if any), indicators of treatment response, and toxicities experienced during treatment.

5. Psychosocial, nutritional and other supportive services provided.

6. Full contact information on treating institutions and key individual providers.

7. Identification of a key point of contact and coordinator of continuing care. Upon discharge from cancer treatment, every patient and his/her primary healthcare provider should receive a written follow-up care plan incorporating available evidence-based standards of care. This should include, at a minimum:

   1. The likely course of recovery from treatment toxicities, as well as the need for ongoing health maintenance/adjuvant therapy.

   2. A description of recommended cancer screening and other periodic testing and examinations, and the schedule on which they should be performed (and who should provide them).

   3. Information on possible late and long-term effects of treatment and symptoms of such effects.

   4. Information on possible signs of recurrence and second tumours.

   5. Information on the possible effects of cancer on marital/partner relationship, sexual functioning, work and parenting, and the potential future need for psychosocial support.

   6. Information on the potential insurance, employment and financial consequences of cancer and, as necessary, referral to counselling, legal aid and financial assistance.

   7. Specific recommendations for healthy behaviours (e.g. diet, exercise, healthy weight, sunscreen use, immunizations, smoking cessation, osteoporosis prevention). When appropriate, recommendations that first-degree relatives be informed about their increased risk and the need for cancer screening (e.g. breast cancer, colorectal cancer, prostate cancer).

   8. As appropriate, information on genetic counselling and testing to identify high-risk individuals who could benefit from more comprehensive cancer surveillance, chemo-prevention or risk-reducing surgery.

   9. As appropriate, information on known effective chemoprevention strategies for secondary prevention (e.g. tamoxifen in women at high risk for breast cancer; aspirin for colorectal cancer prevention).

Box 16.1 (continued) Survivorship care plan

10. Referrals to specific follow-up care providers (e.g. rehabilitation, fertility, psychology), support groups and/or the patient's primary care provider.

11. A listing of cancer-related resources and information (e.g. internet-based sources and telephone listings for major cancer support organizations).

Adapted from the President's Cancer Panel (7).

---

5. Management of psychological, social and spiritual issues.

6. Management of genetic issues.

7. Management of sexuality and fertility issues.

8. Locus of care.

Twelve of the guidelines addressed follow-up and included schedules and recommendations regarding testing. The four most comprehensive guidelines covered five or more of the eight domains assessed above, and originated from government-sponsored guideline groups in Australia, Canada and Scotland. Some conflicting advice can arise about aspects of follow-up care. For example, recommendations on the frequency of follow-up surveillance mammography in breast cancer survivors ranged from yearly to never. In prostate cancer, the CPGs are fewer, and rarely address psychosocial issues or late effects. They all recommend surveillance with Prostate Specific Antigen (PSA) testing and Digital Rectal Examination (DRE), but the frequency varies from every 3 months to yearly. Despite the need for comprehensive management of late and long-term effects, and the existence of recommendations for care plans and health behaviours, very few comprehensive programmes of survivorship care yet exist.

Box 16.2 Life-style guidelines for cancer survivors

Recommendations for Cancer Prevention (after treatment, cancer survivors should follow the recommendations for cancer prevention)

1. Be as lean as possible without becoming underweight.

2. Be physically active for at least 30 minutes every day.

3. Avoid sugary drinks. Limit consumption of energy-dense foods (particularly processed foods high in added sugar or low in fibre or high in fat).

4. Eat more of a variety of vegetables, fruits, whole grains and legumes, such as beans.

5. Limit consumption of red meats (such as beef, pork and lamb) and avoid processed meats.

6. If consumed at all, limit alcoholic drinks to 2 for men and 1 for women a day.

7. Limit consumption of salty foods and foods processed with salt (sodium).

8. Don't use supplements to protect against cancer.

American Institute of Cancer Research, 2007 (30)

Communication challenges in survivorship care

Many barriers to the provision of survivorship care exist both on the part of patients and the care-delivery system. Patient barriers often include a lack of awareness of the late effects of cancer and its treatments. If patients are not aware of their increased risk for late effects, such as osteoporosis or cardiovascular disease, for example, they may be less proactive in seeking appropriate care. Another example pertains to breast cancer survivors' lack of knowledge concerning lymphoedema and the physician's failure to counsel women or provide written information on prevention (16). In addition, only about half of men and women with cancer who were of childbearing age received timely information from their health care providers about their risk of infertility. Often options to preserve or restore fertility come too late to take any preventive measures (17). Similarly, breast cancer survivors often do not recall discussing the reproductive health impact of their treatment, and many report that their concerns are not adequately addressed (18, 19). These examples highlight the importance of communication between care providers and patients regarding possible post-treatment survivorship issues (4).

To add to these difficulties, patient issues around communication can become problematic. Many patients may have literacy issues or are not comfortable conversing in specialized medical terminology, while others originate from different linguistic and cultural backgrounds. As such, communication barriers may arise that relate to sociocultural differences between survivors and their healthcare providers. These may include differences in commonly held attitudes, norms, beliefs, expectations and practices.

Other barriers to communication are illustrated by unmet expectations of survivors regarding follow-up care. For example, a nationwide survey in England found that 19% of survivors reported that doctors and nurses did not spend enough time, or none at all, telling them what to expect when they left the hospital after their first treatment; 26% noted not being given written information about what they should or shouldn't do following their discharge; and 36% were not told about support or self-help groups (20). In another English study of follow-up care, consultations for women with breast cancer were focused on detection of recurrent disease by clinical exams, but little attention was paid to education and psychosocial needs (21). In the US, a poll of cancer survivors by the Lance Armstrong Foundation found that nearly half felt their psychosocial needs were not being met by the health care system (22). Specifically, survivors expressed dissatisfaction with the provision of support in dealing with important issues such as depression, fear of recurrence, chronic pain, ongoing health challenges, infertility, sexual dysfunction, difficulty with relationships and financial or job insecurity. Clearly, providers are not offering the information that patients desire. Unfortunately, many patients may not even be aware of what to ask for if they are ill-informed about long-term and late effects of cancer treatments.

The fragmented care-delivery system is another barrier, which results in a loss of continuity of care. With patients often seeing many different specialists (medical oncologist, surgeon, radiation oncologist) and potentially having care provided in more than one institution or care setting, multiple patient records exist in different, non-compatible systems and no one provider has access to all medical information. This lack of continuity of care can result in sporadic follow-up and the failure of any one care provider to take a leadership role in assuring proper survivorship care. Patients can simply fall through the cracks, as the burden of responsibility is diffused among multiple practitioners, who assume that 'someone else' is attending to the issues. Key strategies to improve the coordination of care as suggested by the Institute of Medicine include: providing educational supports; instituting patient-centred health records, supported by modern information technology; ensuring accountability and defining roles for providers of care; and aligning financial incentives to ensure the delivery of coordinated care (23).

Other issues complicating the delivery of coordinated survivorship care include lack of training of healthcare professionals across the full range of survivorship care needs; lack of communication between, and among, professionals, sites, as well as geographic locations and over long periods of time; lack of agreed-upon standards of follow-up care; and agreement about who is responsible for paying for such care. With the growing interest in survivorship care-planning, there are clear guidelines for survivorship care; the issue now seems to be how to change behaviour and promote the uptake of these suggestions.

Models for survivorship care

Different models for survivorship care-delivery include:

 • shared-care model of follow-up;

 • nurse-led model; and

 • survivorship follow-up clinics.

Shared-care between different clinicians

Shared-care has been defined as 'care which applies when the responsibility for the health care of the patient is shared between individuals or teams who are part of separate organizations, or where substantial organizational boundaries exist' (24). In order for such a model to be successful, good communication between different providers, institutions and the patient must be in place.

Most of the onus in shared-care is placed on the primary care physician; their role is to ensure that all of the patient's health needs are addressed, both physical and emotional. The primary care physician assumes responsibility for:

 • all aspects of chronic disease care that are feasible in the primary care setting;

 • referral of the patient to specialists for periodic re-evaluations and to address issues that require focused expertise; and

 • consultation with specialists on areas of uncertainty.

Specialists are required to communicate findings and recommendations back to the primary care provider, so that the recommendations can be carried out under the supervision of the primary provider. For this type of care to be successful, it is essential that each party understand his or her role, agree to their responsibilities and carry them out as necessary. Shared-care is common in Europe, Canada and Australia. Cancer-related follow-up care can be provided successfully by primary care providers at lower cost than specialists without sacrificing patient satisfaction, but patient anxieties about receiving optimal care need to be addressed (25–27).

Timely and comprehensive communication between providers is the key to the success of shared-care. Professional training of family physicians and general practitioners is imperative in this model. In some countries this requirement becomes problematic due to a shortage of GPs and family physicians. In some communities in Canada, for example, up to 30% of the population is unable to find a general practitioner. Clearly, shared survivorship care would not be feasible if there is a lack of primary care physicians.

Nurse-led survivorship care

The second model, nurse-led follow-up care, has been followed successfully for many years in some childhood cancer centres. Ample evidence exists documenting the success of nurse-led follow-up care in many settings, including rural and remote locations, research settings and for the promotion of continuity-of-care (4). Nurse-led follow-up services prove acceptable, appropriate, effective, and can be an efficient means of maintaining contact with a large group of patients (28). Much like the GP in a shared-care model, this model has nurses coordinating all aspects of survivorship care.

The short supply of nurses in many countries can be a limitation. Nurse-led programmes are often not community-based but work out of hospital settings. Excellent co-operation and communication among care providers are needed, as patients would be referred to specialists as necessary. Specialists must adapt to receiving referrals from nurses and be willing to cooperate fully in this form of shared-care provision. This model has been applied successfully in Europe, but only recently piloted in the United States.

Dedicated survivorship clinics

This third model of specialized survivorship care clinics has been adopted in a few academic medical centres. These clinics integrate needed follow-up care expertise in one location. Such programmes facilitate the application of a holistic and coordinated approach to medical and psychosocial problems. Again, paediatric oncology has been a leader in the development of adolescent survivorship clinics, with upwards of 35 clinics in the US today. These are often run by oncology-trained nurse practitioners, supported by paediatric oncologists. Additional personnel involved usually include social workers, psychologists and other specialists, such as cardiologists, fertility specialists and genetic counsellors. Involvement is often on a case-by-case referral basis. The rehabilitation team recommended by the Association of Community Cancer Centres includes, but is not limited to:

- oncology nursing services;
- psychosocial services;
- physical, occupational and recreational therapy services;
- speech pathology services;
- comprehensive, multidisciplinary lymphoedema services;
- enterostomal therapy services;
- nutritional support services;
- pharmacy services;
- pastoral care services.
- a discharge planner to address home care and community and/or extended care facility services and needs;
- qualified volunteers to provide support and advocacy for cancer patients and their families;
- other complementary services, such as music/art therapy, relaxation, massage and others, in conjunction with rehabilitation disciplines (29).

One potential disadvantage of such survivorship clinics, however, is the separation of survivorship care from other routine care, with the resultant difficulties of communication and coordination. Hence, no matter what model of survivorship care is adopted, the key to success is communication among care providers and patients.

The survivorship consultation—an example of integrated care

Let us consider a typical consultation between a primary care physician and a patient who has recently been through cancer treatment in a shared-care model, currently the most common form of survivorship care. The GP or family physician would ideally have a pre-existing relationship with the patient and have been following her progress through cancer treatment by requesting progress notes from her care team of oncologists and other specialists. This consultation would be greatly facilitated by the provision of the treatment summary and care plan from the treating oncologist, as outlined in Box 16.1. If such a plan is not already available, the primary care physician should request such from the oncology team; if it is not forthcoming, the physician and patient should reconstruct the summary and create a shared care plan, based on clinical practice guidelines that are acceptable to both. The first post-discharge consultation would consist of reviewing or creating the treatment summary and care plan with the cancer survivor, if necessary reviewing relevant clinical practice guidelines for their type of cancer. In preparation for the consultation, the physician should:

- request the treatment summary from the treating oncologist;
- request a survivorship care plan from the treating oncologist or cancer centre;
- review relevant CPGs for the type of cancer and treatments the patient has received;
- obtain lists of referral options in the community for common survivorship issues.

During the consultation, or over multiple visits, clinicians should discuss with patients the following:

- current treatment toxicities, potential late effects and management strategies;
- monitoring plans for signs of possible recurrence or second tumours (e.g. mammography, colonoscopy schedule);
- effects of cancer/treatments on relationships, sexuality, fertility and parenting;
- effects of cancer or treatments on ability to work inside or outside of the home;
- effects of cancer or treatments on mood, anxiety and quality of life;
- recommendations for specific health behaviours (diet, weight control, exercise, smoking cessation, alcohol containment);
- risk of family members and any preventive measures they should be taking (e.g. screening, genetic counselling);
- referrals to specialists or programmes to help with any issues identified.

Discussions and referrals should be summarized in physician notes; referrals to other care providers should include a request for written care summaries to be sent back to the primary physician.

Conclusion

Survivorship is an important phase in the cancer journey, potentially the longest phase that patients will experience. With the advent of increasingly successful acute care, more and more people are moving into this phase of cancer care, and many are finding themselves *Lost in Transition*. Tremendous effort has been put into thinking about this growing cohort and researching their unique problems and needs. Care strategies and plans have been advocated by many governmental bodies and consumer groups; now the care system is at the cusp of implementing a variety of models of survivorship care.

The key issues vary across countries and regions, but what arises as essential is the need for agreement upon the components of survivorship care and the determination of who is responsible for delivering and paying for each component. Care providers have to be willing and able to communicate amongst one another and to see the value of trying to provide continuity of care between cancer specialists, the primary care physician and other subspecialties involved in optimal cancer care provision. Patients must become aware of their risks and care needs beyond acute care, and be proactive in assuring that their needs are met. The system, for its part, has to become more coordinated and receptive to a variety of models of care provision that are capable of meeting these needs. The future for cancer survivors is promising, and resources for treating cancer using models of chronic disease care are rapidly becoming broadly accessible.

Acknowledgements

Dr. Linda Carlson holds the Enbridge Research Chair in Psychosocial Oncology co-funded by the Canadian Cancer Society Alberta / NWT Division and the Alberta Cancer Foundation. Thanks to Joshua Lounsberry for editing assistance.

References

1. Mullan F (1985). Seasons of survival: reflections of a physician with cancer. *New Engl J Med* **313**, 270–3.

2. Welch-McCaffrey D, Hoffman B, Leigh SA, *et al.* (1989). Surviving adult cancers. Part 2: Psychosocial implications. *Ann Int Med* **111**, 517–24.

3. Ries LAG, Melbert D, Krapcho M, *et al.* (2007). SEER Cancer Statistics Review, 1975–2004. Available at: **http://seer.cancer.gov/csr/1975_2004/**. Last accessed 30 April 2008.

4. Committee on Cancer Survivorship (2006). *Improving Care and Quality of Life. From Cancer Patient to Cancer Survivor: Lost in Transition.* Hewitt, M.; Greenfield, S.; Stovall, E. (Eds). Institute of Medicine and National Research Council, Washington, DC.

5. Institute of Medicine (2003). *Childhood Cancer Survivorship: Improving Care and Quality of Life.* National Academy of Sciences, Washington, DC.

6. Centers for Disease Control and Prevention (2004). *A National Action Plan for Cancer Survivorship: Advancing Public Health Strategies.* Department of Health and Human Services, Washington, DC.

7. Reuben SH (2004). *Living Beyond Cancer: Finding a New Balance: President's Cancer Panel 2003–2004 Annual Report.* National Cancer Institute, National Institutes of Health, Department of Health and Human Services, Washington DC.

8. Reuben SH (2006). *Assessing Progress, Advancing Change: President's Cancer Panel 2005–2006 Annual Report.* National Cancer Institute, National Institutes of Health, Department of Health and Human Services, Washington DC.

9. Hewitt M, Ganz PA (2007). *Implementing Cancer Survivorship Care Planning: Workshop Summary.* A National Coalition for Cancer Survivorship and Institute of Medicine National Cancer Policy Forum Workshop In Partnership with The Lance Armstrong Foundation and The National Cancer Institute. National Academy of Sciences, Washington, DC.

10. Rowland JH, Baker F (2005). Introduction: resilience of cancer survivors across the lifespan. *Cancer* **104**(11 Suppl), 2543–8.

11. Aziz NM, Rowland JH (2003). Trends and advances in cancer survivorship research: challenge and opportunity. *Semin Radiat Oncol* **13**, 248–66.

12. Ferrell BR, Grant M (1996). *City of Hope Quality of Life Patient Version.* City of Hope National Medical Centre and Beckman Research Institute, Duarte, CA.

13. Ganz PA, Desmond KA, Leedham B, *et al.* (2002). Quality of life in long-term, disease-free survivors of breast cancer: a follow-up study. *J Natl Cancer Inst* **94**, 39–49.

14. Hewitt M, Rowland JH, Yancik R (2003). Cancer survivors in the United States: age, health, and disability. *J Gerontol Biol Sci Med Sci* **58**, 82–91.

15. Jones LW, Demark-Wahnefried W (2007). Recommendations for health behavior and wellness following primary treatment for cancer. In: Hewitt M, Ganz PA, eds. *Implementing Cancer Survivorship Care Planning Workshop Summary*, pp.166–205. Institute of Medicine, Washington DC.

16. Paskett ED, Stark N (2000). Lymphedema: knowledge, treatment, and impact among breast cancer survivors. *Breast* **6**, 373–8.

17. Canada AL, Schover LR (2005). Research promoting better patient education on reproductive health after cancer. *J Natl Cancer Inst Monogr* **34**, 98–100.

18. Partridge AH, Gelber S, Peppercorn J, *et al.* (2004). Web-based survey of fertility issues in young women with breast cancer. *J Clin Oncol* **22**, 4174–83.

19. Duffy CM, Allen SM, Clark MA (2005). Discussions regarding reproductive health for young women with breast cancer undergoing chemotherapy. *J Clin Oncol* **23**, 766–73.

20. Airey C, Becher H, Erens B, *et al.* (2002). *National Surveys of NHS Patients—Cancer: National Overview 1999/2000*. Department of Health, UK.

21. Beaver K, Luker KA (2004). Follow-up in breast cancer clinics: Reassuring for patients rather than detecting recurrence. *Psychooncology* **14**, 94–101.

22. Lance Armstrong Foundation (2004). *LiveStrong Poll Finds Nearly Half of People Living With Cancer Feel Their Non-Medical Needs are Unmet by the Healthcare System*. LAF, Austin TX.

23. Institute of Medicine (2001). *Crossing the Quality Chasm: a New Health System for the 21st Century*. National Academy Press, Washington DC.

24. Pritchard P, Hughes J (1995). *Shared Care the Future Imperative?* Royal Society of Medicine Press, London.

25. Grunfeld E, Gray A, Mant D, *et al.* (1999). Follow-up of breast cancer in primary care vs specialist care: Results of an economic evaluation. *Br J Cancer* **19**, 1227–33.

26. Grunfeld E, Fitzpatrick R, Mant D, *et al.* (1999). Comparison of breast cancer patient satisfaction with follow-up in primary care versus specialist care: Results from a randomized controlled trial. *Br J Gen Pract* **49**, 705–10.

27. Grunfeld E, Mant D, Yudkin P, *et al.* (1996). Routine follow up of breast cancer in primary care: Randomised trial. *BMJ* **313**, 665–9.

28. Cox K, Wilson E (2003). Follow-up for people with cancer: Nurse-led services and telephone interventions. *J Adv Nurs* **43**, 51–61.

29. Association of Community Cancer Centres (2007). Cancer program guidelines. Available at: **http://www.accc-cancer.org/PUBS/pubs_cpguidelines.asp**. Accessed 5 December 2007.

30. World Cancer Research Fund/American Institute for Cancer Research (2007). *Food, Nutrition, Physical Activity, and the Prevention of Cancer: a Global Perspective*. AICR, Washington DC.

Chapter 17

Dealing with cancer recurrence

Lidia Schapira

When the experience of cancer and its treatment is over, it is easy to 'rewrite history' and think of yourself as having been more wise, mature, and adaptive than indeed was the case. As with childbirth and other traumas, in retelling it you tend to color the experience as you want to remember it, and tell it to others in more acceptable terms.

Kathleen Conway, psychotherapist and survivor of two cancers (1).

Introduction

Cancer survivors often describe the period following their initial diagnosis as a time of heightened awareness and worry. Many describe being unable to enjoy the present for fear of recurrent disease, a condition termed the Damocles syndrome (2). Indeed, sizeable subgroups will have the misfortune to develop recurrence. Personal choices and coping styles determine a person's adaptation to his or her illness, and shape their transition to dealing with recurrence. Cancer clinicians know that there is no set formula for coping; individual resources and coping strengths, collectively referred to as resiliency, vary considerably among individuals.

In this chapter, I will review the central themes and frequent scenarios that physicians, nurses, and therapists need to consider in working with patients with recurrent cancer. In so doing, I rely on knowledge derived from my own clinical experience as a medical oncologist, published biomedical literature, and from extensive reading of patient narratives. Memoirs, diaries, poetry, and works of art give us important insight into the experiential domain of illness and provide inspiration, substance, and meaning to our work.

Patients and clinicians recognize the importance of supportive relationships in the struggle to adapt and live with a chronic illness. Information and good communication help craft sustaining relationships, align mutual expectations, and allow patients and healthcare professionals to gain a sense of common purpose. Before considering the strategies and skills necessary to signal a change in prognosis and support patients and families, let us first take a critical look at the role that language plays in mediating communication.

In the past, the language of physicians and educated laypeople was quite similar. Today, the ubiquitous use of technical jargon, acronyms, and specific adaptations of common phrases make even the simplest communication more problematic (3). Opportunities for misunderstanding are so prevalent that healthcare professionals are summoned to courses on 'plain language' to assist their communication with patients. To complicate matters, the open disclosure of uncertainty and increasing use of qualifiers, such as 'probably' and 'possibly,' now pervasive in medical discourse, can serve to alienate patients (3, 4). Terms routinely employed by physicians may have a completely different meaning for patients and may mistakenly alarm or falsely reassure a patient. A 'negative' biopsy indicates either no tissue or no tumour and thus may have a 'positive' implication for the medical team, but requires an appropriate explanation for an average patient (5). Conversely, a 'positive' lymph node confirms spread of tumour and thus negatively impacts stage and outcome.

A genuine concern for patients motivates oncologists to value opportunities to provide frank and honest information. In my experience, cancer clinicians also greatly value the relationships they form with patients and families over time. With this in mind, we will now examine the special features of communication about a cancer recurrence and review the skills and strategies necessary to provide therapeutic and supportive interventions.

From diagnosis to recurrence: living with uncertainty

To illustrate its prevalence, every year in the US, over one million individuals will be diagnosed with a recurrence of cancer and more than half will die rapidly of their disease (6). In some cases, relapse may still allow hope for a cure, but for many patients it signals the transition to living with an incurable illness. For example, a local or regional recurrence of breast cancer may be managed successfully with surgery or radiation, and it is entirely appropriate for both patient and doctor to remain optimistic about the future. In sharp contrast, visceral metastases portend a shortened survival and the need for lifelong anti-cancer therapy. New advances in cancer therapies now allow many patients living with metastatic cancer to enjoy many years of extended survivorship with a reasonably good quality of life. Since prognostic estimates of life-expectancy at time of recurrence now vary tremendously, depending on tissue type and availability of salvage treatment, I will not attempt to address specific situations, but rather focus on the common challenges facing most patients and physicians dealing with relapse.

Weisman and Worden's classic studies in the early 1980s showed that most people seem to cope surprisingly well with the emotional shock of recurrence (7). Some patients exhibit depressive symptoms, such as the loss of hope for recovery, anxieties and fear of death, resurfacing of unresolved issues, strong attempts to maintain control, and often the urgent need to adapt to living with increasing disabilities (6–8). In a prospective randomized clinical trial, Andersen and colleagues at Ohio State University studied breast cancer patients at the time of recurrent disease (6). Patients reported stress but the news of recurrence was not accompanied by global distress, nor disruption of quality of life. The women's previous experiences with cancer may have harnessed resilience upon hearing the news of relapse (6).

A descriptive study of women with recurrent ovarian cancer examined the meaning of this experience (8). Interestingly, most remembered precisely how the physician had informed them of their recurrence. Many stated that they could tell from the look on their physician's face before they were told, adding that their physician was unusually quiet, looked upset, or seemed distracted and detached (8). Most stated that they could never have been prepared for the shock of cancer recurrence, although they knew it was possible (8).

A Swedish study by Ekwall and colleagues examined the impact of recurrent ovarian cancer on women who had been cancer-free for at least one year before relapsing (9). They spoke of 'being denied one's future', while simultaneously hoping to delay disease advancement (9). Surprisingly, many struggled with a sense of personal failure, guilt, and responsibility for the impact the illness had on family members. They were 'living in limbo' and dealing with important transitions, during which they were particularly vulnerable to loneliness and alienation (9).

Patients experience the news of a recurrence with a sense of shock and disbelief. Oncologists know all too well that patients scrutinize their facial expressions for signs of impending bad news. Patients who have serial determinations of blood tumour markers or imaging studies know that the purpose is to determine signs of early recurrence and are, therefore, trained to expect important news at each visit. In some cases, this preparation may mitigate the blow of hearing bad news. Not all patients will fully grasp the prognostic significance and thus fail to understand that the disease is no longer curable. They anticipate further treatments (e.g. chemotherapy, targeted therapy, or endocrine manipulations) without recognizing that the intention of treatment has evolved from cure to palliation. The tension between the patient's understanding and the medical reality can be a source of frustration for clinicians and is best handled by repeated conversations over many weeks. Patients need time to process the information and come to terms with their predicament. Some interpret the news of a cancer recurrence as an immediate death sentence. They may inquire about a referral to hospice care and an estimate of life-expectancy, a question that causes considerable anguish for medical oncologists and is a scenario too often dramatized in films and soap operas. 'How long do I have to live?' is a question a doctor cannot walk away from, yet is rarely answered to a patient's satisfaction. Patient-centred approaches to address this flesh out each patient's preoccupations and explore the need to know before actually addressing statistical and prognostic information (10–12). Suffice to say that the 'right' answer is determined by context and relationship, and is tailored to meet the individual's needs and their capacity to absorb the material.

Hearing and telling: 'But I thought I was cured'

Experienced doctors are the first to receive bad news such as a test confirming cancer recurrence (13). When the patient and doctor have an established relationship and the news concerns progression of disease or treatment failure, the doctor may also experience a keen sense of disappointment, sorrow, guilt, and frustration (14, 15). If these feelings are not acknowledged and processed, they may undermine the physician's therapeutic potential (16). In an effort to protect the patient, some doctors use euphemisms to soften the blow, potentially adding to the patient's confusion (17, 18). Others wish to minimize the time spent with patients and, in so doing, block the patient's attempts to discuss the implications of the news. Gordon and Dougherty explored the language used to describe the news of advanced disease (19). Physicians used troubling terms such as 'hitting over the head', 'pounding', 'hammering', 'bludgeoning', and 'dumping' to describe their practice of disclosing bad news. This reflects their underlying belief that truth is injurious, the physician abusive, and the practice harmful. It also articulates the unspoken distress experienced by many physicians. Many doctors remember past experiences of delivering bad news as harrowing and describe being overcome by painful memories for many years (20, 21). In order to avoid unnecessary trauma and to improve the effectiveness of junior clinicians, training programmes in medical oncology need to provide both mentorship in, and consolidation of, communication skills training (22).

Hearing bad news sets in motion an emotional and cognitive reaction that needs to be acknowledged, addressed, and supported. Suffering may impair a person's ability to imagine goals for the future, as well as his or her sense of control and self-efficacy (23). In some instances, hearing the news of a cancer recurrence may simply confirm a person's pre-existing worries or suspicions. Since medical decisions often rest on rethinking or regenerating life goals, a process that involves coming to terms with grief, as well as clear reasoning, it is best not to rush into discussions of treatment options (23). Salander's classic studies of patients who received bad news recognized the psychological meaning of 'togetherness' at the time of diagnosis, of a supportive atmosphere, and a personal touch (24). For the clinician, the challenge is to provide a calm and steady presence and to refrain from rushing to fix the problem. For many of us trained to act, this is not always easy to do.

Table 17.1 lists a series of steps and practical tips to help guide these conversations. These are based both on evidence and consensus guidelines for best practice and are not intended to script the dialogue between healthcare professionals and patients. Instead, these talking points can be viewed as aids or props to help sustain a meaningful connection between clinician and patient during times of high emotional stress for both.

Needing to know

Full disclosure of diagnostic and prognostic information, now standard practice in most Western countries, would have shocked our mentors and may even today be considered unnecessarily brutal in many societies (3, 13). Anthropologist Mary-Jo Good wrote that in American oncology practice, hope is primarily conveyed by providing information, in contrast to Europe and Asia, where physicians convey hope primarily by fostering ambiguity (25, 26). The tendency to provide patients with complicated statistics in response to requests for prognostic information has become even more entrenched in the US in recent years. Lawyers and bioethicists have been critical of traditional approaches and favour complete disclosure of information in the name of safeguarding patient autonomy (27). Informing patients allows them to make reasonable therapeutic decisions. The challenge remains to interpret exactly how much information is enough. In practice, patients are often unwilling or unable to share the burden of decision-making; in these circumstances, what ethicists wish for them does not match their agenda (27). Many patients look to their doctors to provide information, as well as direction. They may in fact need and want information, but they also seek guidance in making decisions regarding treatment.

In attempting to develop a guideline addressing just how much information is enough, Christakis argues that patient and doctor may negotiate the amount of information that is helpful (28). Some patients with metastatic disease explicitly ask their physicians not to prognosticate. They find that articulating estimates of life-expectancy is simply unhelpful and depressing. They want their doctor to 'hope with them' for an improvement, an extension, or symptomatic relief. Often physicians dodge questions by simply offering an empathic response. Practices vary considerably and reflect an individual physician's view of what constitutes 'right' or humane practice. If physicians view withholding prognostic information as deceitful, they are likely to favour complete disclosure. On the other hand, if they see withholding prognostic information as an important aspect of fostering hope, they may steer the conversation away from discussion of timelines and projections of future problems (28). As with any therapeutic option, the decision of how much to tell depends on the estimates of risk and benefit (13).

Several convincing studies from the UK, US, Australia, and Northern European countries support a preference for complete disclosure by the majority of respondents. Although estimates vary, we know that between 50 and 97% of patients surveyed wanted to know the truth (29–31). Studies by Butow and Tattersall and their colleagues in Australia provide insight into the decision-making process as it evolves in real time (30–33). Based on analysis of audio-tapes of consultations and patient interviews, they found that most patients were eager for information and valued highly the recommendation of the doctor (30–33).

Ideally, consultations involve the exchange of information in an atmosphere of mutual trust, followed by deliberation, and, finally, a recommendation from the physician based on the patient's goals and preferences. An important and under-utilized communication strategy involves the

Table 17.1 Practical checklist for discussing a cancer recurrence (13, 50, 51, 52, 53, 54)

Strategies	Skills & process tasks	Communication examples
Create setting	Provide a comfortable, safe and private location.	
Introductions and initial assessment	Introduce other team members if present and clarify everybody's role. Note the patient's body language, nonverbal and verbal cues that indicate his or her level of ease or anxiety.	
Perception of illness	Check the patient's present understanding.	'Dr Z. forwarded some test results. Could you tell me what he said about these?'
Setting the agenda	Inform the patient about the objectives of the meeting, time available and how it will be spent.	'Today we'll review further the results of these tests and work out what we need to do.'
Invitation—negotiating agenda with the patient	Address the patient's need to receive and refuse information and clarify the level of detail required in the subsequent information exchange.	'Help me understand your preferences for the level of detail you like in the information I'll give you.' 'Is it all right now for me to tell you the results of the latest scans or blood test?'
Information provision	Present facts that need to be conveyed in order to allow the patient to understand his or her situation and make rational choices regarding treatment.	A warning shot: 'I'm afraid the news is more serious than we suspected.' 'Unfortunately the PET scan showed that the cancer has spread to other organs.'
Empathic response	Words to convey that the clinician acknowledges the importance and possible consequences of this information. An expression of personal disappointment or sorrow may be quite appropriate and therapeutic, accompanied by an invitation to share the sorrow.	'I am so sorry…' 'I too am disappointed and had hoped for a better outcome…' 'This must be very hard to hear…'
Engagement	Partnership statements that promise non-abandonment.	'I want to make it clear that we are here to support and help you.' 'Don't worry alone.'
Sharing uncertainty	Recognize that it is unsettling to face an uncertain future and listen to the patient's concerns and anxieties.	'What are you most concerned about?'
Sorting through options	Help the patient and family to think through available options. Outline the big picture including standard treatment, clinical trials and palliative measures.	'Chemotherapy may stop the growth of this tumour.' 'There is a clinical trial you may wish to consider.' 'We have a terrific team and will work together to control your pain.'
Summary, including goals of future care	Check understanding—review of the medical information and concerns expressed. Summarize the action plan, including the time and place for next contact.	'We need to bring this meeting to an end. Let me take a moment to go over the main points of our conversation…' 'You have an appointment with my colleague in radiation oncology tomorrow at 3 o'clock.' 'I would also like you to call my nurse tomorrow morning to tell her if this medication helped with your pain.' 'We'll meet again in two weeks and see if you're ready for the next treatment.'

discussion of alternatives to the recommended or preferred treatment. Doctors can help patients think through their options, verbalizing what could happen if he or she chose to forego all treatment or used an 'alternative' therapy. In a non-judgmental exchange, the doctor can help his or her patients sort through various possibilities for treatment or observation and imagine the consequences of each decision. This 'active' approach to decision-making is also favoured by patient advocates and facilitates successful coping.

Importantly, many patients and relatives do not wish to be briefed on every aspect of diagnosis and prognosis (27). In situations where the physician's need to inform conflicts with the individual's legitimate request and right not to receive information, physicians often perceive the delivery of bad news as abusive. In practice, we sometimes face competent, educated individuals, who simply do not wish to know detailed side-effects and prefer to skip the explanations of possible harm. They would rather sign the paperwork authorizing treatment without reading it. Case by case, physicians need to decide if the patient's unwillingness to listen invalidates or trivializes the process of obtaining consent for treatment (13).

Patient-centred communication guidelines favour a tailored approach to diagnostic and prognostic information. Dosing information may remain an elusive goal. As we settle into the age of complete disclosure and hurried communication, physicians and nurses need to hone their skills to avoid misunderstandings. Otherwise, patients may find themselves in the very difficult situation of dealing with abundant information and receiving very little guidance, surely a lonely place from which to contemplate a recurrence of cancer.

Hope as a vital sign

> Good doctors know they can't make this go away, they can only hope with me it will continue to move slowly, very slowly.
>
> Patricia Barr, cancer patient and advocate (personal communication).

Studies that address hope within the medical setting recognize that hope can take a variety of forms, ranging from miracle cure to peaceful death. Faced with a dire prognosis, a person may simultaneously hope for cure, while acknowledging and preparing for death. In fact, the ability to wish for a good outcome while facing multiple losses is an expression of an individual's ability to cope with adversity. There are practical and lyrical definitions of hope, yet it remains somewhat difficult to characterize (34–38). Is it an emotion or an attribute? Can it be nurtured and cultivated? Does the absence of hope signal pathology? An irrefutable observation is that the lack of hope is considered a cardinal symptom of depression. Oncology clinicians recognize the lack of hope in their patients and perhaps, at times, even in themselves. This can be described as despair, despondency, misery, and a pervasive bleak feeling that one's life has neither worth nor meaning. In the history of human suffering, we find inspiring examples of persons who were able to transcend physical symptoms, captivity, and cruelty. They found that the will to live flowed from a profound sense of purpose and meaning, perhaps sustained by the memory of a loving relationship (39–41). Manifestations of despair evoke a variety of responses in treating clinicians, some of whom have little experience and tolerance for emotional expression. An empathic response and a promise not to abandon the patient are of great therapeutic value and cannot be omitted from any treatment plan.

Hope evolves and is both vital and dynamic. When first confronted with the news of recurrence, many patients may relate hope to a measurable drop in a tumour marker or shrinkage of tumour on a scan. Oncologists face the difficult challenge of encouraging such expressions of hope, while signalling the need to prepare for a time when treatment may not be available or, indeed, may cause more harm than good. A common pitfall is to encourage 'unrealistic' expectations that do not serve patients or families well in the long haul. An observational study of communication between oncologists and patients with advanced lung cancer by The and colleagues documented many examples of such collusion (42). Although cure was not possible and remissions were expected to be short-lived, physicians hardly ever addressed this, leaving patients to grapple with the disappointment of treatment failure when they were very close to dying (42). Improved communication skills in clinicians, and a growing public acceptance of palliative and hospice care, are needed to transform the current landscape and limit the use of futile treatment. Until that happens, we must support junior staff who find themselves in demoralizing situations, witnessing and participating in medically futile care (43).

Nursing and medical research on hope has traditionally focused on definitions, measurements, and the design of interventions to enhance and foster hope in dying patients and their caregivers (44–49). Indeed, current guidelines recommend that the oncologist balance honest disclosure with sustaining hope (47). Although this goal may not always be within reach, it orients clinicians and guides patients towards the integration of new information into a framework that is ample enough to sustain hope for a better future. Clinicians can begin by exploring the sources of hope, identifying potential obstacles, and shifting to affirming personal attributes and qualities that convey the value of the person (44–49). Encouraging patients to recall uplifting memories and shared experiences will convey respect and foster a sense of connection (48, 49). The most common obstacles to the expression of hope include unremitting pain and physical symptoms, isolation, and fear of abandonment. Clinicians can respond by paying meticulous attention to detail and striving to maintain comfort and dignity to the greatest extent possible. We certainly cannot promise a good outcome, but we need to reaffirm our constancy, support, and respect for our patients, especially when cure is no longer possible.

Advances in cancer medicine over the past decade have led to some truly astonishing improvements. Patients with chronic myelogenous leukaemia or endocrine-sensitive metastatic breast cancer can expect to live many years with their illness, avoid hospitalizations, and enjoy a good quality of life. Contemporary oncologists now face new ethical and communication challenges when patients choose to interrupt therapy in order to have a biologic child or embark on demanding professional quests that will likely remain unfinished. These life-affirming choices may also be interpreted in a broader context as an expression of hope for a better future.

Recurrence of cancer role plays and actor training

Breast cancer scenario

Mary is a 41-year-old married mother of three children, who was diagnosed with breast cancer one year ago. Her tumour did not express oestrogen nor progesterone receptors and involved spread to regional lymph nodes. She was treated with mastectomy, adjuvant chemotherapy, and radiation to her chest wall. She saw her oncologist for a 6-month check-up, at which time she was asymptomatic, but still recovering from the sequelae of her lengthy treatments. Three months later, she developed a persistent cough, and after several weeks, a chest X-ray showed a vague peripheral nodule. Chest CT scan showed pleural-based 'suspicious lesions', as well as two small peripheral pulmonary nodules, each measured at 4 mm. Mary returns to see you for her scan results.

Guide to training the actor

Mary is a well-informed and educated woman, who takes good care of herself and her family (three children, ages 11, 16, and 18). She has great confidence in her medical team. During her adjuvant therapy, she developed a strong working relationship with the nurses and oncologist.

She suspects something is seriously wrong, but is not aware of the dismal prognosis associated with such an early relapse. She will come into the meeting with her husband and expects to hear that she will need more treatment. She may blurt out, 'I thought I was cured' or 'What are we going to do next?' and is not quite prepared for the devastating news she is likely to hear (i.e. that the tumour is incurable). Until this time, she was always eager to hear statistics and detailed information, but now she is really ambivalent. She is terrified, but tries to put on a brave front.

Colon cancer scenario

Barry is a 60-year-old, semi-retired CEO of a biochemical company, who is quite used to giving orders and having the final word. He has a bad marriage and grown children, who don't really like him very much. In fact, he has few close friends and maintains his distance from relatives. He has a passion for photography and often travels by himself to take pictures of wild animals in remote locations. He doesn't really trust the medical establishment and did not participate in routine colonoscopic screening for colon cancer. He was diagnosed three years ago with a node-positive colon cancer and was treated with surgery and adjuvant chemotherapy. His oncologist explained the rationale for periodic surveillance with tumour markers and CT scans in order to identify a possible 'early recurrence', which could still be treated with salvage surgery. Barry's CEA began a slow and steady climb, but his CT scan did not show any disease. However, his PET scan shows multiple liver metastases. Barry has a scheduled appointment to discuss results.

Guide to training the actor

Barry is physically fit and middle-aged. He is gruff, smart, and does not particularly care for small talk. He has built a successful business and is used to giving orders. He is not close to his wife or his grown children, but he is quite civilized. His hobby is wildlife photography and he did, on one occasion, invite his son to accompany him on a photo safari to Africa, where they had a good time together. Barry thinks doctors cannot really 'prevent' disease and only sees his internist when he does not feel well. Prior to his colon cancer, his only exposures to the medical establishment were quite brief and successful: arthroscopic surgery for a torn knee ligament and medical therapy for gastro-oesophageal reflux. Three years ago, he found blood in his stool and this led to a diagnosis of colon cancer. He was rebuked for having 'waited so long' and for not having ever had screening colonoscopies. He saw a brilliant, technical surgeon, who did not care for small talk either and was then referred to the oncologist for adjuvant chemotherapy. He 'endured' the treatments, although never really had much faith that he would derive a personal benefit. He 'went along' with a plan to watch him carefully because he understood that a local recurrence or solitary hepatic metastasis could still be treated (surgically) with curative intent. His oncologist explained that his tumour marker was rising and ordered CT and then PET scans. His CT 'showed nothing'. He thinks that the blood test is probably wrong. Living with this uncertainty does not suit him well. The only acceptable option with a recurrence of cancer would be more surgery with curative intent. He has no more patience for the 'chemo' and no interest in discussing his emotional life with nurses.

As he listens to the latest news, Barry could say: 'Why didn't we pick this up sooner?', 'How long do I have to live?', 'I'm a reasonable man, doctor. I know you keep talking about treatments and responses, but what chance do I have of getting a benefit from any of these drugs?'.

Conclusion

Consultations that deal with recurrence incorporate many of the strategies and skills involved with breaking bad news, discussing prognosis, the use of salvage treatments, providing a supportive framework, sustaining hope, and emphasizing, as appropriate, the chronicity of the illness. Our goal is to tailor information based on knowledge of the patient's coping strengths and limitations, provide empathic support and convey our commitment to care as the journey with cancer unfolds. In integrating all that was covered in earlier training modules, this consultation provides an opportunity to consolidate a crucial set of communication skills.

References

1. Conway K (2007). *Ordinary Life: a Memoir of Illness* (Conversations in Medicine and Society). University of Michigan Press, Ann Arbor, MI.

2. Walker LG (2000). Surviving cancer: does the fighting spirit matter? Inaugural Lecture, 6 November 2000, University of Hull, UK: **http://www.lgwalker.com/inaugural.html**. Accessed 17 April 2009.

3. Schapira L (2004). Shared uncertainty. *J Support Oncol* **2**, 14–18.

4. Diamond J (1998). *Because Cowards Get Cancer too, a Hypochondriac Confronts His Nemesis.* Times Books, New York.

5. Chapman K, Abraham C, Jenkins V, *et al.* (2003). Lay understanding of terms used in cancer consultations. *Psycho-Oncology* **12**, 557–66.

6. Andersen BL, Shapiro CL, Farrar WB, *et al.* (2005). Psychological responses to cancer recurrence. *Cancer* **104**, 1540–7.

7. Weisman AD, Worden JW (1985). The emotional impact of recurrent cancer. *J Psychosocial Oncol* **3**, 5–16.

8. Mahon SM, Casperson DM (1997). Exploring the psychosocial meaning of recurrent cancer: a descriptive study. *Cancer Nurs* **20**, 178–86.

9. Ekwall E, Ternestedt BM, Sorbe B (2007). Recurrence of ovarian cancer—living in limbo. *Cancer Nurs,* **30**, 270–7.

10. Loprinzi CL, Johnson ME, Steer G (2003). Doc, how much time do I have? *J Clin Oncol* **21**(9 Suppl), 5s-7s.

11. Schapira L, Eisenberg PD, MacDonald N, *et al.* (2003). A revisitation of 'Doc, how much time do I have?'. *J Clin Oncol* **21**(9 Suppl), 8s–11s.

12. Stiefel F, Razavi D (2006). Informing about diagnosis, relapse and progression of disease—Communication with the terminally ill cancer patient. *Recent Results Cancer Res* **168**, 37–46.

13. Schapira L (2006). Breaking bad news to patients and families In: L Syrigos, K Nutting, C Roussos, eds. *Tumours of the Chest. Biology, Diagnosis and Management,* 597-605. Springer, New York.

14. Fallowfield L, Jenkins V (2004). Communicating sad, bad, and difficult news in medicine. *Lancet* **363**, 312–19.

15. Mount B (1986). Dealing with our losses. *J Clin Oncol* **4**, 1127–34.

16. Meier DE, Back AL, Morrison S (2001). The inner life of physicians and care of the seriously ill. *JAMA* **286**, 3007–14.

17. Dunn SM, Patterson PU, Butow PN, *et al.* (1993). Cancer by another name: a randomized trial of the effects of euphemisms and uncertainty in communication with cancer patients. *J Clin Oncol* **11**, 989–96.

18. Fallowfield L, Clark AW (1994). Delivering bad news in Gastroenterology. *Am J Gastroenterology* **89**, 473–70.

19. Gordon E, Dougherty CK (2003). Hitting you over the head: oncologists' disclosure of prognosis to advanced cancer patients. *Bioethics* **17**, 142–68.

20. Fallowfield L (1993). Giving bad and sad news. *Lancet* **341**, 476–8.

21. Orlander JD, FinckeBG, Hermanns D, *et al.* (2002). Medical residents' first clearly remembered experiences of giving bad news. *J Gen Int Med* **17**, 825–31.

22. Muss HB, Roenn, J, Damon, LD, *et al.* (2005). American Society of Clinical Oncology ACCO: ASCO core curriculum outline. *J Clin Oncol* **23**, 2049–77.

23. Halpern J (2001). *From Detached Concern to Empathy. Humanizing Medical Practice.* Oxford University Press, Oxford.

24. Salander P (2002). Bad news from the patient's perspective: an analysis of the written narratives of newly diagnosed cancer patients. *Soc Sci Med* **55**, 721–32.

25. Delvecchio Good MJ (1991). The practice of biomedicine and the discourse on hope. *Anthropologies Med* **7**, 121–35.

26. Delvecchio Good MJ, Good BJ, Schaffer C, *et al.* (1990). American oncology and the discourse on hope. *Cult Med Psychiatry* **14**, 59–79.

27. Schneider C (1998). *The Practice of Autonomy Patients, Doctors and Medical Decisions.* Oxford University Press, New York.

28. Christakis NA (1999). *Death Foretold.* The University of Chicago Press, Chicago, IL.

29. Fallowfield L, Ford S, Lewis S (1995). No news is good news: information preferences of patients with cancer. *Psycho-Oncology* **4**, 197–202.

30. Butow P, Kazemi J, Beeney L, *et al.* (1996). When the diagnosis is cancer: patient communication experiences and preferences. *Cancer* **77**, 2630–7.

31. Butow P, Maclean M, Dunn SM, *et al.* (1997). The dynamics of change: cancer patients' preferences for information, involvement and support. *Ann Oncol* **8**, 857–63.

32. Tattersall MH, Butow PN (2002). Consultation audio tapes: an underused cancer patient information aid and clinical research tool. *Lancet Oncol* **3**, 431–7.

33. Tattersall MH, Butow PN, Clayton JM (2002). Insights from cancer patient communication research. *Hematol Oncol Clin North Am* **16**, 731–43.

34. Penson RT, Gu F, Harris S, *et al.* (2007). Hope. *Oncologist* **12**, 1105–13.

35. Mount BM, Boston PH, Cohen SR (2007). Healing connections: on moving from suffering to a sense of well-being. *J Pain Symptom Manage* **33**, 372–88.

36. Groopman J (2004). *The Anatomy of Hope.* Random House, New York.

37. Holland JC (2000). *The Human Side of Cancer, Living with Hope, Coping with Uncertainty.* Harper Collins, New York.

38. Nuland SH (1995). Hope and the cancer patient. In SH Nuland, ed. *How We Die.* First Vintage, New York.

39. Frankl VE (1984). *Man's Search for Meaning,* Touchstone Edition. Simon and Schuster, New York.

40. Hauerwas S (1986). *Reflections on Suffering, Death and Medicine,* pp.23–38. University of Notre Dame Press, Notre Dame.

41. Cassell EJ (1991). *The Nature of Suffering and the Goals of Medicine.* Oxford University Press, New York.

42. The AM, Hak T, Koëter G, *et al.* (2000). Collusion in doctor-patient communication about imminent death: an ethnographic study. *BMJ* **321**, 1376–81.

43. Ferrell BR (2006). Understanding the moral distress of nurses witnessing medically futile care. *Oncol Nurs Forum* **33**, 922–30.

44. Herth K (1992). Abbreviated instrument to measure hope: development and psychometric evaluation. *J Adv Nurs* **17**, 1251–59.

45. Yellen SB, Cella DF (1995). Someone to live for: social well-being, parenthood status, and decision-making in oncology. *J Clin Oncol* **13**, 1255–64.

46. Cella DF (1992). Health promotion in oncology: a cancer wellness doctrine. *J Health Care Chaplain* **4**, 87–101.

47. Clayton JM, Butow PN, Arnold RM, *et al.* (2005). Fostering coping and nurturing hope when discussing the future with terminally ill cancer patients and their caregivers. *Cancer* **103**, 1965–75.

48. Rousseau P (2000). Hope in the terminally ill. *West J Med* **173**, 117–8.

49. Mount BM, Boston PH, Cohen RS (2007). Healing connections: on moving from suffering to a sense of well-being. *J Pain Symptom Manage* **33**, 372–88.

50. Baile WF, Beale EA (2003). Giving bad news to cancer patients: matching process and content. *J Clin Oncol* **21**(9 Suppl), 49–51.

51. Baile WF, Buckman R, Lenzi R, *et al.* (2000). SPIKES- A six step protocol for delivering bad news: applications to the patient with cancer. *Oncologist* **5**, 302–11.

52. Buckman R (1992). *How to Break Bad News: A Guide for HealthCare Professionals.* Johns Hopkins University Press, Baltimore.

53. Clayton JM, Hancock K, Parker S, *et al.* (2007). Sustaining hope when communicating with terminally ill patients and their families: a systematic review. *Psycho-Oncology* 2008, **17**, pages 641–59.

54. Clayton JM, Hancock KM, Butow PN, *et al.* (2007). Clinical practice guidelines for communicating prognosis and end-of-life issues with adults in the advanced stages of a life-limiting illness, and their caregivers. *Med J Aust* **186**(12 Suppl), S77, S79, S83–108.

Chapter 18

Communication about transitioning patients to palliative care

Josephine M Clayton and David W Kissane

Introduction

Despite advances in anti-cancer treatments, most adult cancer patients still eventually die from their disease. For these patients, the goal of care changes from curative to palliative at some point along the disease trajectory. Alternatively, the goal of care may be palliative from the moment of diagnosis in patients presenting with disseminated cancer. Palliative anti-cancer treatments aim to minimize spread of cancer and disease progression, help control symptoms and improve quality of life. Other palliative therapies include medications and interventions to relieve symptoms—including physical, psychosocial and existential issues.

The nature of palliative care

The World Health Organization defines palliative care as:

> ...an approach that improves the quality of life of patients and their families facing the problems associated with life-threatening illness, through the prevention and relief of suffering by means of early identification and impeccable assessment and treatment of pain and other problems, physical, psychosocial and spiritual.

(1)

According to the 'new international framework' for palliative care, 'basic palliative care' refers to the 'standard of palliative care which should be provided by all health care professionals, in primary or secondary care, within their normal duties to patients with life-limiting illness' (2, p.2192). 'Specialist palliative care services' refers to expert multidisciplinary healthcare services whose 'substantive work is with patients who have a life-limiting progressive illness' (2, p.2192, 3). Specialist palliative care services are not available in all parts of the world. In addition, not all patients with advanced, progressive, life-limiting illnesses require specialist palliative care services—some may be cared for most appropriately by their primary healthcare providers (2, 4). Patients may only need to see a specialist palliative care service initially for a limited time to assist in the management of a complex problem, such as uncontrolled pain. As the patient's illness progresses, he or she may need referral to community or home-based palliative care services or to an inpatient palliative care unit for terminal care.

Ideally a palliative approach should be adopted over time as the person's disease progresses—involving a gradual transition rather than a sharp demarcation. Early referral to specialist palliative care services, while the patient is still receiving disease-specific treatments such as chemotherapy and radiotherapy, may enhance symptom control and also reduce any sense of abandonment in patients when chemotherapy is no longer appropriate. Furthermore, early introduction of the palliative care team aids the overall adjustment process (5). Patient preferences favour early referral (6).

In comparison to conventional care, specialist palliative care services improve patient and caregiver satisfaction, provide better pain and symptom control, reduce caregiver anxiety, and increase the likelihood of the patient being cared for during the terminal phase in their place of choice (7).

Discussions about changing treatment goals (from curative to palliative, or from palliation with anti-cancer treatments to symptomatic care only) and referral to specialist palliative care services can be challenging for patients/families and health professionals. Such discussions may evoke fears of impending death, helplessness and abandonment in the patient and their family, if this is not communicated sensitively and effectively by the healthcare team. In this chapter, we conceptualize the process of transitioning patients to palliative care in four distinct ways:

(1) transition to a palliative approach: when the goals of care change from curative to palliative;

(2) referral to specialist palliative care services;

(3) when potentially life-prolonging treatments (including palliative anti-cancer treatments) are no longer effective and symptomatic care only is adopted; and

(4) when the person approaches the terminal phase of their illness.

The timing of these transitions depends on each patient's circumstances and the complexity of their problems.

Communication about transitions in the goals of care

The general objectives when communicating transition from a curative to palliative approach are to guide the patient collaboratively to understand the goals of care relevant to the palliative approach, focusing on optimizing quality of life and gradually developing an acceptance that they have a life-limiting illness, yet sustaining hope about the living that still remains. Importantly, discussions about transitions to palliative care commonly occur over time rather than as a single, one-off communication encounter.

Identifying when to talk about shifting goals of care

Medicare data studied by Joanne Lynn's group in the USA identified a stereotypic trajectory for advanced cancer—slow decline across months, followed by a rapid decline to death in the last two months (8). A clinical dilemma exists as to whether clinicians should protect patients from consideration of dying until this final two months, or prepare them gradually over the preceding time. Patients themselves may also differ in their preference. However, this conceptualization is generally based on a sharp demarcation between active treatment and end-of-life care; we advocate, where possible, for an alternative style through the gradual introduction of the palliative approach.

In studying patients at the end of life, Steinhauser and colleagues found remarkable consistency in the attitudes held by patients, their family caregivers and their physicians over recognition of a person's dignity, receiving excellent symptom control, being able to trust the doctor and being prepared for dying, including being able to say goodbye (9). Physicians, however, seemed unaware how importantly patients rate being mentally aware of one's approaching death, at peace with their God, avoiding being a burden to their family and society, having their funeral planned, helping those around them and feeling that their life is finally complete (9). Offering an open discussion about the transition to palliative and eventually end-of-life care would respond appropriately to these patient preferences.

Another important rationale for effective communication about the transition to palliative care is avoidance of futile care, potentially a major cost to society in times of scarcity of clinical resources and a burden to the patient and their family, who fail to appreciate the reality of their plight. Emanuel and colleagues have pointed out the overuse of chemotherapy in reviewing Medicare data, which shows that one-third of all chemotherapy is administered in the last 6 months of life and 23% in the final 3 months (10). The fact that this administration is similar, irrespective of the responsiveness of the cancer type, suggests its administration is primarily as a source of hope. Another source of data about futile care comes from an analysis of deaths in the intensive care unit. One in five Americans die in an intensive care unit, and ICU expenses account for four-fifths of all terminal inpatient costs (11). An intervention at the Brigham showed that active communication about the goals of care could promote earlier uptake of palliative care and reduce length of stay in the ICU (12).

The challenge of prognostication

Both patients and their physicians err commonly in being too optimistic about the prognosis, contributing to poor understanding of the clinical reality. In one study, only 20% of physician–patient pairs concurred that the doctor had communicated the fatal nature of the illness and an alarming 73% agreed that no discussion of life-expectancy had ever occurred (13). These results are in keeping with the consistent findings that clinicians who feel close to their patients over-estimate survival by a 5- to 6-fold error. Lamont and Christakis found that 23% of physicians would avoid giving any survival estimate, 40% would exaggerate the prospects of survival and only 37% would share their accurate perception (14).

Given how challenging this appears to be, the question arises as to how a physician begins a conversation about dying. Usually this arises in conjunction with a set of investigational results revealing significant disease progression, despite active anti-cancer treatments, and often the presence of substantial tumour burden. Other strong markers of this time having arrived include symptoms such as anorexia, weight loss and cachexia, and changing ECOG status, with greater frailty and increasing dependence on others. Questions from patients, with associated emotional cues indicating their concern, may indicate their readiness for this conversation. A moral obligation may exist for the physician who is aware of the patient's deterioration to inform him or her of their predicament, especially if there is any emergent organ failure.

A set of 'Clinical practice guidelines for communicating prognosis and end-of-life issues with adults in the advanced stages of a life-limiting illness, and their caregivers' (15) was endorsed by the Australian palliative-care community and based on empirical evidence and consensus from an expert advisory group.

What to say to introduce the concept of transitioning to palliative care

In developing guidelines addressing communication at the end of life, Baile and colleagues recommended checking each patient's understanding of recent investigations and treatments to verify a uniform viewpoint or address any misunderstandings and gaps in knowledge (5). Similarly, prior to discussing palliative care with patients, Lo and colleagues suggested a series of open-ended questions to elicit patients' concerns, goals and values (16). This then enables the physician to negotiate new goals of care based upon attitudes that the patient reveals about their quality-of-life expectations. In doing this, clinicians should contrast 'cure' with 'care', introduce the concept of the palliative approach as 'always involving something that can be done to help' and acknowledge, where appropriate, that anti-cancer treatments may continue alongside symptomatic treatments. In contrast, if futile care is being sought, the concept that 'further chemotherapy may do more harm than good' is reasonable. In applying any of these options, great sensitivity to each patient's emotional response is called for, with empathic acknowledgment of the perceived outcome for the patient (17).

The maintenance of morale in the face of disease progression is challenging. Emphasis on living in the present and living life out fully, despite a life-limiting illness, may facilitate patients' wellbeing. Care is needed to avoid lecturing or projecting one's own view about how a patient should be approaching their illness. Avoid giving false or misleading information to try to foster hope, as this can lead to later regret about treatment and life-style decisions that permit best use of the remaining time (18). One approach is to focus the patient upon the common tasks involved in preparation for one's death. These involve not only social and legal acts (wills and advanced directives) but also life review, completion of unfinished business, leaving a legacy, talking about your children's future plans, expressing gratitude for the life you've shared and beginning to say goodbye. One way of opening such discussions is by using a hypothetical question to explore what would be most important to the patient should time be limited. Discussion of hospice care, preferred place of death and wishes about one's funeral can all have a place. It proves helpful to emphasize that the process of farewell is not a final act but rather can extend over several weeks or months and bring many poignant moments to all concerned.

Many patients fear the process of dying. Therefore, to address this actively with medical information and reassurance, permission should be sought as to whether a discussion of this would be helpful. Information herein should be tailored to the specific illness and possible modes of dying for this patient. Extra care is needed to describe the elements of symptom management appropriate for each person.

Open conversation about death and dying can bring considerable relief to patients and their families. However, individual coping styles vary and not all patients want to discuss dying. Positive avoidance is a legitimate way of coping with life's greatest existential threat. Many patients will cope with their dying by drawing upon religious beliefs, finding sources of spiritual peace and using rituals long valued by their cultural or ethnic group. Clinicians do well to affirm each person's involvement with such traditions, inviting support from relevant chaplains or pastoral care workers, as available.

The family of the dying provide fundamental support to their ill relative and have needs of their own as well. Encourage their questions and examine any practical care needs that arise. Affirm the importance of respite to avoid burnout and exhaustion in these carers. Recommend the use of home health aids, visiting nurses or community volunteers, as available.

Early referral to a palliative care service enables key relationships to be established with the patient and their family, while this is still possible. Commitment to care and avoidance of abandonment are crucial. Many physicians understand these principles, but find the burden of end-of-life care challenging. Sharing such healthcare with physicians who choose to specialize in palliative care is entirely appropriate for those who don't enjoy this aspect of medicine. Parallel, shared-care over the latter months of a person's life helps to transition their care into an appropriate palliative care or hospice programme.

In closing any consultation that has covered this process of transitioning to palliative care, taking time to check understanding, answering queries and affirming a focus on continued living is desirable. Expression of your commitment to care and availability, if needed, serves to reassure both patient and family. Informing the team of any agreement reached in the consultation (with appropriate documentation) helps all subsequent care providers to understand the agreed goals of care.

Strategies: typical sequence of steps involved in communicating about the transition to palliative care

The communication goal is to guide the patient to understand the goals of care relevant to the palliative approach, focusing on maintaining quality of life. Based on the Memorial Sloan–Kettering communication skills training module (19), the strategies used to transition a patient from curative to palliative care are shown in Table 18.1.

Table 18.1 Core communication components for discussing the transition to palliative care.

Strategies comprise the sequence of steps used to achieve the communication goal; skills are verbal utterances that assist in the completion of each strategy; process tasks are often non-verbal behaviours or other aids to complete each strategy effectively.

Strategies	Skills	Process tasks
1. Recognize patient's cue or emergent clinical reality.	Declare your agenda items. Negotiate agenda. Check patient understanding.	Ensure setting appropriate to this discussion. Consider goals of care.
2. Establish understanding of disease progression, treatment efficacy and prognosis.	Check patient understanding. Invite patient questions. Make partnership statements.	Deepen understanding of patient's predicament. Correct misunderstandings. Sustain supportive environment. Tailor amount of information to patient's need. Acknowledge reality.
3. Discuss patient's values and priorities; negotiate new goals of care based on the patient's values and priorities as well as the burden versus benefit ratio of available treatments.	Endorse question-asking. Check patient understanding. Reinforce joint decision-making according to the patient's preferred level of involvement.	Introduce palliative approach: ◆ Contrast cure with care. ◆ Emphasize living in the present. ◆ Emphasize 'always something to do to help'. ◆ Commit to continuity of care. Establish quality of life goals of importance. Acknowledge (anti-cancer and palliative treatments can be given simultaneously).
4. Respond empathically to emotion.	Ask open questions about the emotional response and coping. Empathize by clarifying, acknowledging, validating or normalizing emotions.	Promote hope over grief or despair. Emphasize the living over the dying. Discuss difference between the process of saying goodbye and a final farewell.
5. Negotiate the shift to discuss the process of dying.	Make a 'take stock' statement. Check patient understanding. Categorize information. Ask open questions.	Ask permission or check readiness to discuss dying. Describe relevant elements of good symptom control. Provide tailored information.
6. Promote understanding of change and illness transitions.	Validate. Summarize. Praise patient efforts. Express a willingness to help.	Consider patient's response to family. Consider spiritual or religious needs. Address specific cultural needs. Contrast open awareness of end-of-life issues with avoidant coping style. Promote consideration of advantages and disadvantages of treatment choices. Affirm courage.
7. Address caregiver's concerns.	Ask open questions. Endorse question asking. Make partnership statements.	Identify value of respite from caregiver role. Consider role of community volunteers, health aides. Examine instrumental care or nursing care needs.
8. Effect referral to palliative care service whenever appropriate.	Ask open questions. Endorse question asking. Make partnership statements.	Identify value of respite from caregiver role. Consider role of community volunteers, health aides. Examine instrumental care or nursing care needs.
9. Close consultation.	Summarize. Check patient understanding. Endorse question asking. Review next steps.	Remind patient regarding the availability and commitment to care. Affirm progress and focus on continued living. Document discussion and inform team members.

Most patients need to talk about what their disease progression means to optimize their understanding of the medical predicament. An opportunity then exists to establish what aspects of quality of life are important to them. The clinician should educate about the palliative approach, emphasizing that there is always something that can be done medically to reduce suffering and relieve symptoms. As this occurs, empathic support involves acknowledging sadness, before promoting hope alongside grief.

Many will be interested in learning about the process of dying; permission is best sought to talk about this. In educating the patient and caregivers about the possible modes of dying, linkage to the goals of excellent symptom-care promotes confidence in the care plan and peace. Identify any cultural, spiritual or religious needs, while respecting and validating each patient's preferred coping response; affirm courage, when evident.

To address caregiver concerns, examine practical or nursing care needs, the importance of respite from the caregiver role and the contribution of community volunteers or health aides and visiting nurses. Before closing the consultation, summarize the agreed goals of care and any need for parallel, shared care.

There are a number of model statements we can offer to also guide clinicians in their accomplishments of these strategies. These are drawn from a systematic review (20) and consensus-based clinical practice guidelines and are summarized in Tables 18.2 to 18.4 (15).

Commencing or changing disease-specific, anti-cancer treatments

In the setting of an advanced cancer, the main aims of disease-specific, anti-cancer treatments, such as chemotherapy, are to improve the length and quality of life. Patients are helped by a realistic appraisal of the palliative intent of this treatment—that cure is not a treatment goal, but that the treatment can slow disease progression or ameliorate symptoms (see Table 18.2 for useful phrases for the clinician to use). For the patient to be fully informed as a result of this discussion, the clinician seeks to ensure that the patient understands the balance between the potential effectiveness of life-prolonging treatments and their side-effects. Shared decision-making is an imperative here, with the clinician recognizing the patient's desire about their level of involvement (21).

Ceasing disease-specific, anti-cancer treatments

When patients learn about disease progression or the lack of treatment response, clinicians should be ready for the patient to express emotional reactions, such as sadness, anger or disheartenment (32). Empathic support is crucial here, as is the continued availability of the clinical team (see Table 18.3 for useful phrases for the clinician to use). An ongoing focus on expert symptomatic care is a means of sustaining the sense of continuing care.

Discussing referral to specialist palliative care teams

Referral to specialist palliative-care services may not always be needed or feasible for a particular patient, depending on clinical issues, availability and financial or insurance considerations. However, where available, referral may assist through provision of extra support for patients and their families. The expertise of the specialist service can improve quality of life through management of difficult physical, psychosocial or spiritual concerns. Guidelines for making a referral to specialist palliative care services, with useful phrases to facilitate this, are shown in Table 18.4

Table 18.2 Commencing or changing disease-specific treatments

Recommendation	Useful phrases (where applicable)	Evidence Level
◆ Be clear regarding the goals of treatments (e.g. palliative rather than curative) and specifically what outcomes may be improved (e.g. relief of symptoms) and how likely this can be achieved.	'The aim of this treatment is to help make you feel better. We will monitor the benefits and side effects of the treatment and talk about the options if the treatment is not helping you.'	DS (22)
◆ State whether or not survival may be improved by the treatment. ◆ Where applicable, explain that shrinking the cancer will not necessarily prolong survival. ◆ Be proactive for quality of life and avoid recommending toxic treatments if little likely gain will result.	'The aim of this treatment is not to cure but to control the disease for as long as we can. If we control the cancer, it is likely that we will improve some of your symptoms and make you feel better, even if we can't make you live any longer.' 'There is about an x% chance that this treatment will shrink the tumour. That should make you feel better but may only extend your life by a few weeks or months.'	CG (15)
◆ Give clear information about the likely side-effects, costs and time involved to enable patients to make informed decisions in the context of their goals.		DS (6, 23–27)
◆ Ensure that full supportive care will be provided whether or not any disease specific treatment is also given, and provide reassurance to this effect.	'While you receive chemotherapy for your cancer, we will still do everything to support you as a person.' 'There are a number of different people/ services to help you along this cancer journey.'	CG (28)
◆ Encourage the patient to share in decision-making according to their desired level of involvement.	'People vary in how they want to make medical decisions. Some people want to make the decisions themselves, some people want to share decision making with the doctor, and some people want the doctor to make/give a lot of help in making the decisions. What do you prefer?' 'So based on your goal of (e.g. wanting to stay at home as much as possible with your family and friends), I propose that we do the following... What do you think?' 'Given the current situation, our options are as follows... 1... 2... 3...I'm wondering whether option X is the most suitable option for you because.... What are your thoughts?'	DS (29–31)

DS = descriptive studies, CG = consensus guidelines.

Table 18.3 Cessation of disease specific treatments

Recommendation	Useful phrases (where applicable)	Evidence Level
◆ Sensitively explain that his/her disease is no longer responding to the current treatment and that continuing this treatment is likely to cause more side effects than benefit.	'Your disease is no longer responding to the... (e.g. chemotherapy) treatment. To continue this treatment would cause you more harm than good (or will give you tots of side effects but is unlikely to affect the cancer). It is likely that you will have a better quality of life without further.. (type of treatment – e.g. chemotherapy).' 'I wish that more chemotherapy would help this cancer, but unfortunately at this stage it will only make you sicker. Yet there are many other things we can do to help you deal with your condition.' 'Our goal of treatment needs to change from trying to control the cancer to minimizing the symptoms you might get.' 'One of the best predictors of how someone will be able to handle chemotherapy, and how well it will work for them, is how fit and up and about they are while having it. Because you have become quite weak, it is much more likely that the treatment will make you worse, not better.'	CG (28)
◆ Avoid conveying that nothing more can be done. Emphasize that treatments and support will be provided to help them cope with their illness (see section on facilitating hope).	'As you become sicker with this illness we will continue to be there to provide the best available treatments to help control your symptoms and support both for you and your family.' 'Our aim is to optimize your comfort and ability to function as normally as possible.' 'There is nothing more we can do to make this cancer go away but a lot we can do to help you live and cope with it.'	DS (32–33)

CG = consensus guidelines, DS = descriptive studies.

Exemplar clinical scenario to guide role-plays

Emília Tavares is 48-year-old nurse and mother of two teenage children. She has developed advanced ovarian cancer. Chemotherapy and surgery to reduce tumour bulk have contained her disease over 4 years. A partial bowel obstruction has occurred recently, but settled with nasogastric drainage. Emília knows at some level that her days are limited.

Instruction to the patient, Emília Tavares

As a nurse, you remember seeing patients with ovarian cancer die. They seemed to have the worst deaths—feculent vomiting, such suffering. What will your death be like? You lie awake at night thinking about this. Too hard to discuss with your husband! You fear that your death will be horrible. It can only get worse, can't it? And then you think of your children, two fun-loving girls,

Table 18.4 Introducing specialist palliative care services

Recommendation	Useful phrases (where applicable)	Evidence Level
◆ Consider referral to specialist palliative care services, where available and depending on the patient's/caregiver's needs, at any time once the treatment goal changes from curative to palliative (i.e. the patient may still be receiving palliative treatments, such as chemotherapy, aimed at controlling the underlying disease).		CG (34)
◆ Refer to the palliative care health professionals as part of the multidisciplinary team.	'I work closely with the palliative care team in looking after patients such as yourself who have advanced cancer (or lung disease, etc. as appropriate to the underlying illness).'	EO(3)
◆ Raise the topic by being both honest and open, using the term 'palliative care' explicitly.	For the health professional referring to palliative care team: 'The palliative care team can provide extra support to you and your family and help optimise your comfort and level of function.' 'Extra help and support from the palliative care service might be useful now, especially if we are to give you the best and most appropriate care possible.' 'The palliative care team can work closely with you and me in optimizing your comfort and level of function.' For the palliative care professional at time of initial consultation: 'I work closely with the other doctors and nurses caring for you. The aim of palliative care is to ensure that at all stages of your illness, you are kept as comfortable as possible, regardless of what is happening to your (cancer, heart or lungs).'	DS (35)
◆ Clarify and correct misconceptions about palliative care services (particularly that it is not solely for people who are dying or associated with imminent death.)	'What does the term palliative care mean to you?' 'Many people have either not heard of palliative care, or associate it with dying in the very near future.' Then respond to the patient's cues. 'It might be useful for you if I explain what palliative care is really all about?' 'Have you had any experiences with others receiving palliative care?'	CG (36)
◆ Discuss role of the palliative care team, emphasizing expertise in symptom management as well as a wide range of support services, assistance with quality of life, and support for family/partner/children, etc.	'The palliative care team have a lot to offer as support—this includes pain control and the control of other symptoms resulting from the cancer.' 'Palliative care includes a whole range of clinicians who can help support you and your family at this time.' 'The palliative care team works closely with me to help you live life to the full'	CG (28)

Table 18.4 (continued) Introducing specialist palliative care services

Recommendation	Useful phrases (where applicable)	Evidence Level
◆ Explain that the patient can be linked up with palliative care team at same time as receiving treatments directed at the underlying disease (e.g. chemotherapy).	'Our team/service often works very closely with the palliative care team/services whilst giving people treatment X.'	CG (28)
◆ Explain that the patient will still be followed up by the primary health care team (e.g. GP, generalist nurse) and/ or the primary specialist (e.g. oncologist, respiratory physician), where applicable. ◆ Discuss with the patient and/or caregivers what that means in terms of who they should contact for what kinds of issues/ situations.	For general practitioner or primary cancer specialist: 'I will still be your main doctor but the palliative care team will be able to provide extra support or advice with the best medicines for your pain.' For palliative care health professional: 'I will work closely with Dr X. Dr X will still be your main doctor, but we will work together to ensure that you are as comfortable as possible.'	CG(15)

CG = consensus guidelines, EO = published expert opinion, DS = descriptive studies.

13 and 15 years old. How sad to leave them! How unfair this wretched illness is! You sense a deep grief within you as you contemplate this reality. You must talk to someone about your fears. Who can help you with this terrible plight?

Instruction to her husband, Jorge Tavares

You are an accountant whose life was going beautifully until your wife took sick. Now, two surgeries and a batch of chemotherapy treatments later, you are deeply aware of her fear and sad demeanour. You admire her resilience and you do your best to protect her, to keep up a brave front. Yet you also worry about what will happen? How long does she have? She tells you this cancer will kill her. What does the future hold?

Instruction to the oncologist/nurse

Emília is a warm, religious, Latina woman! She has been a pleasure to treat and you sense there is great courage in her. Her recent bowel obstruction has brought a sadness to her demeanour. You want to discuss the role of a venting gastrostomy for drainage in place of her current nasogastric tube. You believe it is time to stop chemotherapy, as her disease has progressed through several regimens. You have a sense that she also wants to talk more about her illness.

Instruction to role-play observers

Discussing the transition to palliative care is a challenging task, in which cultures differ enormously in their approaches, and each clinician approaches it differently. Your task is to add depth to the cultural sensitivity needed in this setting. Take careful note of the conversation, the phrases used in this role-play, so that you can assist the discussion and help strategizing about how to communicate more effectively.

Key tips in training actors as simulated patients

In these simulations, be prepared to ask the clinician frank questions like, 'Am I going to die?' and 'Are you giving up on me, doctor?'. The aim here is to confront the clinician with the inevitability of the cancer's progression and make sure there is potential for the discussion of palliative care. Other useful questions include, 'What is palliative care?', 'Will the drainage tube be permanent?', 'Does a referral to hospice mean that I'm dying, doctor?' and 'Can you promise a peaceful death, doctor?'.

Conclusion

Communication skills training for health professionals has been shown to improve patient outcomes in decision-making with early stage disease. Further research is needed to show whether training for health professionals will improve outcomes for patients and their families during the transition to palliative care. However, it is possible that communicating in the ways above may reduce patient anxiety, help patients to make appropriate decisions and avoid overly burdensome and costly treatments at the end of life. Other objectives include the reduction of barriers to referral to specialist palliative care and the use of timely referrals. Achieving an adaptive adjustment to disease progression and preparation for death is a worthy goal of care.

References

1. World Health Organization (2002). *National cancer control guidelines: policies and managerial guidelines.* Geneva: WHO, **http://www.who.int/cancer/palliative/definition/en/** Accessed 21 May 2008.

2. Ahmedzai SH, Costa A, Blengini C, *et al.* (2004). A new international framework for palliative care. *Eur J Cancer* **40**, 2192–200.

3. Palliative Care Australia (2005). *A guide to palliative care service development: a population approach.* Canberra: Palliative Care Australia. **http://www.pallcare.org.au/Default.aspx?tabid=1221** (accessed May 2007).

4. Palliative Care Australia (2005). *Standards for providing quality palliative care for all Australians.* Canberra: Palliative Care Australia. **http://www.pallcare.org.au/Default.aspx?tabid=1221** (accessed May 2007).

5. Baile WF, Glober GA, Lenzi R, *et al.* (1999). Discussing disease progression and end-of-life decisions. *Oncology* **13**, 1021–35.

6. Hagerty RG, Butow PN, Ellis PA, *et al.* (2004). Cancer patient preferences for communication of prognosis in the metastatic setting. *J Clin Oncol* **22**, 1721–29.

7. Hearn J, Higginson I (1998). Do specialist palliative care teams improve outcomes for cancer patients? A systematic literature review. *Palliat Med* **12**, 317–32.

8. Lunney J, Lynn J, Foley D, *et al.* (2003). Patterns of functional decline at the end of life. *JAMA* **289**, 2387–92.

9. Steinhauser K, Christakis N, Clipp E, *et al.* (2000). Factors considered important at the end of life by patients, families, physicians and other care providers. *JAMA* **284**, 2476–82.

10. Emanuel EJ, Young-Xu Y, Levinsky NG, *et al.* (2003). Chemotherapy use among Medicare beneficiaries at the end of life. *Ann Intern Med* **138**, 639–43.

11. Angus DC, Barnato AE, Linde-Zwirble WT, *et al.* (2004). Use of intensive care at the end of life in the United States: an epidemiologic study. *Crit Care Med* **32**, 638–43.

12. Lilly C, Sonna L, Haley K, *et al.* (2003). Intensive communication: four-year follow-up from a clinical practice study. *Crit Care Med* **31**, S394–99.

13. Fried TR, Bradley EH, O'Leary J (2003). Prognosis communication in serious illness: perceptions of older patients, caregivers, and clinicians. *J Am Geriatr Soc* **51**, 1398–403.

14. Lamont EB, Christakis NA (2001). Prognostic disclosure to patients with cancer near the end of life. *Ann Intern Med* **134**, 1096–105.

15. Clayton JM, Hancock KM, Butow PN, *et al.* (2007). Clinical practice guidelines for communicating prognosis and end-of-life issues with adults in the advanced stages of a life-limiting illness, and their caregivers. *Med J Aust* **186(12 Suppl)**, S77–108.

16. Lo B, Quill T, Tulsky J (1999). Discussing palliative care with patients. *Ann Intern Med* **130**, 744–49.

17. Friedrichsen MJ, Strang PM, Carlsson ME (2000). Breaking bad news in the transition from curative to palliative cancer care–patient's view of the doctor giving the information. *Supp Care Cancer* **8**, 472–78.

18. The AM, Hak T, Koeter G, *et al.* (2000). Collusion in doctor-patient communication about imminent death: an ethnographic study. *BMJ* **321**, 1376–81.

19. Kissane DW, Bylund C, Brown R, *et al.* (2006). *Transition to palliative care.* Communication Skills Training and Research Laboratory, Memorial Sloan-Kettering Cancer Center, New York, NY.

20. Parker S, Clayton JM, Hancock K, *et al.* (2007). A systematic review of prognostic/end-of-life communication with adults in the advanced stages of a life-limiting illness: patient/caregiver preferences for the content, style and timing of information. *J Pain Symptom Manage* **34**, 81–93.

21. National Breast Cancer Centre Advanced Breast Cancer Working Group (2001). *Clinical practice guidelines for the management of advanced breast cancer.* Canberra: NHMRC. **http://www.nhmrc.gov. au/publications/synopses/cp76syn.htm** (accessed May 2007).

22. Norton SA, Talerico KA (2000). Facilitating end-of-life decision-making: strategies for communicating and assessing. *J Geront Nurs* **26**, 6–13.

23. Clayton JM, Butow PN, Arnold RM, *et al.* (2005). Discussing end-of-life issues with terminally ill cancer patients and their carers: a qualitative study. *Support Care Cancer* **13**, 589–99

24. Fallowfield LJ, Jenkins VA, Beveridge HA (2002). Truth may hurt but deceit hurts more: communication in palliative care. *Palliat Med* **16**, 297–303.

25. Gattellari M, Voigt KJ, Butow PN, *et al.* (2002). When the treatment goal is not cure: are cancer patients equipped to make informed decisions? *J Clin Oncol* **20**, 503–13.

26. Clayton JM, Butow PN, Tattersall MH (2005). The needs of terminally ill cancer patients versus those of caregivers for information regarding prognosis and end-of-life issues. *Cancer* **103**, 1957–64.

27. Meredith C, Symonds P, Webster L, *et al.* (1996). Information needs of cancer patients in west Scotland: cross sectional survey of patients' views. *BMJ* **313**, 724–26.

28. Baile WF, Buckman R, Lenzi R, *et al.* (2000). SPIKES—a six-step protocol for delivering bad news: application to the patient with cancer. *Oncologist* **5**, 302–11.

29. Clover A, Browne J, McErlain P, *et al.* (2004). Patient approaches to clinical conversations in the palliative care setting. *J Adv Nurs* **48**, 333–41.

30. Dowsett SM, Saul JL, Butow PN, *et al.* (2000). Communication styles in the cancer consultation: preferences for a patient-centred approach. *Psychooncology* **9**, 147–56.

31. Gattellari M, Butow PN, Tattersall MH (2001). Sharing decisions in cancer care. *Soc Sci Med* **52**, 1865–78.

32. Friedrichsen MJ, Strang PM, Carlsson ME (2002). Cancer patients' interpretations of verbal expressions when given information about ending cancer treatment. *Palliat Med* **16**, 323–30.

33. Morita T, Akechi T, Ikenaga M, *et al.* (2004). Communication about the ending of anti-cancer treatment and transition to palliative care. *Ann Oncol* **15**, 1551–57.

34. Weissman DE, Griffie J (1994). The Palliative Care Consultation Service of the Medical College of Wisconsin. *J Pain Symptom Manage* **9**, 474–79.

35. Dexter PR, Wolinsky FD, Gramelspacher GP, *et al.* (1998). Effectiveness of computer-generated reminders for increasing discussions about advance directives and completion of advance directive forms. A randomized, controlled trial. *Ann Intern Med* **128**, 102–10.

36. Schofield P, Carey M, Love A, *et al.* (2006). Would you like to talk about your future treatment options? Discussing the transition from curative cancer treatment to palliative care. *Palliat Med* **20**, 397–406.

Chapter 19

End-of-life communication training

Tomer Levin and Joseph S Weiner

Introduction

Experience alone is not enough to ensure optimal doctor–patient communication at the end of life—formal communication skills training (CST) is necessary to produce improved outcomes. This chapter outlines the goals and strategies for end-of-life CST, emphasizing common decision-making dilemmas, such as withdrawal of life-extending treatment and do-not-resuscitate (DNR) directives. Common pitfalls seen in training are identified.

The goal of end-of-life communication training: smoother implementation of palliative care

An important rate-limiting step for the implementation of palliative care is clear, empathic clinician–patient–family communication. Although palliative care curricula have been broadly implemented in physician training (1–2), CST is essential given the emotional complexity of the cusp between life and death.

It is burdensome to increase a dying person's suffering with invasive interventions that do not improve length or quality of life, such as cardiopulmonary resuscitation (CPR) (3–5). A minimal use of CPR during end-stage cancer is one proxy measure for effective end-of-life communication. Similarly, the timeliness of discussions clarifying treatment goals near the end of life is another proxy measure. The majority of DNR directives at a national cancer centre were signed the same day that the patient died, suggesting reduced attention to palliative care goals (6).

Discussion of death and dying in oncology should be a predictable process rather than an unexpected crisis. For example, one in five Americans die in intensive care units (ICU) (7) and an estimated 90% of these involve withholding or withdrawing life-extending care (8). The clinical team must guide the family from a position of hope to the reality of impending death as less than 5% of ICU patients are able to participate in these discussions because they are too sick or unconscious (9).

Palliative care outcomes such as patient and family-centred decision-making, emotional, spiritual and practical support, symptom management, length of stay (LOS), family burden (caregiver burnout, depression, post-traumatic stress disorder) and the overall quality of, and satisfaction with, care can be improved by CST (10, 11). The aim is to improve institutional palliative care practices, referred to by von Gunten as 'the way that we do things around here' (12).

Patient-centred communication in cancer care

Patient-centredness is derived from six core functions of clinician–patient communication: 'fostering healing relationships, exchanging information, responding to emotions, managing uncertainty, making decisions and enabling patient self-management' (13). This conceptual model links patient and family needs to clinician–patient–family communication.

The centrality of the family meeting

As discussed in detail in Chapter 15, the family meeting is central to end-of-life decision-making (14, 15) and a key focus of CST. Distress reverberates through the family, making some members second-order patients. (16).

Specific strategies for end-of-life communication

A roadmap for the end-of-life discussion is set out in Table 19.1. This represents a synthesis of expertise (14, 17–22) and our own experience teaching in Memorial Sloan–Kettering Cancer Center's Comskil Laboratory (23).

Important aspects of this roadmap for the end-of-life discussion are discussed below.

Pre-conference clinical team meeting

A multidisciplinary discussion is a prerequisite to reach consensus among team members about prognosis, the goals of care, DNR and treatment withdrawal recommendations, so that the

Table 19.1 Roadmap for the end-of-life patient and family conference (see text for details)

1. Pre-conference Clinical Team Meeting.

2. Opening: introductions and agenda.

3. Gather information about perceived understanding of illness/goals of care:
   - Ask about perceived understanding of illness, likely outcomes and treatment goals.
   - Correct misperceptions, educate about illness/prognosis.
   - Rule: respond to emotions evoked by the discussion.

4. Gather specific information about wishes and thoughts regarding death and dying in one of three ways:
   - Ask directly about thoughts and wishes regarding dying, end-of-life goals of care and DNR directives.
   - Ask about personal experiences in the past with death and dying amongst family or friends and how this impacts on the patient's current dilemma in trying to establish end-of-life goals of care and DNR decisions.
   - Substituted decision-making: If the patient lacks capacity (e.g. unconscious), the family can be asked to share 'who the patient is as a person' with the medical team. As a follow-up, ask the question, 'If the patient could speak to us right now, how might he or she guide us in our decision making?'.
   Note: avoid euphemisms for death, use specific communication techniques (circular, strategic and reflexive questioning, summarizing) to promote consensus, educate patient/family about DNR directives, CPR, prognosis, palliative care and the dying process.

5. Make recommendations for end-of-life care (e.g. DNR directives, withdrawal of life-extending care or hospice referral):
   - Use shared decision making approach to ease burden of responsibility. Consider offering decision delay to facilitate consultation with other family members or empiric trials of further treatment.
   - Reassure: patient will not be abandoned before death, will not suffer, will be comfortable; praise courage and support the decision.

6. Finalize the action plan
   - Summarize plan for end-of-life care and DNR directives.
   - Offer practical assistance and problem solve high priority issues: goals of care, symptom management, spiritual needs, what to expect as death approaches.
   - Set time for next meeting or update, elicit feedback.

patient and family do not receive conflicting messages (14). A quiet room where all participants are seated facilitates open dialogue. If the meeting must be conducted at the bedside, protection of privacy is important. In multi-bed hospital rooms, the discussion could be upsetting to room-mates who cannot help but overhear. Predetermine who is appropriate to attend.

Opening

The meeting is usually led by a senior physician. Every member of the family and clinical team should be introduced by name and role. The agenda is set collaboratively as described in Chapter 15. The family meeting should be normalized: 'We have these discussions with all our patients' (14). Building trust through empathic acknowledgment is crucial.

Gather information about the patient and family's perceived understanding of the illness and goals of care

- ◆ Ask open-ended questions, such as, 'I would like to check how you see the medical situation at the moment…Where do you see things heading?'. When gathering information, listen without interruption to improve rapport. In one study of family meetings, physicians talked 71% of the time and listened only 29%; more listening was correlated with higher family satisfaction (24). Listening is not an easy skill to master and may be contrary to an action-oriented medical culture. A common error seen in CST is for the physician to blurt out his or her analysis of the medical situation, before listening to the patient's understanding.

- ◆ Correct misperceptions. Having first assessed the perceived understanding of the illness and prognosis, the clinician can efficiently correct any misperceptions and educate the patient or family as necessary.

- ◆ Rule: always respond to emotions. CST should model how to address emotions empathically before moving ahead with other agenda items (25). Even experienced clinicians can fail to realize how useful reduction of emotional tension is in improving communication and problem-solving. Eight common ways of addressing emotions are outlined in Table 19.2.

Table 19.2 Eight techniques for responding to emotions in end-of-life communication

Technique	Example
1. Silence	When a person is upset, shared silence is a way of providing safety and saying, 'I understand'.
2. Normalizing/validation	'It is normal to be upset at such a difficult moment… It is understandable that you are angry after all that has happened…'
3. Empathy	'You really have had a rough time…'
4. Name or acknowledge the emotion	'You seem sad…' 'I can see that you are upset…'
5. Gesture or touch	Offering tissues to a tearful patient. Touching the patient's hand.
6. Encourage expression	'Tell me more about how you are feeling …'
7. Paraphrase and repeat back	'If I understand you correctly, you are angry because you were told that your mother's pneumonia would respond to antibiotics…'
8. Praise	'You are very brave…'

Gather specific information about wishes and thoughts regarding death and dying

The patient may have well-crystallized wishes about goals of care (e.g. place of death, DNR directives, hospice.) These views usually evolve over time as the illness progresses. They may or may not have been articulated—cultural or family taboos about discussing death may have kept them covert. Nevertheless, most patients and families are grateful when they can share these with a caring medical team. It is more parsimonious to inquire directly about wishes regarding death and dying, before stating medical recommendations for DNR or palliative care. It aids decision-making if the groundwork for the decision is already under active contemplation rather than assuming a pre-contemplative stance (26).

One strategy that is helpful here is education about palliative care as discussed in Chapter 18. To illustrate, 'What is your understanding of palliative care? …Right, it is used when the cancer cannot be cured and the aim is to maximize quality of life. This approach respects a person's wishes and dignity, so that when their time comes, they can die peacefully and naturally. How does that sound?'. Educational strategies may also be utilized to explain the lack of efficacy of CPR in patients dying of cancer as part of a discussion about DNR directives. Written material can inform families about what to expect during the dying process. A particular CST challenge is helping trainees talk openly about death and dying, rather than using euphemisms. Role-playing with video-feedback is useful to guide trainees to use terms such as 'close to death' and 'dying'.

Many people have experienced prior family deaths, which, in turn, have informed their own preferences. Useful exploratory questions include, 'Have you or anyone in the family ever faced a similar circumstance in dealing with death? What went well when your father went through home hospice? What could have gone better?'. Past experience with a trustworthy hospice service may be reassuring. Negative experiences, such as a painful death, can be used to facilitate discussion of how the dying experience might be improved. The challenge here is the difficulty of talking about past losses at a time of imminent loss. Nevertheless, approaches that build on past experiences have an intrinsic strength.

Substituted decision-making: where there is a lack of capacity to make medical decisions (e.g. the patient is unconscious), invite the family to describe who the patient is and what they would have wished for. The substituted decision by a healthcare proxy serves ethically to preserve the autonomy of an incapacitated patient. A second ethical principle is acting in the best interests of the patient (14, 15). If the patient has an advanced directive, its content is helpful at this point in the roadmap.

Make recommendations for end-of-life care including DNR directives

While respecting the spirit of shared decision-making, the physician should make a clear recommendation, so as to share the burdens and responsibilities of decision-making near the end of life. A useful strategy is offering an empiric trial of seeing what happens in the next 24 hours, and then re-evaluating. Careful reflection also highlights the gravity of end-of-life decision-making. (15, 27)

Fear and doubt are ubiquitous. Stapelton found that specific types of clinician statements were associated with greater family satisfaction:

- assurance that the patient will not be abandoned before death;
- assurance that staff will do everything to maximize patient comfort and minimize suffering; and
- clinician support for the family's decision to withdraw care (28).

After giving these three reassurances, the physician's supportive voice should be heard: 'This is a tough situation, but I think that *we* are making the most reasonable decision given the options…'. Expressing admiration for the patient's and family's strengths and praising their courage in the face of adversity are also useful techniques.

Our roadmap makes communication strategies more transparent, but any barriers to decision-making warrant careful exploration. For instance, a family may worry that they are killing their loved one. Death after a protracted illness will be a relief for some, but others will wonder how they can continue without their relative. Additionally, a patient may express apparently contradictory wishes, such as both wanting to fight and desiring a peaceful death. They may also express different wishes at different times in their illness trajectory (29).

Finalize the action-plan

The end of the meeting is an opportunity to elicit feedback on the discussion, reinforcing a collaborative approach. The discussion should be summarized and the next steps in the action plan specified. Problem-solve any specific practical issues (e.g. hospice, symptom management, spiritual needs). Parameters for the next meeting should be arranged to foster a sense of ongoing support.

Specific strategies for discussing DNR orders

The DNR discussion is not simply a matter of 'getting the form signed' but rather occurs within the broader framework of discussing goals of care, outlined in the roadmap (Table 19.1). Specific elements warrant highlighting.

Clinicians should familiarize themselves with local DNR laws and the relevant forms. This improves confidence with technical aspects of the communication. If a healthcare agent attempts to override a DNR directive signed by the patient, the physician needs the quiet confidence to explain that these laws aim to preserve the incapacitated patient's autonomy and guide caregivers and doctors in substituted decision-making. In general, neither the physician nor the family should override the patient's decision.

A DNR discussion cannot occur without patient education. Terms such as DNR, CPR and palliative care may be intuitive to clinicians, but either foreign or superficially understood by those on the receiving end. Misperceptions are frequent: 'comfort' care may be misunderstood as 'nothing more can be done' (palliative care is actually an active strategy that never ceases to ask, 'What more can be done?'). Legally, DNR laws are shaped by the informed-consent process, where education is a central element. In this respect, patient education may deal with prognosis, treatment alternatives, the low efficacy of CPR if someone is dying from advanced cancer, the human cost of inefficacious treatments at the end of life, palliative care and the centrality of determining what happens to one's own body.

This discussion should be in the spirit of collaborative decision-making and never coercively imposed (see Table 19.3 for examples of coercive reasoning in approaches 4 and 8). Nevertheless, the physician should state a clear medical opinion about DNR directives based on a careful evaluation of the clinical data. Abrogation of the DNR decision entirely to the patient or family is erroneous because the physician denies his or her medical responsibility for the dying process. In a collaborative decision-making process, offering a summary of the conversation further prevents misunderstanding.

A DNR discussion should be held as early as possible, when it is clear that treatments are no longer containing the disease, to maximize the potential for good palliative care. If you reside in a jurisdiction that mandates resuscitation unless a DNR order is in place (e.g. the state of

New York), the roadmap should be followed to achieve understanding of the disease status and the patient's wishes about the goals of care and assistance during their dying.

Conflict over end-of-life communication

Good communication involves the better handling of conflict and use of techniques described in the roadmap aimed at achieving consensus. If, despite clear, empathic communication, a conflict arises, e.g. over whether or not to implement a DNR directive, there may be advantages in respecting the family's wishes (27). Viewing end-of-life communication as a predictable and ongoing process, rather than an emergency, is an important frame of reference. Conflict resolution within this context is aided by time and patience. Other ways to address conflict include second opinions and consultation with social workers, patient representatives, palliative care, psychiatry or the institution's ethics committee, depending upon which resources are available. Consultations promote dialogue, which in turn fosters understanding and builds consensus.

Specific strategies for withdrawal of life-sustaining treatments

Rubenfeld and Crawford (27) argue that withdrawal of life-extending treatment should be carried out with the same meticulous care as for any other medical procedure and outline steps for doing so:

1. Recognize the decision that is needed to withdraw life-extending treatments.
2. Obtain informed consent.
3. Develop an explicit plan for carrying out the procedure and dealing with complications.
4. Move the patient to an appropriate setting for end-of-life care.
5. Provide adequate analgesia/sedation.
6. Carry out plan.
7. Document in medical record.
8. Evaluate outcomes and implement a quality improvement process.

Having a protocol for the withdrawal of life-extending treatment is useful because the 'stuttering withdrawal of care' could otherwise be a way to avoid uncomfortable communication with the family or the perceived linkage between the clinicians' actions and death (27, 30).

Transferring the dying patient to a private room or hospice setting, with less medical technology, is desirable on one level, but carries its own communication challenges. Although stopping electronic monitoring allows a focus on the person, rather than physiological parameters, both family and staff may struggle to forgo identification with intensive treatment modalities (27). This change may evoke abandonment anxiety. Clarification that 'the withholding of life-sustaining treatment' does not equate to 'the withdrawal of care' helps to alleviate this anxiety. Education about the rationale for these changes and what may be expected is a vital pre-emptive communication strategy (14, 31).

Care in the last hours of life is a core competency that includes attending to the grief and bereavement of the family (31). Their perception of care is an important quality indicator (32).

Specific strategies for discussing requests to die sooner

Patient's requests to die sooner should not be blocked reflexively by saying that euthanasia is illegal or not your practice. Clinicians should instead explore these statements in an empathic manner. At one end of the spectrum, such requests for hastened death may represent fluctuating existential distress, an attempt to come to terms with an impending death. At the other end, they may reflect demoralization, depression, suicidal ideation or poorly controlled pain, all of which are potentially treatable (33). As such, they are an opportunity to engage the patient in their palliative care planning (34).

Invitations such as, 'I'd like to hear more about your desire for me to help you die. Tell me what's on your mind,' are helpful to elicit the reasons for the request. More specific questions can elicit suffering: 'What is the hardest part about what you are going through?'; this can then be addressed by the physician.

End-of-life communication and health outcomes

Preliminary evidence is emerging that better communication improves health outcomes. One randomized, controlled study examined the traumatizing effect of an ICU death on the emotional health of families across 22 hospitals (35). The communication intervention consisted of structured objectives for an end-of-life meeting (Value and appreciate what family members say; Acknowledge emotions; Listen; Understand who the patient is as a person; and Elicit questions from family). The family received an educational brochure about what to expect from death and bereavement. Ninety days after the death, family members in the intervention group reported significantly lower post-traumatic symptoms and anxiety/depression scores. Better preparation for loss may reduce later symptoms of distress.

Another study examined the effect of a standardized family meeting within 72 hours of ICU admission, in which prognosis, values regarding dying and the acceptability of invasive treatments were discussed (36). A care plan was agreed upon with clear markers for success or failure. Prior to the intervention there were 0.3 meetings/patient, but afterwards a 5-fold increase occurred, which was sustained at 4-year follow-up. LOS decreased significantly by 25%, which was also sustained 4 years later.

Another study examined the impact of transferring dying patients from the ICU to a high-support medical room and found significantly reduced ICU LOS in patients with multi-organ failure and fewer clinical interventions (37). Overall, hospital LOS was similar. Similarly, an automatic, proactive ethics consultation prompted by mechanical ventilation for more than 96 hours showed significantly greater documented communication, more DNR directives, increased withdrawal of life-extending care and reduced ICU LOS (38).

In contrast, the multi-centre, multi-million dollar SUPPORT study failed to show that a dedicated nurse, who facilitated palliative care communication, increased the rate of advanced directives or reduced the rate of CPR (39). This study taught that complex problems demand multimodal solutions, including system change—the study nurse was not well-integrated into the treatment team, eliminating an effect on physician communication (40).

Barriers to end-of-life communication that can be targeted by communication skills training

Skill deficits clearly impede good end-of-life communication (41). They may further result in loss of clinical confidence, avoidance of emotionally-charged issues and inefficient decision-making. For example, one physician who was asked to 'do something more' by the distraught family of a ventilated, moribund, cancer patient, responded by ordering more chemotherapy (42).

Deficits in clinical communication may also cause iatrogenic harm to patients and their proxies (43). For instance, the mother of a dying daughter felt traumatized by the physician's repeated discussion of DNR directives: 'She hounded me day and night to sign the DNR and when I said that I was not ready, she sent in another team to harass me.' Correcting skill deficits, forms a large part of communication training. An analysis of common communication errors is presented in Table 19.3.

Table 19.3 Common mistakes in end-of-life communication and alternative approaches

Approaches to avoid	Why this approach is problematic	Alternative approaches
1. There is nothing more that can be done.	Although chemotherapy may no longer be helpful, other treatments can improve quality of life.	'Although we cannot shrink the cancer, we can improve your quality of your life. Could I discuss this with you further?'
2. He needs to gain more weight and then we can give him more chemotherapy.	Goals of care for end-of-life are deferred under the illusion that the cancer is curable. The patient is coerced to eat more and, when overwhelmed by cachexia, may be blamed for not trying hard enough. Family focus is on eating rather than palliative care.	'Your father has lost considerable weight because, despite our best treatments, the cancer has spread. Chemotherapy will not help him at this time but we have many other ways of helping so that he can be home and functional for as long as possible.'
3. If your heart stops, would YOU want us to do everything?	Cardiac arrest is disconnected from multi-organ failure, its usual association in dying cancer patients and is described as an isolated mechanical problem. Responsibility for the DNR decision is placed squarely on the patient ('you'), in contradiction to the philosophy of shared decision-making. The poor efficacy of resuscitation in end-stage cancer patients is not discussed, although in the physician's mind, implied; 'To do everything' is a euphemism for attempting CPR. The patient is unlikely to fully understand the illusion of this 'choice'.	'What do you know about CPR in general? Have you known of anyone who required CPR? What was that experience like?' (Ascertaining the patient's knowledge about CPR facilitates patient education and correction of CPR misperceptions.) 'Although CPR can help people with heart attacks who are otherwise pretty healthy, it generally causes more harm than good for people such as yourself when cancer is advanced.' (This could be followed by quiet listening for the patient's thoughts and feelings.?) 'May I share my thoughts about how useful CPR might be for you? My recommendation is that CPR would not be helpful. It will not reverse the cancer and if you survived, you would be so sick that you would have to be treated in the ICU on a breathing machine. Ultimately, it would also be counter-productive to allowing you to have a peaceful and natural death, when your time comes.'
4. If your heart were to stop, you would not want us to institute heroic measures, would you?	The opposite of heroism is cowardice. No one would want cowardly measures instituted so this question has a coercive tone. On another level, 'heroic measures' is a medical euphemism for ineffectual CPR in a dying patient. The patient may not understand this hidden meaning.	'What are your thoughts about the spread of your cancer? Do you ever think about dying?' (Talk openly about death and use the term 'dying' rather than a euphemism.)
5. His illness has progressed. His cancer is advanced.	The words 'progressed' and 'advanced' have positive connotations in our society, however, in this context, progress and advancement are medical euphemisms for dying.	'I am afraid that he has entered the dying phase of his illness.'

Table 19.3 (continued) Common mistakes in end-of-life communication and alternative approaches

Approaches to avoid	Why this approach is problematic	Alternative approaches
6. He has failed third-line treatment.	The patient should not be blamed for the failure of treatment.	'The third-line treatment did not work. This cancer is very aggressive.'
7. If I talk about end-of-life planning, the patient will give up hope.	There is no evidence that talking realistically about death results in loss of hope, provided that the patient is open to this discussion. It is more likely that talking about it will allow the patient to prepare and feel more supported. By contrast, not talking about dying causes a 'conspiracy of silence', often resulting in isolation and demoralization.	'Now that your cancer has progressed, it is important for us to consider what you can hope for, besides a cure.'
8. CPR is likely to result in them pounding on your chest to restart your heart. They could crack your ribs. Then they would shove a big plastic tube down your throat.	This approach is coercive, traumatizing and not in the spirit of shared-decision making or patient-centered care.	'CPR was not designed for dying patients and will not extend your life. It will more likely prolong your suffering and interfere with our goal of a peaceful death.'
9. This patient is in denial.	Labelling patients as being 'in denial' sets them up as adversaries who must be convinced of imminent death. This erodes trust, making decision-making more complicated.	'What is your understanding of your cancer? Where do you see things going? Have you given thought to what might happen if things don't go in that direction?' The clinician approaches decision-making as a process of discovery that will evolve over time.

Knowledge deficits, whether on the side of the physician or the patient, can seriously impede end-of-life communication. The patient refusing a palliative intervention may not understand the goals of care. S/he may have lacked prior exposure to hospice or have been shielded from the experience of death. Using a stages-of-change model, the pre-contemplative person may particularly benefit from learning about palliative care (26). Watching an educational DVD on hospice care may serve to demystify dying and facilitate the process of decision-making. Physicians may also benefit from an educational approach.

The clinician's emotional reaction to end-of-life communication can also present a barrier to palliative care communication and patient care (41, 43). To illustrate, an attending physician may think, 'There is nothing that I can offer this patient,' and feel sad. As a consequence s/he may avoid visiting the patient, sending a junior staff member instead. Communication training could reframe this distorted belief by helping the learner to explore alternative ways of looking at the dilemma. The physician might be invited to reflect on ways to help the patient besides curing the cancer—the patient might be grateful for good palliative care and the family appreciative, if the death was peaceful.

Discussion of death and dying in the real world or in training programmes can be a painful reminder of the clinician's own losses and this can, in turn, influence communication, often in subtle ways. Communication training, if properly carried out, can be a safe environment for personal reflection and growth. One training programme has been designed to focus primarily on the clinician's emotional reaction to improve cancer communication (44). Similarly, mindfulness may help overcome barriers as a thoughtful being is hypothesized to be more teachable (44).

Standardized role-play scenarios

Role plays are tailored to the learner's clinical setting. Table 19.4 presents a role-play scenario where a physician is asked to talk to the family of an incapacitated cancer patient about end-of-life goals of care and the utility of a DNR directive. When constructing a role-play scenario, a more detailed version is created for the simulated patient. This can contain prompts to test the learner's response to various challenges. Examples of such prompts are:

- ◆ A very ill patient becomes visibly upset and does not say anything for 20 seconds.
- ◆ The patient asks: 'Isn't there anything more that you can do?'.
- ◆ The patient asks: 'How much time do I have left?'.

In each instance, the clinician's empathy and exploratory abilities are practiced with statements such as 'I wish there was more I could do' (20).

Table 19.4 An example of a content-focussed standardized role-play scenario

	Family meeting: Discussing DNR directives in the setting of palliative goals of care
Patient	Mary Carpenter (ventilated in ICU)
Daughter (healthcare proxy)	Regina Davies
Son-in-law	Henry Davies
Overview	Meeting with family, one of whom is the healthcare proxy, of a ventilated patient who is dying in an ICU from a refractory, metastatic solid tumor. The physician's task is to speak to the family about DNR directives and appropriate goals of care.
Scenario	Mrs Carpenter, aged 77 years, a widow and retired personal assistant with widely metastatic stomach cancer has continued to deteriorate despite several treatment regimens. She now has brain metastases. She underwent surgery three weeks previously for ischaemic bowel with multiple complications including sepsis and shock. She has been on vasopressor support and ventilated in the ICU since surgery. She is now in anuric renal failure and you must make a decision regarding continuous renal replacement therapy (CRRT). You have conferred with your colleagues. Her MPM prognostic score is 98.4%. It seems likely that she will die within days. Yesterday, you met with the family to talk about the altered prognosis and end-of-life goals of care. Today, Mrs Carpenter's condition continues to worsen. Your task is to now talk to the family about DNR, not initiating CRRT and capping care at the present level as part of changing the focus of care towards a peaceful death.

Conclusion

Attempts to integrate patient-centred CST into real-world settings, thereby improving health outcomes, are gaining momentum (13). Investing in such training and research is important, because better communication may lead to improved palliative care outcomes.

There are limitations to the current research literature. Firstly, there is a paucity of rigorous, randomized, controlled trials, in part because of the expense and sophistication needed to mount such studies (46). Secondly, complex problems require multifaceted interventions which, in turn, create difficulty measuring cause and effect. The challenge facing end-of-life CST is to move beyond the lessons learned from the SUPPORT study and continue to design, test and disseminate multifaceted interventions.

References

1. Weissman DE, Ambuel B, von Gunten CF, *et al.* (2007). Outcomes from a national multispecialty palliative care curriculum development project. *J Palliat Med* **10**, 408–19.

2. Robinson K, Sutton S, von Gunten CF, *et al.* (2004). Assessment of the Education for Physicians on End-of-Life Care (EPEC) Project. *J Palliat Med* **7**, 637–45.

3. Vitelli C, Cooper K, Rogatko A, *et al.* (1991). Cardiopulmonary resuscitation and the patient with cancer. *J Clin Oncol* **9**, 111.

4. Wallace SK, Ewer MS, Price KJ, *et al.* (2002). Outcome and cost implications of cardiopulmonary resuscitation in the medical intensive care unit of a comprehensive cancer centre. *Support Care Cancer* **10**, 425–9.

5. Reisfield GM, Wallace SK, Munsell MF, *et al.* (2006). Survival in cancer patients undergoing in-hospital cardiopulmonary resuscitation: a meta-analysis. *Resuscitation* **71**, 152–60.

6. Levin TT, Li Y, Weiner JS, Lewis F, Bartell A, Piercy J, Kissane DW (2008). How do-not-resuscitate orders are utilized in cancer patients: timing relative to death and communication-training implications. *Palliat Support Care* 6(4):341-8.

7. Angus DC, Barnato AE, Linde-Zwirble WT, *et al.* (2004). Use of intensive care at the end of life in the United States: an epidemiologic study. *Crit Care Med* **32**, 638–43.

8. Prendergast TJ, Luce JM (1997). Increasing incidence of withholding and withdrawal of life support from the critically ill. *Am J Respir Crit Care Med* **155**, 15–20.

9. Prendergast TJ, Luce JM (1997). Increasing incidence of withholding and withdrawal of life support from the critically ill. *Am J Respir Crit Care Med* **155**, 15–20.

10. Mularski RA, Curtis JR, Billings JA, *et al.* (2006). Proposed quality measures for palliative care in the critically ill: a consensus from the Robert Wood Johnson Foundation Critical Care Workgroup. *Crit Care Med* **34**, S404–11.

11. Curtis JR, Engelberg RA (2006). Measuring success of interventions to improve the quality of end-of-life care in the intensive care unit. *Crit Care Med* **34**, S341–7.

12. von Gunten CF (2007). Culture eats strategy for lunch. *J Palliat Med* **10**, 1002.

13. Epstein RM, Street RL, Jr (2007). *Patient-Centred Communication in Cancer Care: Promoting Healing and Reducing Suffering.* National Cancer Institute, Bethesda, MD.

14. Curtis JR (2004). Communicating about end-of-life care with patients and families in the intensive care unit. *Crit Care Clin* **20**, 363–80, viii.

15. Prendergast TJ, Puntillo KA (2002). Withdrawal of life support: intensive caring at the end of life. *JAMA* **288**, 2732–40.

16. Rait D, Lederberg MS (1989). The family of the cancer patient. In: Holland JC, Rowland JH, eds. *Handbook of Psychooncology. Psychological Care of the Patient with Cancer,* pp.585–97. Oxford University Press, New York.

17. von Gunten CF, Weissman DE (2002). Discussing do-not-resuscitate orders in the hospital setting: part 1. *J Palliat Med* **5**, 415–7.

18. von Gunten CF, Weissman DE (2002). Discussing do-not-resuscitate orders in the hospital setting: part 2. *J Palliat Med* **5**, 417–8.

19. Baile WF, Buckman R, Lenzi RR, *et al.* (2000). SPIKES-A six-step protocol for delivering bad news: application to the patient with cancer. *Oncologist* **5**, 302–11.

20. Back AL, Arnold RM, Baile WF, *et al.* (2007). Efficacy of communication skills training for giving bad news and discussing transitions to palliative care. *Arch Int Med* **167**, 453–60.

21. Lorin S, Rho L, Wisnivesky JP, *et al.* (2006). Improving medical student intensive care unit communication skills: a novel educational initiative using standardized family members. *Crit Care Med* **34**, 2386–91.

22. Curtis JR, Engelberg RA, Wenrich MD, *et al.* (2002). Studying communication about end-of-life care during the ICU family conference: development of a framework. *J Crit Care* **17**, 147–60.

23. Levin TT, Brown R, Bylund C, *et al.* (2007). *Shared Decision-Making About DNR Orders.* Comskil Laboratory, Memorial Sloan–Kettering Cancer Centre, New York.

24. McDonagh JR, Elliott TB, Engelberg RA, *et al.* (2004). Family satisfaction with family conferences about end-of-life care in the intensive care unit: increased proportion of family speech is associated with increased satisfaction. *Crit Care Med* **32**, 1484–8.

25. Cohen-Cole S (1991). *The Medical Interview: the Three-Function Approach.* Mosby, St. Louis: CV.

26. Prochaska J, DiClemente C (1992). Stages of change in the modification of problem behaviors. *Prog Behav Modif* **28**, 183–218.

27. Rubenfeld GD, Crawford SW (2001). Principles and practice of withdrawing life-sustaining treatment in the ICU. In: Curtis JR, Rubenfeld GD, eds. *Managing Death in the ICU: the Transition from Cure to Comfort.* Oxford University Press, New York.

28. Stapleton RD, Engelberg RA, Wenrich MD, *et al.* (2006). Clinician statements and family satisfaction with family conferences in the intensive care unit. *Crit Care Med* **34**, 1679–85.

29. Hsieh HF, Shannon SE, Curtis JR (2006). Contradictions and communication strategies during end-of-life decision making in the intensive care unit. *J Crit Care* **21**, 294–304.

30. Gianakos D (1995). Terminal weaning. *Chest* **108**, 1405–6.

31. Ferris FD, von Gunten CF, Emanuel LL (2003). Competency in end-of-life care: last hours of life. *J Palliat Med* **6**, 605–13.

32. Teno JM (2005). Measuring end-of-life care outcomes retrospectively. *J Palliat Med* **8**(Suppl 1), S42–9.

33. Hudson PL, Schofield P, Kelly B, *et al.* (2006). Responding to desire to die statements from patients with advanced disease: recommendations for health professionals. *Palliat Med* **20**, 703–10.

34. Back AL, Starks H, Hsu C, *et al.* (2002). Clinician–patient interactions about requests for physician-assisted suicide: a patient and family view. *Arch Int Med* **162**, 1257–65.

35. Lautrette A, Darmon M, Megarbane B, *et al.* (2007). A communication strategy and brochure for relatives of patients dying in the ICU. *New Engl J Med* **356**, 469–78.

36. Lilly CM, Sonna LA, Haley KJ, *et al.* (2003). Intensive communication: four-year follow-up from a clinical practice study. *Crit Care Med* **31**(5 Suppl), S394–9.

37. Field BE, Devich LE, Carlson RW (1998). Impact of a comprehensive supportive care team on management of hopelessly ill patients with multiple organ failure. *Chest* **96**, 353–6.

38. Dowdy MD, Robertson C, Bander JA (1998). A study of proactive ethics consultation for critically and terminally ill patients with extended lengths of stay. *Crit Care Med* **26**, 252–9.

39. Teno J, Lynn J, Wenger N, *et al.* (1997). Advance directives for seriously ill hospitalized patients: effectiveness with the patient self-determination act and the SUPPORT intervention. SUPPORT Investigators. Study to Understand Prognoses and Preferences for Outcomes and Risks of Treatment. *J Am Geriat Soc* **45**, 500–7.

40. Teno JM (1999). Lessons learned and not learned from the SUPPORT project. *Palliat Med* **13**, 91–3.

41. Weiner JS, Cole SA (2004). ACare: a communication training program for shared decision making along a life-limiting illness. *Pall Support Care* **2**, 231.

42. Kissane DW (2007) A case of a dying patient ordered chemotherapy in the ICU. Personal communication. New York.

43. Weiner JS, Roth J (2006). Avoiding iatrogenic harm to patient and family while discussing goals of care near the end of life. *J Palliat Med* **9**, 451–63.

44. Favre N, Despland JN, de Roten Y, *et al.* (2007). Psychodynamic aspects of communication skills training: a pilot study. *Support Care Cancer* **15**, 333–7.

45. Zoppi KK, Epstein RM (2002). Is communication a skill? Communication behaviors and being in relation. *Family Med* **34**, 319–24.

46. Weiner JS, Arnold RM, Curtis JR, *et al.* (2006). Manualized communication interventions to enhance palliative care research and training: rigorous, testable approaches. *J Palliat Med* **9**, 371–81.

Section C

A specialty curriculum for oncology

Section editor: Phyllis N Butow

This section expands on the core curriculum through the addition of important elective topics and a range of special issues that arise in cancer and palliative care. Whether in the use of the internet or unproven therapies, the communication of genetic risk, the effects of reconstructive surgeries or enrolment in clinical trials, the practice of oncology brings unique challenges. Careful attention is needed to culture and ethnicity, as well as a willing openness to discuss all the potential outcomes of anti-cancer treatments, such as their impact on sexuality and fertility. Herein we present the state of the science in grappling with these more technical communication challenges.

Chapter 20

Enrolment in clinical trials

Richard Brown and Terrance L Albrecht

Introduction

Despite recent advances, the 5-year survival rates for many cancers remains low, and there is a continued need for research to improve cancer outcomes. Clinical trials represent the gold-standard approach to providing evidence for advances in treatment. Clinical trials are research studies designed to improve cancer prevention, diagnosis, treatment and survivorship. This research base necessarily involves enroling cancer patients and others (e.g. family members for genetic linkage studies, healthy community volunteers to serve as matched controls) into clinical trials.

As with any research enterprise, patients and others voluntarily enrol and maintain their status as participants in these trials. Unfortunately, many medical and surgical oncology trials have insufficient accrual rates, a problem that has plagued the implementation of clinical trials for many years. Low accrual severely hinders progress in cancer prevention and treatment (1–3).

The goal of this chapter is to outline issues involved in recruitment to clinical trials, to describe the ethical principles underlying informed consent and to provide suggested strategies to aid communication between healthcare providers and patients about clinical trials.

Types of cancer clinical trials

According to the US National Cancer Institute, cancer clinical trials are generally categorized into one of the following phases of research:

- Phase I trials are initial studies with humans that usually enrol limited numbers of people. Their main purpose is to evaluate dosage safety, and the frequency and method by which new drugs should be administered (e.g. either orally, or by injection into the bloodstream or muscle).

- Phase II trials are designed to further evaluate drug and dosage safety and to begin assessing the impact of drugs in treating specific types of cancer.

- Phase III trials test new drugs, new drug combinations or new surgical procedures by comparing them against current standards of care. A participant will usually be randomly assigned to the standard (control) group or the new treatment group. Phase III trials often require, by design, large numbers of enrolees and data may be collected at multiple clinical sites across a nation and abroad (4).

Accrual to clinical trials

Patients are typically offered the opportunity to enrol in a clinical trial as a treatment option by their oncologists. The base rate of accrual at a cancer centre depends on the number of trials available to eligible patients at a given point in time. As noted above, low accrual rates have been reported in the literature and can be attributed to many factors, including the communication process that occurs when oncologists talk to patients (and families or companions, if present) about joining clinical trials (1, 3, 5). Albrecht and colleagues suggest from their data at two cancer centres that low rates may be partially due to the extent to which physicians do, and do not, explicitly offer trials to their patients, and, in turn, are partially due to the extent to which patients understand that they have, or have not, been offered enrolment in a trial.

The challenge to physicians lies in the multiple, and sometimes conflicting, communication goals they face in communicating with patients and their families/companions in the outpatient clinic setting. Physicians must establish relational trust in the encounter, provide high-quality care, ensure that patients are sufficiently informed to authentically provide 'informed consent' or 'informed refusal' in making treatment choices and enrol patients in clinical trials (accrual rates are actually performance measures for physicians at some institutions). Through this process, physicians are mandated to honour ethical and scientific principles of neutrality and full disclosure to protect their patients (6). This is a tall order; the full range of ethical concerns associated with clinical trials is described below.

Ethical concerns

Beneficence and the move from paternalism

These two concepts of beneficence and paternalism became linked in the *Corpus Hippocraticum*, with the doctors of ancient Greece undertaking to 'come for the benefit of the sick, remaining free of all intentional injustice and of all mischief', while at the same time withholding the patient's diagnosis and prognosis, and diverting the patient's attention away from the illness and treatment. (7). The notion of beneficent paternalism persisted in the medical tradition through to the eighteenth century when philosopher/physicians attempted to regulate professional conduct by formulating and publishing codes of conduct aimed at establishing medicine in an ethical framework (8).

The principle of beneficence remains a fundamental ethical principle guiding medical practice; however, the traditional paternalistic role of the doctor has become increasingly unacceptable in the light of changes in patient attitudes towards medical practice in the late-twentieth century. Individuals no longer presume that the doctor knows best and many prefer an approach that involves greater patient involvement in decision-making and respect for individual autonomy. An examination of trends in physician behaviour over four decades suggests that physicians have shifted away from paternalistic styles, characterized by withholding information from patients about their prognosis, diagnosis and treatment options in the belief that such information would be beyond patients' comprehension and cause them excessive fear, anxiety and loss of hope, thus worsening patient outcomes (9). Contemporary medical practitioners acknowledge the importance of providing accurate information to patients (9). Various reasons have been offered to account for this shift, including an increased fear of litigation among physicians, legal requirements and the publication of guidelines for the disclosure of diagnoses (10), and an improvement in therapies for cancer patients through technological advancement. Importantly, the law has been vital in promoting the concept of informed consent to standard and experimental treatments (11).

Active participation in the consultation requires negotiation between the physician and the patient that is discouraged by the traditional paternalistic model. Patients are now seeking information to enable them to make decisions about treatment options, to understand prognostic issues and to be clear about treatment side-effects.

Autonomy

Autonomy in general refers to the individual's right to self-determination. According to Faden and Beauchamp (7), an individual acts autonomously if three conditions are satisfied, i.e. the individual acts:

+ intentionally (in accordance with a plan or one's inner knowledge);
+ with understanding; and
+ free from controlling influences.

The autonomy of an individual must be differentiated from autonomous actions, as to choose to act in a non-autonomous fashion; for example, transferring decision-making to a third party can form part of an individual's autonomy (8).

The extreme view of patient autonomy suggests that patients make their own decision about treatment, while the doctor adopts a passive role. A more reasonable view argues in favour of the physician who inquires about the patient's preferences and values, thus developing an understanding of the patient as a person, before a treatment decision is reached that maximizes the patient's treatment goals (12).

In the experimental context, particularly the case of the randomized clinical trial, Kodish *et al.* argue that patient autonomy can only be ensured if the patient is 'free to choose any therapy which they might have received by participating in the RCT and is equally free to choose the randomization alternative' (13). Moreover, they emphasize the right of a patient to make the choice to refuse any treatment, even when a treatment is proven, as an essential component of autonomous decision-making (13). However, this is a perspective that may overvalue patient autonomy and is clearly at odds with current medical practice. That is, for ethical reasons, patients are currently offered experimental treatments only on trial. And, in serious illnesses such as cancer, the possibility of taking the 'no treatment' option may be discussed; however, the treating doctor often actively discourages this option.

Equipoise

Individual equipoise

Equipoise is defined as the point at which a rational and well-informed person has no preference between two (or more) available treatment options (14). Thus, a physician who is convinced that one treatment option offers a better possibility of benefit for his/her patients than another, cannot ethically recommend random allocation as a means of making a treatment choice. The potential benefit to the patient must be the paramount consideration in the treatment decision. On the other hand, if the physician is uncertain about the difference in potential benefit between two (or more) treatments offered in a clinical trial, it is ethically acceptable to defer control of the treatment decision to the randomization process (15). However, the practical application of equipoise as a means of justifying the selection of randomization, as an ethical means of making treatment decisions, remains controversial.

Equipoise has also been named the 'uncertainty principle', reflecting the prominence of the physician's inability to choose (based on lack of evidence) between comparative treatment benefits. Critics of equipoise question the degree of uncertainty physicians apply to the process of choosing between known and experimental treatments, and recent articles have added qualifiers such as 'reasonably', 'substantially' and 'genuinely' to uncertainty to try and further describe the physician's belief about the treatment options. However, this raises the question of who decides what counts as reasonable or substantial uncertainty (16). This seems largely left to the conscience of the physician.

Collective equipoise

Clearly, from the physician's perspective, reaching individual equipoise, weighing up uncertainty, is a difficult process. However, another level of complexity is added by the introduction of the concept of collective equipoise. According to Chard *et al.* (16) collective equipoise relates to the uncertainty of a profession as a whole, about a particular treatment modality. While individual equipoise may not be achieved (i.e. there is a preference for a particular treatment), this is balanced by others in the profession holding the opposing view (a preference for the alternate treatment). Thus, overall the profession is in collective or clinical equipoise. Clinical equipoise recognizes that it is the community of physicians that establishes best practice standards and not the individual physician (17).

Supporters of the primacy of collective equipoise have suggested that in a case where clinical equipoise exists, a randomized controlled trial is an ethical imperative to avoid retaining ineffective modes of treatment. In this situation, collective equipoise should override the physician's individual equipoise; thus, even if the physician has a preference for a particular treatment (of those being compared), s/he would be expected to recruit patients to the trial (17). Conversely, while clinical equipoise appears to offer a neat solution for the physician committed to research but conflicted by degrees of clinical uncertainty, there are a number of compelling arguments suggesting that equipoise is inherently unethical as a justification for randomized trials. Enkin (18) and others point out that, if moral authority is granted to the medical community as a whole, the individual responsibility of physicians is devalued and the needs of the patient for guidance are overlooked (19). While the medical community may be certain about the effectiveness of a treatment at one time, this certainty can change and the preferences of individuals do count. In addition, clinical equipoise may pose a threat to the transparency of the doctor–patient relationship (16). If the physician is participating in a trial justified by collective equipoise and does not disclose a particular treatment preference, then a basic ethical tenet has been violated (20). Again, this poses a dilemma for the physician who must balance his/her clinical opinion, enthusiasm for research, the weight of clinical uncertainty and the best interest of the patient, in order to make an ethical treatment recommendation.

Justice

The ethical principle of justice refers, in the current context, to the application of rules of fairness and equality to the clinical trial process. This can be realized as:

- fairness in the distribution of the harm and benefit of trial treatments; and
- equitable criteria for the inclusion of potential trial participants.

In the first instance it is argued that injustices occur when individuals are advantaged through medical research at the expense of others (21). Marquis (22) clarifies this point in noting that few would condone a society in which people are sacrificed for their functioning organs in order to benefit the needs of the society in general. However, ethical conflicts can arise and ethical principles surrounding individual versus social benefit need to be recognized and balanced. Trial patients (particularly those participating in Phase I studies) are commonly treated with promising new treatments that are not guaranteed to provide any personal benefit but which may benefit others in the future. The crucial difference between Marquis' example and the plight of trial patients, is that trial patients are routinely informed of the uncertainty of treatment benefit prior to trial entry; thus, gaining informed consent guards against such an ethical problem. However, as the quality of information provision about trials is variable and as patients can misunderstand this information, it is possible to question the validity of the safeguard of informed consent.

Informed consent

Informed consent can be defined as an autonomous action taken by a patient giving permission for a doctor to undertake a medical plan (23). Informed consent became part of United States law in 1914 (23). However, while this legal instruction instituted patient authorization as part of the treatment process, it did not define the nature of the information that should be provided to the patient about their illness or possible treatments.

Gert *et al.* (24) provide a considered view of the bioethics of the consent process (both for clinical trials and standard treatments). They differentiate between the moral rules governing this situation, which are more or less compulsory and governable by law (including provision of adequate information, lack of coercion and assessment of patients' competence to make a choice), and moral ideals, to which doctors aspire but cannot necessarily fulfil in all instances; for example, providing information about alternative treatments in a way that does not over-emphasize the attractiveness of one or belittle another. The consent process involves the doctor presenting information to the patient about their illness and the options for treatment, and making an appraisal about the patient's response to the information, including the degree to which the patient understands the information provided (24). The rationale underlying the doctrine of informed consent is to protect patient autonomy and to ensure that patients have an active role in making treatment decisions (23, 25).

Barriers to recruitment

Physician barriers

Gaining informed consent to clinical trials is problematic for doctors. Many doctors experience problems initiating clinical-trial discussions and find the dual roles of caring physician and experimenter difficult to resolve (26). Prospective studies have reported that 70–80% of non-accrual is attributable to the doctor (27, 28). Doctors' reasons for not accruing patients to trials include concerns over:

- damaging the doctor–patient relationship;
- acknowledging the uncertainty of treatment benefits; and
- practical issues, such as rigid protocol designs, patient inconvenience and extra work for physicians (3, 29).

These results suggest that efforts to improve doctors' participation in clinical trials need to address communication difficulties experienced by doctors when recruiting patients to trials.

Patient barriers

Many eligible patients who are invited to participate in a trial, decline (though estimates widely vary from 23 to 50%) (28). Reasons for trial refusal by eligible patients include concerns regarding experimentation, and uncertainty and loss of control over treatment decisions (29). Many patients, and the general community, do not understand the role of randomization in avoiding bias in treatment selection (30). Other barriers have been identified as objections to being an experimental subject (31), race, gender and lack of knowledge of the requirements of trial participation (32) and the possibility of receiving a placebo.

Improving the recruitment process of patients to clinical trials

Physician communication

Patients' decisions about enrolling in trials are affected by *what* physicians tell them about the clinical trial and *how* physicians tell them the information. Content messages are what physicians tell patients about the trial. These include legally proscribed aspects of the study protocol (essentially the information on the consent document), and the potential adverse effects (side-effects) that the patient is likely to experience from the drug therapies. Albrecht and colleagues have added three additional types of content messages that they have found important for patient understanding of clinical trials. These include messages of reassurance and support, specifically regarding the patient's experience of each potential side-effect, reassurance and support regarding the patient's decision to enrol in the clinical trial (whether he/she decides for or against enrolment) and discussion regarding the benefits and drawbacks of clinical trial participation.

Finally, perhaps the most important content message from the physician is to recommend to a patient that he/she enrol in a trial. Such recommendations do influence patients' decisions (33). In observing clinical offers, Eggly and colleagues have shown that most physicians do recommend the trials that they are offering to their patients. Indeed, in contrast to the equipoise principle, many do so in a directive, not a general, manner, such as saying, 'I recommend this trial for you' as opposed to saying 'I recommend this trial'.

The patient's perspective: improving the decision process

From the patient's perspective, the decision of whether to enrol in a clinical trial is complicated by the reasons used to arrive at the conclusion, and the affective and cognitive aspects of the decision as it is made, and afterwards. Reasons for the decision made (and the relative weight given to each) vary widely and include personal factors (perceived quality of life, length of survival), family members and significant others' opinions, perceptions of the potential side-effects and whether they seem manageable, and perceptions of the financial costs (related to coverage and out-of-pocket) involved in enrolling in the trial. Physician communication behaviours also factor in to patients' judgments, especially how well they seemed to listen and answer questions, how the patient perceived the way the physician interacted with his/her family/companions, and how well explanations were given and the level of empathic support provided.

Cognitive and affective aspects of the decision involve the degree to which the patient is confident in the decision he/she is making, the extent of agreement shared with the physician and family/companions regarding the nature of the decision, and the level of positive relational affect perceived with the physician, and the family/companion as they face the decision and the treatment process together (34).

Communication about clinical trials

The development of communication skills training has been suggested as a promising way forward to aid clinicians in the difficult task of clinical trial recruitment. Brown *et al.*, in a series of articles, have developed and pilot-tested an informed consent communication skills workshop. The results of this programme of research revealed four areas where communication training could aid physician–patient communication (5, 35, 36). These included:

- shared decision-making strategies;
- the sequence of moves in the consultation;
- the type and clarity of the information provided; and
- disclosure of controversial information and coercion.

These themes reflect the clinical judgment and theoretical perspectives of linguists, psycho-oncologists, ethicists and oncologists involved in the analysis.

Shared decision-making strategies

Participation in treatment decision-making, at the patient's preferred level of involvement, was identified as an essential component of seeking informed consent to the clinical trial. Shared decision-making promotes:

- autonomy in making treatment choices; and
- positive psychological outcomes for the patient once a decision has been reached (37).

Fourteen strategies contributing to a collaborative decision-making framework were identified. They are summarised in Box 20.1.

Importantly, language that portrays the patient as an active agent in the process of deciding about, and enacting, their own healthcare, encourages the sense of an autonomous self among patients. Grades of agency occur; the most active participant is portrayed as the doer, decider. The least active participant is portrayed as the person or object 'done to' (the one who is treated, told, organized).

Sequence of moves in the consultation

The analysis led to an understanding of the importance of sequence in the interaction. Thus, the consultation data were categorized into a series of phases, and an ideal sequence of these phases was identified. This model was developed to promote patient understanding of information, to ensure equal weight was given to the discussion of standard and experimental treatments, and to avoid potential coercion (see Fig. 20.1)

Bearings

The first phase, Bearings, ensures that the doctor and patient have a shared understanding of the patient's illness. If this is not established, further discussion can be at cross-purposes.

Box 20.1 Strategies for doctors to encourage collaborative decision making

- Introduce joint decision-making process.
- Use language that realizes and reflects patient autonomy.
- Check preferred decision-making style (involved or not).
- Check information preferences of patient.
- Invite questions and comments.
- Check medical knowledge of patient.
- Check patient understanding.
- Explicitly offer choice of treatment.
- Acknowledge uncertainty of treatment benefits.
- Declare professional recommendation.
- Provide opportunity for amplification of patient voice.
- Provide time and opportunity to discuss patient concerns in detail.
- Offer decision delay.
- Offer ongoing decision support/ answers to future questions.

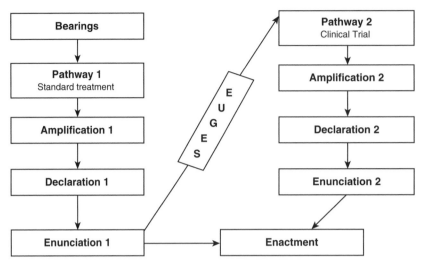

Fig. 20.1 The recommended sequence of moves.

Pathway 1

The next phase, Pathway 1 (the discussion of standard treatment), should be discussed in enough detail for the patient to be clear about the standard treatment available off the trial. It was considered essential to provide a description (if applicable) of the range of standard treatments available; including their potential benefits, side-effects and appropriateness.

Amplification 1

There are three components that occur after an explanation has been provided. First, Amplification 1 involves giving the patient an opportunity to express their reactions to the treatment options presented, if they have not already done so—what it will mean for them in their own individual circumstances—and to begin to weigh up the benefits and costs of each of these.

Declaration 1

Second, within this model the doctor should make their treatment recommendation explicit because, if it is implicit, then it is more likely to be coercive. This does not disallow patient choice. Rather it clarifies which option the doctor thinks is optimal, with an opportunity provided for the patient to declare their view also.

Enunciation 1

This is a move in which the patient articulates their decision, not merely accedes to/agrees to the doctor's framing of a decision. It is important that the decision is actually voiced, firstly, to enhance patient autonomy and, secondly, to provide an opportunity for the doctor to assess whether or not to move on to a discussion of a clinical trial.

Segue

It is also important before moving to Pathway 2 (the discussion of a clinical trial) to acknowledge that the trial is another treatment option that will add a further level of complexity to the discussion and gain the patient's agreement to move on to that phase. This phase is called the Segue. If this phase is not included, the patient can become overwhelmed and confused about the standard and clinical trial options.

Pathway 2

During Pathway 2, the clinical trial is presented as another treatment option, which compares the standard treatment against an experimental treatment. It is important to clearly delineate that the treatment choice is between receiving standard treatment and treatment on trial. A general explanation of trials, including a description of the rationale for clinical trials, usefully precedes a detailed explanation of the current trial on offer. This explanation can include a description of the ethical rationale for the trial, including equipoise, beneficence, non-maleficence and issues of justice and autonomy. The patient then has a framework that may make it easier to subsequently consider the advantages and disadvantages of the specific trial.

Amplification 2

Amplification 2 provides an opportunity for patients to talk about their attitudes towards, and understanding of, clinical trials, based on their own or others' experience.

Declaration 2

During Declaration 2, the doctor can emphasize that the patient's choice will not influence his or her relationship with the doctor and other staff or their medical care, and also that the patient can withdraw from the trial at any time. As in Declaration 1, it is important that the doctor makes a treatment recommendation, which may be that both standard treatment and treatment on the trial are acceptable options, with the trial from the doctor's view, having the added advantage of contributing to knowledge. This is an important step, in order to make explicit, rather than leave covert, the doctor's view.

Enunciation 2

Finally, in Enunciation 2 the patient is given an opportunity to declare their decision about participation in a clinical trial. Again, this may involve a choice to defer the decision to a subsequent consultation.

Enactment

After all that has been achieved, the doctor needs to implement the decision or describe the next steps; this is called Enactment. The logistics of the decision are then set out and the implementation is begun.

Type and clarity of information

Within Pathways 1 and 2, a number of facts need to be communicated in order for the patients to give ethical informed consent. However, merely including these facts will not necessarily ensure understanding. The fullness and clarity of the explanation needs also to be considered. Intervention studies designed to facilitate understanding of complex information in medical consultations have identified a number of useful strategies to ensure clarity including: avoiding jargon, and repeating and summarizing information (38, 39).

Disclosure and coercion

It is clear from audio-tape analysis of consultations in which consent is sought, that some issues are commonly not disclosed to patients (7). These include:

- that in many instances the participating doctors may be investigators on the trial and thus have a potential conflict or duality of interest;

+ the accessibility of trial treatments after the trial has ceased;
+ the availability of other potentially suitable trials.

It is not known whether disclosure of such information is ethically required or rather would need-lessly complicate the consent interview and overwhelm the patient.

Words used by doctors, who may be quite unaware of their ramifications, may encourage or perhaps coerce patients into participating in clinical trials. These are outlined below.

Doctor preferences

If the doctor does not state explicitly their views on clinical trial participation, while acknowledging patient choice, patients may feel unspoken pressure to participate. Preferences may be covertly suggested in many ways; for example, by spending more time talking about the trial treatment versus standard treatment, by minimizing versus maximizing side-effects and/or benefits of one or other treatment, or by differential use of agency (patient active in one treatment, passive in the other) and proximity (patient will be part of the team if they join the trial, or offered standard treatment). Another subtle example of this is where probabilities are presented as group statistics in one treatment and as personalized in another. For example, 'most patients will lose their hair on this treatment' (group) versus 'it is most likely that you will lose your hair on this treatment' (personalized). Subtle differences such as these may influence patient decisions.

Terms

Doctors commonly use the term 'you are eligible for this trial'. This phrase, however, can imply that the patient is 'lucky' to have been selected, or should be hopeful that their disease status allows them to participate in the trial. We suggest using the phrase 'the trial is suitable for you'. This is a subtle yet powerful delineation. Making it clear that a trial is 'suitable' for the patient objectifies the trial and does not imply the patient should aim to meet a set of criteria.

Appealing to altruism

A common motivation for patients to enter clinical trials is a sense of making a contribution to medical knowledge that will benefit others, or altruism. Finding the balance between recognizing and appreciating patient altruism, and using it in a coercive fashion, can be difficult. Once again, the terms used can make a difference. Thus the use of terms such as '*You* can benefit future generations' is perhaps more coercive than 'This will help us find the answer to this question'.

Framing

Coercion may also occur when the potential value of a clinical trial treatment is presented with a positive frame versus negative framing for the standard treatment (or visa versa). Patient preferences for framing of prognostic information should be negotiated. Research suggests that some patients prefer positively framed information ('you have a 70% chance of cure'), as this encourages a positive outlook, while others prefer negatively framed information ('you have a 30% chance of the cancer coming back'), as this emphasises the importance of additional treatment.

Summary and conclusions

Seeking informed consent to cancer clinical trials presents a significant communication challenge for oncologists and patients. Improving this communication may lead to increased accrual to clinical trials. Strategies aimed to aid this communication focus on four areas designed to ensure a transparent dialogue, underpinned by ethical informed consent and free from coercion.

The authors continue to pursue research agendas that explore gaps in communication about clinical trials and factors that effect decision-making about clinical trials. In addition, the authors are evaluating the utility of interventions that aid both physicians and patients in

---

Box 20.2 Scenario for communication skills training

Beth Robinson – Colon Medical

Shared Decision Making

Character history

Beth Robinson, 44, lives in Westchester with her husband Mark, and four kids: Josh, 15, twins Caroline and Matthew, 11, and Samuel, 9. Mark is an executive vice-president at a Madison Avenue advertising agency. Beth used to work in public relations, but quit working full-time after the twins were born. When Samuel started kindergarten four years ago, Beth began working part-time as a special events coordinator for the Mayor's Office in Scarsdale.

Beth's mother lives about an hour away, and Mark's parents and his brother and his family live in New Jersey. They are a fairly close, extended family; the grandparents attend the kids' baseball and soccer games, music concerts, and the family usually celebrates holidays together.

Disease history

Due to family history (Beth's father died of colon cancer), Beth has been having regular colonoscopies since the age of 40. Her last colonoscopy was normal. Over the past two months, Beth became conscious of increased flatulence, probable bright blood and slight mucous per rectum. She was referred to a surgeon for a follow-up colonoscopy that was performed under a GA (general anaesthesia) last week. The surgeon biopsied a suspicious area of mucosal thickening and ulceritis in the low sigmoid colon (the S-shaped section of the colon that connects to the rectum). The area measured 2.5 × 3 cm approximately. The biopsy showed a high-grade adenocarcinoma with penetration into the muscular layer of the colon (a fast-moving cancer that begins in cells that line certain internal organs and that have gland-like properties). The results showed cancer, and the surgeon had her in for surgery within days. When the pathology results came back, it showed that the cancer had already begun to spread to two lymph nodes in the pelvic area. Beth was referred to a medical oncologist to discuss treatment options. Beth is coming in today to meet with the doctor for the first time.

The doctor's task today is to discuss with Beth the different treatment options that she has, including the likelihood of a clinical trial (Beth does not know what a clinical trial is).

Beth's physical symptoms

Increased flatulence, blood in stool, slight mucus in stool.

Beth's concerns

Taking care of family.

What will the long-term effects be?

How to tell husband and family.

Ability to keep working?

communicating about trials. Box 20.2 shows a scenario which could be used for roleplaying a clinical trial consent.

References

1. Albrecht, T.L., L.A. Penner, and J.C. Ruckdeschel, Understanding patient decisions about clinical trials and the associated communication processes; a preliminary report. *Journal of Cancer Education*, 2003. **18**(210 – 4).

2. Albrecht, T.L., J.C. Ruckdeschel, J.C. Riddle, *et al.*, Communication and decision making about cancer clinical trials. *Patient Education and Counseling*, 2003; **50**: 39–42.

3. Fallowfield, L., D. Ratcliffe, and R.L. Souhami, Clinicians' attitudes to clinical trials of cancer therapy. *European Journal of Cancer*, 1997; **33**: 2221–9.

4. **http://cancer.gov/clinicaltrials/learning.what-is-a-clinical-trial.html**

5. Brown, R.F., P. Butow, F. Boyle, *et al.*, Seeking informed consent to cancer clinical trials: evaluating the efficacy of communication skills training. *Psycho-oncology*, 2007; **16**(6): 507–516.

6. Wilcox, D.P. and H.A. Thompson, From informed consent to informed refusal. *Tex Med*, 1990; **86**(5): 38–40.

7. Hippocrates, *A History and Theory of Informed Consent*, ed. R.R. Faden and T.L. Beauchamp. 1986, New York: Oxford University Press, ch 3, pp.60–61.

8. Lord, R.S.A., Informed consent in Australia. *Australian and New Zealand Journal of Surgery*, 1995; **65**: 224–228.

9. Novack, D.H., E.J. Freireich, and S. Vaisrub, Changes in physician attitudes towards telling the cancer patient. *Journal of the American Medical Association*, 1979; **241**: 897–890.

10. Reiser, S.J., Words as scalpels: Transmitting evidence in clinical dialogue. *Annals of Internal Medicine*, 1980; **92**: 837–842.

11. WMA, World Medical Association; Declaration of Helsinki: Ethical Principles for Medical Research Involving Human Subjects, in *Bulletin of the World Health Organisation*, 2001: 373–374.

12. Thomasma, D.C., Beyond medical paternalism and patient autonomy; a model of physician conscience for the physician-patient relationship. *Annals of Internal Medicine*, 1983; **98**: 243–248.

13. Kodish, M., J.D. Lantos, and M.D. Siegler, Ethics of randomised clinical trials. *Cancer*, 1990; **65**(Supplement No 10): 2400–2405.

14. Lilford, R.J. and J. Jackson, Equipoise and randomisation. *Journal of the Royal Society of Medicine*, 1995; **88**: 552–559.

15. Weijer, C., S.H. Shapiro, and K.C. Glass, clinical equipoise and not the uncertainty principle is the moral underpinning of the randomised clinical trial. *British Medical Journal*, 2000; **321**: 756–758.

16. Chard, J.A. and R.J. Lilford, The use of equipoise in clinical trials. *Social Science and Medicine*, 1998; **47**(7): 891–898.

17. Freedman, B., Equipoise and the ethics of clinical research. *New England Journal of Medicine*, 1987; **317**: 141–145.

18. Enkin, M.W., Clinical equipoise and not the uncertainty principle is the moral underpinning of the randomised controlled trial. *British Medical Journal*, 2000; **321**: 756 -758.

19. Hellman, S., Editorial: randomised clinical trials and the doctor–patient relationship. An ethical dilemma. *Cancer Clinical Trials*, 1979; **2**: 189–93.

20. Johnson, N., R.J. Lilford, and W. Brazier, At what level of collective equipoise does a clinical trial become ethical. *Journal of Medical Ethics*, 1991; **17**: 30–4.

21. Belmont, *The Belmont Report; The National Commission for the Protection of Human Subjects of Biomedical and Behavioural Research*. 1979, US Govt Printing Office: Washington DC.

22. Marquis, D., Leaving therapy to chance. *Hastings Centre Report*, 1983; **13**: 40–47.

23. Finklestein, D., M. Karsh-Smith, and R. Faden, Informed Consent in Medical Ethics. *Archives of Opthamology*, 1993; **111**: 324–326.

24. Gert, B., C.M. Culver, and K.D. Clouser, *Bioethics: a Return to Fundamentals*. 1997, New York: Oxford University Press.

25. Kirby, M.D., Informed consent: what does it mean. *Journal of Medical Ethics*, 1983; **9**: 69–75.

26. Fallowfield, L., Can we improve the professional personal fulfilment of doctors in cancer medicine. *British Journal of Cancer*, 1995; **71**: 1132–1133.

27. Lee, J.Y. and S.R. Breaux, Accrual of radiotherapy patients to clinical trials. *Cancer*, 1983; **52**: 1014–1016.

28. Martin, J.F., W.G. Henderson, and L.G. Zacharski, Accrual of patients into a multi hospital cancer clinical trial and its implications on planning future studies. *American Journal of Clinical Oncology*, 1984; **7**: 173–182.

29. Hancock, B.W., M. Aitken, C. Radstone, *et al.*, Why don't cancer patients get entered into clinical trials? Experience of the Sheffield Lymphoma Group's collaboration in British National Lymphoma Investigation studies. *British Medical Journal*, 1997; **314**: 36–37.

30. Ellis, P., S.M. Dowsett, P.N. Butow, *et al.*, Attitudes to randomised clinical trials among outpatients attending a medical oncology clinic. *Health Expectations*, 1999; **2**: 33–43.

31. Barofsky, I. and P.H. Sugarbaker, Determinants of patient non participation in randomised clinical trials for treatment of sarcomas. *Cancer Clinical Trials*, 1979; **2**: 237–246.

32. Cunny, K.A. and H.W. Miller, Participation in clinical drug studies: motivations and barriers. *Clinical Therapy*, 1994; **16**: 273–282.

33. Eggly, S., T.L. Albrecht, F.W.K. Harper, *et al.*, Oncologists recommendations of clinical trial participation to patients. *Patient Education and Counselling*, 2008; **70**(1): 143–148.

34. Albrecht, T.L., S.S. Eggly, M.E.J. Gleeson, *et al.*, Influence of clinical communication on patients' decision making on participation in clinical trials. *Journal of Clinical Oncology*, 2008; **26**: 2666–2673.

35. Brown, R.F., P.N. Butow, D.G. Butt, *et al.*, Developing ethical strategies to assist oncologists in seeking informed consent to cancer clinical trials. *Social Science and Medicine*, 2004; **58**: 379–390.

36. Brown, R.F., P.N. Butow, P. Ellis, *et al.*, Seeking informed consent to cancer clinical trials: describing current practice. *Social Science and Medicine*, 2004; **58**(12): 2445–2457.

37. Gattellari, M., P.N. Butow, and M.H. Tattersall, Sharing decisions in cancer care. *Social Science and Medicine*, 2001; **52**(12): 1865–1878.

38. Kupst, M., K. Dresser, J.L. Schulman, *et al.*, Evaluation of methods to improve communication in the physician-patient relationship. *American Journal of Orthopsychiatry*, 1975; **45**(3): 420–429.

39. Ley, P., Primacy, rated importance and the recall of medical statements. *Journal of Health and Social Behaviour*, 1972; **19**: 311–317.

Chapter 21

Working as a multidisciplinary team

Jane Turner

What is a multidisciplinary team?

A multidisciplinary team has been described as: 'A collection of individuals who are interdependent in their tasks, who share responsibility for outcomes, who see themselves and are seen by others as an intact social entity embedded in one or more larger social systems' (1). Although there are emerging descriptions of the composition of multidisciplinary teams in cancer care, there is a paucity of research data to guide recommendations about the particular strategies that are likely to be of benefit in promoting optimal team functioning.

Why do we need multidisciplinary teams?

Cancer treatment is becoming increasingly complex, and internationally there is an acceptance that care is optimally delivered in the context of a multidisciplinary team. In the absence of multidisciplinary care, there is a risk that treatment options offered are confined to the area of expertise of the individual practitioner, with the potential for key issues, such as psychosocial care, to be overlooked (2). This is of particular importance in view of clear evidence about the benefit of psychosocial interventions in reducing distress and improving wellbeing of patients with cancer and their families (3).

What is the composition of a multidisciplinary team?

In addition to the 'obvious' members of a team, such as pathologist, radiologist, surgeon, medical oncologist and radiation oncologist, the presence of allied health professionals enhances capacity for comprehensive treatment of patients. For example, the morbidity associated with concurrent chemotherapy and radiotherapy for patients with head and neck cancer is considerable, and input from speech pathologists and dieticians can prevent the development of some problems such as aspiration, and restore better function through nutritional advice. Similarly, patients with lymphoedema or difficulties with mobility require assessment and treatment by physiotherapists, or occupational therapists. In the treatment of patients with brain tumours, the inclusion of a neuropsychologist is especially valuable, as they can provide guidance about functional capacity, including ability to resume roles and occupations after treatment.

Advantages of a multidisciplinary approach

Evidence has been emerging over the past 10 years or so about the clinical impact of care delivered by multidisciplinary teams. Some of the data comes from general medicine and surgery, with increasing evidence from cancer care. A review of studies of the effectiveness of multidisciplinary teams concluded that their advantages include: decreased unplanned admissions to hospital; improved access to healthcare; enhanced continuity of care; and improved clinical outcome (4).

Other evaluations cite the following advantages of a multidisciplinary approach.

Survival

A Cochrane review of stroke patients who received inpatient care in a dedicated stroke unit delivering multidisciplinary care, found that these patients were more likely to be alive, independent and living at home one year later (5).

Information for patients

Women treated for breast cancer by a multidisciplinary team in which there is a breast care nurse are more likely to receive hospital fact sheets (6). Given the clear evidence about the benefit of appropriate information in reducing distress and improving adjustment, it appears that it is advantageous for women with breast cancer to be treated by a multidisciplinary team (3).

Evidence-based treatment

Advances in treatment may be more likely to be implemented in a multidisciplinary context in which knowledge is shared. For example, one study reviewed treatment recommendations made for women with breast cancer by a single clinician, comparing these recommendations with those made subsequently when a multidisciplinary team had been established (7). The study examined the case notes of 75 women, and in 43% of cases, the recommendation of the team differed from that of the solo practitioner. In 13 such cases, the team recommended breast-conserving surgery, rather than mastectomy, which has clear implications for longer term adjustment of the woman in terms of body image and sexuality.

Clinical trials

In Australia, when a breast care nurse is included in the team, women with breast cancer are more likely to participate in clinical trials (6). In the UK also, patients attending a multidisciplinary clinic for treatment of lung cancer have higher rates of recruitment into trials (8). This may reflect the 'culture' of the team, but it is also likely that logistic factors are important, such as availability of staff to explain randomization, and take an active role in recruitment.

Cost effectiveness

Especially if there is clarity of role definition, there is reduced duplication and potential for reduction in hospital inpatient stay (9). Furthermore, incorporation of members of a team with psychosocial expertise has cost implications, as demonstrated by a meta-analysis in which 90% of studies reported a decrease in medical service utilization following a psychological intervention (10).

Patient satisfaction

Inclusion of a nurse in a supportive and informational role is highly acceptable to patients, and the support offered, for example, by a breast care nurse, is associated with increased patient satisfaction (11).

Impact on health professionals

Enhancement of knowledge and skills

There are some inherently difficult tasks facing health professionals working in oncology. Although breaking bad news is often cited as a major stressor, even more challenging is raising discussion about transition from curative to palliative goals of treatment, or cessation of active treatment, and clinicians may feel guilty and helpless when faced with this clinical situation (12). High distress is experienced by 40% of family members in this context, exacerbated if they perceived that the physician was less willing to explore their feelings (13). Team members bring a diverse range of knowledge and expertise, and this is likely to promote discussion and provide opportunities for learning (14). Being able to draw on the expertise and support of team members trained in psychosocial care is likely to be of considerable assistance for health professionals facing challenging clinical problems, leading to reduced distress for patients and increased professional satisfaction.

Stress and burnout

A UK study of 72 multidisciplinary breast cancer teams analysed team composition and processes, and the mental health of members. The prevalence of minor psychiatric morbidity was substantially lower amongst team members than that documented for members of the NHS workforce generally (14).

Characteristics of well-functioning teams:

It is self-evident that the goal of a multidisciplinary team is to provide the best patient care possible, using a coordinated approach (15). Initiatives at various institutions have resulted in the development of over-arching principles of multidisciplinary care. Common central themes are the need for effective communication, and the creation of a nurturing and collaborative environment of trust and respect (16). A central, but often not articulated, issue is that members have confidence about their own roles and skills, and the capacity to acknowledge what is beyond their scope (17). The key features of effective teams can be summarized as follows (18):

- Clear purpose—relevant to patients and linked to the organization.
- Goals—need for members to agree and describe these in measurable terms.
- Good leadership—leaders need to set and maintain structure, manage conflict, coordinate tasks and provide feedback.
- Regular patterns of communication, clear well-written records.
- Cohesion—sense of camaraderie and involvement generated by working together over time.
- Mutual respect—open to talents and beliefs of each person in addition to their professional contribution.

What is the evidence about communication in teams?

Evaluation of team communication is complex, and it is hard to capture subtle aspects of teamwork and information-sharing. In many instances, surrogate measures such as burnout or personal satisfaction are used. Research into healthcare teams lags behind current models in the organizational behaviour literature (19), and there are few critical evaluations of routine practice.

Inter-professional communication

Receiving a timely discharge letter is essential for the health professional involved in ongoing care; however, a review of 55 observational studies revealed that 25% of discharge summaries never reached the primary care physician (20), with obvious implications for quality of continuing care. Working in different clinical settings poses a challenge for communication, but even when staff work in the same environment, there is not always clear communication. In a postal survey of 130 Resuscitation Training Officers, 67% reported that there was no communication between team members prior to attending a cardiac arrest, and 33% of those who did communicate described this as 'informal' or 'fortuitous' (21).

An observational study of eight physicians in a general medical unit in the UK documented communication episodes. For the five 'busiest' physicians, a communication event occurred every 11.6 minutes (22). There was a bias towards direct communication with other staff in preference to use of information technology or other resources, with the potential for these frequent interruptions to impact adversely on clinical care.

Clarity of role

A survey of multi-disciplinary teams in UK revealed that, although clinic nurses perceived themselves as having a major role in discussions about test results and psychosocial concerns, this was not acknowledged by other team members (23). This lack of awareness of the role and activities of other team members can lead to duplication of effort and inefficient use of resources, and pose the risk that patients, who are already anxious, will perceive inconsistencies or differences in emphasis in information that is provided. The other risk is that coverage of information is not comprehensive, because of the assumption that other team members will provide the information (24).

Impact of poor communication

Although difficult to quantify, there is some research examining the impact of poor communication within multidisciplinary teams on outcomes.

Adverse patient outcome

It is self-evident that poor communication can cause dissatisfaction for patients who perceive that their care is not coordinated, or that contradictory advice is offered (17).

A surgical review of 444 malpractice claims from 4 liability insurers in the USA evaluated 258 errors that led to patient injury. A single communication breakdown was cited in 72% of cases, in 23% of cases there were two communication breakdowns, and in 5% there were three or more (25).

The most extreme adverse outcome is patient death. The National Confidential Enquiry into Patient Outcomes and Death, established in the United Kingdom, released a report into perioperative deaths in 2002 (26). In addition to many specific surgical, medical or anaesthetic issues, the report raised, in strong terms, the risks posed when highly skilled health professionals function autonomously, rather than collaborating as part of a team, with consequent issues for patient safety. The report noted that 'Individual clinicians are becoming transient acquaintances during the patient's surgical passage through illness rather than having responsibility for continuity of care'.

Impact on family and carers

In the absence of a well-functioning team, patients and family members bear the burden of repeatedly informing different health practitioners about changes in treatment plans and medication, with the potential for errors that are compounded over time (27).

Staff stress

This appears to be a significant issue; more than one-third of nurses surveyed in an Australian study reported dissatisfaction with the degree to which they felt part of a team (28). Poor communication amongst team members has been described as leading to loss of confidence in members (29).

Nurses report that they feel stressed if their communication with physicians about patients is sub-optimal, because this affects their ability to best function in their professional capacity (30). In the case of patients with advanced cancer, oncology nurses report that they find it especially stressful if the physician does not communicate with them about a patient's poor prognosis or clarify the goals of treatment, as this limits their ability to support the patient (31). 'In some high-pressure settings, such as ICU, poor communication about goals of care may lead to nurses experiencing a sense of abandonment as 'doctors make the decisions, but nurses have the burden of carrying them through' (32). In addition to the obvious implications for staff burnout, it is difficult to imagine that any such tension would not be tacitly conveyed to patients and their relatives.

What underpins communication difficulties?

The culture

Traditional training in medicine has promoted an 'apprenticeship' style of medical education, encouraging students' aspirations to be part of a close-knit professional group, with the inherent risk that they becoming increasingly inward-looking (33). Furthermore, there is an emphasis on expertise and responsibility, which are linked strongly with autonomy, these characteristics conflicting with the more collaborative approach in a multidisciplinary team (34). However, imposition of the need for a more collaborative approach can lead to tension (35).

The defined hierarchy of seniority and expertise of traditional medicine can lead to communication difficulties, as junior staff assume that they would not be listened to if they expressed concerns. Their reticence to discuss concerns is compounded by anxiety that to discuss problems may make them appear incompetent to those who assess them (36). In some settings, there is an entrenched culture of blame, such that under-reporting of problems is the 'safest option' (37).

However, education may not be solely to blame for stereotyped attitudes about status and roles. Formal assessment of healthcare students reveals that, even on entry into their education, they have defined attitudes towards different health professional groups; for example, perceiving some as more caring than others (38).

Role definition

Variation in role definition leads to stress, and many staff enter a team with pre-conceived ideas about status and superiority (39). Novice nurses express that their greatest anxiety is talking to physicians (40), perhaps because of the perception of professional inequality in status. If this is not overtly addressed, more 'junior' staff members will remain reluctant to discuss important clinical issues.

Training

Exploration of perceptions about nurse–physician communication has revealed that physicians feel that nurses are often disorganized, making it more difficult to follow the information provided, and nurses are perceived as lacking ability to respond to questions (40). For their part, nurses express concern about the capacity of tired doctors on night shift to focus on discussion, and their reluctance to discuss the goals of care. This is consistent with the finding that nurses' expression of concern about medical orders leads to these orders being changed by the physician in a third of communications (40). Differences in emphasis and style of training can thus lead to difficulties in having one's concerns about patients understood by another professional group. Hence expecting different professional groups to seamlessly become 'team players' is unrealistic without additional support and explicit training.

The organization

Whilst it is accepted that hospitals will often be large centres comprised of specialist departments, the ways in which these can be accessed and the preferred method of communication are often poorly described or not articulated at all. If an intern is concerned that a patient might be depressed but feels uncertain about how to access the social worker or other psychosocial professional, there is real potential for the patient's need to go unmet. Often the system designed for inpatients is different from that for outpatients (41).

The ethos of the organization can also be affected by budgetary restraints, and focus on the 'bottom line', rather than quality care, inevitably affecting the ability of a team to function.

Concerns about time

Delivery of quality care for patients with cancer is increasingly demanding as patients survive for longer, and receive complex and potentially toxic treatments with the risk of error. When staff feel under pressure to provide care, making allowances for 'extra' commitments, such as attendance at a team meeting, may seem very difficult and 'not worth it'.

Not true believers

An inclusive approach to multidisciplinary treatment is not always embraced. For example, whilst health professionals are aware of support services, fewer than 60% recommend these to their patients, or feel that they are helpful (42). Physicians, in some instances, are concerned that patients may be exposed to bias or misinformation in support groups, undermining coping and satisfaction with decision-making (43). If psychosocial care is considered by health professionals to be based on 'soft science' rather than research-derived evidence, this will inevitably affect communication within the team.

Geographic isolation

Patients often prefer to receive their treatment in a location close to their home, family and supports. However, this necessitates the development of a referral network by the local health professional, who may encounter logistic difficulties in forging these links (44).

Personality style and personal issues relating to team members

Team members inevitably will have different personality styles, some being more amenable to discussion than others (45). Furthermore, health professionals are not immune from the use of immature personality defences, such as projection and displacement, which are likely to adversely affect team-functioning. Members of a poorly functioning team may unconsciously scapegoat a team member who is different by virtue of training and experience, sex or race, leading to escalating tension, the development of factions and further deterioration in team function.

Of especial concern is evidence that professionals working in oncology have high levels of stress. A UK study found that 31% of oncologists had high levels of exhaustion (46). The study did not explore sources of support for these oncologists, nor consequences for team-functioning, but there is potential for those burdened by the caring role to withdraw not only from the patient, but also from effective communication with other staff (47).

General problems with meetings

Direct application of business models of meetings is not necessarily appropriate to healthcare settings; however, some themes are generic, such as the need to have an agenda, time-frame for the meeting, method of arriving at decisions and implementing these, and facilities adequate in size (48).

Improving communication in multidisciplinary teams

Whilst the general ideals described at the beginning of this chapter are useful in clarifying the mission for a clinical service, there remains a dearth of research examining ways in which this environment can be created. It is naïve to assume that historical boundaries and hierarchical structures will magically dissipate on formation of a multidisciplinary team, and these issues are likely to require specific attention (49).

The following recommendations are based on the best-available evidence, and grounded in clinical experience in an oncology setting.

Communication skills training

Staff who have participated in workshops involving role-plays designed to enhance awareness of the roles of other members of the team, rate this as valuable and self-report increased listening (50). This study also reported a trend of decreased staff turnover. This is consistent with results of another study involving staff in a neonatal intensive care unit. Staff participated in a one-day course to enhance interpersonal communication skills, following which, twice-weekly team meetings were scheduled. The entire intervention was phased in over a 3-month period. Follow-up measures confirmed that, following the intervention, the mean level of problems with emotional exhaustion significantly decreased (51).

Training of staff in the operating theatre has resulted in improved communication with a direct impact on patient care, a significant number of patients receiving prophylactic antibiotics earlier and more patients receiving prophylaxis for deep vein thrombosis (52).

Few training workshop reports have defined core content of training; however, the following themes are considered to be important (53):

◆ The potential for blurring of roles.

◆ Group skills.

◆ Communication skills.

◆ Conflict resolution.

◆ Leadership skills.

This group described an intervention in a palliative care unit to promote enhanced clinical roles of nurses, combined with a more explicit pattern of communication with the physician. The intervention was associated with greater nurse confidence and physicians also reported high satisfaction (53).

Staff orientation and policy development

A resource that describes the roles of team members may be instructive for other team members, and provide valuable information for patients. Establishment of a 'directory' of staff expertise to supplement existing service directories can involve direct contributions of the staff members, in order to provide accurate information about skills, referral processes and roles. This may seem excessively bureaucratic; however, whilst verbal introductions and orientation programmes have the value of imparting much practical 'real-world' information, they carry the inherent risk that stereotypes or prejudices are perpetuated, as they are handed down from one generation of staff to another.

Although most institutions have mission statements about the importance of care of patients, few acknowledge the status of staff and their inter-relationships, and as multidisciplinary teams become even more established, explicit statements about roles and patterns of communication may be incorporated into mission statements. Similarly, descriptions of position statements and duties usually delineate responsibilities and lines of reporting for the individual, but there is potential to expand these to include statements about expectations of inter-professional communication and respect of roles.

Practical strategies

Use of structured proformas

One hospital developed an intervention to assist nurses to communicate with physicians in the clinical setting, using the following prompts (40):

S—Situation, e.g. what prompted this call? Does the doctor know the patient, or does the doctor need background information?

A—Assess—what is the nurses' primary concern?

F—Findings and Figures—what are the pertinent results, e.g. BP, PR, temperature?

E—Express and Expect—what the nurse thinks is wrong with the patient, request for review, investigation, etc.

R—Read back—read back any telephone orders received.

There are no published evaluations of this intervention, which would probably not be replicated across teams, but it does provide a practical example of specific steps that can be taken to rectify communication difficulties.

Defining core content

Similarly, there has been some work examining the level of detail that is useful in written correspondence between team members. For example, referring surgeons and family doctors want information regarding the proposed treatment, expected outcomes and any psychosocial concerns, yet these are commonly omitted (54).

Innovative use of IT

Case conferencing by video-link has been demonstrated to be highly acceptable to team members, and has the potential to overcome geographic impediments to effective team communication (55).

Simulated patients are commonly used in medical education, and there is potential to expand and modify these technologies to give students in different institutions the opportunity to assume different professional roles and communicate with colleagues about a simulated patient (56). Early evaluation suggests that the technology helps students learn to define the domains of different specialties and to improve their inter-professional communication.

The disruption caused by frequent contact from other staff members and the attendant risk that calls are disregarded, or given low priority, may be reduced if staff are encouraged and trained to use technology to glean information, where possible, rather than 'calling a friend' when in doubt.

Review of focus

Discussion of problems and resolution of difficult clinical issues are important, but reflection on successes is likely to promote team pride and optimism. However, in most teams there is an emphasis on identification of problems, rather than reflection on what has worked, and the factors that have contributed to a good outcome (57).

Interdisciplinary education

Traditional education in 'silos' may reduce the capacity of health professionals to communicate. In contrast, inter-professional training can lead to increased professional confidence in communication with other team members (53). One study of inter-professional education involved students studying medicine, nursing, physiotherapy and pharmacy. Knowledge and understanding of the sharing of roles improved. Interestingly, student rating of their own inter-professional skills dropped post-education, perhaps because of heightened awareness of personal gaps and the complexities of team communication (58).

After initial resistance, it appears that most learners approach inter-professional learning positively, but as yet there is little clear evidence about the impact of this on subsequent inter-disciplinary communication (59).

Promoting status and confidence

Staff may be reluctant of offer information or comments in team meetings because of the perception that their opinion will be seen as less valuable than that of someone from a different professional group. Building confidence about engaging in team meetings and the importance of contributions from all members is important (60).

Inclusive approach

Consider all members of the team. Clerical staff do not treat patients, but they represent the 'front line' and the receptionist who constantly warns patients that 'the doctor is very busy' may engender anxiety (61). Many could assist the team in practical ways, e.g. improving the design of a reception area, but their opinion will have to be invited, as typically they have experienced strongly hierarchical management systems (62).

Recognition of the emotional dimensions

There is a body of research on stress and burnout, and whilst these terms are popularly used, there is often little acknowledgement of the emotional demands of working in oncology. Validation of the grief and sadness inherent in the care of patients with cancer is an important step, as is giving staff the chance to reflect on their personal context (47).

Realistic approach

Accept that personality differences will occur and have clear professional boundaries (45).

Practical exercises

- ◆ You have been asked to design a brochure for patients being treated by your multidisciplinary team. Your task is to list the different disciplines and describe their contributions to patient care, and indicate the clinical context in which the patient might have contact with each team member.

- ◆ Construct a template to assist a family doctor to provide the information needed in a referral letter about a new patient to a multidisciplinary cancer clinic.

- ◆ List the information that would be required for an initial consultation by a surgeon, medical oncologist, radiation oncologist.

- Imagine that you are a patient who has recently undergone surgical treatment for cancer. Your task is to write to the hospital administration congratulating them on the excellent nursing care provided in their institution, giving specific examples.

- You are assuming the role of radiation therapist giving a lecture to nurses about radiotherapy treatment of patients with head and neck cancer. Provide details to the nurses about the information you would want them to provide if they wanted you to review a patient with severe desquamation.

- Write a paragraph to be included in the patient information brochure above describing the importance of psychosocial care for patients with cancer and their families.

Clinical exercises

- Lynda is a 43-year-old woman who has three young children. She has advanced breast cancer, which has progressed despite extensive chemotherapy. She has been admitted to hospital for management of pain, related to liver metastases, but there has been no open discussion about her prognosis.

  - Imagine that you are one of the nurses caring for her. How could you discuss with her oncologist your concerns about Lynda, especially as she keeps saying: 'Things will work out, I know I'll beat this'?

  - Imagine that you are the oncologist who has been treating her since her original diagnosis of breast cancer 4 years ago. Describe to your house officer how it feels to have a patient develop progressive disease despite your best efforts.

- Lionel is a 26-year-old single man undergoing treatment for a germ cell tumour.

  - Imagine that you are the house officer or oncologist treating him. How could a social worker or psychologist assist? How would you raise possible referral with this patient? How could you respond if he was resistant to referral?

  - How would you respond to his criticism of other staff?

References

1. Cohen SG, Bailey DE. (1997). What makes teams work: group effectiveness research from the shop floor to the executive suite. *J Manage* **23**, 239–290

2. Zorbas H, Barraclough B, Rainbird K, *et al.* (2003). Multidisciplinary care for women with early breast cancer in the Australian context: what does it mean? *MJA* **179**, 528–531.

3. National Breast Cancer Centre and National Cancer Control Initiative (2003). *Clinical practice guidelines for the psychosocial care of adults with cancer.* National Breast Cancer Centre, Camperdown, NSW.

4. Mickan SM (2005). Evaluating the effectiveness of healthcare teams. *Australian Health Review* **29**, 211–217.

5. Stroke Unit Trialists' Collaboration. (2001). Organized inpatient (stroke unit) care for stroke. *Cochrane Database of Systematic Reviews*, **3**.

6. National Breast Cancer Centre's Specialist Breast Nurse Project Team (2003). An evidence-based specialist breast nurse role in practice: a multicentre implementation study. *European Journal of Cancer Care* **12**, 91–97.

7. Chang JH, Vines E, Bertsch H, *et al.* (2001). The impact of a multidisciplinary breast cancer center on recommendations for patient management. The University of Pennsylvania experience. *Cancer* **91**,1231–7.

8. Magee LR, Laroche CM, Gilligan D (2001). Clinical trials in lung cancer: evidence that a programmed investigation unit and a multidisciplinary clinic may improve recruitment. *Clin Oncol* **13**, 310–311.

9. Friedman DM, Berger DL (2004). Improving team structure and communication. *Arch Surg-Chicago* **139**, 1194–1198.

10. Chiles JA, Lambert MJ, Hatch AL (1999).The impact of psychological interventions on medical cost offset: a meta-analytic review. *Clin Psychol-Sci Pr* **6**, 204–220.

11. McArdle JMC, George WD, McArdle CS, *et al.* (1996). Psychological support for patients undergoing breast cancer surgery: a randomised study. *BMJ* **312**, 813–816.

12. Back AL, Arnold RM, Baile WF, *et al.* (2005). Approaching difficult communication tasks in oncology. *Cancer* 55, 164–177.

13. Morita T, Akechi T, Ikenaga M *et al.* (2004).Communication about the ending of anticancer treatment and transition to palliative care. *Ann Oncol* 15: 1551–1557.

14. Haward R, Amir Z, Borrill C, *et al.* (2003). Breast cancer teams: the impact of constitution, new cancer workload, and methods of operation on their effectiveness. *Brit J Cancer* **89**, 15–22.

15. Bokhour BG (2006). Communication in interdisciplinary team meetings: what are we talking about? *Journal of Inter-professional Care* **20**, 349—363.

16. Ohlinger J, Brown MS, Laudert S, *et al.* on behalf of the CARE group (2003). Development of potentially better practices for the neonatal intensive care unit as a culture of collaboration: Communication, accountability, respect, and empowerment. *Pediatrics* **111**, e471-e481.

17. Henneman EA, Lee JL, Cohen JI (1995). Collaboration: a concept analysis. *J Adv Nurs* **21**, 103–109.

18. Mickan SM, Rodger SA (2005). Effective healthcare teams: a model of six characteristics developed from shared perceptions. *Journal of Inter-professional Care* **19**, 358—370.

19. Freund A, Drach-Zahavy A (2007).Organizational (role structuring) and personal (organizational commitment and job involvement) factors: do they predict inter-professional team effectiveness? *Journal of Inter-professional Care* **21**,319—334

20. Kripalani S, LeFevre F, Phillips CO, *et al.* (2007). Deficits in communication and informationtransfer between hospital-based and primary care physicians. implications for patient safety and continuity of care. *JAMA* **297**, 831–841.

21. Pittman J, Turner B, Gabbott DA (2001). Communication between members of the cardiac arrest team—a postal survey. *Resuscitation* **49**, 175–177.

22. Coiera E, Tombs V (1998). Communication behaviours in a hospital setting: an observational study. *BMJ* **316**, 673–676.

23. Jenkins VA, Fallowfield LJ, Poole K (2001). Are members of multidisciplinary teams in breast cancer aware of each other's informational roles? *Quality in Healthcare* **10**, 70–75.

24. Catt S, Fallowfield L, Jenkins V, *et al.* (2005). The informational roles and psychological health of members of 10 oncology multidisciplinary teams in the UK. *Brit J Cancer* **93**, 1092–1097.

25. Greenberg CC, Regenbogen SE, Studdert DM, *et al.* (2007). Patterns of communication breakdowns resulting in injury to surgical patients. *J Am Coll Surg* **204**, 533–540.

26. National confidential enquiry into patient outcome and death (2002). Functioning as a team? **www.ncepod.org.au/pdf/2002/02sum.pdf**

27. Street A, Blackford J (2001). Communication issues for the interdisciplinary community palliative care team. *J Clin Nurs* **10**, 643–650.

28. Barrett L, Yates P. (2002). Oncology-haematology nurses: a study of job satisfaction, burnout, and intention to leave the specialty. *Australian Health Review* 25,109–121.

29. Fallowfield L, Jenkins V (1999). Effective communication skills are the key to good cancer care. *Eur J Cancer* **35**, 1592–1597.

30. Barnard D, Street A, Love AW (2006). Relationships Between Stressors, Work Supports, and Burnout among cancer nurses. *Cancer Nurs* **29**, 338–345.

31. Turner J, Clavarino A, Yates P, *et al.* (2007). Oncology nurses' perceptions of their supportive care for parents with advanced cancer: challenges and educational needs. *Psycho-Oncol* **16**, 149–157.

32. Puntillo KA, McAdam JL (2006). Communication between physicians and nurses as a target for improving end-of-life care in the intensive care unit: challenges and opportunities for moving forward. *Crit Care Med* **34**[Suppl.],S332–S340.

33. Lester H, Tritter JQ (2001). Medical error: a discussion of the medical construction of error and suggestions for reforms of medical education to decrease error. *Med Educ* **35**, 855–861.

34. Davies C (2000). Getting health professionals to work together. *BMJ* **320**, 1021–1022.

35. Moss F (2004). The clinician, the patient and the organization: a crucial three- sided relationship *Qual Saf Healthcare* **13**; 406–407.

36. Sutcliffe KM, Lewton E, Rosenthal MM (2004). Communication failures: an insidious contributor to medical mishaps. *Acad Med* **79**,186–194.

37. Scott-Cawiezell J, Vogelsmeier A, McKenney C, *et al.* (2006). Moving from a culture of blame to a culture of safety in the nursing home setting. *Nursing Forum* **41**, 133–140.

38. Lindqvist S, Duncan A, Shepstone L, *et al.* (2005). Development of the 'Attitudes to Health Professionals Questionnaire' (AHPQ): A measure to assess inter-professional attitudes. *Journal of Inter-professional Care* **19**, 269—279.

39. Dreachslin JL, Hunt PL, Sprainer E, *et al.* (1999). Communication patterns and group composition: Implications for patient-centered care team effectiveness. *J HealthC Manage* **44**, 252–268.

40. Dixon JF, Larison K, Zabari M (2006). Skilled communication: making it real. *Advanced Critical Care* **17**, 376–382.

41. Wyatt JC, Sullivan F (2005). ABC of health informatics. Communication and navigation around the healthcare system. *BMJ* **331**, 1325–1327.

42. Matthews BA, Baker F, Spillers RL (2002). Health professionals' awareness of cancer support services. *Cancer Pract* **10**, 36- 44.

43. Steginga SK, Smith DP, Pinnock C, *et al.* (2007). Clinicians' attitudes to prostate cancer peer-support groups. *BJU International* **99**, 68–71.

44. Tulloh BR, Goldsworthy ME. (1997). Breast cancer management: a rural perspective. *MJA* **166**, 26–29.

45. Birmingham J (2002). The science of collaboration. *TCM* **13**, 67–71.

46. Ramirez AJ, Graham J, Richards MA, *et al.* (1995). Burnout and psychiatric disorder among cancer clinicians. *Brit J Cancer* **71**, 1263–1269.

47. Meier DE, Back AL, Morrison RS (2001). The inner life of physicians and care of the seriously ill. *JAMA* **286**, 3007–3014.

48. Myrsiades L (2000). Meeting sabotage: Met and conquered. *The Journal of Management Development* **19**, 870–884.

49. Fleissig A, Jenkins V, Catt S, Fallowfield L (2006). Multidisciplinary teams in cancer care: are they effective in the UK? *Lancet Oncology* **7**, 935–943.

50. Amos MA, Hu J, Herrick CA (2005). The impact of team building on communication and job satisfaction of nursing staff. *Journal for Nurses in Staff Development* **21**, 10–16.

51. Sluiter JK, Bos AP, Tol D, *et al.* (2005). Is staff well-being and communication enhanced by multidisciplinary work shift evaluations? *Intens Care Med* **31**,1409–1414.

52. Awad SS, Fagan SP, Bellows C, *et al.* (2005). Bridging the communication gap in the operating room with medical team training. *Am J Surg* **190**, 770–774.

53. Hall P, Weaver L, Gravelle D, *et al.* (2007). Developing collaborative person-centred practice: A pilot project on a palliative care unit. *Journal of Inter-professional Care* **21**, 69–81.

54. McConnell D, Butow PN, Tattersall MHN (1999). Improving the letters we write: an exploration of doctor-doctor communication in cancer care. *Brit J Cancer* **80**, 427–437.

55. Wilson SF, Marks R, Collins N, *et al.* (2004). Benefits of multidisciplinary case conferencing using audiovisual compared with telephone communication: a randomized controlled trial. *J Telemed Telecare* **10**, 351–354.

56. Sijstermans R, Jaspers MWM, Bloemendaal PM, *et al.* (2007). Training inter-physician communication using the Dynamic Patient Simulator®. *Int J Med Inform* **76**, 336–343.

57. Friedman LH, Bernell SL (2006). The importance of team level tacit knowledge and related characteristics of high-performing healthcare teams. *Healthcare Manage Rev* **31**, 223–230.

58. McNair R, Stone N, Sims J, *et al.* (2005). Australian evidence for inter-professional education contributing to effective teamwork preparation and interest in rural practice. *Journal of Inter-professional Care* **19**, 579–594.

59. Priest H, Sawyer A, Roberts P (2005). A survey of inter-professional education in communication skills in healthcare programmes in the UK. *Journal of Inter-professional Care* **19**, 236–250.

60. Norris E, Alexander H, Livingston M, *et al.* (2005). Multidisciplinary perspectives on core networking skills. A study of skills: and associated training needs, for professionals working in managed clinical networks. *Journal of Inter-professional Care* **19**,156–163.

61. Boyle FM, Robinson E, Heinrich P, *et al.* (2004). Cancer: Communicating in the team game. *ANZ J Surg* **74**, 477–481.

62. Bateman H, Bailey P, McLellan H (2003). Of rocks and safe channels: learning to navigate as an inter-professional team. *Journal of Inter-professional Care* **17**, 141–150.

Chapter 22

Communicating genetic risk

Elizabeth Lobb and Clara Gaff

Background

As cancer is common, many people have a family history of one or more relatives with a cancer diagnosis. The nature and extent of a family history of a specific cancer influences each family member's risk of developing the cancer: this component of an individual's cancer risk is called their genetic risk. Broadly speaking, individuals can be classified into three risk categories for a specific cancer: average risk, moderate risk and high risk (1, 2).

- Individuals at average risk either do not have a family history of cancer or the cancers in the family are 'spontaneous', i.e. the cancer can be attributed to cumulative chance events and environmental factors. Their lifetime risk of developing a cancer is the same as the population risk of that cancer.

- Individuals at moderate risk have some relatives affected with the same type of malignancy, usually diagnosed at a similar age to the age of onset in the general population. The causes of these 'familial cancers' are not usually apparent but are likely to be due to multiple interacting factors, clusters of spontaneous cancer or multiple gene mutations with a weak effect. The individual's lifetime risk of developing a cancer will depend on the number and age of diagnosis of affected relatives and is determined from epidemiological data.

- Individuals at high risk have a number of closely related affected family members, often with an earlier age of onset than the general population. These family histories are suggestive of an inherited cancer syndrome, caused by mutations in genes regulating DNA repair, cell growth and cell division. Usually, these are inherited in a dominant fashion, with an affected parent having a 50% chance of passing the mutation on to each child. Most hereditary cancer syndromes result in cancer predisposition, i.e. the lifetime risk of a person who carries the mutation is more than the population risk but less than 100%. The degree of risk will depend on the hereditary cancer syndrome and the specific cancer. For instance, in hereditary breast/ovarian cancer (HBOC), the average cumulative risks in BRCA1-mutation in carriers by age 70 years is 65% for breast cancer and 39% for ovarian cancer. For BRCA2 the corresponding estimates are 45 and 11% (3). Genetic testing to identify a causative mutation may be offered to an affected member of a high-risk family. If such a mutation is found, then predictive testing can be offered to other at-risk family members to determine if they have inherited the cancer causing mutation or a normal copy of the gene. Information about specific hereditary cancer syndromes can be found in Trepanier *et al.* (2).

Individuals with a family history of cancer may seek advice about their risk of developing cancer from their general practitioner (primary healthcare physician) or a cancer specialist. Seeking advice about the risk of developing cancer is by no means the only motivation for seeking advice. Other reasons broadly include concerns about family members' risks, in particular their children's risk, seeking information about risk-reduction options, genetic testing and following a medical practitioner's advice (4–6).

The first task of the health professional is to determine in which genetic risk category the individual lies. While the nature of the information communicated and the responses of individuals to different risk categories may vary, the principles of risk communication are broadly the same. Similarly, the process of risk communication to those who have had a cancer themselves is conceptually the same as to those who have not had cancer, although the content and impact may be different. People who have been diagnosed with cancer usually seek information about their risk of developing a second primary cancer, of their cancer having been caused by a hereditary predisposition and/or the risk of their relatives developing the same cancer (7). For simplicity, in this chapter we will assume the person attending the clinic, the consultand, has not had cancer and has a high risk family history. Individuals at high risk of developing cancer are usually seen in specialized multidisciplinary cancer genetic services, staffed by genetic counsellors, medical geneticists and/or cancer specialists.

From the information above it can be inferred that an individual concerned about their 'risk of developing cancer' is in fact required to integrate a number of different risks:

(1) the likelihood that there is a genetic susceptibility to cancer in the family;

(2) the risks at an individual level of inheriting or transmitting a predisposing mutation present in the family; and

(3) the risk of developing the disease, depending on the individual's personal genetic status (8).

In addition to these genetic risks, for some hereditary cancer syndromes there is the additional challenge of considering reductions in risk associated with preventative surgery (e.g. prophylactic mastectomy or oophorectomy) and early detection options (e.g. colonoscopy).

Risk communication has been described as 'the open, two-way exchange of information and opinion about risk, leading to better understanding and better (clinical) decisions' (9), i.e. risk communication is more then the act of telling the consultand a risk figure, it also encompasses the personal meaning that is made of that information. In summarizing 20 years of research and process in risk perception and communication, Fischoff suggests that risk communication requires summarizing the relevant science, analysing recipients' decisions, assessing their current beliefs, drafting messages, evaluating their impact and repeating the process, as needed. Accomplishing these tasks, he concludes, can significantly reduce the chances of producing messages that go against good practice in communication (10).

Little is known of how genetic specialists, such as medical geneticists and genetic counsellors, communicate risk in actual practice. Sachs and colleagues (2001) observed that they find it difficult to communicate risk information in a way that the consultand can interpret (11) and there appears to be variability in the approach of different practitioners (11–13). In addition, risk communication does not occur in isolation. The consultants bring their beliefs about their risk to the consultation and there is a process of relationship-building between the health professional and consultant before communication occurs.

After discussing genetic risk communication, we discuss the implications for family members, the knowledge, behavioural, psychological and psycho-social outcomes that may be anticipated from good communication of genetic risk and the variability in the approach of different practitioners (12, 13). In the absence of specific evidence-based recommendations for genetic risk communication, we have drawn on genetic counselling texts, practice recommendations and the communication literature more broadly to provide the following strategies for communicating genetic risk.

Risk perception, beliefs and information processing

As responses to information are influenced by pre-existing perceptions (14), and risk perception may be an important motivator of health-related behaviour (15), it is important to have an understanding of how individuals construct their perception of risk. Perceived risk has been defined as one's belief about the likelihood of personal harm (15). This may be expressed qualitatively ('It is inevitable that I will get cancer') or quantitatively ('My chance of getting cancer is 60%'). Despite a plethora of studies that require participants to enumerate their perceived genetic risk, risk appears to be experiential and not something that individuals can easily quantify (16).

Risk perceptions are 'built up over time, are informed by personal experiences and social networks and are shaped by behavioral norms and media reporting' (17, p.17). Different levels of exposure to breast cancer, different consequences (medical, somatic and psychosocial) and different degrees of identification with the affected relative will all influence an individual's own perception of their risk and their emotional response to these experiences (18). Thus, two women with the same objective risk of developing breast cancer but different experiences of breast cancer in their family, social networks and exposure to the media, are likely to respond differently to genetic risk information. It seems reasonable to assume that this is true of hereditary cancer more broadly.

When communicating risk information, the health practitioner needs to be aware of the ways in which this information is processed. A number of theoretical models have been proposed to describe how representations of illness are developed, how risk information is processed and how these influence decisions and behaviour (16–19).

Of particular relevance is the Heuristic-Systematic Model (20), which proposes that risk information can be processed cognitively and/or affectively when a decision is being made. Systematic processing involves careful examination and analysis of the content of the information provided, such as cancer risks and the management options discussed in a cancer genetics consultation. Consequently it requires considerable cognitive effort. Heuristic processing is more intuitive, using rules-of-thumb or 'shortcuts' to make sense of information. The use of heuristics has been demonstrated in cancer genetics (21). The belief that physical or temperamental similarity with an affected individual confers higher risk for cancer (22) is an example of a 'representativeness' heuristic: information about similarity and stereotypes is used to make a judgment, in this case about personal risk. Heuristic processing requires relatively little effort and is more likely to occur when, *inter alia*, the information has low personal relevance, there is time pressure, the person is experiencing an affective response to risk such as worry, and when there is ambiguity in the information (19). Informed decision-making is assumed to be the result of systematic processing and it has been argued that the provision of genetic risk information should be given in conditions that promote systematic processing; for example, with sufficient, unambiguous information and without time constraints (19).

Communicating risk

Conveying genetic risk must cover a great conceptual distance—from probabilities based on mathematics derived from populations, to the communication of individual risk, and then to the interpretation and meaning made of personal risk by individuals. Accurate risk comprehension among participants in genetic counselling programmes may be critical to their decision-making about whether to have a genetic test and, among those who test positive, to their decision-making about risk management (16).

Considerable effort is expended prior to a cancer genetic consultation to ensure that a comprehensive, accurate risk assessment has been performed and risk figure calculated. Perhaps unsurprisingly, the literature on communication of genetic risk in cancer focuses on numerical probability (16), as numerical risks appear to present precise information regarding the probability that a health problem will occur and convey authority (23). When clinicians present numerical probability information, they rely on the premise that people will respond to a given probability in a consistent manner. That is, a 10% risk should be interpreted as a 10% risk, regardless of whether it is presented as a percentage, or an odds ratio or whether it is presented as numerically or pictorially (24).

Despite the appearance of precision inherent in numerical presentation, in fact studies of different populations and subgroups show that people presented with the same numerical figure have divergent estimates of cancer genetic risk (25, 26). People make errors when asked to transform percentages into proportions and vice versa, and they confuse information about the frequency of an event with its rate of occurrence. Thus it would appear that people cannot reliably understand and interpret numerical probability statistics (27).

An alternative expression of risk is verbal probability, e.g. there is a high risk. This is often used by doctors to express uncertainty, or when there is a lack of information from empirical research or conflicting results from published studies (28). Budescu argues that most lay people understand words better than numbers and typically handle uncertainty by means of verbal expressions, e.g. 'I think that...', 'chances are...', 'it is unlikely that' (29). He argues that words are perceived as more flexible and less precise in meaning. Studies in genetic counseling settings have shown that, when provided with numerical estimates, people appear to spontaneously transform their probability information into discrete categories, e.g. high or low risk (30, 31), supporting a notion that words are easier and more comfortable to process than numbers.

The provision of risk information may be simplified by asking the consultand for his/her preferences relating to the format of the risk information (words, numbers or both) and the type of risk information sought (e.g. lifetime risk, 10-year risk). Publications have typically failed to support this premise, however (32–34). For example, Lobb *et al.* (34) found that there was no association between the way genetic risk was communicated in familial cancer consultations and women's accuracy of risk recall or satisfaction with the consultation. Women who were given risk information, both as words and numbers or in their preferred format, were not more accurate or satisfied than those who were not. These findings suggest that risk is a difficult concept to grasp, and that it may be important spending time in the consultation exploring women's understanding of risk in different contexts and formats (34).

A 'contextually based approach' is recommended by cancer genetic risk assessment and counselling guidelines (2), and appears to be applied in practice (12). This approach is consistent with findings that people are more likely to base their judgement on concrete, case-based information than on abstract, statistical information (35, 36). Information is conveyed in a manner that assists the consultand to understand the personal implications of a given health risk. Of necessity, this requires interaction between the health practitioner and consultand, as described above, to develop an understanding of the ways in which the experiences and health condition perceptions of the consultand contribute to his or her risk perception and, critically, the decisions that he or she may make in relation to that risk. People are interested in information about cause, severity and prevention or treatment options. This contributes to their mental model or beliefs about the health risk. Genetic information has the potential to affect the consultands' beliefs about the cause of a disease and consequently its controllability, thereby affecting emotional adjustment and motivation to engage in behaviour that might reduce risks. For example, in one study, provision of DNA-based genetic risk information about hereditary heart disease resulted in an increased belief in the genetic causation of heart disease, leading to a reduced expectation that behavioural change (e.g. diet) would be effective in reducing risk, and an increased expectation that biological means (e.g. medication) would be effective (37).

Clearly, the communication of genetic risk is a potentially complex task, but one that can be facilitated by focusing on the lived experience of the person at risk and the meaning they make of information provided. Emotional disturbances, such as misplaced anxiety, that may prevent at-risk individuals seeking appropriate care (38–40), can become apparent during this process. Addressing these may facilitate the systematic processing of information and decision-making (19). Decision aids (41), risk communication aids (42) and shared decision-making programmes that include information on risk may also facilitate communication and can produce higher knowledge scores, lower decisional conflict and more active patient participation in decision-making (43).

Risk communication in families

In most areas of medicine, the risks discussed are relevant only to the person in the consultation. However, inherited risk is shared within families, and the genetic risk status of one family member has implications for the others. Consultations about genetic risk, therefore, consider the relevance of the information to relatives of the consultand. For example, if a known cancer-predisposing mutation is identified, then at-risk relatives can be tested for this mutation. The consultand will be advised of this in the consultation and asked to inform those now eligible for testing. As a desire to have genetic testing for cancer predisposition is related to a desire to help family members (44–46), it is rare that the consultand will refuse to inform relatives (47). Nonetheless, it is also rare that all at-risk relatives in a family are informed about the availability of genetic testing (48). Thus, familial risk communication is a potentially important determinant of decision-making and testing outcomes.

A number of strategies may be needed to assist individuals to communicate with family members. A key step is to explore family dynamics to identify and gently challenge assumptions underlying any communication barriers. Forrest et al. (49) describe failure to inform as having either a positive motivation (i.e. a desire to protect from harm), a negative motivation (failure to overcome barriers) or being neutral (perceiving that nothing is needed). Identifying which of these are preventing communication with family members can assist counseling. In some families there is a 'pivotal person' who takes on family communication about genetics as their mission. Studies have shown that this person is usually female (50) and often a mutation carrier (51). Identifying and engaging this person may be helpful. Alternatively, intermediaries may be recruited to assist with informing specific family members (52).

Adjuncts to verbal dissemination of risk information within families include audio-tapes, video-tapes, written summaries and leaflets. Audio-tapes of oncology consultations have been found facilitate family communication about the illness (53). However, studies in genetic counseling on the use of audio-tapes found that few women listened to their audio-tape and even fewer shared it with family members (54).

Written summaries of genetic consultations have been found to be beneficial for facilitating family communication and improving understanding and recall (55). However, a combination of verbal and written communication with family members results in more relatives contacting genetic services about their risk than either form of communication alone (56). Strategies and exemplars to facilitate risk communication are given in Table 22.1.

Table 22.1 Key risk communication strategies

Goal	Exemplar
Clarifying consultand's expectations and setting the agenda	'Before I start, perhaps you could tell me what you would like to find out today?'
Goal-setting	'I can talk about the chances of you developing cancer and, although we cannot completely prevent breast cancer, I can talk about the options for reducing your risk. Would that be helpful?'
Explaining the process	'A while back, you sent me information about the cancers in your family. I'll go through that now and check that I have the facts straight, then talk to you about the likelihood that cancer might be inherited in your family and what your chance of developing cancer is. Then we can talk about what you might be able to do about that risk..'.
Identifying consultand's belief and perceptions	'Before I start talking about our interpretation of what is happening in your family, could you tell me what you believe has caused the cancers in your family?'
Checks individual's genetic knowledge	'There is a lot about "genes" in the news nowadays and everyone has some idea of what this means. Could you tell me what you imagine when I talk about a gene.'
Check information preference	'Is that something you want to know?'
Check concerns	'Is that something that concerns you?'
Checks understanding	'I've given you a lot of information today and I know you want to talk to your family about this. What do you think you might say to them?'
Invites questions	'Please ask me any questions...interrupt me...if I use any words that don't make sense tell me "I just didn't understand that" and we'll go back.'
Validate the individual	'You seemed to have picked that up really well, is that fairly clear?'
Begin to personalize the information	'So, on the basis of three people in your family having developed .... cancer, closely related to one another, and with these two people at the younger end. ...we'd certainly be very suspicious that there's an inherited predisposition to .... cancer.'
Ask consultand's opinion	'Is that something that you've considered/thought all along?'
Explain medical terminology	'Now if we find an alteration, the technical term is a mutation, in one of those two genes BRCA1 or BRCA2.'
Use a diagram	
Check preference for risk information?	'Did you want the numbers on that?'
Re-frame	'So to put that another way.....'
Discussing family history to minimize distress	'Explain the process, take note of special dates, e.g. date of diagnosis or death of other family member, explore emotional concerns, identify individual beliefs and perceptions, and validate the individual's experiences.'

Box 22.1 Case Study: a young woman at potentially high risk of hereditary bowel cancer

Jane Brown is 32 years old and has been married to Peter for 10 years. They have a daughter, Mia 5 years, and Jane works part-time as a sales assistance in a Department store. Jane and Peter met while still at school and Peter has a management position in a bank. His work is quite stressful and takes him away from home on a regular basis.

Jane moved to the city when she married, but her mother Glenda and a sister still live in the country. Jane is the youngest of three children. She has a 38-year-old sister, Jean, and a brother, Michael who is 35. Jane's father David, was diagnosed with advanced bowel cancer at 38, and died 2 years later leaving Glenda to raise the three children.

Jane was 10 years old at the time of her father's illness and has strong memories of trips to the hospital at the time of her father's treatment. Her mother was weepy and tired. The father's diagnosis and death are not discussed in the family and Glenda has subsequently re-married.

Jane has one paternal aunt (Monica) who has recently been diagnosed with bowel cancer at 52, another paternal aunt (Joanne) was affected by endometrial cancer at 48 and has subsequently passed away. One maternal cousin of Jane (Bob) was also diagnosed with bowel cancer in his 40s, has completed treatment and remains well.

Since her cousin's diagnosis, Jane has become increasingly anxious about her own risk of bowel cancer. She has attended for colonoscopy and has had polyps removed. She is attending the familial cancer clinic to discuss her own risk of developing bowel cancer.

Conclusion

As described above, in the past there has been a focus on the impact of interventions such as decision aids, audio-taped consultations, written summaries and genetic counselling consultations, on shifting inaccurate baseline risk perceptions (57). However, more recent studies suggest that a more meaningful outcome relates to one of the goals of genetic counselling, facilitating adjustment (58) In this context, adjustment to living at increased risk of cancer may be achieved by exploring the personal meaning of that risk and its implications. Current models of risk communication suggest that this will have a positive effect on social and medical decision-making. The case study in Box 22.1 provides an opportunity to try out some of these strategies.

References

1. Hampel H, Sweet K, Westman JA, Offit K, Eng C. Referral for cancer genetics consultation: a review and compilation of risk assessment criteria. *J Med Genet.* 2004 Feb; **41**(2): 81–91.

2. Trepanier A, Ahrens M, McKinnon W, Peters J, Stopfer J, Campbell Grumet S, *et al.* Genetic Cancer Risk Assessment and Counseling: Recommendations of the National Society of Genetic Counselors. *J Genet Couns.* 2004; **13**(2): 83–114.

3. Antoniou A, Pharoah PDP, Narod SA, Risch HA, Eyfjoprd JE, Hopper JL, *et al.* Average risks of breast and ovarian cancer associated with BRCA1 or BRCA2 mutations detected in case series unselected for family history: A combined analysis of 22 studies. *Am J Hum Genet.* **72**(5): 1117–30, 2003 May. 4.

4. Brain K, Gray J, Norman P, Parsons E, Clarke A, Rogers C, *et al.* Why do women attend familial breast cancer clinics? *J Med Genet.* 2000; **37**: 197–202.

5. Hopwood P, Evans G, Howell A. Women at high risk of breast cancer: risk perception and counselling needs. *Cancer Detect Pre.* 1993; **17**(50): Abs 009/02.

6. Collins V, Halliday J, Warren R, Williamson R. Cancer worries, risk perceptions, and associations with interest in DNA testing and clinic satisfaction in a familial colorectal cancer clinic. *Clin Genet.* 2000; **58**: 460–8.

7. Cappelli M, Surh L, Humphreys L, Verma S, Logan D, A H, *et al.* Psychological and social determinants of women's decisions to undergo genetic counselling and testing for breast cancer. *Clinical Genetics.* 1999; **55**: 419–30.

8. Huiart L, Eisinger F, Stoppa-Lyonnet D, Lasset C, Nogues C, Vennin P, *et al.* Effects of genetic consultation on perception of family risk of breast/ovarian cancer and determinants of inaccurate perception after the consultation. *J Clin Epidemiol.* 2002; **55**: 665–75.

9. Ahl A, Acree J, Gipson P, McDowell R, Miller L, McElvaine M. Standardisation of nomenclature for animal health risk analysis. *Review of Scientific and Technical Office.* 1993; **12**(4): 1045–53.

10. Fischhoff B. Risk perception and communication unplugged: Twenty years of process. *Risk Analysis.* 1995; **15**(2): 137–45.

11. Sachs L, Taube A, Tishelman C. Risk in numbers--difficulties in the transformation of genetic knowledge from research to people--the case of hereditary cancer. *Acta Oncologica.* 2001; **40**(4): 445–53.

12. Lobb E, Butow P, Barratt A, Meiser B, Tucker K. Differences in individual approaches: Communication in the familial breast cancer consultation and the effect on patient outcomes. *J Genet Couns.* 2005; **14**(1): 43–54.

13. Ellington L, Baty BJ, McDonald J, Venne V, Musters A, Roter D, *et al.* Exploring genetic counseling communication patterns: the role of teaching and counseling approaches. *J Genet Couns.* 2006 Jun; **15**(3): 179–89.

14. Marteau TM. Communicating genetic risk information. *Brit Med Bull.* 1999; **55**(2): 414–28.

15. Weinstein ND. Reducing unrealistic optimism about illness susceptibility. *Health Psychol.* 1983; **2**: 1–10.

16. Sivell S, Elwyn G, Gaff C, Clarke A, Iredale R, Shaw C, *et al.* How risk is perceived, constructed and interpreted by clients in clinical genetics, and the effects on decision making: A systematic review. *J Genet Couns.* **17**(1): 30–63, 2008 Feb.

17. Berry D. Risk, Communication and Health Psychology in Health Psychology, in Health Psychology, Series Editors: Payne S, Horne S, p.17. Maidenhead: Open University Press; 2004.

18. Rees G, Fry A, Cull A. A family history of breast cancer: women's experiences from a theoretical perspective. *Soc Sci Med.* 2001 May; **52**(9): 1433–40.

19. Etchegary H, Perrier C. Information processing in the context of genetic risk: implications for genetic-risk communication. *J Genet Couns.* 2007 Aug; **16**(4): 419–32.

20. Chen S, Chaiken S. The Heuristic-Systematic Model in its broader context. In: Chaiken S, Trope Y, editors. *Dual-Process theories in social psychology.* New York: The Guilford Press; 1999 pp 73–96.

21. Kenen R, Ardern-Jones A, Eeles R. Family stories and the use of heuristics: women from suspected hereditary breast and ovarian cancer (HBOC) families. *Sociol Health Ill.* 2003 Nov; **25**(7): 838–65.

22. Scott S, Prior L, Wood F, Gray J. Repositioning the patient: the implications of being 'at risk'. *Soc Sci Med.* 2005 Apr; **60**(8): 1869–79.

23. Zimmer AC. Verbal vs numerical processing of subjective probabilities. In: Scholtz RW, editor. *Decision-making under uncertainty.* Amsterdam, North-Holland; 1983. p. 159–82.

24. Rothman AJ, Kiviniemi MT. Treating people with information: An analysis and review of approaches to communicating health risk information. *JNCI Monograph.* 1999; **25**: 44–51.

25. Hallowell N, Green JM, Statham H, Murton F, Richards MPH. Recall of numerical risk estimates and counselees' perceptions of the importance of risk information following genetic counselling for breast and ovarian cancer. *Psychol Health.* 1997; **2**(2): 149–59.

26. van Dijk S, Otten W, van Asperen CJ, Timmermans DR, Tibben A, Zoeteweij MW, *et al.* Feeling at risk: how women interpret their familial breast cancer risk. *Amer J Med Gen.* 2004 Nov 15; **131**(1): 42–9.

27. Schwartz LM, Woloshin S, Black WC, Welch HG. The role of numeracy in understanding the benefit of screening mammography. *Annals Inter Med.* 1997; **127**: 966–72.

28. Timmermans D. The roles of experience and domain of expertise in using numerical and verbal probability terms in medical decisions. *Med Decis Making.* 1994; **14**: 146–56.

29. Budescu DV, Weinberg S, Wallsten TS. Decisions based on numerically and verbally expressed uncertainties. *J Exp Psychol, Human Perception and Performance.* 1988; **14**: 281.

30. Bottorff JL, Ratner PA, Johnson JL, Lovato CY, Joab SA. Communicating cancer risk information: The challenges of uncertainty. *Patient Education and Counseling.* 1998; **33**: 67–81.

31. Palmer CG, Sainfort F. Toward a new conceptualization and operationalization of risk perception within the genetic counseling domain. *J Genet Counsel.* 1993; **2**: 275–94.

32. Halpern DF, Blackman S, Salzman B. Using statistical information to assess oral contraceptive safety. *Appl Cognitive Psych.* 1982; **3**: 251–60.

33. Harding CM, Eiser JR, Kristiansen CM. The representation of mortality statistics and the perceived importance of causes of death. *J Appl Soc Psychol.* 1982; **12**: 169–81.

34. Lobb E, Butow P, Meiser B, Barratt A, Gaff C, Young M, *et al.* Women's preferences and consultants' communication of risk in consultations about familial breast cancer: impact on patient outcomes. *J Med Genet.* 2003; **40**(e56).

35. Kelly PT. Informational needs of individuals and families with hereditary cancers. *Seminare in Oncology.* 1992; **8**(4): 288–92.

36. Rook KS. Effects of case history versus abstract information on health attitudes and behaviours. *J Appl Soc Psych.* 1987; **17**: 533–53.

37. Marteau TM, Weinman J. Self regulation and the behavioural response to DNA risk infromation: a theoretical analysis and framework for future research. *Soc Sci Med.* 2006; **62**(6): 1360–8.

38. Lerman C, Daly M, Sands C, Balshem A, Lustbader E, Heggan T, *et al.* Mammography adherence and psychological distress among women at risk for breast cancer. *JNCI.* 1993b; **85**(13): 1074–80.

39. Kash KM. Psychological distress associated with genetic breast cancer risk. In: Eeles RA, Ponder BAJ, Easton DF, Horwich A, editors. *Genetic predisposition to cancer.* London: Chapman & Hall; 1996. p. 282–9.

40. Alexander NE, Ross J, Sumner W, Nease R, Littenberg B. The effect of an educational intervention on the perceived risk of breast cancer. *J Gen Inter Med.* 1996; **11**(2): 92–7.

41. Wakefield CE, Meiser B, Homewood J, Pete M, Taylor A, Lobb EA, *et al.* A randomized control of a decision aid for women considering genetic testing for breast and ovarian cancer risk. *Br Ca Res & Treat.* 2008; **107**: 289–301.

42. Lobb EA, Butow PN, Moore A, Barratt A, Tucker K, Kirk J, *et al.* Development of a communication aid to facilitate risk communication in consultations with women from high risk breast cancer families: A Pilot Study. *J Gen Counsel.* 2006; **15**(5): 393–405.

43. O'Connor AM, Rostom A, Fiset V, Tetroe J, Entwistle V, Llewellyn-Thomas A, *et al.* Decision aids for patients facing health treatment or screening decisions: Systematic review. *BMJ.* **319**(7212): 731–4, 1999 Sep 18.

44. Lerman C, Daly M, Masny A, Balshem A. Attitudes about genetic testing for breast-ovarian cancer susceptibility. *J Clin Onc.* 1994; **12**(4): 843–50.

45. Bluman LG, Rimer BK, Berry DA, Borstelmann N, Inglehart JD, Regan K, *et al.* Attitudes, knowledge and risk perceptions of women with breast and/or ovarian cancer considering testing for BRCA1 ads BRCA2. *J Clin Onc.* 1999; **17**(3):1040–6.

46. Esplen M, Madlensky L, Butler K, McKinnon W, Bapat B, Wong J, *et al.* Motivations and psychosocial impact of genetic testing for HNPCC. *Amer J Med Genet.* 2001; **103**(1): 9–15.

47. Clarke A, Richards M, Kerzin-Storrar L, Halliday J, Young MA, Simpson SA, *et al.* Genetic professionals' reports of nondisclosure of genetic risk information within families. *Eur J Hum Genet.* 2005 May; **13**(5): 556–62.

48. Edwards A, Sivell S, Dundon J, Elwyn E, Evans R, Gaff C, *et al. Effective Risk Communication in Clinical Genetics—a systematic review.* Department of Health: Genetics Research Program. Cardiff: Cardiff Centre for Health Sciences Research; 2006. Report No.: ISBN 0–9550975–2–5 Contract No.: Document Number|.

49. Forrest K, Simpson SA, Wilson BJ, van Teijlingen ER, McKee L, Haites N, *et al.* To tell or not to tell: barriers and facilitators to family communication about genetic risk. *Clin Genet.* 2003; **64**: 317–26.

50. Richards M. Families, kinship and genetics. In: Marteau T, Richards M, editors. *The troubled helix: Social and psychological implications of the new human genetics.* Cambridge: Cambridge University Press; 1996. p. 249–73.

51. Peterson SK, Watts BG, Koehly LM, Vernon SW, Baile WF, Kohlmann WK, *et al.* How families communicate about HNPCC genetic testing: findings from a qualitative study. *Am J Med Genet.* 2003 May 15; **119**C(1): 78–86.

52. Wakefield CE. Meiser B. Gaff CL. Barratt A. Patel MI. Suthers G. Lobb EA. Ramsay J. Mann GJ. Issues faced by unaffected men with a family history of prostate cancer: a multidisciplinary overview. *Journal of Urology.* 2008. **180**(1): 38–46.

53. McClement SE, Hack TF. Audio-taping the oncology treatment consultation: a literature review. *Pt Educ Counsel.* 1999; **36**: 229–38.

54. Lobb EA, Butow P, Meiser B, Barratt A, Kirk J, Gattas M, *et al.* The use of audiotapes in consultations with women from high risk breast cancer families: A randomised trial. *J Med Genet.* 2002; **39**(9): 697–703.

55. Hallowell N, Murton F. The value of written summaries of genetic consultations. *Pt Educ Counsel.* 1998; **35**: 27–34.

56. Suthers GK, Armstrong J, McCormack J, Trott D. Letting the family know: balancing ethics and effectiveness when notifying relatives about genetic testing for a familial disorder. *J Med Genet.* 2006 Aug; **43**(8): 665–70.

57. Edwards A, Gray J, Clarke A, Dundon J, Elwyn G, Gaff C, et al. Interventions to improve risk communication in clinical genetics: Systematic Review. *Pt Educ Counsel.* 2008 **71**(1): 4–25.

58. Resta R, Biesecker BB, Bennett RL, Blum S, Hahn SE, Strecker MN, *et al.* A new definition of Genetic Counseling: National Society of Genetic Counselors' Task Force report. *J Genet Counsel.* 2006; **15**(5): 77–83.

Chapter 23

Rehabilitative and salvage surgery

Andrea Pusic, Rachel Bell, and Diana Harcourt

Introduction

Mastectomy can have devastating affects on a patient's body image, sexuality and view of herself as a woman. Although breast reconstruction is not a panacea for the problems that breast cancer patients face, it is an option that should be explored in detail with them. The plastic surgeon and other care providers play a crucial role in communicating these options, benefits and risks, and also in managing patients' appearance-related expectations (1).

This chapter will discuss current breast reconstruction techniques, issues surrounding the timing of reconstruction and provide some examples of helpful statements to use with patients. For non-plastic surgeons involved in the care of breast cancer patients, this information may provide a solid foundation to facilitate individual patient counselling and support. We will also address the impact of breast reconstruction on quality of life and how patient expectations may shape perceptions of outcome.

Communicating breast reconstruction options

Most women who have had a mastectomy are candidates for breast reconstruction. In the United States, these operations are considered reconstructive and are covered by medical insurance (2). The plastic surgeon should explain a woman's options, particularly the advantages and disadvantages of each choice, but ultimately it is the woman who must decide—will she have reconstruction, and if so, when and by what method?

In the counselling process, it is important to convey to patients that reconstruction does not affect the detection of future tumours, nor does it impact on recurrence or survival in any way (3, 4). In addition, patients need to be reassured that it is valid for them to have appearance-related concerns whilst fighting their cancer. Although reconstruction is a personal choice, and some women may want to defer reconstruction decisions until they have finished treatment, women should know that it is typical to want to feel and look the same after mastectomy, as they did before the diagnosis of breast cancer.

Timing of reconstruction

Immediate versus delayed reconstruction

Reconstruction can occur at the same time as mastectomy, 'immediate reconstruction', or may begin later, weeks or even years after the mastectomy, 'delayed reconstruction'. The optimal timing for any woman depends on a number of factors including the stage of breast cancer, the patient's medical history, her psychological and social situation, and the potential need for post-operative radiotherapy.

Advantages of immediate reconstruction

◆ Psychological issues. Can reduce psychological trauma associated with feeling 'different' or even 'disfigured' after a mastectomy.

◆ Reduces number of operations. Decreases number of anaesthetics and hospital stays.

◆ Improved aesthetics. Skin-sparing mastectomy may be carried out, which results in smaller incisions, smaller scars and preserves the normal contours of the breast.

Disadvantages of immediate breast reconstruction

◆ Decision-making. Many patients choose to delay breast reconstruction because they are overwhelmed by the number of decisions they are required to make around the time of diagnosis and initial mastectomy. Others feel they need to focus on their cancer first before they are psychologically and physically ready to proceed with restoring their breast.

◆ Increased risk of surgical complications. The risks of surgical complications, although rare, are slightly greater primarily due to the increased operative times and complexity of the operation, e.g. infection, seroma (fluid collection under the skin), haematoma (blood collection under the skin) and deep venous thrombosis (blood clots in leg veins).

◆ Timing of reconstruction and the implications of radiation. Post-operative radiation therapy is common amongst mastectomy patients and can have significant effects on the cosmetic outcome of reconstruction (5), the most important of which is fibrosis (scarring) of the skin. Scarring associated with radiation therapy can prevent adequate skin expansion and is associated with an increased incidence of capsular contracture (scarring around implants).

In counselling patients, it is important to convey that decisions about the timing of breast reconstruction are individual. While immediate reconstruction may offer the advantages of few surgical procedures and a potentially better final result, the patient must be completely committed to the process before beginning. If patients are having difficulties making a decision about reconstruction, delayed reconstruction may be preferable. It is a choice requiring careful consideration; if a woman is already feeling overwhelmed about her diagnosis, the pending surgery and other anxieties, then decision making can be very difficult. Acknowledgement of this can be helpful. For example:

> Now, I want to raise another issue which is going to add more complexity. In addition to deciding if and when you would like to undergo breast reconstruction—we also need to decide on the type of reconstruction. I know that you have had a lot of information to take in and think about already. Would you like to discuss the types of reconstruction now?

Type of reconstruction

There are two main approaches to breast reconstruction: using a breast implant or using a woman's own tissue. In this section, we will discuss these different techniques and their relative benefits and disadvantages.

Reconstruction using breast implants

Women with small breasts that do not sag are the best candidates for implant reconstruction, whilst women with large breasts who have implant reconstruction on one side often need a reduction or a lift of the opposite breast in order to match the reconstructed breast. Of note, women who have received radiation therapy in the past may not always be candidates for reconstruction using implants alone because of the increased risk of complications.

Box 23.1 Breast implants: how it is done?

For most women, implant reconstruction is performed in two stages. First, a tissue expander is placed under the skin and muscle of the chest wall. The expander, which is similar to a saline implant, is a deflated plastic bag that can be gradually filled with fluid to stretch the remaining skin to create a breast mound. Beginning about 2 weeks after surgery, a small amount of fluid is introduced using a needle through the skin into the tissue expander. This expansion procedure is repeated weekly over the course of 6–8 weeks. Approximately 4 weeks after the last expansion, the tissue expander is replaced with a permanent implant under general anaesthesia and the expanded skin is used to create the final breast shape.

It is important for care providers to address possible safety issues with breast implants. Breast implants have been safely used for reconstruction for over 30 years, nevertheless, two specific issues should be considered in patient counselling:

Implant leakage

Implants have a silicone shell that can be filled with either saline or silicone. Like all man-made devices, implants eventually wear out; however, the majority last at least ten years. In the past, there was speculation that leaking silicone gel may be associated with autoimmune disorders; however, several large, multicentre trials have failed to find any significant association (6, 7). Silicone implants have thus recently been re-approved in the United States by the Food and Drug Administration.

Capsular contracture

As a normal response to any artificial material, the body normally forms a capsule or layer of scar tissue around the implant. In most instances the capsule remains thin and soft; however, in some women it becomes unusually strong, resulting in a breast that is firm to the touch. Occasionally, a capsular contracture may be so strong that it causes pain and distorts the shape of the reconstructed breast; surgery may be needed to relieve these symptoms. In some cases, breast reconstruction with implants must be abandoned.

Reconstruction using the patient's own tissue

This method creates a breast mound with tissue 'borrowed' from another part of the patient's body. Breasts reconstructed in this way are soft and have a more natural shape and, although this involves a longer and more complicated procedure initially, the reconstructed breast ages much like a natural breast and is generally better matched to the opposite breast than those restored using implants. The most common type of tissue reconstruction is called a TRAM (transverse rectus abdominis myocutaneous) flap, which moves skin and fat from the lower abdomen to the chest to create a breast shape. Other less commonly used 'donor' sites include the buttocks and thighs.

Flap loss

The main risk of the free flap (TRAM or DIEP) technique is that in a small percentage of patients, microsurgery fails to re-establish circulation to the transplanted tissue ('complete flap loss'). Women who smoke, are obese or have conditions such as diabetes are at a slightly greater risk for microsurgery failure.

Box 23.2 Own tissue: how is it done?

In a pedicled TRAM flap, the abdominal tissue is moved by sliding it underneath the skin to the site of the mastectomy. The tissue remains attached to one of the abdominal muscles, which is loosened enough to allow the tissue to move upwards towards the chest. The abdominal muscle supplies blood to the skin and fat tissue that will form the new breast, but this may lead to abdominal weakness.

In a free TRAM flap, the surgeon completely detaches the abdominal tissue, moves it to the chest, and then reattaches it using microsurgery to reconnect the blood vessels. Only a small part of one abdominal muscle is used with this technique. In some cases, the free TRAM flap can be performed without sacrificing any of the abdominal muscle. This procedure is referred to as a free DIEP (Deep Inferior Epigastric Perforator) flap or simply a 'perforator flap', since the tissues that are transferred are based only on the perforating vessels that travel through the rectus muscle. These different methods are compared in Table 23.1.

Abdominal complications and scars

With any method of TRAM flap reconstruction, there is the potential for complications in the abdominal area. In approximately 10% of patients, abdominal weakness, bulge or hernia may occur (8). Although this method will remove excess fat from the abdomen, it will not make the abdomen completely flat, nor will the patient's waist measurement necessarily become smaller. In addition, patients can expect a long, lower abdominal scar at a level midway between the navel and pubic hair area.

Reconstruction with a combination of patient's own tissue and breast implants

Sometimes a combination of techniques is required for breast reconstruction. This situation most commonly arises in women who have previously undergone breast radiation and who now

Table 23.1 Comparison of tissue reconstruction techniques

	Pedicled TRAM	Free TRAM	DIEP flap
Surgery	No microsurgery	Microsurgery required	Microsurgery required Most difficult dissection
General anesthesia	3–5 hrs	4–6 hrs	6–8 hrs
Hospitalization	4–5 days	4–5 days	4–5 days
Recovery period	4–6 weeks	4–6 weeks	3–4 weeks
Risk of fat necrosis	Slightly Higher	Lowest	Low
Risk of partial flap loss	Slightly Higher	Lowest	Low
Risk of complete flap loss	Lowest (<1%)	Low (1%)	Slightly Higher (1–3%)
Risk of abdominal weakness	Slightly higher	Moderate to Low	Lowest risk
Risk of abdominal bulge/hernia	Slightly higher (10%)	Low	Lowest risk
Breast shape/form	Natural/soft	Natural/soft	Natural/soft

require breast reconstruction. In these cases, reconstruction with tissue expanders and implants alone is usually not advisable due to high rates of complications, such as capsular contracture. In these cases, the latissimus muscle from the back can be used to provide coverage for a tissue expander/implant and to bring tissues that have never been radiated to the breast.

Comparison of different techniques

The best method of reconstruction depends on several factors, including the size and shape of the patient's breasts, the amount of body tissue that the woman has in potential donor sites, such as the abdomen, and whether or not the patient has had, or will receive, radiation therapy. The plastic surgeon should recommend one or more options based on these factors. If more than one method is suitable, the patient can choose which one they prefer. It is important that patients understand the major advantages and disadvantages of each method. Table 23.2 presents a brief comparison of the techniques.

Table 23.2 Comparison of implants and tissue reconstruction

	Implant/expander reconstruction	**Tissue reconstruction**
Surgery	2–3 operations	1–2 operations
General anesthesia	Yes	Yes
Hospitalization	2–3 days	4–5 days
Recovery period	2–3 weeks	4–6 weeks
Need for multiple office visits for expansion	Yes	No
Scars	Mastectomy scar only	Mastectomy and donor site scar
Shape and consistency	No natural sag; may be firm	Soft, very natural shape
Matching opposite breast	More modifications	Fewer modifications
Occasional problems	Breast hardening with a change in breast shape; Rippling of the skin	Abdominal weakness or bulge (TRAM); Partial breast hardening; Flap loss
Blood transfusion	None	Rare

Reconstruction of the nipple and areola

Nipple/areola reconstruction is usually performed 2 to 3 months after any final adjustment is made to the reconstruction, and for most women, the procedure involves very little discomfort. Although there are several nipple-reconstruction techniques, it is usually made from the skin and fat of the reconstructed breast and the areola can be made from a skin graft taken from the upper inner thigh. It is important to communicate to patients that, regardless of procedure, the nipple will have no sensation. The finishing touch in nipple/areola reconstruction is a 'tattoo' procedure to match the color of the woman's natural nipple and areola.

Matching the opposite breast

A reconstructed breast will not precisely match the patient's natural breast. If the woman has large breasts or breasts that sag, she may need a reduction or lift of the natural breast to improve shape and establish symmetry. A patient with small breasts may choose to augment her natural breast with an implant and reconstruct the missing breast to match this larger size. The surgeon may say:

> As you can see, there are risks and benefits to each of the different reconstruction options. Many women tell me that the best thing about having a reconstruction is that they feel comfortable and feminine in clothing. It is important to know that no matter which option you choose we will not be able to exactly match your breasts and you will have some permanent scarring. You may want to take some time to look over some information and pictures and talk with others before deciding.

Exploring patient expectations

The over-riding goal of breast reconstruction is to restore a woman's body image and to fulfill her personal expectations regarding the results of surgery (9). Studies in other surgical areas have shown that unrecognized or unfulfilled expectations may more strongly predict dissatisfaction than even the technical success of the surgery (10). In breast reconstruction surgery, such expectations are particularly central; two patients with uncomplicated surgery and unremarkable wound healing may have vastly different perceptions of their reconstructive result depending on their preoperative expectations.

Patients can derive information from a variety of sources, including the internet and television; however, this information may be misleading and contribute to unrealistic expectations for patients. For most patients, the most important source of knowledge is their surgeon. Despite this, in a busy practice, most surgeons are forced to limit their patient consultations to discussions about procedural information and potential problems. By focusing on complications, surgeons may ironically find that their patients are well-informed about uncommon adverse events, but do not know what to expect when all goes well. For example, a breast reconstruction patient who has just undergone reconstruction with implants may be disconcerted to hear audible fluid shifts during the early post-operative period. Similarly, she may look forward to nipple reconstruction without realizing that the new nipples will have no sensation.

A common concern for women is the desire to look 'normal' in clothing. Without breast reconstruction this can only be achieved with an external breast prosthesis, which can be cumbersome. Some women are concerned about the potential for the prosthesis to shift or become dislodged when they are around others. Reconstruction eliminates the need for an external breast prosthesis, which seems to be the most satisfying aspect of breast reconstruction for many women (11). Despite the shortcomings of breast reconstruction, most women express satisfaction with their results. Many find they can wear all types of clothing, including more revealing styles, with complete confidence.

Quality of life issues

Discussing body image and appearance concerns

Physical appearance has been understood to impact on self-esteem, depression and tendency to social isolation; however, many women may try to suppress their appearance-related concerns during their battle with cancer (12). In fact, some may even feel embarrassed to discuss body image concerns when their life is at risk. However, women who have had a mastectomy are not only dealing with cancer, they may also be grieving the loss of their previous appearance and trying to incorporate changes into an adjusted body image. It is important for surgeons to normalize body issue concerns and to open up discussion about such concerns, not just reassure the patient.

Understanding the impact on body image

Any form of surgery can have an enduring impact on body image. Delayed breast reconstruction has the potential to restore a positive body image for women who have been struggling with their post-mastectomy body. For women who choose immediate reconstruction, breast reconstruction may prevent some of the stress associated with the appearance-related effects of mastectomy and can help a woman maintain an intact body image.

Research has shown that breast reconstruction has proven benefits in terms of improved body image and quality of life for many women who have undergone mastectomy (13, 14). However, it is not a universal remedy for all the challenges and distress associated with loosing a breast (15). Although women often report being satisfied with their decision to undergo reconstruction (13, 16) they can still experience difficulties adjusting to their new appearance and incorporating their reconstructed breast(s) into the internal representation they have of their body.

Objective vs subjective assessment of outcomes

Evidence within the field of appearance research has found little correlation between objective and subjective assessment of appearance. Objective measures of appearance, such as length of scars, do not predict levels of psychosocial distress, such as social anxiety. A patient's perception of the visibility of scarring to others is typically a better predictor of levels of psychosocial distress (17).

A patient's assessment of the aesthetic outcome of reconstructive surgery might not agree with that of her significant others or her surgeon. Whilst a surgeon might be keen to perform further procedures, e.g. to tidy up scar tissue, the patient might be satisfied with the outcome of surgery and not want to undergo any further operations. Similarly, it should not be surprising that patients might sometimes be unhappy with the results of surgery that their surgeon is very pleased with. Such disparity could result from differing pre-surgical expectations about the likely outcome of surgery. These expectations will have been influenced by the information and communication between patient and surgeon during the decision-making period. If a surgeon has not ascertained what the patient hopes to achieve from reconstruction, then they are unlikely to have a good understanding of their expectations and wishes.

Scarring

Scarring (particularly at the donor site), asymmetry of the two breasts, complications and the need for additional procedures have all been identified as areas of dissatisfaction amongst breast reconstruction patients (18). Whilst all women will have some permanent scarring due to the mastectomy and breast reconstruction, it can be difficult to predict the personal impact of scarring.

When the reconstruction is carried out using the patients own tissue, scarring at the donor site can be significant. Scars on the stomach, back, thigh and buttocks can often be easily covered in clothing; however, there is the potential for some women to feel very conscious of the area of the body that was used for a flap. Women who have undergone TRAM flap procedures have reported feeling dissatisfied with the scarring across their abdomen and being unprepared for this (19). Women reported that it would have been useful to meet patients who had previously had the procedure, rather than merely viewing photographs of outcomes. Although scarring is unavoidable, the patient is likely to be better prepared for the outcome if they have realistic expectations about the likely location and appearance of scars.

Partners and intimacy

Mastectomy and reconstruction presents challenges for both single women and women in committed relationships. For single women, new relationships come with concerns about how and when to tell one's partner about their cancer/mastectomy and what their reaction may be. For partnered women, concerns about how a partner will react to their mastectomy and whether they are still physically attractive come to the fore. Overall women may question their femininity and attractiveness, which can have detrimental effects on intimacy and other parts of a relationship. Patients and their partners must adjust to the woman's altered appearance and this often involves a process of acceptance of the new breast/s. Reconstructive surgery may decrease distress about the appearance of one's breasts but may not change a woman's overall body image (20).

Many women, let alone their partners, are unprepared for the impact that mastectomy and breast reconstruction may have on her body image and couple intimacy (21). Partners and other family are often the main providers of support; however, they will also be dealing with their own worries and reactions to the patient's cancer and new appearance (12) and may find it difficult to provide all the support that the woman is seeking. Partners play an important and often beneficial role in women's experiences of breast cancer and its treatment (22–25); however, partners are often absent from consultations with plastic surgeons and may not be aware of the complications related to breast reconstruction.

Both women and their partners have sometimes reported a loss of sexual desire after surgery (26), and some women have reported feeling sexually and physically unattractive up to 5 years after reconstruction (27, 28). Male partners have reported concerns that touching the reconstructed breast might be painful for their partner and worries that they might reopen surgical wounds (29). Although this reluctance is driven by concern for their partner, a woman who is conscious of her altered appearance and is looking for reassurance that she is still attractive to her partner might easily misinterpret this lack of contact. This has the potential to create difficulties within the relationship that open communication between both parties could alleviate.

Partners can find it awkward to be present during consultations, and find it difficult to discuss their feelings and concerns since the focus of healthcare staff, family and friends is, understandably, upon the patient (29). Unfortunately, such feelings create barriers to good communication between the partner and patient, and also between the partner and the breast care team. In addition to the potential benefits of providing support and information about the impact of reconstruction on intimacy and sexual functioning as part of standard care, couples with ongoing difficulties could benefit from referrals for further support. Some partners might value the opportunity to discuss issues with other partners, possibly through online discussion boards, which might be more appealing and accessible than face-to-face support groups. Even couples who had a strong intimate relationship before surgery will likely have to renegotiate their intimate relationship, at least in the short term. For Instance:

> We often focus on the medical aspects of reconstruction, but I don't want to ignore the impact on quality of life. Mastectomy and reconstruction can have an affect on your body image and intimate relationships. Reconstruction can help some women feel normal again, but this is a process that takes time. I want to encourage you to involve your partner, as it is also important for him/her to know what to expect. Would you like to invite your husband/partner to join us in our discussion?

Facilitating decision-making

Making the decision for or against breast reconstruction after mastectomy can be difficult and daunting for patients; new and complex information, particularly regarding the type and timing of surgery must be considered. Whilst some women find it very easy to make this decision quickly, a small group find it very difficult (16). Decision aids can decrease decisional conflict and increase satisfaction with the decision making process (30).

Women might perceive themselves to have relatively little time to make their decision because they are keen for the cancer treating surgery to take place as soon as possible and fear that delaying their decision could have implications for their health (16). A major challenge for healthcare staff is how to give potential breast reconstruction patients sufficient information and time to make their decision within the confines of a busy hospital service.

The process of decision-making about reconstruction can be especially difficult when the choices are presented soon after the diagnosis of cancer, and the possibility of mastectomy has just been raised. Understandably, women's ability to consider the details of breast reconstruction at this stage may be hampered by their concerns about their cancer diagnosis and treatment options (31). Furthermore, the decision may be influenced, consciously or unconsciously by others, especially partners (26, 29).

Generally, patients feel more comfortable making a decision when they feel they are fully informed. In addition to having multiple open discussions, information should be available in a variety of formats and should address both the possible physical and psychosocial consequences of surgery. Patient handouts, educational sessions, photos, interactive computer programs and audio-tapes (32) can all help to meet individuals' information needs.

Surgeons and specialist nurses have essential roles in ensuring patients have sufficient and appropriate information (33) to meet individual needs and to give informed consent. There is considerable variation in the type and extent of information that women want before feeling able to make a choice; those who prefer detailed, in-depth information have been classified as 'monitors' and those preferring not to engage with more than the basic facts have been identified as 'blunters' (34).

Images in surgical textbooks can be hard to relate to; ideally, a surgeon would have a library of photographs of their own patients. Photographs of women of diverse ethnicity, age, physique and at various stages in their post-surgical recovery can help women make their decision. Although images of less successful aesthetic outcomes may be upsetting for some women, it is important to provide a range of photos (33).

The opportunity to meet a patient who has already had a similar type of breast reconstruction to what the current patient is considering can facilitate their decision-making. Unlike their medical appointments in which there is a power differential and the doctor or nurse spends most of the consultation discussing items on their agenda, meeting another patient is an opportunity to meet someone who is not an expert but has experience to share. This can provide a personal point of view and may also help remind the patient that they are not alone in their experience.

Women have described how the use of emotive language, such as 'disfigured or deformed', by healthcare professionals can influence the decision to have reconstruction. Some aspects of the outcome of surgery, e.g. physical sensation after surgery, are particularly difficult to predict and describe to those contemplating reconstruction. What is considered to be 'mild tingling' to one woman could be 'persistent pain' to another. The use of language to convey these experiences accurately is an incredibly difficult task for healthcare professionals who have not experienced the surgery themselves.

Increasingly, women are seeking information about reconstruction from a variety of sources, including the mass of information and personal accounts currently available on the internet and online discussion forums (35). These can be very powerful and useful resources, but women might also be overwhelmed by graphic accounts and the amount of information available. Patients can benefit from their surgeon addressing their concerns and anxieties, clarifying ambiguities, establishing realistic expectations and from being directed towards 'credible' websites.

Providing patients with accurate and realistic information, specifically with regards to possible outcomes and side-effects, may reduce the likelihood and extent of regret about their decision at a later stage. Women who report lower levels of satisfaction with information are more likely to experience moderate to strong regret about their decision, compared to those experiencing no regret. Patients have reported the most dissatisfaction with information provided in a written format, information about sensations, expected outcomes, risks and side effects, and the timing of information provision (36).

Consultations about breast reconstruction can take considerable time and need to be handled with sensitivity and care in order that women are to be enabled to make a fully informed decision that is best for them as an individual (37). Examples of questions that can help this process are outlined in Box 23.3.

Given the complexity of the surgery and the range of options available, women need time to make their decision and are likely to benefit from more than one consultation (31, 38). This enables women to process the first consultation, seek additional information and speak to other people, e.g. loved ones and other patients, before clarifying any remaining queries with their surgical team.

Unfortunately, current pre-operative teaching may fail to address many issues that are also significant to patients. Patients are rarely asked about their surgical goals, expectations and requests. In under-estimating the significance of patient expectations, surgeons may fail to appreciate that patient viewpoints can differ considerably from their own. Since patient expectations at least partially determine perceptions of surgical outcome, surgeons overlook the importance of expectations at their own peril. Understanding patient expectations can promote shared decision-making and identify misconceptions that may lead to dissatisfaction (10).

Until recently, surgeons have largely decided what information is, or should be, important to patients. However, there is now greater recognition that discussions about breast reconstruction procedures and complications are not enough; surgeons need to explore patient's expectations,

Box 23.3 Suggested discussion topics

What do you hope breast reconstruction will achieve?

How do you think it will affect your life, if at all? Will it impact on your work/hobbies/choice of clothing/relationships/intimacy?

How do you think the reconstructed breast(s) will compare to your breast(s) before surgery? (e.g. scarring, sensation).

Why do you want to have it at this point in time?

Have you considered different types of reconstructive procedures?

Have you discussed your decision with anyone else, e.g. your partner/family?

If yes, what do they think about it? If no, why not?

Is there anything that worries or bothers you about having breast reconstruction? (e.g. reactions of others, aesthetic outcome, recovery).

Have you considered using a prosthesis rather than having reconstruction? What do you think of breast prosthesis?

Do you know, or have you met, anyone who has had breast reconstruction? Have you discussed it with them?

discuss body image, sexuality and intimacy. The decision to have a breast reconstruction can be difficult for women who are already dealing with a cancer diagnosis. The plastic surgeon plays an important role in helping patients with their decisions and needs to recognize that clear communication during consultations can impact on patient's satisfaction with the outcome of reconstruction, perhaps even more than what happens in the operating room.

References

1. Rankin N, Newell S, Sanson-Fisher R, *et al.* (2000). Consumer participation in the development of psychosocial clinical practice guidelines: opinions of women with breast cancer. *Eur J Cancer Care* **9**(2): 97–104.
2. US Department of Labor. Women's Health & Cancer Rights Act 1998.
3. Patel RT, Webster DJT, Mansel RE. (1993). Is immediate postmastectomy reconstruction safe in the long-term? *Eur J Surg Oncol* **19**: 372–5.
4. Langstein HN, Cheng MH, Singletary SE, *et al.* (2003). Breast cancer recurrence after immediate reconstruction: patterns and significance. I.Feb; **111**(2): 712–20.
5. Cordeiro PG, Pusic AL, Disa JJ, *et al.* (2004). Irradiation after immediate tissue expander/implant breast reconstruction: outcomes, complications, aesthetic results, and satisfaction among 156 patients. *Plast Reconstr Surg* **113**(3): 877–81.
6. Noone RB. (1997). A review of the possible health implications of silicone breast implants. *Cancer* **79**: 1747–56.
7. Silverman BG, Brown SL, Bright RA, *et al.* (1996). Reported complications of silicone gel breast implants: an epidemiologic review. *Ann Internal Med* **124**(8): 744–56.
8. Nahabedian MY. (2007). Secondary operations of the anterior abdominal wall following microvascular breast reconstruction with the TRAM and DIEP flaps. *Plast Reconstr Surg* **120**(2): 365–72.
9. Sarwer DB, Whitaker LA, Pertschuk MJ, *et al.* (1998). Body image concerns of reconstructive surgery patients: an underrecognized problem. *Ann Plast Surg* **40**(4): 403–7.
10. Mancuso CA, Salvati EA, Johanson NA, *et al.* (1997). Patients' expectations and satisfaction with total hip arthroplasty. *J Arthroplasty* **12**(4): 387–96.
11. Contant CM, van Wersch AM, Wiggers T, *et al.* (2000). Motivations, satisfaction, and information of immediate breast reconstruction following mastectomy. *Patient Educ Couns* **40**(3): 201–8.
12. Rumsey N, Harcourt D. (2004). Body image and disfigurement: Issues and interventions. *Body Image* **1**(1): 83–97.
13. Al-Ghazal SK, Sully L, Fallowfield L, *et al.* (2000). The psychological impact of immediate rather than delayed breast reconstruction. *Eur J Surg Oncol* **26**(1): 17–9.
14. Al-Ghazal SK, Fallowfield L, Blamey RW. (2000). Comparison of psychological aspects and patient satisfaction following breast conserving surgery, simple mastectomy and breast reconstruction. *Eur J Cancer* **36**(15): 1938–43.
15. Harcourt D, Rumsey N. (2001). Psychological aspects of breast reconstruction: a review of the literature. *J Adv Nurs* **35**(4): 477–87.
16. Harcourt D, Rumsey N. (2004). Mastectomy patients' decision-making for or against immediate breast reconstruction. *Psychooncology* **13**(2): 106–15.
17. Rumsey N, Harcourt D. *The Psychology of Appearance*. Buckingham: Open University Press; 2005.
18. Holly P, Kennedy P, Taylor A, Beedie A. (2003). Immediate breast reconstruction and psychological adjustment in women who have undergone surgery for breast cancer: a preliminary study. *Psychol, Health Med* **8**(4): 441–52.
19. Abu-Nab Z, Grunfeld EA. (2007). Satisfaction with outcome and attitudes towards scarring among women undergoing breast reconstructive surgery. *Patient Educ Couns* **66**(2): 243–9.

20. Sarwer DB, Wadden TA, Whitaker LA. (2002). An investigation of changes in body image following cosmetic surgery. *Plast Reconstr Surg* **109**(1): 363–9.

21. Yurek D, Farrar W, Andersen BL. (2000). Breast cancer surgery: comparing surgical groups and determining individual differences in postoperative sexuality and body change stress. *J Consult Clin Psychol* **68**(4): 697–709.

22. Segrin C, Badger T, Dorros SM, *et al.* (2006). Interdependent anxiety and psychological distress in women with breast cancer and their partners. *Psychooncology* **16**(7): 634–43.

23. Hinnen C, Hagedoorn M, Sanderman R, *et al.* (2007). The role of distress, neuroticism and time since diagnosis in explaining support behaviours in partners of women with breast cancer: results of a longitudinal analysis. *Psycho-Oncology* **16**(10): 913–9.

24. Northouse L. (1989). The impact of breast cancer on patients and husbands. *Cancer Nurs* **12**(5): 276–84.

25. Pistrang N, Barker C. (1995). The partner relationship in response to breast cancer. *Soc Sci Med* **40**: 789–97.

26. Marshal C, Kiemle G. (2005). Breast reconstruction following cancer: its impact on patients' and partners' sexual functioning. *Sexual and Relationship Therapy* **20**(2): 155–79.

27. Rowland JH, Desmond KA, Meyerowitz BE, *et al.* (2000). Role of breast reconstructive surgery in physical and emotional outcomes among breast cancer survivors. *J Natl Cancer Inst* **92**(17): 1422–9.

28. Sheehan J, Sherman KA, Lam T, Boyages J. (2008). Regret associated with the decision for breast reconstruction: The association of negative body image, distress and surgery characteristics with decision regret. *Psychol Health* **23**(2): 207–219.

29. Sandham C, Harcourt D. (2007). Partner experiences of breast reconstruction post mastectomy. *Eur J Surg Oncol* **11**: 66–73.

30. Waljee JF, Rogers MA, Alderman AK. (2007). Decision aids and breast cancer: do they influence choice for surgery and knowledge of treatment options? *J Clin Oncol* **25**(9): 1067–73.

31. Frierson GM, Andersen BL. Breast Reconstruction. In: Sarwer DB, Pruzinsky T, Cash TF, *et al.*, eds. *Psychological aspects of reconstructive and cosmetic plastic surgery: clinical, empirical and ethical perspectives.* Philadelphia: Lippincott Williams & Wilkins; 2006.

32. Takahashi M, Kai I, Hisata M, Higashi Y. (2006). The association between breast surgeons' attitudes toward breast reconstruction and their reconstruction-related information-giving behaviors: a nationwide survey in Japan. *Plast Reconstr Surg* **118**(7): 1507–14; discussion 15–6.

33. Wolf L. (2004). The information needs of women who have undergone breast reconstruction: Part 1: decision-making and sources of information. *Eur J Oncol Nurs* **8**: 211–23.

34. Miller SM. (1995). Monitoring versus blunting styles of coping with cancer influence the information patients want and need about their disease. *Cancer* **76**: 167–77.

35. Losken A, Burke R, Elliott F, *et al.* (2005). Infonomics and breast reconstruction: are patients using the internet? *Ann Plast Surg* **54**(3): 247–50.

36. Sheehan J, Sherman KA, Lam T, *et al.* (2007). Association of information satisfaction, psychological distress and monitoring coping style with post-decision regret following breast reconstruction. *Psychooncology* **16**(4): 342–51.

37. Rosenqvist S, Sandelin K, Wickman M. (1996). Patients' psychological and cosmetic experience after immediate breast reconstruction. *Eur J Surg Oncol* **22**(3): 262–6.

38. Harcourt DM, Rumsey NJ, Ambler NR, *et al.* (2003). The psychological effect of mastectomy with or without breast reconstruction: a prospective, multicenter study. *Plast Reconstr Surg* **111**(3): 1060–8.

Chapter 24

Discussing unproven therapies

Penelope Schofield, Justine Diggens, Sue Hegarty,
Catherine Charleson, Rita Marigliani, Caroline Nehill,
and Michael Jefford

Introduction

The use of unproven therapies or complementary and alternative medicine (CAM) continues
to evoke strong debate and diverse views within the medical community. Many doctors are
concerned about the lack of scientifically credible research to support the claims of CAM proponents (1). However, a large and growing number of cancer patients use CAM (2, 3). Evidence
indicates that clinicians neglect to appropriately discuss issues surrounding CAM use with their
patients (4–6). Improving CAM-related communication between clinicians and cancer patients
has been widely advocated by researchers, medical practitioners, CAM practitioners and
patients (2, 4, 6).

CAM comprises a very heterogeneous group of practices, health systems and products; used
with different motivations and anticipated benefits, ranging from promoting psychological
well-being to curing cancer. Hence, communication strategies will be influenced by each unique
situation. While this complexity is challenging, assisting clinicians to initiate and engage patients
in discussions about CAM is an essential contribution to improving health-related communication. Implications for improving the ways in which doctors discuss CAM use with their patients
are wide-reaching, impacting directly upon the medical and psychological well-being of patients.
This chapter presents a definition of CAM, the rationale supporting the need to improve communication about CAM and evidence-based guidelines about how to discuss CAM in a conventional oncology setting. The practical application of the guidelines is then described through
the development and implementation of a communication skills workshop for training health
professionals.

Defining complementary and alternative medicines

Defining what constitutes CAM has been the subject of much debate. The US National Center for
Complementary and Alternative Medicine (NCCAM) defines CAM as 'a group of diverse medical
and health care systems, practices, and products that are not presently considered to be part of
conventional medicine' (7). What constitutes CAM changes continually as new CAMs are introduced and as therapies with scientifically demonstrated safety and efficacy are integrated into
conventional care (7).

There are a number of different, but overlapping, terms that fall under the CAM umbrella:

- Complementary treatments are used together with conventional medicine. There may or may
  not be evidence of safety or effectiveness. The anticipated outcomes may be improved quality
  of life, reduced side-effects and/or survival benefits.

- Alternative medicine is used in place of conventional medicine. Often, the anticipated outcome is a benefit in survival. Unproven therapies usually refer to treatments that have not been rigorously tested for safety or efficacy.
- Integrative or integrated medicine combines CAM for which there is some high-quality evidence of safety and effectiveness with treatments from conventional medicine.

The need for improving communication about CAM

Many cancer clinicians struggle with discussions around CAM, which is perhaps not surprising given the complexity inherent in the area. Some cancer patients invest considerable amounts of time, money and energy pursuing CAM with uncertain benefit, that may even be harmful (8–10). People with cancer rely on their doctors for information and guidance regarding treatment decisions (11). Physicians' knowledge of commonly used CAM has been found to be low in studies from Australia (12), Canada (13), Israel (14) and Italy (15). A further recent US study found few physicians felt comfortable discussing CAM with patients, and the majority (84%) thought they needed to learn more about CAM to adequately address patient concerns (16).

Patients and doctors do not routinely discuss CAM use (17–20). By analysing 314 initial oncology consultations, Schofield and colleagues (4) found CAM use was referred to in just 29% of consultations, with patients and kin initiating the bulk of these discussions. Moreover, approximately a third of patient-raised CAM references were ignored or glossed over by the doctor (4). Clinicians may simply not know how to respond to questions about CAM, supporting the need for clear and accepted guidelines in this area. Compared to patients with cancer, oncologists are less likely to believe that CAM use may improve immunity, quality of life, cure disease or prolong life (21). These discrepant views are likely to contribute to the communication gap.

Guidelines for discussing CAM in conventional oncology settings

A set of guidelines have been developed by the authors on this topic. The aim of these guidelines was to articulate a set of evidence-based recommendations to enable clinicians to have respectful, well-informed and balanced discussion with patients about CAM. A systematic review of the relevant literature was conducted to develop the recommendations for effectively discussing CAM in an oncology consultation (see Table 24.1). The principles presented in the Guidelines are discussed below.

Understand

Elicit the patient's understanding of their situation before asking about CAM use. This will provide the clinician with insights about the patient's perceptions of their situation, which will assist the clinician in responding to the issue of CAM use (4). Effective communication between health professional and patient assists coping, aids decision-making and is the most effective protection against harmful CAM use (22). Ask open questions with a psychological/existential focus to determine their concerns and goals. Understanding an individual's concerns and hopes for the future assists understanding of the reasons underpinning interest in CAM.

Respect

Respect cultural and linguistic diversity and different belief systems. Attitudes towards conventional Western medicine and CAM may be influenced by a person's belief systems and their cultural background. Some people may believe that external forces, such as spirits, caused cancer.

Table 24.1 Recommended steps for effectively discussing CAM

Recommended step	Working with the patient	Example of question to ask
Understand	Elicit the patient's understanding of their situation and clarify their information preferences, before asking about CAM use.	What is your understanding of things at this point? What have you been told about the test results?
	Ask open questions with a psychological/ existential focus to determine their concerns and goals.	What concerns you most about your illness? What are your hopes for the future?
Respect	Respect cultural and linguistic diversity and different belief systems.	What do you believe might have caused your illness?
Ask	Ask questions about CAM use often and at crucial points in the illness trajectory.	Are you currently doing or considering doing anything else for this condition/the side-effects you're experiencing/your overall health or well-being?
	Adopt an inquisitive, open-minded approach, as appearing judgmental or dismissive will reduce disclosure.	It's really important for me to know what other things you are doing to address your illness so I can help you in the best way possible.
Explore	Explore details of CAM use and actively listen.	Can you tell me more about <this CAM> please? What does it involve? How often do you use it? What are you hoping for from <this CAM>? Do you know if there has been any research done on the effects of <this CAM>?
	Provide balanced evidence-based advice in relation to the CAM.	In Western medicine, a therapy is considered effective if a large group of patients who receive the therapy show an improvement compared with those who did not receive the therapy. It sounds like the effectiveness of <this CAM> is based on individual cases.
	Help respond to advice from family and friends.	Others want the best for you, let's talk about these suggestions. What do you think of these suggestions?
Respond	Respond to the person's emotional state, and express empathy. Support the desire for hope and control.	This is a pretty tough time; I can understand you want to do everything possible. It's natural that you feel the need to explore all possible options to help you survive this disease; I fully support you in that.
Discuss	Discuss relevant concerns about the CAM while respecting the patient's belief systems. Concerns may include: ♦ unknown effect and unknown quality; ♦ high financial or time cost; ♦ potential for psychological harm.	Might the time involved prevent you from doing other things you would like to do? Is this cost going to cause financial hardship for you or your family? How do you think you might feel if you followed this advice but did not achieve the outcome you had hoped for?
	Discuss a trial period, what might be a reasonable time-frame to assess benefit/efficacy.	How long would you expect it to take to see a benefit from <this CAM>?

Table 24.1 (continued) Recommended steps for effectively discussing CAM

Recommended step	Working with the patient	Example of question to ask
Advise	Encourage use of CAM that may be beneficial and, if appropriate consider making a referral to a CAM practitioner.	I'd encourage you to use <this CAM>; the evidence suggests it could really help you.
	Accept use of CAM for which there is no evidence of physical harm or benefit. Support the patient's decision, even if it conflicts with your private view.	We don't know much about <this CAM>. It doesn't seem to be harmful and it may even be helpful. I respect that's what you wish to do.
	Discourage use of CAM where there is good evidence it will be unsafe or harmful.	I respect and support your right to make this decision. However, as we have discussed I firmly believe that you have a better chance of a good outcome if you follow this treatment plan.
	Balance advice with an acknowledgment of the patient's right for self-determination and autonomy.	While there is little evidence for us to know if <this CAM> will be helpful, of course, the decision is yours and I will support your right to choose.
Summarise	Summarise main points of discussion, check their understanding and for final questions. Provide evidence-based information sources.	We have covered a lot today. Just so that I can check I've explained things properly, can you summarise what we have discussed? If you like I am happy to have a discussion with your <CAM provider>.
Document	Document discussion in medical records.	
Monitor	Follow up discussion about CAM at the following consultation.	

Others may blame themselves for getting cancer because of life-style factors, such as exercise, diet, stress or even their thought patterns. It is a popular belief that changing life-style or thought patterns, particularly being positive, can influence survival (25). Patients are not necessarily looking for clinicians' belief in, or endorsement of, a particular CAM, but value characteristics such as open-mindedness, respect and active listening (5).

Ask

Ask questions about CAM use often and at critical points in the illness trajectory. By asking about CAM, clinicians indicate that this is an acceptable topic of conversation (1, 24). It is recommended that enquiries about CAM be part of routine initial history-taking (5, 25, 26), and again raised at critical times in the illness trajectory, such as the commencement of a new treatment regimen or after the diagnosis of recurrence (5). It is also important to consider CAM as a possible explanation for unusual side-effects or test results (27, 28).

Adopt an inquisitive, open-minded approach—being judgmental or dismissive is likely to inhibit disclosure. Similarly, terms such as 'complementary', 'alternative' or 'unproven' can be considered value-laden, may be interpreted differently by different patients or may sound dismissive (2, 26).

Explore

Explore details of CAM use and actively listen. Clinicians should ask direct, probing questions about their patients' CAM use, as well as follow-up questions to elicit motivations for pursuing, and expectations of, CAM use (29). It is critical that motivations and expectations are understood. Active listening facilitates accurate understanding to provide advice that supports patient choice and minimises risk (22).

Provide balanced, evidence-based advice in relation to the CAM. It may be useful to describe the Western medical approach to acquiring and implementing research findings. Discussion may be needed to help some patients to understand this approach and outline how conventional therapies are evaluated to allow a discussion about scientific evidence and unproven treatments (24).

Help respond to advice from family and friends. Patients may be recommended to pursue CAM by friends and family members, who may also offer anecdotal evidence of benefit (2). Patients may, therefore, need assistance from their health professional on how to respond to advice from family and friends.

Respond

Respond to the person's emotional state and express empathy. Given that the motives for using CAM often arise from the hope of a cure when a cure is not possible (4), or in the setting of illness-related physical or emotional distress (30), it is important to explore the person's emotional state, and respond appropriately. Empathic comments are also helpful by illustrating interest and understanding of the person's situation.

Support the desire for hope and control. It appears that many people use CAM in an effort to gain hope and control. Research has found that patients with advanced disease who raised CAM with their oncologist, linked CAM use with the desire to explore all possibilities of a cure, to increase their survival time or to improve their quality of life (4). Offering to answer questions about CAM and being willing to personally talk to CAM practitioners, may support hope in this context.

Discuss

Discuss relevant concerns about CAM, while respecting the person's belief systems. It is important to indicate clearly throughout discussions that the patient will not be abandoned, even if the patient's beliefs regarding CAM differ from the clinician's own (1, 32). If there are reasonable concerns that the CAM practitioner may be behaving unethically, it is important to explore this issue with the patient and suggest seeking more information about the practitioner.

Concerns may include:

- Safety and efficacy. It may be advisable for the clinician to conduct an objective assessment of available evidence related to efficacy and safety. Then, discuss possible adverse effects (pharmacological or due to possible contaminants) and whether CAM may worsen the patient's condition or interact with standard therapy.

- Financial, time and psychological costs. Encourage patients to consider how much time, money and hope they are willing to invest in the CAM. Even for CAM for which there is no evidence of physical harm, there may be potential psychological risks. Beliefs linking a positive thinking or fighting spirit and survival represent this type of risk. For a patient who holds this belief and whose cancer advances, they may feel at least partially responsible for this poor outcome (23). In the event of a patient forgoing conventional treatment, it is critical to discuss with patients the potential opportunity cost that is, the possibility that the conventional treatment may not be successful if adopted at a later time.

- Discuss a trial period. For some CAM, close follow-up may be warranted, particularly if the CAM risks being potentially harmful (28). When CAM use commences, use of a symptom diary may help determine whether the therapy is beneficial or harmful or has no effect for the individual patient (28).

Advise

It is reasonable to encourage or discourage the use of a particular CAM based on the relative risk or benefit that is likely to ensue (2, 28).

- Encourage. A number of therapies classed as CAM have been shown to be safe and efficacious, and might reasonably be recommended (28). It may be appropriate to make a referral to a qualified CAM practitioner.

- Accept use of CAM for which there is no good evidence of physical harm or benefit. Support the patient's decision, even if it conflicts with your private view.

- Discourage. It is reasonable for clinicians to discourage treatment by unlicensed professionals, the injection of substances not approved by regulatory bodies and any CAM that might delay or potentially impair conventional treatments with proven efficacy (28). If the patient is rejecting potentially curative treatment in favour of an unproven CAM, a short document—written and signed by the treating health professional and outlining the recommended conventional treatment options—could be offered. However, the health professional should avoid any implication of abandoning the patient (1).

- Balance advice with an acknowledgment of the patient's right for self-determination and autonomy. A model of shared decision-making about CAM between physician and patient is recommended, with the physician providing information about the possible risks and benefits and the patient providing information about their values (21, 22). Patients should be able to participate in decision-making according to their own preference for involvement.

Summarize

Summarize main points of discussion and check understanding. A summary is a useful way to ensure there are no misperceptions, and signals the end of the consultation. Refer patients to credible resources to get up-to-date, evidenced-based CAM information (7). Advice should be reiterated and, if there is reasonable evidence of potential for harm, reiterate concerns for the patient's safety.

Document

Document the discussion. A summary of the consultation should be documented in the patient's medical record. In addition, members of the person's broader treatment team should be informed about the discussion, especially if the CAM use is potentially harmful.

Monitor

Follow up discussion about CAM at the next consultation. It is critical that any discussions about CAM, particularly use of potentially harmful CAM, is followed up in subsequent consultations.

How to structure learning

Intensive workshops combining facilitated discussions drawing on evidence-based communication research and clinical experience, and the use of role-play with simulated patients and structured feedback have been demonstrated to achieve the greatest learning gains. This section describes the communication training module that we developed to teach effective communication about CAM in a conventional oncology setting.

The Cancer Council Victoria (an Australian state-based cancer charity) through its Victorian Cancer Clinicians Communications Program (VCCCP) has developed a workshop 'Effectively discussing complementary and alternative medicine with cancer patients, their families and friends' in collaboration with the National Breast and Ovarian Cancer Centre and Peter MacCallum Cancer Centre. This training programme adds to a suite of communication skills training modules.

Format of the workshop

The format of the CAM workshop follows the standard VCCCP format. VCCCP implements evidence based, small-group, interactive workshops that promote active learning through role-play. Workshops comprise a maximum of ten participants, two trained health professional co-facilitators and a trained actor, playing the role of a patient. Participants are encouraged to consider the difficulties and challenges they encounter in clinical situations, share these issues in discussion and work on them during the role-play. A relaxed and secure environment is encouraged to allow participants to experiment with techniques and approaches they may not normally use. There are two facilitators: a psycho-social expert, who is familiar with facilitation of small groups and relevant communication skills; and a clinical specialist, who can discuss relevant clinical information.

In general, workshops run for four and a half hours and commence with a short presentation on background research evidence, followed by a DVD modelling ideal communication, then a group discussion of the verbal and non-verbal skills displayed in the DVD. Evidence-based communication guidelines on the topic are then presented and compared to the group observations. The simulated 'patient' is then introduced to the group (an 'open chair' discussion between 'patient' and participants). A brief medical history of the 'patient' is provided and then each participant asks one question of the 'patient' to obtain a social history. Each learner then participates in a series of role-plays with the simulated patient over 10 to 20 minutes. The role-play is individually tailored to the participant's learning goals. Role-plays can be stopped at any time by the participant who is encouraged to seek assistance from the group. Otherwise, role-plays are stopped after 3 to 4 minutes by the facilitators, who then lead a constructive group discussion and seek suggestions for alternative strategies to be tried by the learner.

Actor training and setting up the scenario

VCCCP have a pool of professional actors who have undertaken both simulated patient training, as well as module specific training. The actors are provided with a detailed case scenario, including the illness narrative, detailed personal history and characterization. For the CAM module, the actors were provided with information about the use of CAM in the cancer population and participated in an interactive discussion with a behavioural science researcher (PS); medical oncologist (MJ) and a cancer survivor who had used CAM during her treatment (RM). This assists the actor to understand the feelings and emotions of a patient and motivations around CAM usage. To create the scenarios in the CAM workshop, we managed the complexity inherent in a CAM discussion by using three strategies. First, each of the participants were surveyed prior to the workshop to determine under what circumstances they have CAM discussions, what were common challenges or difficulties, and what were their learning goals for the workshop. We also enquired about learning objectives at the beginning of the workshop. Second, we limited the range of patient and CAM variation. We specified a particular time in the patient's illness trajectory (advanced, incurable cancer, having chemotherapy with palliative intent) and limited possible CAM use to four—highly restrictive diet, Reiki, microwave therapy and high-dose vitamin C. These were chosen as they allowed us to quite quickly create scenarios that incorporated a great range of challenges in communication around CAM. Third, the facilitators and actor met prior to the workshop to tailor and practice the pre-arranged scenarios to meet the learners' needs and ensure that all scenarios felt realistic.

Developing a DVD and workshop manuals

Based upon the above guidelines and other communication recommendations, workshop manuals for both facilitators and participants have been developed that support implementation of this workshop and act as an ongoing resource for participants. The facilitator's manual provides all of the necessary tools and materials (including PowerPoint slides) for facilitators to run an interactive workshop effectively, and includes a suggested workshop outline that can be adjusted to reflect their personal style or participant needs. A DVD was also created to complement the workshop. Two scenes were devised and scripts were drafted drawing on the recommended guidelines articulated in Table 24.1. The first scene focuses on a patient (Barry) taking multivitamins and herbal preparations, whilst having pre-operative chemotherapy and radiation for curable rectal cancer. The second scene involves the same patient four years later. The patient now has advanced incurable disease and is contemplating a range of CAM therapies, whilst also considering palliative chemotherapy. Table 24.2 displays the dialogue for the second scene and links the doctor's responses to the recommended guidelines.

Table 24.2 A discussion between a medical oncologist (MEDONC) and a patient (BERRY) about complementary and alternative medicine (script for a DVD scene):

Barry was a 65-year-old married man when he first experienced symptoms of bleeding from the bowel, four years ago. His general practitioner organised a colonoscopy, which showed that Barry had a rectal cancer. Barry was advised to have pre-operative chemoradiation followed by surgery. He completed this treatment and a further four months of post-operative adjuvant chemotherapy. He has been well for the subsequent three and a half years, but has recently been diagnosed with advanced, incurable disease. He has been told that the average (median) survival for people in this circumstance is about 20 months. He is thinking about pursuing alternative treatments, but also wishes to try conventional chemotherapy, that he has been told has a very good chance of improving his survival, though cannot cure his disease.

Character	Dialogue	Recommendation addressed
BARRY	So let me get this straight, the most you can guarantee with the chemo is 24 months, assuming all goes well.	
MEDONC	24 is an average. 50% of people will live longer than that; some for many years. I have one patient who was in a very similar situation to you still coming in to see me 3 years down the track.	Supporting hope
BARRY	OK, and the other 50%?	
MEDONC	Yes, could be less as well. It's not a lot, I know.	Empathy

Table 24.2 (continued) A discussion between a medical oncologist and a patient about complementary and alternative medicine: script for a DVD scene

Character	Dialogue	Recommendation addressed
BARRY	No. I need to do everything I can. There are some other things I'm considering as well. There's an interstate clinic that offers a range of treatments. I want to hit it from every angle.	
MEDONC	I can understand that. Can I ask, what sorts of things are they offering?	Ask about CAM
BARRY	I haven't brought the papers in... ozone treatment I think, Hoxsey diet, some sort of hyperthermia or something—as you people say, a real cocktail. Have you heard of them?	
MEDONC	I've heard of some of them. What are you hoping these treatments will offer you?	Explore expected outcome
BARRY	More time, 24 months isn't much On their website they say some people have lived for years and years. Look, they're not being irresponsible and promising cure, but there are lots of satisfied customers, and I wouldn't mind being one of them. I thought that maybe I should do this before the chemo. What do you think?	
MEDONC	Well I'm not an expert on these treatments but your question is a really important one and I can understand you'd want to look into every option possible. It would be good to talk a little about what they are offering, and how they work. What do you know about the treatments, for example, what do they involve?	Open, inquisitive approach and exploring details
BARRY	It'd involve me going up there for 3 or 4 months—I'd stay with my son. I think it's pretty intensive, daily treatment, so I don't think I'd be able to have chemo at the same time—so I'm wondering about maybe chemo before or after?	
MEDONC	It sounds to me that if you started this you would'nt be able to start chemo for 3 to 4 months?	Active listening
BARRY	That's right.	
MEDONC	I'd be really reluctant for you to go interstate for 3 or 4 months and delay having the chemotherapy, which has good evidence behind it. If these other treatments don't work, your health may in fact deteriorate over the next 3 or 4 months, and your body might not be able to tolerate the chemotherapy if that happens. The chemotherapy is based on many international studies that involve thousands of people. That means we can be confident in knowing that the chemo is the best available treatment we can offer.	Discuss concerns and provide evidence-based advice
MEDONC	What do you know about these other treatments? Have they been studied in the same way, or are they basing outcomes on individual cases?	Explore evidence underpinning CAM

(continued)

Table 24.2 (continued) A discussion between a medical oncologist and a patient about complementary and alternative medicine: script for a DVD scene

Character	Dialogue	Recommendation addressed
BARRY	To be honest I don't know... My son's been badgering me. He really thinks I should try this first.	
MEDONC	I'm sure he wants the best for you. However my concern is that we don't know much about the chances of these treatments working for you.	Discuss concerns
BARRY	Hmm. Maybe I should look into it more closely.	
MEDONC	Could you bring any information in to our next appointment? We could look at it together. I'm also wondering how much this treatment is going to cost.	Explore cost of CAM
BARRY	I don't know. I'm not particularly concerned about the money, but I'm not going to throw it at nothing—I could be spending my time in the Bahamas!	
MEDONC	That raises issues about how you want to be spending your time. I think this is something else that needs to be weighed up.	Discuss concerns
BARRY	Yeah, there's a lot for me to think about, and I don't want to miss out on the chemo but I really like the sound of these other treatments.	
MEDONC	When you bring in the information at the next appointment, do you want to see if your wife and son can come along and anyone else that you would like?	Revisit and monitor
BARRY	I know that Barbara would probably like that. I'll see.	
MEDONC	OK great. Of course the decision is ultimately yours and I understand that you need to explore all options, but I'd like to be sure that you understand I do have some serious concerns about the evidence behind these treatments, their side effects and that it may delay the chemotherapy. We need to look at this closely to make sure you're making the right decision. Ultimately I'll support you whatever you decide.	Balanced advice acknowledging patients right for self-determination
BARRY	Thanks, sure.	
MEDONC	There are a number of good web-sites and written resources you might be interested in. Can I give you some written information to take away?	Provide evidence-based information sources
BARRY	Yes thanks (medical oncologist hands the literature)	
MEDONC	Barry we've covered a lot today. Do you have any other questions or is there anything else you'd like to discuss?	Check for final questions
BARRY	No. I don't think so. I just want to get the best outcome. What you've said makes sense but I guess I need to think about it.	

References

1. ASCO. The Physician and Unorthodox Cancer Therapies. *Journal of Clinical Oncology* [ASCO Special Article]. 1997; **15** (1): 401–6.

2. Eisenberg DM, Davis RB, Ettner SL, *et al.* Trends in alternative medicine use in the United States, 1990–1997: results of a follow-up national survey. *Jama* 1998 Nov 11; **280** (18): 1569–75.

3. Flannery M, Love M, Pearce K, *et al.* Communication about complementary and alternative medicine: perspectives of primary care clinicians. *Alternative Therapies in Health & Medicine* 2006; **12** (1): 56–62.

4. Schofield PE, Juraskova I, Butow PN. How oncologists discuss complementary therapy use with their patients: an audio-tape audit. *Support Care Cancer* 2003 Jun; **11** (6): 348–55.

5. Adler SR, Fosket JR. Disclosing complementary and alternative medicine use in the medical encounter: a qualitative study in women with breast cancer. *Journal of Family Practice* 1999 Jun; **48** (6): 453–8.

6. Tasaki K, Maskarinec G, Shumay DM, *et al.* Communication between physicians and cancer patients about complementary and alternative medicine: exploring patients' perspectives [see comment]. *Psychooncology* 2002; **11** (3): 212–20.

7. NCCAM. Time to talk: ask your patients about their use of complementary and alternative medicine. http://nccam.n.h.gov/timetotalk/forphysicians.htm. 2007.

8. MacLennan AH, Wilson DH, Taylor AW. Prevalence and cost of alternative medicine in Australia. *Lancet* 1996 Mar 2; **347** (9001): 569–73.

9. Lowenthal R. Public illness: how the community recommended complementary and alternative medicine for a prominent politician with cancer. The *Medical Journal of Australia* 2005; **183** (11/12): 576–9.

10. Markovic M, Manderson L, Wray N, *et al.* Complementary medicine use by Australian women with gynaecological cancer. *Psychooncology* 2006 Mar; **15** (3): 209–20.

11. Degner L, Sloan F, A J. Decision-making during serious illness: what role do patients really want to play? *Journal of Clinical Epidemiology* 1992; **45** (9): 941–50.

12. Newell S, Sanson-Fisher RW. Australian oncologists' self-reported knowledge and attitudes about non-traditional therapies used by cancer patients. The *Medical Journal of Australia* 2000 Feb 7; **172** (3): 110–3.

13. Bourgeault IL. Physicians' attitudes toward patients' use of alternative cancer therapies. *Canadian Medical Association Journal* 1996 Dec 15; **155** (12): 1679–85.

14. Giveon SM, Liberman N, Klang S, *et al.* A survey of primary care physicians' perceptions of their patients' use of complementary medicine. *Complementary Therapies in Medicine* 2003 Dec; **11** (4): 254–60.

15. Crocetti E, Crotti N, Montella M, *et al.* Complementary medicine and oncologists' attitudes: a survey in Italy. *Tumori* 1996; **82** (6): 539–42.

16. Corbin Winslow L, Shapiro H. Physicians want education about complementary and alternative medicine to enhance communication with their patients. *Archives of Internal Medicine* 2002 May 27; **162** (10): 1176–81.

17. Oldendick R, Coker AL, Wieland D, *et al.* Population-based survey of complementary and alternative medicine usage, patient satisfaction, and physician involvement. South Carolina Complementary Medicine Program Baseline Research Team. *Southern Medical Journal* 2000 Apr; **93** (4): 375–81.

18. Giveon SM, Liberman N, Klang S, *et al.* Are people who use 'natural drugs' aware of their potentially harmful side effects and reporting to family physician? *Patient Education and Counseling* 2004 Apr; **53** (1): 5–11.

19. MacLennan AH, Myers SP, Taylor AW. The continuing use of complementary and alternative medicine in South Australia: costs and beliefs in 2004. The *Medical Journal of Australia* 2006 Jan 2; **184** (1): 27–31.

20. Begbie SD, Kerestes ZL, Bell DR. Patterns of alternative medicine use by cancer patients. *Med J Aust* 1996 Nov 18; **165** (10): 545–8.

21. Richardson MA, Masse LC, Nanny K, *et al.* Discrepant views of oncologists and cancer patients on complementary/alternative medicine. *Support Care Cancer* 2004 Nov; **12** (11): 797–804.

22. Zollman CV, A. ABC of complementary medicine: complementary medicine and the doctor. *British Medical Journal* 1999; **319**: 1557–61.

23. Schofield P, Ball D, Smith JG, *et al.* Optimism and survival in lung carcinoma patients. *Cancer* 2004 Mar 15; **100** (6): 1276–82.

24. Mackenzie G, Parkinson M, Lakhani A, *et al.* Issues that influence patient/physician discussion of complementary therapies. *Patient Education and Counselling* 1999 Oct; **38** (2): 155–9.

25. Richardson MA, Sanders T, Palmer JL, *et al.* Complementary/alternative medicine use in a comprehensive cancer center and the implications for oncology. *Journal of Clinical Oncology* 2000 Jul; **18** (13): 2505–14.

26. Steyer TE. Complementary and alternative medicine: a primer. *Family Practice Management* 2001 March: 37–42.

27. Eisenberg D. Advising patients who seek alternative and complementary medical therapies. *Annals of Internal Medicine* 1997; **127** (1): 61–9.

28. Weiger WA, Smith M, Boon H, *et al.* Advising patients who seek complementary and alternative medical therapies for cancer. *Annals of Internal Medicine* 2002 Dec 3; **137** (11): 889–903.

29. Burstein H. Editorial: discussing complementary therapies with cancer patients: what should we be talking about? *J Clin Oncol* 2000; **18** (13): 2501–4.

30. Molassiotis A, Fernadez-Ortega P, Pud D, *et al.* Use of complementary and alternative medicine in cancer patients: a European survey. *Annals of Internal Medicine* 2005 Apr; **16** (4): 655–63.

31. Herbert CP, Paluck E. Can primary care physicians be a resource to their patients in decisions regarding alternative and complementary therapies for cancer? *Patient Education and Counselling* 1997; **31**: 179–80.

32. Frenkel M, Ben-Arye E, Baldwin CD, *et al.* Approach to communicating with patients about the use of nutritional supplements in cancer care. *Southern Medical Journal* 2005 Mar; **98** (3): 289–94.

Chapter 25

The effect of internet use on the doctor–cancer patient relationship

Carma L Bylund and Jennifer A Gueguen

Cancer patients' use of the internet for cancer information and support

Seeking information

According to the latest Pew Internet and American Life Project (1), 80% of adult internet users seek health information from the internet. Consequently, given that 70% of adults report being online (1), more than half of US adults (113 million people) have used the internet to seek out health information and it is likely that a similar proportion of people use the internet in this way in other developed countries. In studies examining cancer patient populations from academic or community medical centres, four studies using heterogeneous cancer populations report 31–60% of cancer patients or caregivers to have used the internet to search for information about cancer (2–5). In similar settings, 48% of prostate cancer patients, 42% of breast cancer patients, 39% of melanoma patients and 44% of gastrointestinal cancer patients reported using the internet to access cancer information (6–9). Clearly, the internet has significantly transformed the way in which patients meet their health-related information needs. Patients cite the constant availability of information, the anonymity and the wealth of information as the internet's greatest strengths as a tool (10).

Patients who search for cancer-related internet information differ considerably from those who do not. Studies of mixed groups of cancer patients find that patients who do search for internet information tend to be younger, own a computer, have internet access at home and have a higher education level than cancer patients who do not search for cancer-related internet information (2, 3, 11). In studies of lung and breast cancer patients, education and income were positively correlated with the likelihood of using the internet to search for cancer-related information (6, 12). Although younger age has been correlated with internet use in prostate cancer and melanoma (7, 8), this is not the case in breast cancer (6). The role of the internet in information-seeking by ethnic minority patients with cancer is currently an issue being explored. While some studies have not found race/ethnicity to be associated with internet use for information-seeking about cancer (11), a number of studies report the internet to be used less frequently as a source of information by racial/ethnic minority patients (6, 8, 13). Cancer-related internet information is also accessed by those caring for loved ones with the disease. Caregivers who seek cancer-related information on the internet can also expose patients who do not themselves use the internet to this information. In a group of melanoma patients, 30% reported using the internet for information about their disease and another 9% reported having someone else do so (7). Some studies have found that more caregivers than patients access the internet directly for information about cancer (2, 13). However, patients in turn are being exposed to this information as it is provided to them by their caregivers.

Seeking support

Studies suggest that support-seeking is highest for diseases such as cancer, which can be viewed as stigmatizing; living with cancer and all that it entails is a social experience, one that influences a patient's relationships with others and one that is influenced by those same relationships (14). Support groups are a way for patients with cancer to talk to and learn from others who have had similar experiences, perhaps the only people who can really understand what a patient is going through (10). The literature about cancer support groups has suggested that participation in such groups can positively affect patients' adaptation to illness, including decreasing feelings of alienation, anxiety, isolation and misinformation (15).

Cancer-specific support groups were first reported in the 1970s, but the number of patients with cancer who are turning to the internet for support and the number of internet-based cancer support groups has risen dramatically in recent years (16, 17). The internet has allowed the cancer support group to evolve, becoming resistant to several of the obstacles experienced by traditional in-person support groups, including unpredictable attendance patterns and inconvenient meeting times, while increasing the probability that patients will come into contact with others who have had similar experiences (10, 18). Online cancer support groups offer patients social support, information, shared experience, role models, professional support, advocacy and empowerment (18). Participation in these groups has also been shown to reduce social isolation and negative moods including depression and cancer-related trauma (17).

Web forums have been used as a point of entry for many researchers interested in information- and support-seeking behaviour differences between men and women with the disease. In general, men are thought to turn to internet-based cancer support groups for information-seeking reasons and women for encouragement and support-seeking reasons (17). The themes of men's postings to web forums often include concerns about treatment information, healthcare providers and procedures, while the themes of women's postings include the exchange of emotional support and the impact of the illness on others (19). Additionally, a study of postings to an online cancer support group found that these trends hold for information- and support-provision patterns as well: men were more than twice as likely to give information and women more than twice as likely to give encouragement and support (18).

Far less is known about the support-seeking behaviour than the information-seeking behaviour of patients with cancer. A literature review performed by Klemm *et al.* (16) revealed a limited research base on the topic predominated by female Caucasian patients with often-studied cancer types (e.g. breast cancer). The authors suggest an agenda for future research of support-seeking behaviour that includes male patients, ethnic minority patients, patients with diverse cancer types and patients of various age groups.

Benefits and drawbacks of cancer-related internet information

There are several reported benefits of cancer patients reading cancer-related internet information. As noted above, many patients find support through online cancer support groups. Further, health-related internet searches can empower patients who are seeking to become active participants in their care. Caregivers have reported that using the internet for information has played a fundamental role in helping them provide care to their sick family members (11). In a study of mixed-type cancer patients, 62% reported that cancer-related internet information made them feel more hopeful (11). One potential of the internet in helping cancer patients and their caregivers lies in its ability to provide a wealth of information from various sources about topics that they frequently misunderstand. For example, while cancer clinical trials are critical to cancer patient care and outcomes, participation is low and patient understanding about the topic is limited (20). The potential is there for websites on clinical trials to have a positive impact.

However, other research has pointed out some of the detrimental effects of patients searching out cancer-related information on the internet. After reading cancer-related internet information, some patients become overwhelmed, aware of conflicting medical information, and more nervous, anxious and confused (7, 11, 21). In contrast, of oncologists who reported thinking that internet information makes patients more hopeful, 38% see this as a bad thing (22).

The impact of the internet on the doctor–patient relationship

Patients' ability to search for cancer-related information on the internet has the potential to significantly influence doctor–patient communication and relationships. The internet has provided patients access to information that was previously either unavailable or difficult to access. This has also had a levelling effect on the power imbalance in the doctor–patient relationship, specifically in terms of expert power (23, 24). Studies report that 36% of melanoma patients have stated that they intended to discuss internet information with their physician (7), while 40% of mixed cancer-type patients reported already discussing internet information with their physician (11). These percentages of cancer patients, who have discussed cancer-related internet information with their doctors, are fairly similar to general population statistics (25–28).

Forty-four per cent of oncologists report having difficulty with discussions about internet information (22). Studies have shown several reasons why these discussions can be challenging for both doctors and patients. Some oncologists find internet-informed patients have a harmful effect on the doctor–patient relationship, particularly when patients directly challenge them or when patients have too much information (29). Oncologists also report that internet information can lead to unnecessary discussion during a consultation that may consequently result in conflict (29). Further, internet discussions may result in longer consultations (22), which can be frustrating for doctors who have limited time with each patient. The literature also demonstrates that doctors and patients do not always agree about the characteristics of internet information, and it is easy to see how this lack of concordance may lead to challenging doctor–patient consultations. For example, cancer patients often make judgments about the accuracy of information that they find on the internet, and many perceive it to be quite accurate (11). Ninety-two per cent of radiation oncology patients found cancer-related internet information to be reliable (5). However, oncologists report concern with the accuracy of cancer-related internet information, with 91% of oncologists in one study reporting that the internet had the potential to cause harm to patients (29, 30). Additionally, although some patients report feeling empowered by internet information (21), internet information is only empowering to the extent that the oncologist is receptive to the patient being involved in the decision-making process (31).

Communication about internet information

Since cancer patients and their caregivers are increasingly using the internet to find health information (2), some healthcare professionals in oncology advocate that clinicians should consider providing guidance in helping patients find reliable information on the internet and engaging them in conversations about what they have found, so as to help them interpret this information. There is reason to believe that this guidance and support may increase patient satisfaction and enhance doctor–patient communication (10).

However, to date, little research has attempted to examine the actual process of communication about internet information between doctors and patients. In considering this process, it is helpful to consider a theoretical perspective. Fundamentally, doctor–patient communication is interpersonal communication. Thus communication theory may help us understand why doctor–patient conversations about internet information can be difficult. Facework theories (32–34) are a useful guide. *Face* is defined by Cupach and Metts (35) as 'the conception of self that each person displays in particular interactions with others' (p.3). These theories explain that in interpersonal communication, an individual's communication may threaten his or her face, which is called a face-threatening act (33). The conversational partner may respond in a manner that further threatens the other person's face or works to support the other person's face.

In our previous work, we have conceptualized the patient's act of introducing internet information into a doctor–patient consultation as a face-threatening act (36). The doctor may feel her face is threatened by the patient looking for information elsewhere. Or the patient may feel his face is threatened by acknowledging that he has looked elsewhere. Because the focus in this chapter is on training doctors to better communicate in these situations, we focus on the potential face threat to the patient. How a doctor responds to the patient raising the internet information, and the course of the discussion that follows, can prove to either support the patient's face (by validating the patient's efforts or taking the information seriously) or further threaten the patient's face (by warning the patient about the dangers of the internet or being dismissive of the information without any validation of efforts). Based on this theoretical framework and our previous work, we expect that face-saving, or supporting comments and discussion from doctors, will lead to higher patient satisfaction and lower patient anxiety.

Our pilot work in this area focused specifically on describing these discussions (37). Cancer patients and their caregivers (family or friends) were asked to recall a conversation with their oncologist about internet cancer information, and 74 participants responded. Participants introduced the internet information in a variety of ways. A little more than half reported asking a question to the oncologist (e.g. 'I read some information on the internet about a new drug called Arimidex and that it has fewer side-effects than Tamoxifen. Is that true?'); 28% reported making a statement of fact (e.g. 'Doctor, I heard there is a new drug to help lung cancer'); and 13% made an assertive statement (e.g. 'I went to the internet and learned there was brachytherapy radiation for breast cancer. I would like to be referred for this treatment.'). The majority of oncologists used face-saving responses, such as taking the information the patients presented seriously (61%) or showing active interest (13%), while 28% disagreed with the information or the patient's request, responses that have the potential to be face-threatening. This pilot work also examined how oncologists' responses to internet information affected patient satisfaction. Preliminary analyses show that cancer patients were more satisfied when the doctor took the information they had read seriously ($P<0.05$), with a trend toward them being less satisfied when the doctor disagreed with the information ($P = 0.06$).

We have also conducted a much larger study with a similar methodology, although not in a cancer-specific population. This study found that provider disagreement with internet information results in lower patient satisfaction (36). Certainly, providers will disagree with information that their patients bring in, and it is unreasonable to expect them not to do so in order to improve patient satisfaction. Therefore, we focused on understanding which additional strategies might moderate disagreement; in other words, which strategies might provide a face-saving effect. Our data showed that when a provider disagrees with the internet information, a demonstration that she is taking the information seriously significantly improves patient satisfaction with the interaction.

However, patients often choose not to talk with their clinicians about the health-related internet information that they have read. Imes, Bylund and colleagues examined reasons for not talking with a healthcare provider about internet health information (38). In this study, 714 patients (non-cancer specific) listed reasons why they had not talked with their provider about internet health information they had found: 29% of the reasons given were an attribution the patient had made about the information—low quality, repetitive, or non-relevant; 20% of the reasons listed had to do with healthcare systems or personal circumstances, such as not having a doctor at the time or not having enough time in the visit to discuss the information; 14% of the reasons were categorized as patient perceptions of clinician attributions about the information. For example, some patients reported that their clinician did not listen, was dismissive, uninterested or not open to the information because it came from the internet. Thirteen per cent of respondents' reasons were 'turf-related', meaning that the patient did not talk because he or she felt that would be invading the provider's turf, or the respondent thought that the clinician would feel offended, threatened or intimidated by the patient's attempt to discuss health-related internet information. Eight per cent of the reasons listed by patients were related to the patient wanting to save face. In other words, the patients reported not discussing the internet health information because they feared being embarrassed, laughed at, seen negatively or seen as overly concerned. The authors conclude that the majority of reasons patients gave for not talking about internet information indicated that respondents felt that they could not discuss their internet research with their clinicians. The authors note that, 'When patients make decisions to not discuss information because of these issues, they may miss important opportunities to both inform and learn from their healthcare provider about the information that they have found' (p.545).

Improving clinician–patient communication about internet health information

Suggested guidelines

To the best of our knowledge, there has not been a module specifically developed on discussing internet information with patients. In our training programme at Memorial Sloan–Kettering Cancer Center, we occasionally instruct simulated patients to refer to the internet during a particular workshop (e.g. in a Discussing Prognosis module, a simulated patient might say that she had read about her prognosis on the internet). However, the foci of other modules do not generally allow for discussion and practice about discussing internet information with patients. We have developed some preliminary guidelines for clinician–patient discussions about internet health information. These could be applied to a workshop focused particularly on discussing internet information or could be adapted for such discussions that are raised in other workshops (Box 25.1).

Explore the patient's experience with internet information

This strategy would likely be used after a patient introduces internet information. Another suggestion would be to recommend that clinicians use this strategy routinely to begin such a discussion with new patients. Communication skills that might be useful in achieving this strategy include asking open questions, clarifying and restating.

Box 25.1 Guidelines

1. Explore the patient's experience with internet information.
2. Respond empathically to patient's experience.
3. Acknowledge patient efforts.
4. Correct misunderstandings.
5. Provide guidance.
6. Reinforce clinician–patient partnership.

Exemplary statements:

'I'd just like to take a minute and talk about internet health information, as I do with all my patients. Tell me about your experience with looking up information on your cancer on the internet.'

'You mentioned that you had found some information on the internet. It's helpful for me to understand your experiences with looking up information about your cancer on the internet.'

Respond empathically to patient's experience

If a patient discloses emotions surrounding the experience of reading internet information, the clinician should respond empathically (39). Empathic communication skills include: acknowledging, validating or normalizing the patient's emotion or experience and encouraging the patient to express feelings.

Exemplary statements:

'I'm glad to hear that you've found some websites that have been helpful for you.'

'Yes, finding conflicting information on different websites can be really frustrating.'

Validating patient's efforts

Research on this topic has indicated that validating a patient's efforts in searching for information is important (36, 39). It is expected that this validating can create a buffer of sorts if the information found was incorrect and the clinician will need to explain this.

Exemplary statements:

'It's great that you are actively searching for information about your options for treating your cancer.'

'You've done your homework! That's great!'

Correct misunderstandings or incorrect information

It may be necessary to correct a patient's misunderstandings or incorrect information that the patient has found. We recommend that this is done after validating efforts (Box 25.1, 3). Communication skills that may be helpful in achieving this include: previewing information, inviting patient questions and checking patient understanding. At times, you may need to defer the patient's questions about internet information, and using the skill of negotiating the agenda might be useful.

Exemplary statements:

'There are a couple aspects of this information you found on the internet that I think we should talk about. First…'

'What do you see as the difference between what you read and what you and I have talked about?'

'I am happy to answer the questions about the information you found on that website; however, I think my answers might make more sense to you after I explain the treatment options.'

Provide guidance

Providing guidance to patients about internet information may not be comfortable for all clinicians. Those who are familiar with the internet, have found useful websites, or have developed effective strategies for searching for internet health information may feel comfortable providing guidance. Encouraging the use of credible internet sources for medical information and providing recommendations of such sites can be very helpful for patients (39).

Exemplary statements:

'One of the web sites that some of my patients have found useful is…'

'Our institution's web page gives some internet resources for patients with breast cancer. Have you looked at those?'

Reinforce the clinician–patient partnership

At the end of the discussion about the internet information, it may be helpful to reinforce the clinician–patient partnership. This strategy can set a foundation for the future of this relationship by advocating for the open sharing of information. To do this, a clinician may use communication skills such as making a partnership statement or endorsing question asking.

Exemplary statement:

'I think it's very important that we talk about the information that you are reading on the internet about your cancer. In our future visits, please let me know if you have questions about what you have been reading.'

Clinical scenarios and actor training

The following brief clinical scenario offers two variations on the theme of internet discussions that could be used in a small group communication role-play session. The first variation could be used in a module that is specifically focused on practicing the internet discussion. The second variation could be used in a module on Shared Treatment Decision-Making, where one learning goal is to practice discussions about internet information.

We have found it useful in working with actors to actually go online and search terms about cancer and give those printouts to the actors. This takes a little bit of background work in finding materials and working with the actor to integrate them into the role-plays; however, we find that this improves the believability of the scenario.

Instructions to learner

Today, you are meeting with a new patient, Christopher Palmer. Mr Palmer, age 55, is a high school history teacher who presents to you with an elevated PSA of 11 ng/ml. After biopsy, he was diagnosed with localized prostate cancer with a Gleason Score of 7.

(Facilitator: Allow the learner and patient to engage in a brief, 1 or 2 minute beginning to the consultation in order to establish rapport). You have decided that with each new patient you meet, you will take some time during the discussion to talk about the patient's experience with finding information on the internet.

Variation A: (fast forward).

You have now completed the discussion about treatment options with the patient. Christopher has said that he is leaning toward having a radical prostatectomy. You feel that now would be a good time to initiate a discussion about cancer-related internet information with the patient.

Instructions to patient: In this variation, the patient should say that he has spent 1–2 hours reading internet information about prostate cancer on the internet, and he should have brought with him some examples such as:

- a couple of printouts of material of things that he found were conflicting;

- a printout of an alternative or complementary therapy that he would like to try.

Variation B

You are meeting with Christopher for the first time today and need to discuss treatment options with him.

Instructions to patient: During the treatment discussion, the patient should volunteer information that he's found on the internet and have a few questions prepared (even pulling out printed out copies) to discuss with the doctor.

References

1. Fox S. Online Health Search 2006. 2006, Pew Internet & American Life Project.

2. Basch E, Thaler H, Shi W, *et al.* Use of information resources by patients with cancer and their companions. *Cancer* 2004; **100**: 2476–83.

3. Monnier J, Laken M, Carter C. Patient and caregiver interest in Internet-based cancer services. *Cancer Practice* 2002; **10**: 305–10.

4. Ranson S, Morrow G, Dakhil S, *et al.* Internet use among 1020 cancer patients assessed in community practices: a URCC CCOP study. *Proceedings/Annual Meeting of the American Society of Clinical Oncology* 2003; **22**: 534.

5. Metz J, Devine P, DeNittis A, *et al.* A multi-institutional study of internet utilization by radiation oncology patients. *International Journal of Radiation Oncolog –Biology–Physics* 2003; **56**: 1201–05.

6. Fogel J, Albert SM, Schnabel F, *et al.* Use of the internet by women with breast cancer. *Journal of Medical Internet Research* 2002; **4**: e9.

7. Sabel MS, Strecher VJ, Schwartz JL, *et al.* Patterns of Internet use and impact on patients with melanoma. *Journal of the American Academy of Dermatology* 2005; **52**: 779–85.

8. Smith R, Devine P, Jones H, *et al.* Internet use by patients with prostate cancer undergoing radiotherapy. *Urology* 2003; **62**: 273–77.

9. Yakren S, Shi W, Thaler H, *et al.* Use of the Internet and other information resources among adult cancer patients and their companions. *Proceedings/Annual Meeting of the American Society of Clinical Oncology* 2001; **20**: 398a.

10. Penson RT, Benson RC, Parles K, *et al.* Virtual connections: internet healthcare. *Oncologist* 2002; **7**: 555–68.

11. Helft PR, Eckles RE, Johnson-Calley CS, *et al.* Use of the internet to obtain cancer information among cancer patients at an urban county hospital. *Jorunal of Clincal Oncology* 2005; **23**: 4954–62.

12. Peterson M, Fretz P. Patient use of the Internet for information in a lung cancer clinic. *CHEST* 2003; **123**: 452–57.

13. James N, Daniels H, Rahman R, *et al.* A study of informaiton seeking by cancer patients and their carers. *Clinical Oncology* 2007; **19**: 356–62.

14. Davison KP, Pennebaker JW, Dickerson SS. Who Talks? The social psychology of illness support groups? *American Psychologist* 2000; **55**: 205–17.

15. Klemm P, Reppert K, Visich L. A nontraditional cancer support group: the internet. *Computers in Nursing* 1998; **16**: 31–36.

16. Klemm P, Bunnell D, Cullen M, *et al.* Online cancer support groups: a review of the research literature. *Computers, Informatics and Nursing* 2003; **21**: 136–42.

17. Im E, Chee W, Liu Y, *et al.* Characteristics of cancer patients in internet cancer support groups. *Computers, Informatics and Nursing* 2007; **25**: 334–43.

18. Klemm P, Hurst M, Dearholt S, *et al.* Cyber solace: Gender differences on internet cancer support groups. *Computers in Nursing* 1999; **17**: 65–72.

19. Seale C, Ziebland S, Charteris-Black J. Gender, cancer experience and internet use: a comparative keyword analysis of interviews and online cancer support groups. *Social Science and Medicine* 2006; **62**: 2577–90.

20. Carden CP, Jefford M, Rosenthal MA. Information about cancer clinical trials: an analysis of Internet resources. *European Journal of Cancer* 2007; **43**: 1574–80.

21. Fleisher L, Bass S, Ruzek S, *et al.* Relationships among internet health information use, patient behaviour and self-efficacy in newly diagnosed cancer patients who contact the National Cancer Institute's (NCI) Atlantic Region Cancer Information Service (CIS). in AMIA Annual Fall Symposium 2002.

22. Helft PR, Hlubocky F, Daugherty CK. American oncologists' views of Internet use by cancer patients: a mail survey of American Society of Clinical Oncology members. *Journal of Clinical Oncology* 2003; **21**: 942–47.

23. Bylund CL, Sabee C, Imes R, *et al.* Exploration of the construct of reliance among patients who talk with their providers about internet information. *Journal of Health Communication* 2007; **12**: 17–28.

24. Makoul G. Perpetuating passivity: reliance and reciprocal determinism in physician-patient interaction. *Journal of Health Communication* 1998; **3**: 233–59.

25. Diaz JA, Griffith RA, Ng JJ, *et al.* Patients' use of the internet for medical information. *Journal of General Internal Medicine* 2002; **17**: 180–85.

26. Diaz JA, Sciamanna CN, Evangelou E, *et al.* Brief report: What types of internet guidance do patients want from their physicians? *Journal of General Internal Medicine* 2005; **20**: 683–85.

27. Fox S, Rainie L. *Vital decisions: how internet users decide what information to trust when they or their loved ones are sick.* 2002, Pew Internet and American Life Project: Washington, D.C.

28. Murray E, Lo B, Pollack L, *et al.* The impact of health information on the internet on the physician-patient relationship. *Archives of Internal Medicine* 2003; **163**: 1727–34.

29. Broom A. Medical specialists' accounts of the impact of the internet on the doctor/patient relationship. *Health* 2005; **9**: 319–38.

30. Newnham G, Burns W, Snyder R, *et al.* Attitudes of oncology health professionals to information from the Internet and other media. *Medical Journal of Australia* 2005; **183**: 197–200.

31. Broom A. Virtually he@lthy: The impact of internet use on disease experience and the doctor–patient relationship. *Qualitative Health Research* 2005; **15**: 325–45.

32. Miller K. *Communication theories: perspectives, processes, and contexts.* 2002, Boston: The McGraw-Hill Companies.

33. Brown P, Levinson S. *Politeness: some universals in language use.* 1987, Cambridge: Cambridge University Press.

34. Goffman E. *The presentation of self in everyday life.* 1959, Garden City, NY: Doubleday.

35. Cupach W, Metts S. *Facework.* 1994, London: Thousand Oaks.

36. Bylund CL, Gueguen JA, Sabee CM, *et al.* Provider-patient dialogue about internet health information: An exploration of strategies to improve the provider-patient relationship. *Patient Education and Counseling* 2007; **66** 346–52.

37. Bylund CL, Gueguen JA. Physician–patient conversations about internet cancer information. *Psycho-Oncology* 2006; **15**: S189.

38. Imes RS, Bylund CL, Routsong T, *et al.* Patients' reasons for refraining from discussing internet health information with their healthcare providers. *Health Communication* 2008; **23**: 538–547.

39. Wald H, Dube C, Anthony D. Untangling the web—the impact of internet use on healthcare and the physician–patient relationship. *Patient Education and Counseling* 2007; **68**: 218–24.

Chapter 26

Promoting treatment adherence

Kelly B Haskard and M Robin DiMatteo

Overview of patient adherence in the context of cancer treatment

Patient adherence (also termed compliance or concordance) involves the degree to which a patient carries out, correctly and completely, the medical regimen recommended by the patient's health professional. The regimen can involve medications, screenings, appointment-keeping, dietary management, and/or other treatments and life-style changes. Persistence refers to following a course of treatment for the entire period of time it is prescribed. In the context of cancer care, patients may be required to adhere to adjuvant hormonal therapy, faithfully attend all chemotherapy or radiation appointments, appear for regular follow-up screenings, and/or make recommended changes in diet and exercise patterns. Although adherence has important documented effects on cancer outcomes, many factors influence whether or not patients adhere. This chapter details the following:

- the importance of adherence, as well as the reasons why adherence may be difficult for patients;
- the value of providers' awareness of their patients' non-adherence, and their open discussion and collaboration to help their patients achieve adherence; and
- the communication process that facilitates adherence.

We also delineate specific strategies within healthcare provider-patient communication that can be used to promote adherence.

Rates of adherence

Meta-analytic work suggests that across medical conditions and regimens, the average rate of patient adherence is about 75%; thus, a quarter of all patients, on average, fail to follow their treatment recommendations (1). In this meta-analysis, across 65 studies of different types of cancer, adherence was slightly above average, with 79.1% of cancer patients following recommended treatments (1). More specifically, rates of adherence to Tamoxifen treatment for breast cancer have been found to range from 69 to 79% (focusing on adherence and persistence over 5 years of treatment) (2–4). Lung cancer patients' adherence to adjuvant chemotherapy has been assessed at 84% for four of six cycles and 50% for all six cycles (5). Other findings on adjuvant chemotherapy for lung cancer patients demonstrate that only about 50% of patients follow through with all recommended cycles of chemotherapy (6). Studies of adjuvant chemotherapy treatment for colon cancer show approximately 78% adherence (7). In a study of skin cancer patients, 84% of those who survived melanoma conducted self-examinations at least once a year, although a smaller number (59%) wore sunscreen (8).

Outcomes of non-adherence

Non-adherence matters if it affects health outcomes. The literature identifies important consequences of non-adherence to patients' health status and disease outcomes, including poor symptom control, disease recurrence, and/or shortened survival time. Ending treatment early could increase the risk of disease recurrence and metastasis (9). Other outcomes of patient non-adherence are relevant as well, such as the economic costs of unused prescriptions and unnecessary, unproductive, or wasted medical visits. Non-adherence can also erode trust in the physician–patient relationship, contributing to frustration for both parties.

Outcomes are also affected when patients fail to consistently attend their scheduled appointments, such as for chemotherapy or radiation treatments. In one study of patients undergoing breast conservation therapy and radiation, survival was worse when patients failed to adhere to their radiation protocol (10). Other research exploring the predictors of survival from breast cancer found that missing appointments was a key predictor of shorter survival time (11), and research on colon cancer has shown increased risk of mortality when patients fail to complete treatment (7). Critical thresholds for adherence may be essential to better outcomes, such as in HIV care, where patients who are more than 95% adherent to their protease inhibitor medication regimen have significantly better outcomes than those with lower rates of adherence (12). Some standards of care in cancer require a level of at least 80% adherence (12).

The reasons for improved outcomes when patients adhere to recommended treatments may be complex (13). More favourable outcomes may occur because adherent patients benefit from the direct therapeutic effects of their treatments, or possibly also because of 'non-specific' therapeutic effects of adhering (14, 15). That is, benefits may accrue both through biological or pharmacological effects and through psychological and behavioural mechanisms, such as provider and patient expectations, optimism, or engaging in other positive health behaviours (16, 17). The beneficial effects of patient adherence on health outcomes have been shown to occur both when treatment is an active medication and when it is a placebo (14), further demonstrating that expectations of healing or engaging in positive health behaviours may benefit health in numerous ways.

Barriers to adherence in cancer

Patients' success at adhering to the complex treatment regimens for cancer can be multifaceted, and influenced by a wide variety of factors. Many elements in the patient's life that predict his or her ability to adhere have been elucidated in the theoretical and empirical adherence literature. Some barriers to adherence can signal patients' intentional non-adherence, whereas others may be unintentional. Such a distinction recognizes the multifactorial nature of adherence. Intentional non-adherence in the context of cancer, for example, could result from a patient's choice not to continue adjuvant medication treatment, with its attendant side-effects, in order to prevent recurrence and increase chances for survival. A patient might also purposely miss follow-up appointments, or take partial doses of a regimen because they feel asymptomatic or do not understand or believe in the purpose of the treatment. Unintentional non-adherence, on the other hand, involves misunderstanding the regimen (e.g. timing or dosing), or forgetting to follow through because of a chaotic life-style, family responsibilities, or lack of necessary resources.

Patient factors

A simple model of predictors of adherence

A perfect model to explain adherence to treatment does not exist, and many predictors have been offered in the research literature, but a useful model involving three broad groups of factors provides a framework for understanding why patients may not adhere. This model describes, respectively, the cognitive, motivational, and resource-related factors that influence adherence. Very simply, a patient must: (a) know what to do to adhere, (b) want to adhere, and (c) be able to adhere (18).

Cognitive

A primary factor in determining patients' adherence is their knowledge and understanding of the treatment. In the process of cancer care, patients usually must process a great deal of information about their disease and treatment interventions, including how to follow medication regimens properly, how to cope with side-effects, the importance of regular screenings, and how to follow a diet and exercise plan that will promote healing. Many patients forget what they have been told by their physicians and healthcare providers, and especially when they are stressed or distressed, the chances of forgetting may be significantly increased (19). Some research has indicated that health literacy is a strong predictor of adherence. A study of impoverished early stage breast cancer patients being treated with radiation therapy found that only 36% of patients were fully adherent, and predictors of non-adherence that approached traditional significance levels included patients' level of literacy (10).

Motivation

Patients also must possess the motivation to adhere. Their beliefs, attitudes, and perceptions all contribute to enhancing motivation. Patients with more confidence in their abilities to discuss their treatment with their healthcare providers are more adherent (20). Research on patient health beliefs has found that discontinuation of Tamoxifen was associated with patient beliefs that the risks of treatment outweighed the benefits (21, 3). Patients who cope with the challenges of illness in a proactive manner, such as by seeking support and information, actively solving problems, and expressing concerns, may be more motivated to adhere than those who avoid the challenges of the illness and treatment (22).

Resources

Having necessary resources (e.g. finances, time, and access to care) can be crucial to adherence. Research in breast cancer, for example, suggests that patients may miss appointments for reasons including work commitments and poor transportation options (11). Social support also matters; patients who possess less tangible and emotional support and have less cohesive families are at greater risk of non-adherence (23). Theoretical models of the relationship between social support and health suggest that patients may be encouraged to adhere better by supportive social networks, subsequently affecting their physiology and disease risk (24). Studies have suggested that greater social support is associated with better adherence to both breast cancer screening (25) and chemotherapy treatment for colon cancer (7).

Mental health

Each predictor of adherence described above can be affected by 'distressed psychological states', such as depression, anxiety, or stress (26), which often attend a serious illness such as cancer. As many as one-third of cancer patients experience mild or moderate depression, and up to one-fourth experience major depression (27). Many patients also experience guilt, fear, anxiety, stress, pain, lowered quality of life, and fatigue; and there is evidence that these can affect their adherence. Emotional distress can reduce adherence to strategies for cancer detection. The utilization of preventive health services, such as colon cancer screening and mammography, occurs significantly less frequently in distressed older adults than in their non-distressed counterparts (28). Further, patients with worse adherence to immunosuppressive medication after transplant have been found to self-report greater levels of distress (29). Such distressed states can also influence health behaviours such as diet, exercise, sleep, and use of alcohol and tobacco (30).

Severity of disease

Although not falling neatly into the simple model of adherence predictors listed above, severity of disease may also influence adherence. A recent meta-analysis found that in more serious diseases, including cancer, patients who self-reported poorer health were significantly less likely to be adherent (31). According to objective measures of disease severity (e.g. blood pressure), in less serious diseases (e.g. hypertension), patients in poorer health were more likely to be adherent. However, in more serious diseases such as cancer or HIV, patients who were objectively more seriously ill (such as those with later stages of the disease, or who had a serious abnormality, or those with higher viral load and lower CD4 cell count) were less likely to be adherent to their regimens (31). These findings suggest that the difficulties faced by the most severely ill cancer patients may interfere with their adherence for a variety of reasons, including their doubts about the efficacy of treatment, or being physically and psychologically overwhelmed with the demands of the disease. In such situations, adherence represents another difficult task among the many challenges of dealing with a potentially life-threatening illness.

Interaction or system-level factors

Regimen complexity

Clinically, it is important that adherence not be unduly difficult for the patient, and treatment must fit into the patient's life-style if it is to be successful. Adherence is compromised when the regimen is complex or when there are side-effects (20). In chemotherapy, side-effects that harm physical, social, and emotional functioning contribute to discontinuing the regimen before it has been completed, leading to the failure to achieve optimum health benefits (32). In breast cancer, for example, adjuvant therapy can be accompanied by side-effects such as hot flashes and joint pain (33). For the treatment of many cancers, patients must regularly attend radiation therapy appointments, which can be physically and emotionally draining and accompanied by distressing side-effects. Chemotherapy can compromise immune functioning resulting in fatigue, as well as social isolation to reduce the risk of infection. Indeed, patients in collaboration with their doctors may make a thoughtful choice to not begin a treatment or to discontinue it prematurely because of effects on quality of life. In such situations, non-adherence is clearly intentional but is a reasonable choice on the part of patients.

Communication and interactional dynamics

Effective physician–patient communication, or communication that occurs in the context of a collaborative, trusting relationship, can improve adherence and health outcomes (34). (See Box 26.1 for key physician health care provider adherence-related communication skills.) Some research, for instance, has indicated that greater support from physicians and more patient involvement in decision-making increases adherence (2). Further, patients are more likely to adhere to screening when they are encouraged to do so by their healthcare providers (35). Research on cancer screening in a group of low-income women has indicated that the predictors of follow-through with screening recommendations included a longer, more satisfying relationship with a healthcare provider (36). A survey of oncology healthcare providers indicated that more than 85% believed effective communication enhanced patient adherence (37). In practice, however, such a therapeutic partnership does not always occur. A study of oncologist–patient communication about adjuvant hormonal therapy for breast cancer revealed that many issues related to medication-taking, difficulties in adherence, and difficulties persisting with the regimen in the long term were not ever discussed by physicians and patients (38). Efforts to improve the larger interaction-level barriers to patient adherence require recognition of the importance of a therapeutic physician–patient relationship in ensuring the efficient transfer of information. These efforts also depend upon creating provider–patient partnerships, focusing on the patient's quality of life, and addressing other barriers that patients may face.

Effective communication as a means to promote adherence

Overview

Effective communication in the medical visit involves both verbal and non-verbal behaviour, including voice tone, eye contact, facial expressions, use of touch, gestures, and body orientation or 'synchrony'. Such communication focuses on affective or psychosocial aspects of care, as well as the tasks of the medical visit, such as exchange of information. Particularly in the context of treatment of a serious illness such as cancer, communication is more 'high stakes', as it involves giving bad news to patients, making major decisions about treatment, discussing participation in clinical trials, navigating communication with family members, and developing rapport. Communication about adherence itself can be particularly difficult, but is absolutely necessary because of the implications for patient outcomes. Research shows that healthcare providers do not accurately predict their patients' adherence (17). They may also be unaware of patients' circumstances, such as lack of social support or lack of adequate resources, that can increase their risk of non-adherence (39). Thus, provider–patient communication requires openness about expectations of treatment, help in coping with the challenges of adherence, and assistance with strategies to enhance adherence. Therapeutic discussions aimed at breaking down barriers to adherence should not focus on blame but rather on providing opportunities and encouragement for the open transfer of information and collaboration to improve patients' adherence, health outcomes, and quality of life.

One of the most important steps to achieving adherence involves the development of rapport in a therapeutic, collaborative relationship. Open communication and the sharing of goals and hoped-for outcomes are essential to promoting adherence. From the first visit, a partnership between provider and patient must be fostered and then strengthened over future visits, throughout the course of illness and treatment. Demonstrating empathy for patients involves the provider's awareness of the perspective of the patient, understanding the patient's point of view, and communicating that perception to the patient. This empathic behaviour should extend toward understanding the difficulties of disease management and medication-taking, and should view solving the challenges of adherence from the patient's perspective.

It is important that oncology healthcare providers and their patients be concordant in their communication with one another and share their perceptions of the treatment plan and progress. One study found that physicians and cancer patients were very disparate in their reports of their discussion about how treatment would affect the patient's quality of life (40). Patients had reported this was one of the most important topics of communication with their physician. Providers' failure to discuss something so important to patients as their quality of life and its potential compromise could decrease patients' adherence to treatment (40).

Exchange of information

Patients may vary in the amount of medical information they want to receive, and physicians also vary in how much they feel comfortable giving. Information is a form of social support that can give cancer patients knowledge about their disease (41), and it is likely that greater knowledge could translate into better adherence to treatment. Communication that is initiated by physicians

Box 26.1 Key physician/healthcare provider adherence-related communication skills

1. Help patients to know and understand their treatments and how to follow them.
   - Summarize or clarify the patient's understanding of the details of the regimen. For example: 'Why don't you repeat back to me your understanding of how to take this medication so we can be sure that I have been clear?'
   - Request that the patient ask questions. For example: 'I encourage you to ask me all of your questions about the treatment process during our visit today.'
   - Encourage patients to take written information that is provided. For example: 'I think it would be helpful if you use this checklist, and as we talk you can check off any relevant issues (side-effects, strategies to deal with them, etc.). Then before you leave today, you can take some of the printed materials the office has put together related to those checked items.'

2. Motivate patients to believe in the treatment, and want to adhere to it.
   - Discuss the relationship between adherence and outcomes. For example: 'The evidence from the studies that have been done indicates that when patients take this drug for five years the chances of recurrence are greatly reduced.'
   - Converse about the risks and benefits of treatment as well as alternative treatment options. For example: 'As with any treatment, there may be some side-effects of this treatment, but the long-term benefits may likely outweigh those.' 'It seems like you're thinking this might not be the best treatment for you. Why don't we talk about it, as well as about some of the possible alternatives?'
   - Encourage problem-focused and proactive coping. For example: 'Many patients have difficulty remembering to take their medication at the same time every day. Let's talk about some things that may help you to remember so that we can plan for that challenge in advance.'
   - Promote positive expectations about the outcomes of treatment. For example: 'I am hoping for a very good outcome, and I feel confident that your following the treatment precisely will very much improve the chances.'

3. Recognize barriers to adherence and help patients follow treatment. Focus on the following:
   - Patient's views about duration and costs of regimen. For example: 'I know that it will be a life-style change to fit the radiation appointments into your schedule each week but I think it will be very beneficial for you. Perhaps you can think of this as a way to do something important to take care of yourself.'
   - Patient's support system/resources and building social support. For example: 'How has your husband's response to the cancer been for you?' 'Do you think it might be helpful for you to join a support group so that you could talk with other women who are having similar experiences?'
   - Patient's mental health. For example: 'Tell me about how your moods have been. Sometimes when patients are feeling particularly distressed, they have difficulty taking their medication as prescribed for a number of different reasons. Let's talk about some of the ways you might handle that.'

> **Box 26.1 (continued) Key physician/healthcare provider adherence-related communication skills**
>
> ◆ Available resources. For example: 'Do you have a way to get to and from the clinic for your chemotherapy appointments?'
>
> ◆ Helpful reminder methods. For example: 'It can be really helpful to put your medication next to the coffee pot or tea kettle. Then you remember to take it regularly every morning as you have your cup of coffee or tea.'

and involves discussing the disease and treatment, fosters patients' perceptions that they have choice, and enhances their satisfaction with care (42). In providing information about adherence, physicians may benefit their patients most by refraining from use of excessive medical jargon. Instead, they can promote adherence by writing down important information, and checking to be sure that patients understand (43).

Partnership, involvement, and shared decision-making

Although there may be some variation among patients in their desire to be involved in decision-making, evidence indicates that they do value and want to be involved in decision-making (44). If patients are not encouraged to be involved, their rates of adherence suffer, as shown in a study of adherence to Tamoxifen (2). Similarly, breast cancer patients who possess self-efficacy in talking to their doctors about issues relevant to their disease have been found to be more likely to be adherent (20). Achieving concordance in the management of medication regimens in cancer involves understanding what matters to patients, recognizing the importance of quality of life, keeping track of symptoms, and communicating with all members of the healthcare team (45). Shared decision-making can be implemented by understanding the patients' desires regarding decision-making, the physician giving all possible information about the decision to be made and drawing out the values of the patient, and the two working together to come up with a plan (43).

Communication about psychological state and resources

One major barrier to adherence may be patients' mental health. Understanding and memory, motivation and attitudes, and social support and resources can all be negatively affected by poor mental health. Patients' distressed psychological states can impede their ability to adhere. Thus, it is important for physicians and healthcare providers to be aware of, and inquire about, symptoms and behaviours that may indicate that a patient is struggling with depression or distress.

It is also important to discuss resources, including the financial burden of treatment, and the availability of tangible resources and emotional support from loved ones. Both types of resources, social and economic, can have a major impact on a patient's willingness and ability to follow through with recommended treatments.

Communication and the healthcare team

All members of the patient's healthcare team may be able to exert influence in communicating about adherence. (See role-play below.) The majority of the empirical research on this topic has focused on physicians, although nurses, pharmacists, and others also have significant opportunities to answer patients' questions, give information, and counsel patients about adherence. Training programmes that focus on improving oncology nurses' communication skills find that confidence in their communication with patients does improve as a result of training (46), although adherence was not measured. Nurse-led interventions involving nurse-directed reminders to patients have positive effects in encouraging patients to engage in cancer screening and in reducing perceived barriers (47). Nurses can also be involved in patients' follow-up care after surgery, such as in the case of colorectal cancer (48).

Strategies to increase memory and simplify adherence

Difficulties in understanding and remembering medication regimens can threaten adherence; therefore, memory aids (e.g. reminders, cues, lists, calendars, pillboxes, timers, etc.) can play an important role in helping patients to remember to take their medications correctly. Healthcare providers can suggest such tools to their patients and can even be involved in providing reminders, such as for appointments. Studies show that patients find written information about their treatment to be helpful (49). In practice, of course, it can be challenging to assist large numbers of patients with the support and reminders that are needed to help them adhere. One innovative study involved the development of a computer database tracking system for cervical and colon cancer screening (50). The database kept track of lab results, generated letters to patients telling them of their results, and sent appointment reminder information; this system resulted in significant increases in screening.

Interventions to improve communication about adherence

Effective communication may not be easy, but it is a trainable skill; intervention studies show that training in communication skills works. Such skills as information-giving and effective listening can be improved, and the positive effects of training can persist over time (51). Although few communication skills training programmes have explored the outcome of patient adherence, some have demonstrated that improved communication skills, as a result of training, do improve patient satisfaction with care (52), and that more satisfied patients are typically more adherent (53). A meta-analysis of interventions to improve patient adherence, including adherence to cancer treatments (54), showed that cancer patients had longer survival times and lower recurrence rates because of the effects of adherence-enhancing interventions.

Conclusion

Improving provider–patient communication and reducing patient barriers are important steps toward improving cancer patient adherence. Research on specific communicative behaviours in oncology and their relationship to adherence is somewhat sparse. There is a need for more specific research focused on describing the communication behaviours that are most beneficial to adherence. Follow-up research should then assess the design of interventions to improve those behaviours. In practice, healthcare providers can help patients improve adherence by communicating openly with them, collaborating in making decisions about treatment, and being aware of the challenges to adherence. Developing a trusting relationship focused on making a treatment regimen part of the patient's life is a key to promoting adherence in cancer patients.

Roleplay

Jane Mason is a 41-year-old woman with early stage oestrogen-receptor positive breast cancer. She is a mother of two daughters, Lily who is 14 and Taylor who is 11; she is divorced from their father. Jane and her sister own a small accounting business, which they run from a home office. Jane had a lumpectomy and radiation therapy; her oncologist is now recommending adjuvant hormonal therapy to prevent recurrence of her cancer. Jane is hesitant because of what she has heard about the side-effects of the recommended medication and the five-year duration of the medication seems daunting to her. She has a busy schedule as a single mother and businesswoman, and she worries the medication will interfere too much with her life. She doubts that the benefits will outweigh the drawbacks. Jane has also been struggling with depression since her diagnosis and feels that she doesn't want to burden her sister or young daughters with talking about her feelings.

Jane's oncologist sits down with her to discuss the efficacy of the medication and its' relationship to the outcomes of her cancer. They also discuss the likelihood of various potential side-effects and some strategies to cope with them and reduce their severity if they do occur.

The nurse talks with her about ways to fit the medication schedule into her busy life-style and about memory aids to help remind her when a dose should be taken.

The social worker talks with Jane about seeking professional help for her depression, suggesting that it might help to have someone to talk with outside of her family.

Acknowledgements

This work was supported by a Robert Wood Johnson Foundation Investigator Award in Health Policy Research (PI: M. Robin DiMatteo), by a grant from the National Institute on Aging 5R03AG27552–02 (PI: M. Robin DiMatteo), and by the Committee on Research of the U.C. Riverside Academic Senate. The views expressed in this paper are those of the authors alone and do not imply endorsement by the funding sources.

References

1. DiMatteo MR (2004). Variations in patients' adherence to medical recommendations: a quantitative review of 50 years of research. *Med Care* **42**, 200–9.
2. Kahn KL, Schneider EC, Malin JL, *et al.* (2007). Patient centered experiences in breast cancer: predicting long-term adherence to tamoxifen use. *Med Care* **45**, 431–9.
3. Lash TL, Fox MP, Westrup JL, *et al.* (2006). Adherence to tamoxifen over the five-year course. *Breast Cancer Res Treat* **99**, 215–20.
4. Partridge AH, Wang PS, Winer EP, *et al.* (2003). Non-adherence to adjuvant tamoxifen therapy in women with primary breast cancer. *J Clin Oncol* **21**, 602–6.
5. Dediu M, Alexandru A, Median D, *et al.* (2006). Compliance with adjuvant chemotherapy in non-small cell lung cancer. The experience of a single institution evaluating a cohort of 356 patients. J BUON **11**, 425–32.
6. Alam N, Shepherd FA, Winton T, *et al.* (2005). Compliance with post-operative adjuvant chemotherapy in non-small cell lung cancer. An analysis of National Cancer Institute of Canada and intergroup trial JBR.10 and a review of the literature. *Lung Cancer* **47**, 385–94.
7. Dobie SA, Baldwin LM, Dominitz JA, *et al.* (2006). Completion of therapy by Medicare patients with stage III colon cancer. *J Natl Cancer Inst* **98**, 610–9.
8. Manne S, Lessin S (2006). Prevalence and correlates of sun protection and skin self-examination practices among cutaneous malignant melanoma survivors. *J Behav Med* **29**(5), 419–34.
9. Andersen BL, Kiecolt-Glaser JK, *et al.* (1994). A biobehavioural model of cancer stress and disease course. *Am Psychol* **49**, 389–404.
10. Li BD, Brown WA, Ampil FL, *et al.* (2000). Patient compliance is critical for equivalent clinical outcomes for breast cancer treated by breast-conservation therapy. *Ann Surg* **231**, 883–9.
11. Howard DL, Penchansky R, Brown MB (1998). Disaggregating the effects of race on breast cancer survival. *Fam Med* **30**, 228–35.
12. Paterson DL, Swindells S, Mohr J, *et al.* (2000). Adherence to protease inhibitor therapy and outcomes in patients with HIV infection. *Ann Intern Med* **133**, 21–30.

13. DiMatteo MR, Giordani PJ, Lepper HS, *et al.* (2002). Patient adherence and medical treatment outcomes: a meta-analysis. *Med Care* **40**, 794–811.

14. Horwitz RI, Horwitz SM (1993). Adherence to treatment and health outcomes. *Arch Intern Med* **153**, 1863–8.

15. Epstein LH (1984). The direct effects of compliance on health outcome. *Health Psychol* **3**, 385–93.

16. Czajkowski SM, Chesney MA, Smith AW (1990). Adherence and the placebo effect. In: Shumaker SA, Schron EB, Ockene JK, (1st edn). *The handbook of health behaviour change*, pp. 515–534. Springer, New York.

17. Haskard KB, DiMatteo MR, Williams SL (in press). Adherence and health outcomes: How much does adherence matter? In: Shumaker SA, Ockene JK, Riekert K, ed. *The handbook of health behaviour change* (3rd edn). pp. 771–784. Springer, New York.

18. DiMatteo MR, DiNicola DD (1982). *Achieving patient compliance: the psychology of the medical practitioner's role.* Pergamon, Elsmford, NY.

19. Mystakidou K, Tsilika E, Parpa E, *et al.* (2005). Assessment of anxiety and depression in advanced cancer patients and their relationship with quality of life. *Qual Life Res* **14**(8), 1825–33.

20. Demissie S, Silliman RA, Lash TL (2001). Adjuvant tamoxifen: predictors of use, side-effects, and discontinuation in older women. *J Clin Oncol* **19**, 322–8.

21. Fink AK, Gurwitz J, Rakowski W, *et al.* (2004). Patient beliefs and tamoxifen discontinuance in older women with estrogen receptor–positive breast cancer. *J Clin Oncol* **22**, 3309–15.

22. Holahan CJ, Moos RH, Holahan CK, *et al.* (1997). Social context, coping strategies, and depressive symptoms: an expanded model with cardiac patients. *J Pers Soc Psychol* **72**, 918–28.

23. DiMatteo MR (2004). Social support and patient adherence to medical treatment: a meta-analysis. *Health Psychol* **23**, 207–18.

24. Uchino BN (2006). Social support and health: a review of physiological processes potentially underlying links to disease outcomes. *J Behav Med* **29**, 377–87.

25. Katapodi MC, Facione NC, Miaskowski C, *et al.* (2002). The influence of social support on breast cancer screening in a multicultural community sample. *Oncol Nurs Forum* **29**, 845–52.

26. DiMatteo MR, Lepper HS, *et al.* (2000). Depression is a risk factor for noncompliance with medical treatment: meta-analysis of the effects of anxiety and depression on patient adherence. *Arch Intern Med* **160**, 2101–7.

27. Spiegel D, Giese-Davis J (2003). Depression and cancer: mechanisms and disease progression. *Biol Psychiatry* **54**, 269–82.

28. Thorpe JM, Kalinowski CT, Patterson ME, *et al.* (2006). Psychological distress as a barrier to preventive care in community-dwelling elderly in the United States. *Med Care* **44**, 187–91.

29. Achille MA, Ouellette A, Fournier S, *et al.* (2006). Impact of stress, distress and feelings of indebtedness on adherence to immunosuppressants following kidney transplantation. *Clin Transplant* **20**, 301–6.

30. Katon WJ (2003). Clinical and health services relationships between major depression, depressive symptoms, and general medical illness. *Biol Psychiatry* **54**, 216–26.

31. DiMatteo MR, Haskard KB, Williams SL (2007). Health beliefs, disease severity, and patient adherence: a meta-analysis. *Med Care* **45**, 521–8.

32. Richardson JL, Marks G, Levine A (1988). The influence of symptoms of disease and side-effects of treatment on compliance with cancer therapy. *J Clin Oncol* **6**(11), 1746–52.

33. Cella D, Fallowfield LJ (2007). Recognition and management of treatment-related side-effects for breast cancer patients receiving adjuvant endocrine therapy. *Breast Cancer Res Treat* 107(2): 167–180.

34. Stewart M, Brown JB, Boon H, *et al.* (1999). Evidence on patient-doctor communication. *Cancer Prev Control* **3**, 5–30.

35. Castellano PZ, Wenger NK, Graves WL (2001). Adherence to screening guidelines for breast and cervical cancer in postmenopausal women with coronary heart disease: an ancillary study of volunteers for hers. *J Womens Health Gend Based Med* **10**, 451–61.

36. O'Malley AS, Forrest CB, Mandelblatt J (2002). Adherence of low-income women to cancer screening recommendations. *J Gen Intern Med* **17**, 144–54.

37. Roberts C, Benjamin H, Chen L *et al.* (2005). Assessing communication between oncology professionals and their patients. *J Cancer Educ* **20**,113–8.

38. Davidson B, Vogel V, Wickerham L (2007). Oncologist-patient discussion of adjuvant hormonal therapy in breast cancer: results of a linguistic study focusing on adherence and persistence to therapy. J Support Oncol **5**, 139–43.

39. Bickell NA, LePar F, Wang JJ, Leventhal H (2007). Lost opportunities: physicians' reasons and disparities in breast cancer treatment. *J Clin Oncol* **25**, 2516–21.

40. Meropol NJ, Weinfurt KP, Burnett CB, *et al.* (2003). Perceptions of patients and physicians regarding phase I cancer clinical trials: implications for physician–patient communication. *J Clin Oncol* **21**, 2589–96.

41. Maly RC, Leake B, Silliman RA (2004). Breast cancer treatment in older women: impact of the patient-physician interaction. *J Am Geriatr Soc* **52**, 1138–45.

42. Liang W, Burnett CB, Rowland JH *et al.* (2002). Communication between physicians and older women with localized breast cancer: implications for treatment and patient satisfaction. *J Clin Oncol* **20**, 1008–16.

43. Lee SJ, Back AL, Block SD, *et al.* (2002). Enhancing physician–patient communication. *Hematology Am Soc Hematol Educ Program*, 464–483.

44. Martin LR, Williams SL, Haskard KB, *et al.* (2005). The challenge of patient adherence. *Ther Clin Risk Manag* **1**, 189–199.

45. Chewning B, Wiederholt JB (2003). Concordance in cancer medication management. *Patient Educ Couns* **50**, 75–8.

46. Wilkinson SM, Leliopoulou C, Gambles M, *et al.* (2003). Can intensive three-day programmes improve nurses' communication skills in cancer care? *Psychooncology* **12**, 747–59.

47. Foley EC, D'Amico F, Merenstein JH (1995). Five-year follow-up of a nurse-initiated intervention to improve mammography recommendation. *J Am Board Fam Pract* **8**, 452–6.

48. Knowles G, Sherwood L, Dunlop MG, *et al.* (2007). Developing and piloting a nurse-led model of follow-up in the multidisciplinary management of colorectal cancer. *Eur J Oncol Nurs* **11**, 212–223.

49. Silliman RA, Dukes KA, Sullivan LM, *et al.* (1998). Breast cancer care in older women: sources of information, social support, and emotional health outcomes. *Cancer* **83**(4), 706–11.

50. Bock GW, Kwan BM (2007). Encouragement of patient self-management and adherence through use of a computerized tracking system for cervical and colon cancer screening. *J Am Board Fam Med* **20**(3), 316–9.

51. Fallowfield L, Jenkins V, Farewell V, *et al.* (2003).Enduring impact of communication skills training: results of a 12-month follow-up. *Br J Cancer* **89**,1445–9.

52. Stewart M, Brown JB, Hammerton J, *et al.* (2007). Improving communication between doctors and breast cancer patients. *Ann Fam Med* **5**, 387–94.

53. Bultman DC, Svarstad BL (2000). Effects of physician communication style on client medication beliefs and adherence with antidepressant treatment. *Patient Educ Couns* **40**, 173–85.

54. Roter DL, Hall JA, Merisca R, *et al.* (1998). Effectiveness of interventions to improve patient compliance: a meta-analysis. *Med Care* **36**, 1138–61.

Chapter 27

Communication strategies and skills for optimal pain control

Melanie Lovell and Frances Boyle

Pain is a significant cause of suffering for cancer patients. The onset of pain can herald a host of fears of death, disability, disfigurement, dependence and distress. The role of the healthcare professional (HCP). is to offer competent pain management with compassion and commitment to excellence, central to which is facilitating communication with the patient.

Pain is not an event in isolation. It occurs in a personal and physical environment influenced by the social, cultural, spiritual and biological inheritance of the patient (1). The experience of pain, therefore, has a unique impact on, and meaning for, each individual. At the time of assessment, factors such as associated fatigue, depression and anxiety may result in the pain becoming overwhelming (2). Assessing the pain involves not only measuring the level of pain and determining the nature of the pain, so as to diagnose the aetiology and mechanism of pain, but also exploring the 'deeper level of pain experience'. Failure to do so can result in poor pain control and a lost opportunity for transformation of the experience and healing of the individual (3).

Pain prevalence and impact

Pain is a problem on a large scale for patients with cancer. A meta-analysis of prevalence studies showed the prevalence of pain rates in patients at all stages of disease was 53% (CI 43–63%). and of those, one-third graded their pain as moderate or severe (4). Patients with pain may have more than one pain; in one survey of patients with advanced cancer and pain, patients had a median of three pains (5). Some groups have been shown to be at higher risk of poor pain control. These include paediatric patients, the elderly, cognitively impaired patients, those with a past history of substance abuse and minority groups (6, 7).

Patients with unrelieved severe pain have reduced function and quality of life (8), and increased levels of anxiety and depression (9, 10). Pain also has a significant impact on caregivers (11, 12). Despite these research findings, and the fact that most pain in cancer responds to analgesics and adjuvant therapies, there is evidence from many studies that cancer pain is frequently undertreated (13), and there are many barriers that may contribute to sub-optimal pain management.

Barriers to optimal pain control

The American Pain Society (APS) identified contributing barriers due to lack of patient, professional and public knowledge, lack of institutional commitment, regulatory concerns and limited access to, or reimbursement for, interdisciplinary care. The APS further recommends addressing these barriers to improve pain managmnent through physician leadership and a multilevel approach addressing healthcare providers, institutions and patients and their families. Crucial prongs in the approach include quality improvement activities, evidence-based pain management practice and patient involvement in decision-making (14).

Knowledge barriers can be broadly classified as those associated with myths regarding morphine and other opioids, and a failure in communication to counter these, and those associated with communicating about the pain experience (15, 16). Patients and their caregivers may be afraid of injections, becoming addicted to morphine, becoming tolerant to its effects, or that morphine may put them at risk of unpleasant side-effects or even death. These fears have been longstanding, cross-cultural and pervasive, and relate to confusion concerning the therapeutic use of morphine versus the deleterious effects of morphine as a drug of abuse (17). Despite clinical evidence that these fears are unfounded (18), these barriers persist and are common (7, 19–23). Fear of addiction can affect as many as 75% of oncology outpatients (23). Barriers may be higher in minority cultural groups (7) and may result in failure to take the recommended analgesic regimen (24).

Interventions to reduce barriers directed at patients

There is evidence from randomized controlled trials that educating patients about pain and its management can reduce these barriers and, in some studies, reduce pain levels (25–31). The nursing interventions studied that have reduced pain levels include targeted interventions tailored to individual patient needs (25, 31). For example, in one study, a pain education programme, consisting of a tailored information session (meeting knowledge, attitude and skill gaps identified by questionnaires), of 30–60 minutes was audio-taped and sent home with patients accompanied by a pain brochure. Patients were also instructed how to register their pain intensity and given information about what should be done in the event of uncontrolled pain (29).

Other studies have used a standardized intervention (such as a video, an information session, use of a pain diary or access to a health professional to adjust the medication) for each patient without taking into account the patient's pre-existing knowledge or attitudes. Some of these have shown improvements in pain levels (27, 32).

The palliative care trial (33) that examined the impact of a patient educational visit or general practitioner educational visit, showed that a single case conference or patient educational visit, conducted when the patient's performance status had deteriorated to the point of needing a caregiver, maintained higher function by 5–10%, compared to the control group, and reduced hospital admissions. Independent educational visitors observed the educators during visits (34). Brief education sessions for minority groups have not been shown consistently to improve pain control (35). However, in one study, patient coaching, involving addressing individual patient misconceptions about pain control and rehearsing patient–physician dialogue, resulted in reduced pain in the intervention group (36).

Other measures that have been shown to be effective in a meta-analysis of psycho-educational interventions, include relaxation-based cognitive behavioural techniques and supportive counselling (37).

Interventions to improve pain control directed at healthcare professionals (HCPs)

The most common professional barrier to pain control is knowledge about how to assess and treat pain (38). A systematic review of studies looking at interventions aimed at health professionals showed such interventions may have an impact on attitude and knowledge, without having much impact on pain scores (39). Introduction of a pain-management protocol may improve pain control, although in one study, only one of two intervention groups showed a benefit (40). A systematic review of institutional interventions designed to improve pain and its management in hospitalized patients revealed that no study showed consistent improvement in pain levels;

however, some studies showed routine pain assessment resulted in improvement in patient and staff satisfaction. (41). Meta-analysis of studies of involvement of specialist palliative care teams has shown improved pain control and patient satisfaction (42).

Measuring and describing pain

Pain is a subjective experience (43) and its management is dependent on patient reporting of pain experience. A numeric rating scale is a valid, reliable tool for accurately measuring the intensity of an individual's pain (see Fig. 27.1) (44).

A proportion of patients will find this difficult to use and they may be able to use categorical scales (none, mild, moderate or severe). Patients who are unable to communicate verbally, such as paediatric patients or those with dementia, must be assessed by the HCP using a scale such as the faces scale (45).

Patients should be advised on how to use a pain diary to record pain scores, triggers and relieving factors, and response to analgesia. There are a number of validated pain diaries, example.g. Maunsell's (46). It has been shown that a pain diary can help a patient cope with pain (47).

Descriptors that are reliable for neuropathic pain are a matter of ongoing research. In one study, those which most significantly correlate with neuropathic pain, include pain evoked by stroking the skin, bedclothes against the skin or heat, sensations of pins and needles, pricking, jumping-bursting, stabbing-shooting (48). McQuay offers a pragmatic definition of neuropathic pain that is shooting and/or burning pain that is poorly responsive to conventional analgesics (49).

Consensus from this evidence about the goal of each clinical encounter and guidelines to complete it, including strategies that form key steps in achieving this goal

The goal of the clinical encounter is diagnosis of aetiology and mechanism of pain and optimal management of the pain in the context of the whole patient. This includes the goal of empowering the patient (33). The patient is thereby able to more effectively communicate about, and manage, pain, with a concomitant reduction in pain. There are a number of key messages that need to be understood by both HCP and patient to enable this:

- The majority of cancer pain can be safely, quickly and effectively relieved (6).
- Pain can be measured effectively using rating scales.
- Pain can be monitored effectively using a daily pain diary.
- It is important to screen patients for pain at each visit.

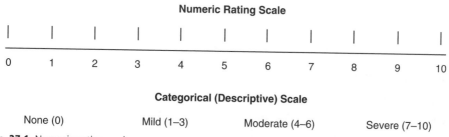

Fig. 27.1 Numeric rating scale.

- Patients should be encouraged to report pain.
- Common myths about pain and pain control should be explored and discussed.
- Addiction and tolerance are rarely a problem when opioids are used for cancer pain management.
- Patients should be instructed how to communicate effectively about their pain (6).
- It is important to treat the pain early and get the best control possible.
- Side-effects of opioids can be managed.
- Patients should be provided with written instructions about pain relief.

Key communication skills and process tasks

Listed below are key communication skills and process tasks important to the completion of each strategy, with model statements for use by clinicians to exemplify each skill.

Screening for pain

'It is very important to know if you are experiencing pain so we can manage it early.'

'Can you tell me how severe your pain is now using a scale of 0–10, where 10 is the most severe pain you can imagine and 0 is no pain?'

'What was your pain score when it was at its worst in the last 24hours?'

Identifying presence of pain(s) and likely aetiology and underlying mechanism

Site

'Can you point with one finger to where the pain is worst?'

'Do you have other pains?'

'Where is each one worst?'

Temporal factors

'How long ago did you first get the pain?'

'When did it get worse?'

'Is it constant or does it come and go?'

'How often do you get the pain?'

'How long does each episode last?'

Exacerbating and relieving factors

'Does there appear to be a trigger causing the pain?'

'What makes the pain worse?'

'What makes the pain better?'

Response to treatment

'What are you doing or taking for the pain?'

'On our rating scale what number does that change the pain from/to?'

'How long does it take to work and how long does it work for?'

To determine if pain is neuropathic

'Can you describe the pain?'

'Is the pain worse when the skin is stroked, touched by the bedclothes or touched by something warm?'(48).

Breakthrough pain

'Do you ever get a flare of the pain?'
Above questions should also be applied to any breakthrough pain.

Documenting the pain in a daily diary

Using a form similar to Fig. 27.2, please rate your pain on a scale 0–10, 0 being no pain and 10 being the worst pain imaginable. Please note your **average** pain for the preceding 24 hours at the same time each evening, say 7:00pm and also if you have breakthrough pain (a flare of your pain).

Determining the impact of pain

'What effect does the pain have on your ability to sleep/walk/work/your mood and your relationships?'

Determining the meaning of pain

'What do you think the pain means?'

'What do you think is the cause of the pain?'

'What do you expect will happen now with respect to the pain?'

Day	Time	Pain level	Pain relief – dose	Pain level 1 hour later	Comments
Thursday					
Friday					
Saturday					
Sunday					
Monday					
Tuesday					
Wednesday					

Fig. 27.2 Pain diary.

Identifying beliefs that may act as barriers to pain control

Beliefs regarding pain and pain communication that are potential barriers to pain relief, include: fear of progressive disease, fear of distracting the doctor from curing or treating the cancer, stoicism, fatalism, fear of death or disability:

'Some people feel they want to be brave and put up with pain—does that describe you?'

'Do you feel pain is an expected part of living with cancer?'

It is important to reassure patients:

'Managing pain is a crucial part of your overall cancer treatment.'

Identifying patient related barriers to opioid use.

Addiction

'Some people believe that they will get addicted to this type of medication—are you afraid that might happen to you?'

The key message is:

'Addiction is not a problem when morphine is used for cancer pain management.'

Tolerance:

'Some people are afraid that they might get used to the medication and they will need more and more for it to work or that there will not be anything strong enough if the pain gets worse.'

It can be explained as follows:

'If the pain gets worse the dose can be increased as needed and if the pain gets better, for example in response to anti-cancer treatment, the dose can be decreased.'

Side-effects

'Are you concerned about potential side-effects of the medication?'

'Morphine does cause some side-effects which can be managed.'

Fear that morphine will hasten death

'Some people think that starting morphine is the beginning of the end—Morphine is the best strong pain reliever we have and many people are on it for months or years.'

Fear of masking the pain

'Are you concerned that treating the pain will mask what is going on in your body?'

Identifying cultural issues affecting pain communication

'Are there beliefs in your culture about pain.'

This needs to be explored with sensitivity and without preconceptions. This is discussed in greater depth in Chapters 32 and 33.

Spiritual issues affecting communication

'How do you see your pain with respect to your faith?'

Dealing with difficult pain communication situations

History of substance abuse

This is a special situation and previous substance abusers are at risk of poor pain control (50). Kirsh and Passik suggest a number of strategies: involve the multidisciplinary team; take a full non-judgemental history, explaining that it is important for the clinician to know previous drug use to prevent withdrawal and to prescribe adequate analgesia; set realistic goals recognizing that abstinence and compliance may not be realistic, providing social, emotional support and setting limits; evaluate and treat comorbid psychiatric disorders; consider the therapeutic implications of tolerance, reassessing regularly and involving significant others; use written agreements; be clear that no extra medication or prescription will be supplied for missed appointments or unaccounted-for missing home drug supplies; try to identify family members who will be a source of strength or support, or conversely may attempt to buy or sell the patient's medications. The aim is a therapeutic alliance with the patient, supporters or family members and clinicians.

Paediatric patients

The key to assessing pain in children is observing behaviour (6). There is one tool developed specifically for hospitalized children, age 2–6 with cancer pain called the Douleur E'chelle Gustave-Roussy (DEGR(R)) instrument (51). It evaluates chronic pain behaviours, such as appearing depressed or withdrawn.

Older persons

Pain is a common problem in the elderly and assessment can be difficult as older patients may be more reluctant to report pain. Sensory or cognitive impairment may make communication difficult (52).

Cognitively impaired

Communication with this group is discussed in Chapter 47. Behaviour in this group may indicate that pain is present (see Box 27.1). Changed behaviour should also trigger an assessment for pain (52).

It is also helpful to get a history from carers to determine behaviour in response movement such as turning.

Instructing patients in pain control

Patients should be given written instructions about how to use the medication, including for break-through pain, how to deal with side-effects and when and how to call the healthcare professional. Patients may also be taught how to communicate effectively with clinicians. In a randomized controlled trial, the following script was shown to be an effective tool for this purpose (26).

> Hello, Dr___, this is____. I'm calling to talk with you about the pain I'm having. Over the past week, my pain has been____on a 0–10 rating scale. The pain has been so severe that I have not been able to sleep, do my usual activities, or visit with my friends. I've been taking my pain medicine as you pre-scribed it. I've also been taking ___ additional doses of medicine every day. The medicine isn't working. Can we change the pain medicine so I can get better pain control?

Exemplary clinical scenarios across the range of common cancers to guide role-plays

Breast cancer and bone metastases

Elizabeth is a 40-year-old woman who had early breast cancer four years ago, treated with surgery, chemotherapy, radiotherapy and tamoxifen (daily tablet, ongoing). This week she lifted her

Box 27.1 Common pain behaviours in cognitively impaired elderly persons

Facial expressions:

- ◆ Slight frown; sad, frightened face.
- ◆ Grimacing, wrinkled forehead, closed or tightened eyes.
- ◆ Any distorted expression.
- ◆ Rapid blinking.

Verbalizations, vocalizations:

- ◆ Sighing, moaning, groaning.
- ◆ Grunting, chanting, calling out.
- ◆ Noisy breathing.
- ◆ Asking for help.
- ◆ Verbally abusive.

Body movements:

- ◆ Rigid, tense body posture, guarding.
- ◆ Fidgeting.
- ◆ Increased pacing, rocking.
- ◆ Restricted movement.
- ◆ Gait or mobility changes.

Changes in interpersonal interactions:

- ◆ Aggressive, combative, resisting care.
- ◆ Decreased social interactions.
- ◆ Socially inappropriate, disruptive.
- ◆ Withdrawn.

Changes in activity patters or routines:

- ◆ Refusing food, appetite change.
- ◆ Increase in rest periods.
- ◆ Sleep, rest pattern changes.
- ◆ Sudden cessation of common routines.
- ◆ Increased wandering.

Mental status changes:

- ◆ Crying or tears.
- ◆ Increased confusion.
- ◆ Irritability or distress.

Note: Some patients demonstrate little or no specific behaviour associated with severe pain.
Table used with permission from the American Geriatrics Society (Table 3, 52).

5-year-old son and felt severe pain in her mid-thoracic spine. She has been resting and taking simple analgesia, but the pain has not been controlled. The pain is in the middle of her back, constant and aggravated by movement, and radiates around the right side of her ribs, with a burning quality and paraesthesiae. Differential diagnosis includes crush fracture, benign (e.g. low bone density from hormonal therapy) or malignant or, less likely, a disc prolapse. When seen, she is splinting her movement, trying to down play the severity for fear or an ominous diagnosis, and very anxious.

◆ Key examination: local tenderness, rule out spinal cord compression (sensation, reflexes, plantar responses).

◆ Key investigations: X-ray, MRI or CT.

◆ Key communication issues: measuring pain, breaking bad news of possible relapse, ensuring acute analgesia with short acting opioid, whilst investigating urgently.

◆ For the actor: trying to suppress both anxiety and movement cause a rigid thorax and shallow breathing. No hair loss.

Bowel cancer and pre-sacral mass

Alan is a 65-year-old man who had rectal cancer threeyears ago treated with radiotherapy, chemotherapy and surgery. One year ago he relapsed locally in the pelvis, with pain in the sacral area, radiating to both thighs. He has had further chemotherapy with some initial improvement, but is now suffering from increasing pain, which limits activity at home. His partner rings to say that he is not sleeping but will not take his medication (long-acting oral opioid) due to poor efficacy and constipation, but has not been 'telling the truth' at his visits. He is also 'very grumpy and irritable' with her.

◆ Key communication issues: eliciting fears about pain and analgesia, communicating about interference with sleep and ADL, eliciting symptoms of depression, negotiating alternative approaches to analgesia with lower side-effects (e.g. adding co-analgesics, fentanyl patch, spinal pump).

◆ For the actor: move slowly to the chair, as if legs unsteady. Avoid eye contact, short answers and little spontaneous speech. Hard to convince that there are better ways, and not at all convinced that he is depressed (not that kind of guy). He would not have hair loss.

Bone marrow transplant patient with mucositis pain

Graham is a 19-year-old in hospital for a bone marrow transplant. Chemotherapy was given last week and marrow reinfused 3 days ago. His mouth and throat are becoming very painful, his anxiety is increasing, and he is almost hysterical with pain '20 out of 10.'

◆ Key communication issues: separating anxiety from pain, explaining cause (mucositis from chemo), establishing confidence with IV analgesia with patient control, negotiating a pain scale.

◆ For the actor: lots of movement and anxiety, but muffled speech as if mouth is sore. Need to conceal hair.

Possibility of substance abuse

Steve is a 30-year-old male with metastatic melanoma, in hospital to have radiotherapy to a mass of lymph nodes in the groin. His pain in the leg and back is described as 'severe', but at times he is seen up, walking outside to smoke and laughing with friends, and staff are concerned that his pain is not 'real'. He has been an injecting heroin addict in the past, although claims to have been clean for several years.

- ◆ Key communication issues: cross-checking reports of pain with other interference measures, e.g. sleep. Assessing tolerance for opioids when he is given short-cting break through doses, i.e. checking pain response. Using co-analgesics to spare opioids. Opening an honest conversation.

- ◆ For the actor: casual dress and a slightly evasive manner covering up real concern that he is not being taken seriously. No hair loss. Walks with a limp.

In summary

Patients and families can hope for a number of benefits: improved pain control, improved knowledge about pain and its management, improved communication with HCP, patients empowered to be more involved in their own pain control, improved quality of life, improved function, and reduced caregiver stress.

References

1. Lickiss NJ (2003). Approaching death in multicultural Australia. *Medical Journal of Australia* **179**: S14–S6.

2. Twycross R (1994). *Pain relief in advanced cancer.* London: Churchill Livingstone.

3. Kearney M (1992). Palliative medicine—just another specialty? *Palliative Medicine* **6**: 39–46.

4. van den Beuken-van Everdingen MHJ, de Rijke JM, Kessels AG, *et al.* (2007). Prevalence of pain in patients with cancer: a systematic review of the past 40 years. *Annals of Oncology* **18**(9): 1437–49.

5. Twycross R, Harcourt J, Bergl S(1996). A survey of pain in patients with advanced cancer. *Journal of Pain & Symptom Management* **12**(5): 273–82.

6. Miaskowski C, Cleary J, Burney R, *et al.* (2005). *Guideline for the management of cancer pain in adults and children.* Glenview: American Pain Society.

7. Juarez G FB, Borneman T (1999). Cultural considerations in education for cancer pain management. *Journal of Cancer Education* **14**(3): 168–73.

8. Ferrell BR, Grant MM, Rhiner M, *et al.* (1992). Home care: maintaining quality of life for patient and family. *Oncology* **6**(2 Suppl): 136–40.

9. Massie M, Holland J (1992). The cancer patient with pain: psychiatric complications and their management. *Journal of Pain and Symptom Management* **7**: 99–109.

10. Mystakidou K, Tsilika E, Parpa E, *et al.* (2006). Psychological distress of patients with advanced cancer: influence and contribution of pain severity and pain interference. *Cancer Nursing* **29**(5): 400–5.

11. Ferrell B, Borneman T, and Juarez, G(1998). Integration of pain education into home care. *Journal of Palliative Care* **14**(3): 62–8.

12. Ferrell BR, Rhiner M, Cohen M, *et al.* (1991). Pain as a Metaphor for Illness Part I: Impact of Cancer Pain on Family Caregivers. *Oncology Nursing Forum* **18**(8): 1303–09.

13. Cleeland CGR(1994). Pain and its treatment in outpatients with metastatic cancer. *New England Journal of Medicine* **330**: 592–6.

14. Gordon D, Dahl J, Miaskowski C, *et al.* (2005). American pain society recommendations for improving the quality of acute and cancer pain management: American Pain Society Quality of Care Task Force. *Archives of Internal Medicine* [Review] **165**(14): 1574–80.

15. Potter VT, Wiseman CE, Dunn SM, *et al.* (2003). Patient barriers to optimal cancer pain control. *Psycho-Oncology* **12**(2): 153–60.

16. Ward SE GN, Miller-McCauley V, Mueller C, *et al.* (1993). Patient-related barriers to management of cancer pain. *Pain.* 52: 319–24.

17. Hanks G, De Conno F, Cherny N, *et al.* (2001). Morphine and alternative opioids in cancer pain: the EAPC recommendations. *British Journal of Cancer* **84**(5): 587–93.
18. McQuay H (1999). Opioids in pain management. *Lancet Oncology* **353**: 2229–32.
19. Gunnarsdottir S DH, Serlin RC, Voge C, *et al.* (2002). Patient-related barriers to pain management: the Barriers Questionnaire II (BQ-II). *Pain* **99**: 385–96.
20. Lin C Ward S. (1995). Patient-related barriers to cancer pain management in Taiwan. *Cancer Nursing* **18**(1), 16–22.
21. Yates P, Aranda S, Edwards E, Nash R, Skerman H, Mc Carthy A(2004). Family caregivers' experiences and invovement with cancer pain management. *J Pall Care* **20**(4), 287–96.
22. Aranda S Yales P, Edwards H, Nash R, *et al.* (2004). Barriers to effective cancer pain management: a survey of Australian family caregivers. *European Journal of Cancer Care* **13**(4): 336–43.
23. Potter VT Wiseman CE, Dunn SM, Bogle FM. (2003). Patient barriers to optimal cancer pain control. *Pscho-oncology* **12**(2): 153–60.
24. Miaskowski C, Dodd MJ, West C, *et al*(2001). Lack of adherence with the analgesic regimen: a significant barrier to effective cancer pain management. *Journal of Clinicla Oncology* **19**(23): 4275–9.
25. Yates P Edwards E, Nash R, Aranda S, *et al.* (2004). A randomized controlled trial of a nurse-administered educational intervention for improving cancer pain management in ambulatory settings. *Patient Education and Counselling* **53**:227–37.
26. Miaskowski C, Dodd M, West C, *et al.* (2004). Randomized clinical trial of the effectiveness of a self-care intervention to improve cancer pain management. *Journal of Clinical Oncology* **22**(9): 1713–20.
27. Clotfelter CE (1999). The effect of an educational intervention on decreasing pain intensity in elderly people with cancer. *Oncology Nursing Forum* **26**(1): 27–33.
28. Oliver JW, Kravitz RL, Kaplan SH, *et al.* (2001). Individualized patient education and coaching to improve pain control among cancer outpatients. *Journal of Clinical Oncology* **19**(7): 2206–12.
29. De Wit R, van Dam F, Loonstra S, *et al.* (2001). Improving the quality of pain treatment by a tailored pain educatin programme for cancer patients in chronic pain. *European Journal of Pain* **5**: 241–56.
30. Rimer B Keints MK, Levy M, Engstrom PF, *et al.* (1986). Cancer pain management: a clinical trial of an education program for patients. *Advances in Cnacer Control: Healthcare Financing and Research* 311–7.
31. Ward S, Donovan H, Owen B, *et al.* (2000). An individualized intervention to overcome patient-related barriers to pain management win women with gynecologic cancers. *Research in Nursing and Health* **23**: 393–405.
32. Vallieres I, Aubin M, Blondeau L, *et al.* (2006). Effectiveness of a clinical intervention in improving pain control in outpatients with cancer treated by radiation therapy. *International Journal of Radiation Oncology, Biology, Physics* **66**(1): 234–7.
33. Abernathy A, Currow D, Hunt R, *et al.* (2006). A pragmatic $2 \times 2 \times 2$ factorial cluster randomized controlled trial of educational outreach visiting and case conferencing in palliative care—methodology of the Palliative Care Trial [ISRCTN 81117481]. *Contemporary Clinical Trials* **27**: 83–100.
34. Shelby-James T (2007). Palliative care trial. [Date 21 April 2008]. Available from: **http://www.caresearch.com.au/home/Nationalprogram/Palliativecaretrial/tabid/677/Default.aspx.**
35. Anderson K, Mendoza T, Payne R, *et al.* (2004). Pain education for underserved minority cancer patients: a randomized controlled trial. *Journal of Clinical Oncology* **22**(24): 4918–25.
36. Kalauokalani D, Franks P, Oliver J, *et al.* (2007). Can patient coaching reduce racial/ethnic disparities in cancer pain control? Secondary analysis of a randomized controlled trial [see comment]. *Pain Medicine* **8**(1): 17–24.
37. Devine EC (2003). Meta-analysis of the effect of psychoeducational interventions on pain in adults with cancer. *Oncology Nursing Forum* **30**(1): 75–89.

38. Von Roenn J, Cleeland C, Gonin R, *et al.* (1993). Physician attitudes and practice in cancer pain management. A survey from the Eastern Cooperative Oncology Group. *Annals of Internal Medicine* **119**(2): 121–6.

39. Allard P, Maunsell E, Labbe J, *et al.* (2001). Educational interventions to improve cancer pain control: a systematic review. *Jopurnal of Palliative Medicine* **4**(2): 191–203.

40. Cleeland C Portenoy R, Rue M, Mendoza TR, *et al.* (2005). Does an oral analgesic protocol imiprove pain control for patients with cancer? An intergroup study coordinated by the Eastern cooperative Oncology Group. *Annals of Oncology* **16**: 972–80.

41. Goldberg G, Morrison R (2007). Pain management in hospitalized cancer patients: a systematic review. *Journal of Clinical Oncology* **25**(13): 1792–801.

42. Higginson I, Finlay I, Goodwin D, *et al.* (2003). Is there evidence that palliative care teams alter end-of-life experiences of patients and their caregivers? *Journal of Pain & Symptom Management* **25**(2): 150–68.

43. Ferrell B, Rhiner M, Ferrell B (1993). Development and Implementation of a Pain Education Program. *Cancer Supplement* **72**(11): 3426–32.

44. Jensen MP KP, Braver S(1986). The measurement of clinical pain intensity. *Pain* **27**: 117–26.

45. Wong D, Baker C (1988). Pain in children. *Pediatric Nursing* **14**(1): 9–17.

46. Maunsell E, Allard P, Dorval M, *et al.* (2000). A brief pain diary for ambulatory patients with advanced cancer: acceptability and validity. *Cancer* **88**(10): 2387–97.

47. De Wit R, van Dam F, Hanneman M, *et al.* (1999). Evaluation of the use of a pain diary in chronic cancer pain patients at home. *Pain* **79**(1): 89–99.

48. Bennett M (2001). The LANSS pain scale: the Leeds assessment of neuropathic symptoms and signs. *Pain* **92**: 147–57.

49. McQuay H (2002). Neuropathic pain: evidence matters. *European Journal of Pain* **6**(Suppl A): 11–8.

50. Kirsh K, Passik S (2006). Palliative care of the terminally ill drug addict. *Cancer Investigation* **24**(4): 425–31.

51. Gauvin-Piquard A, Rodary C, Rezvani A, *et al.* (1999). The development of the DEGR(R): a scale to assess pain in young children with cancer. *European Journal of Pain* **3**(2): 165–76.

52. AGS panel on persistent pain in older persons (2002). The management of persistent pain in older persons. *Journal of the American Geriatrics Society* **50**(s6): 205–24.

Chapter 28

Discussing adverse outcomes with patients

Thomas H Gallagher and Afaf Girgis

Introduction

Few communication challenges are as difficult for healthcare providers as talking with patients about adverse events, especially when the adverse event was due to a medical error. Ethicists and professional organizations have long endorsed open communication with patients about adverse events and errors in their care. Recently, however, there has been a substantial increase in attention being paid to transparent communication with patients. Many countries, including Australia, the United Kingdom, and Canada have undertaken major disclosure initiatives. The Joint Commission, the body responsible for the accreditation of most US healthcare facilities, now requires that patients be informed of all outcomes in their care, including 'unanticipated outcomes' (1).

Yet there is increasing evidence of a significant gap between expectations for open communication with patients and actual clinical practice. Several studies in a variety of countries suggest that less than one-third of adverse events due to errors are disclosed to patients (3–6). Other research suggests that when these conversations do take place, they often fall short of meeting patient expectations (7, 8). Healthcare workers endorse the general concept of disclosure, but struggle with how to turn this principle into practice, especially when it comes to choosing their words when talking with patients about adverse events (9, 10). Significant fear persists among both healthcare workers and institutions that more open disclosure of adverse events and errors could increase the likelihood of a medical malpractice suit being filed (11).

Communication dilemmas associated with disclosure of adverse events and errors to patients exist at multiple levels, ranging from the individual patient–provider encounter, to issues of national health policy. In this chapter, we will consider what is currently known about patients' and providers' attitudes and experiences with disclosure, explore the special aspects of disclosure in the oncology context, consider disclosure in an inter-professional context, discuss how healthcare institutions are responding to calls for greater transparency, what is known about the impact of disclosure on outcomes including litigation, and present some of the health policy challenges associated with disclosure. The chapter concludes by considering a disclosure case study, and discussing next steps for disclosure in oncology.

Adverse events and errors in the oncology context

Discussions about disclosing adverse events and errors to patients are often plagued with unclear use of terminology. It is important to distinguish between 'adverse events', 'unanticipated outcomes', and 'medical errors' (12). An adverse event is defined as any harm that is caused by medical management and that results in measurable disability. Adverse events are relatively common, and the vast majority of them are not caused by medical errors. (Similarly, an unanticipated outcome is defined as any unexpected result from any aspect of diagnosis or treatment that may or may not be associated with an error—a broad definition that it is not particularly useful.) While finding an ideal definition for the concept of medical error has proven elusive, the most commonly used definition is from the US Institute of Medicine: 'The failure of a planned action to be completed as intended or the use of a wrong plan to achieve an aim' (12). As strictly defined here, medical errors are, in fact, quite common. But just as most adverse events are not due to errors, the vast majority of errors do not cause harm to the patient, and are not associated with an adverse event. Those medical errors that could have caused the patient harm but did not, either by chance or timely intervention, are known as near misses.

There is a general expectation that healthcare workers will communicate openly with patients about all adverse events, whether due to medical error or not (4, 13). However, talking with patients about adverse events not due to error is more straightforward than talking with patients about adverse events due to error. Therefore, the remainder of this chapter will focus on the challenges associated with disclosing adverse events that were due to medical errors, also known as 'harmful medical errors', to patients.

While disclosing harmful medical errors to patients can be difficult in any clinical context, the oncology environment poses special challenges (14). Oncology care is fraught with uncertainty, and it can be difficult to know whether a medical error occurred and, if so, whether the error was associated with harm. This is further complicated by the toxic nature of most oncology therapies, where adverse events are commonplace. The psychological burdens associated with cancer make oncology patients especially vulnerable, but the consequences of medical errors in oncology can also be severe for the provider, with emotional distress among oncologists being common (15). In addition, medico-legal issues associated with oncology can pose difficult challenges. Delayed diagnosis of cancer, and breast cancer in particular, is one of the most frequent precipitants of medical malpractice lawsuits in the US (16).

Despite these challenges, the oncology community is ideally positioned to take a leadership role within the medical profession in enhancing the disclosure of adverse events and errors to patients. The oncology community has led in developing a knowledge base and set of practical skills for a related communication dilemma, namely the delivery of bad news to patients. There is good reason to believe that ten years from now, healthcare workers will approach the disclosure of harmful medical errors to oncology patients very differently than they do at present.

International developments in disclosure

Important developments related to disclosure have been taking place across the world. In 2001, the Joint Commission, the United State's organization that accredits hospitals and healthcare organizations, required that hospitals and healthcare organizations disclose all outcomes of care to patients including 'unanticipated outcomes', leading many hospitals and healthcare institutions to develop formal disclosure policies (27). By 2005, nearly 70% of healthcare organizations in the US had established disclosure policies (28).

In July 2003, the Australian Council for Safety and Quality in Healthcare issued its Open Disclosure Standard, a national standard for open communication in public and private hospitals following an adverse event in healthcare. The goal of the standard was to ensure open, honest, and timely communication with patients following adverse events, not only to meet the needs of the affected patient but also as an important aspect of improving patient safety. Extensive educational material was developed to help implement this standard, and the Department of Human Services provided funding to enable over 42 sites to participate in a national pilot project to evaluate the impact of this standard. Results of these pilot projects are expected soon.

In the United Kingdom, the National Patient Safety Agency of the National Health Service issued a similar policy in 2003 that led to a programme entitled 'Being Open'. As in Australia, extensive educational material for healthcare organizations, providers, and patients have been developed and pilot projects are underway to determine the impact of this new policy. To our knowledge, however, outcomes data from either Australia's Open Disclosure or the UK's Being Open projects have not been published.

Considerable activity related to disclosure has been taking place in Canada. The Canadian Patient Safety Institute recently issued its 'Canadian Disclosure Guidelines'. These guidelines focus on the disclosure of adverse events, and emphasize that healthcare providers and organizations have an obligation to communicate to a patient about any harm that has occurred in their care. The Canadian guidelines articulate a thoughtful approach to disclosure and encourage an expression of regret following adverse events. However, the Canadian guidelines, as with the disclosure programmes in Australia and the UK, highlight an important area of persistent ambiguity that complicates the disclosure process. The Canadian guidelines emphasize the importance of 'avoiding the use of "error" in the context of disclosure'. They note that while healthcare provider error may appear to be the most obvious contributing factor to an adverse event, there are often system breakdowns and other latent conditions that are more important contributors. On the other hand, the guidelines call for patients to be informed about 'the facts' of the event, and 'actions taken as a result of internal analysis that have resulted in system improvements'. The guidelines do note that 'if applicable, and when all the facts are established, a further expression of regret that may include an apology with acknowledgement of responsibility for what has happened as appropriate' can be included in the disclosure. It can be difficult for providers and organizations to know how best to comply with the dual requirements for open and transparent communication about adverse events that were clearly due to error, while not admitting fault or using 'error' language.

Patients' and physicians' attitudes and experiences regarding disclosure

Several studies over the past six years have shed considerable light on patients' preferences for disclosure (7, 9, 10, 17). Patients uniformly desire the disclosure of all harmful errors in their care, even when the harm was relatively minor. Patients also desire a consistent set of information about harmful errors, including an explicit statement that an error occurred, an explanation of what the error was and its implications for their health, why the error occurred, and how recurrences will be prevented. These last two pieces of information (why the error occurred and how recurrences will be prevented) are highly valued by patients, as they show that a lesson has been learned from the event and that recurrences are less likely. Patients also value an apology as recognition of the emotional impact of the error on them personally.

Recent research has also shed new light on how healthcare workers approach disclosure. Several large survey studies of physicians suggest that they strongly endorse the general concept of disclosure, but struggle with how to turn this principle into practice (9). One study compared the disclosure attitudes of physicians in the US and in Canada, countries with significantly different malpractice climates (10). The US and Canadian physicians' disclosure attitudes and experience were much more similar than different, suggesting that the external malpractice environment may not be as powerful a determinant of physicians' disclosure attitudes as once thought. However, despite this general support for disclosure, many physicians struggled with what words to say to patients following harmful errors. The study also showed that healthcare workers may disclose less information about errors that would be unapparent to the patient, and that medical and surgical physicians approached disclosure differently. Another study of how surgeons would approach disclosure also showed that many surgeons failed to use recommended skills (18). For example, only 8% of surgeons mentioned anything to the hypothetical patients involved in this study about prevention of error recurrences.

Impact of disclosure on outcomes

Emerging research is beginning to clarify the impact disclosure has on litigation and other outcomes, and many commentators have suggested that effective disclosure may enhance such outcomes (19–21). This assertion stems in part from research that has found that patients who sue often cite both the perception that the truth was hidden from them, as well as deficient communication skills, as important reasons for why they filed a lawsuit. Several survey studies have also suggested that full disclosure may reduce patients' intention to sue and promote faster settlements and lower awards (19, 21). The relationship between disclosure and litigation, however, continues to be a complex and contentious issue. The vast majority of patients injured by medical care never sue, which may in part reflect their lack of awareness that a medical error caused their injury. If this is true, open disclosure could stimulate rather than mitigate lawsuits (11). Even in those studies that have shown a generally positive relationship between open disclosure and intent to sue, this relationship is often diminished for the most serious errors. Such uncertainty about the impact of disclosure on litigation is likely to persist for the foreseeable future.

Despite this uncertainty, several US institutions have developed programmes for open disclosure of adverse events and errors, and reported favourable impacts on their litigation experiences. The first of these programmes, at the Lexington, Kentucky Veterans Hospital, which encouraged full disclosure of harmful errors and facilitation of compensation in selected circumstances, did not appear to have a deleterious impact on volume or payouts of the institution's malpractice claims (22). More recently, the University of Michigan reported that their programme for open disclosure and early compensation had a dramatic positive impact on their number of malpractice claims, time to resolution, and payouts (23). The best-known disclosure and compensation programme in the private sector has been developed by COPIC Insurance Company (24). Their '3Rs' programme encourages open disclosure following unanticipated outcomes and provides compensation for patients' lost time and other out-of-pocket expenses up to $30,000. The 3Rs programme has important exclusion criteria, including patient death, attorney involvement, written demand for payment, gross negligence, or complaint to the medical board. However, since the programme's inception in 2000, COPIC has handled over 3200 cases through the 3Rs programme, with average payments of only $5,400. None of the 3Rs cases has proceeded to a full jury trial. While the generalizability of these case reports is uncertain, they do provide some support for the concept that at least a subset of adverse events and errors can be effectively handled through such programmes.

Inter-professional issues in error disclosure

Up to this point, disclosure has primarily been conceptualized as a conversation between an individual patient and his or her physician. However, the patient safety movement has done much to highlight the role that system breakdowns play in most medical errors. Rarely is an individual healthcare worker solely responsible for the occurrence of a medical error. In the field of oncology, delivery of healthcare by teams of providers is the norm, including physicians as well as nurses, therapists, technicians, dieticians, and psychologists. When harmful errors happen to patients in the setting of inter-professional care, multiple team members may discuss the event with one another, and may or may not discuss the event with the patient. Yet no clear standards currently exist for how inter-professional healthcare teams should discuss errors among themselves and with patients.

A few studies have begun to explore the perspectives of nurses on disclosure. In one study, nurses were found to be less likely than physicians to disclose errors to patients, particularly cognitive versus medication errors (25). These authors suggested that nurses may believe that disclosing a cognitive error to a patient would be equivalent to denouncing their physician colleagues. Others have suggested that nurses may hesitate to disclose errors due to their reluctance to admit human frailty or their lack of knowledge about how to disclose errors skilfully, as well as the lack of support that institutions generally provide to healthcare workers who have made a serious error (26). A recent focus group study of nurses found that nurses supported the importance of disclosure overall but questioned disclosure to anxious patients and litigious families, as well as disclosure of minor errors. In this study, nurses emphasized the team dimensions of disclosure, and described many episodes of poor communication among team members about what patients had been or would be told, which resulted in nurses responding to patients' and families' questions with deception or avoidance. Nurses wanted to be involved in the error disclosure process, in part to avoid being blamed for errors, yet reported lacking adequate knowledge and experience to skilfully discuss errors. These nurses also highlighted the critical role that their nurse managers played in operationalizing institution disclosure policies on the patient care floors.

Considerable work has yet to be done about the optimal inter-professional approach to disclosure. Team disclosure conversations naturally involve a planning phase, where the team members discuss the event, and plan whether and how to disclose the event to the patient. Once this team discussion and planning process is complete, the team discloses to the patient and/or the family. Given the inherent power differentials present on such teams, strong communication and conflict resolution skills are required to discuss the event and its disclosure in a mutually supportive and blame-free way. There is also considerable work yet to be done regarding the roles different team members play in the disclosure process. Often the physician will lead the disclosure process, and may or may not want additional members of the healthcare team present for the disclosure. While nurses have expressed an interest in participating in disclosures, it is unclear how to structure team disclosures in ways such that they support rather than overwhelm the patient. Furthermore, the role of the physician in disclosing events that were strictly nursing errors to the patients has yet to be determined. The oncology community, with its considerable experience in inter-professional healthcare delivery, is ideally positioned to explore inter-professional best practices in the disclosure of harmful errors to patients.

Institutional factors promoting disclosure

Until recently, transparency and the willingness to disclose harmful medical errors to patients were seen primarily as properties residing within the character of individual healthcare providers. However, just as the patient safety movement has emphasized the system components that contribute to most harmful errors, transparency is increasingly being conceptualized as a property of a system. In other words, aspects of the institution in which healthcare workers practice can either facilitate or inhibit the disclosure of harmful medical errors to patients. Institutional factors associated with transparency take a number of forms, the most obvious of which are the institutions' policies and procedures related to disclosure. Yet few institutional disclosure policies provide specific guidance in how disclosure of harmful errors to patients should be carried out. Furthermore, in many institutions healthcare workers receive mixed messages about disclosure: formal institutional policies encourage disclosure, even as institutional risk managers advise and promote caution.

Institutions looking to expand their policies and procedures around disclosure can draw on the 2006 US National Quality Form (NQF) Safe Practice on disclosure (29). This national disclosure guideline represents an advance in a number of areas. It requires the disclosure of all serious unanticipated outcomes to patients, and provides specific guidance on the information to be disclosed. Most notably, the Safe Practice requires that patients be informed whether the unanticipated outcome was due to an error or system failure. The Safe Practice requires that patients be informed of the results of event analysis and error prevention plans in sufficient detail to support informed decision-making. The Safe Practice also requires an expression of regret for all serious unanticipated outcomes, and a formal apology when unanticipated outcomes were due to clear-cut errors or system failures.

Most importantly, the Safe Practice articulates the key components of an institutional disclosure support system. The support system includes training in disclosure for healthcare workers, emotional support for patients and healthcare workers following unanticipated outcomes, and the availability of disclosure coaching around the clock to assist healthcare workers with disclosure tasks. The Safe Practice requires hospitals to integrate their risk management, patient safety, and quality improvement programmes, and calls for the application of performance improvement tools to the disclosure process. Finally, many major healthcare purchasing coalitions in the US now use these Safe Practice guidelines as standards in their pay for performance programmes, and hospital-specific compliance with the Safe Practices for over 1,300 hospitals is currently published on the internet.

Legislative approaches to promoting disclosure and apology

Recognition of current inadequacies in the disclosure and apology process has led many countries to take legislative action. Healthcare workers' and institutions' fear of litigation is a frequently cited barrier to disclosure and apology (13). Thus, one common legislative strategy to promote disclosure and apology has been to adopt laws protecting some aspects of the disclosure and apology process from being considered admissions of liability. In the US, states have used two approaches to promote disclosure and apology (2). Thirty-five US states and the District of Columbia have enacted 'apology laws' that protect portions of these conversations from being used as evidence of liability. Nine US states have adopted 'disclosure laws' that typically mandate that serious unanticipated outcomes be disclosed. Apology laws have also been adopted in other countries including Australia, Canada, and the United Kingdom.

The variety of US apology laws reflects the range of apology laws that have been enacted elsewhere in the world. While these laws represent important endorsements of transparency, analysis of the US apology laws highlights their significant limitations. Twenty-five of the US apology laws protect only an expression of regret and not explanations of the event or admissions of fault. These laws suggest that statements acknowledging the injury, but not causation or explanation ('I'm sorry this happened'), will be protected, while portions of a statement explaining or acknowledging fault or responsibility ('I'm sorry I hurt you,' or 'I'm sorry I made a mistake when I administered the wrong medication') could be used in litigation. Four US states with apology laws protect the entire disclosure statement, allowing a provider to express remorse and admit fault to the patient without concern that the information disclosed could be used in court as evidence of fault. Even in these few US states that protect admissions of fault, the act of communicating this information might still stimulate a lawsuit. Given these limitations, many physicians, healthcare institutions, and risk managers are likely to remain concerned about the legal risks associated with disclosure and apology.

Communication strategies

Communication training has an important role to play in improving the disclosure process. Most physicians report that they have not had formal training in disclosure, and lack confidence in their disclosure communication skills. Physicians frequently cite these communication skills deficits as important barriers to having these conversations with patients. Fortunately, physicians' experience in related communication dilemmas, such as breaking bad news to patients, can be a helpful starting point when considering how to approach disclosure of harmful medical errors. But there are important differences between disclosure of harmful errors and breaking bad news; for example, when the physician may be partly responsible for the event having taken place. Therefore, physicians should not assume that their bad news delivery skills transfer directly to the disclosure of adverse events.

Disclosure conversations have two key components: information sharing and emotion handling. Both must be attended to if a disclosure conversation is to be successful. If healthcare workers focus only on what information to disclose to the patient without carefully considering the patient's emotions, the patient may feel well-informed about the event but perceive the healthcare worker as aloof and cold. If a healthcare worker focuses primarily on responding to the patient's emotions, the patient may feel well-supported but confused about exactly what happened. Other sections of this book cover the topic of empathic communication in detail. Therefore, the remainder of this chapter will focus on the information-sharing dimensions of disclosure.

There are several core principles healthcare workers should keep in mind when approaching disclosure. First, disclosures will typically take place over more than one conversation. Disclosure conversations can be uncomfortable enough that some healthcare workers might wish to have the conversation once and be done with it. Yet breaking a disclosure into several conversations has a number of advantages. First, information about the event's cause and plans for preventing recurrences often take time to develop. Waiting to tell the patient about a harmful error until a full analysis has been completed would result in a delay that many patients would consider excessive. Therefore, an initial conversation should be held with the patient as soon as the event is discovered. This conversation can then be followed up with subsequent conversations, as additional information about the event becomes apparent. Breaking disclosure conversations into multiple discussions also allows patients time to digest the information and ask questions, as well as providing the opportunity to attend to any breaches in the patient/provider relationship the error may have caused.

Error disclosure can be thought of as involving four key steps.

Step one: get help

The emotional distress that accompanies harmful medical errors can distort healthcare workers' judgment about what happened, as well as judgment about whether and how to disclose the event to the patient. Therefore, it is essential that healthcare workers avail themselves of institutional resources to assist them in the disclosure process. Patient safety analysts and quality officers are key resources who can assist in conducting a thorough analysis to determine whether the event in question was an error and to help formulate plans for prevention. Other important sources of help include risk managers, medical directors, department chairs, or other supervisors. Careful consultation with these institutional disclosure support resources can help ensure patients receive accurate information about the event. Those providing such support to frontline clinicians should be cognizant of the emotional impact these events have on providers and be prepared to offer support services as needed.

Step two: plan the initial disclosure conversation

Consultation with the disclosure support resources should allow for careful discussion of whether the event should be disclosed and, if so, what should be said. Breakdowns in the disclosure process often occur because of lack of such planning. It is especially important to anticipate patients' likely questions about the event and consider thoughtful responses. When the harmful error involved a healthcare team, the entire team should be involved in the disclosure planning, with careful consideration given to the roles of each team member in the disclosure process, and how to respond to questions the patient is likely to ask about the event.

Step three: hold the initial conversation

The initial conversation should be held within the first 24 hours after the event is discovered. Relatively little may be known about the event at this point, and so it is important not to speculate about whether the event was an error, what caused the error, or who was responsible. Often these initial conversations consist of letting the patient know that an adverse event has taken place, what the event was and its implications for the patient's health, clinical steps that have been taken to mitigate the event, and that the event will be thoroughly investigated and the results shared with the patient. An expression of regret is appropriate during the initial conversation for all adverse events. The initial conversation concludes with the opportunity for the patient to ask questions.

Step four: follow-up conversation

The follow-up conversation provides the opportunity for healthcare workers to share with patients new information about the event, whether it was due to an error and, if so, how recurrences of the event will be prevented. If a formal event analysis reveals that the adverse event was due to a medical error, a formal apology should be provided. The follow-up conversation also provides an additional opportunity for patients to ask questions, and healthcare workers should ensure that patients know how to contact them if they have future questions. This is also often the proper time to introduce discussions of compensation, as appropriate. Such discussions are typically conducted by the institutional risk manager or other administrator, and clinicians should generally avoid addressing compensation issues with patients unless explicitly authorized to do so by the institution.

Some organizations emphasize the importance of taking responsibility as part of the disclosure process. While patients appreciate an explicit statement of acceptance of responsibility, there are numerous unanswered questions about how best to incorporate accepting responsibility into disclosure discussions. Attending physicians may feel uncomfortable accepting responsibility when leading disclosure of events in which they only played a small role. In some organizations, senior administrators make statements of responsibility on behalf of the institution to the patient. It is unclear what specific obligations flow from a healthcare worker or institution accepting responsibility for an error. Individual clinicians, for example, may feel powerless to affect a change in the systemic factors that led to the event. Additional research is needed to explore how to best meet patients' needs for acceptance of responsibility around harmful errors in ways that are comfortable for both healthcare workers and institutions.

Other organizations are focusing primarily on the apology dimensions of the disclosure process. These organizations seek to follow the lead of scholars who advocate that an 'authentic' apology is one that 'acknowledges the legitimacy of the violated rule, to admit fault for its violation, and three, expresses genuine remorse and regret for the harm caused by the violation' (30). An authentic apology 'invites forgiveness, which is the door to reconciliation'. This view of apology contrasts sharply with an 'expression of regret,' in which the healthcare worker tells the patient, 'I'm sorry this happened to you' but does not admit fault or seek forgiveness. While substantial theoretical considerations support some dimensions of this push towards 'authentic apologies', there is only limited empirical evidence about how patients perceive specific apology strategies. Patients may be most interested in whether an apology seems sincere to them, rather than about what specific words were used in the apology itself. How best to integrate apology into the disclosure process is another important area of future research.

Role-play scenario

As with any other communication dilemma, practicing error disclosure is critical if healthcare workers are to improve their skills in this area. An error disclosure case with possible roles for different health professionals to adopt is provided below.

Frank Jones is a 63-year-old with metastatic non-small cell lung cancer who was admitted to the Intensive Care Unit with seizures. Head CT shows a large mass, presumably another metastasis. In the ICU he is treated with a loading dose of Dilantin, 300 mg three times daily, then switched to Dilantin 300 mg. once daily when his Dilantin levels are therapeutic. He is being transferred to the floor, and the physician writing transfer orders mistakenly writes for the patient to receive Dilantin 300 mg. three times daily rather than the once daily dose the patient was currently receiving. This medication error is not noticed by the floor nurses or by the pharmacist. Two days later, the patient experiences Dilantin toxicity and becomes confused, disoriented, and falls on their way to the bathroom, striking their head on the sink. A Dilantin level at the time of the fall was very elevated at 30. A head CT after the fall shows a new but small subdural haematoma.

Physicians: Mr Jones has returned from his CT scan, and wants to know why he fell. He presumes he must have had another seizure.

Nurses: The physician has just given Mr Jones a brief explanation of what happened that emphasized the fall as a result of the Dilantin level being a little high, but did not explicitly tell the patient that the high Dilantin level was the result of a medication error.

Social workers: The physician tells you that he did not explicitly disclose the error to the patient because he thought that it was in the patient's best interest not to know the details of the event, given his extremely poor prognosis from his underlying disease. The nurse agrees that full disclosure would do more harm than good for the patient. You wonder how to help the healthcare team with next steps.

Conclusion

The gap between expectations that harmful errors be disclosed to patients and current clinical practice should prompt healthcare workers, institutions, professional organizations, and policy makers to adopt new approaches to communicating with patients following these events. The oncology community's expertise in sharing bad news with patients makes it an ideal group to take a leadership role in developing enhanced standards for disclosure conversations as well as to undertake research on the impact of different disclosure strategies on important patient outcomes such as trust and satisfaction in the cancer care setting.

References

1. The Joint Commission. *Hospital Accreditation Standards, 2007.* Oakbrook Terrace, IL: Joint Commission Resources; 2007.

2. Baker GR, Norton PG, Flintoft V, *et al*. The Canadian Adverse Events Study: the incidence of adverse events among hospital patients in Canada. *CMAJ* 2004; **170**(11): 1678–1686.

3. Blendon RJ, DesRoches CM, Brodie M, *et al*. Views of practicing physicians and the public on medical errors. *N Engl J Med* 2002; **347**(24): 1933–1940.

4. Brennan TA, Leape LL. Adverse events, negligence in hospitalized patients: results from the Harvard Medical Practice Study. *Perspect Healthc Risk Manage* 1991; **11**(2): 2–8.

5. Vincent C, Neale G, Woloshynowych M. Adverse events in British hospitals: preliminary retrospective record review. *BMJ* 2001; **322**(7285): 517–519.

6. Mazor KM, Simon SR, Yood RA, *et al*. Health plan members' views about disclosure of medical errors. *Ann Intern Med* 2004; **140**(6): 409–418.

7. The Kaiser Family Foundation/Agency for Healthcare Research & Quality/Harvard School of Public Health. National survey on consumers' experiences with patient safety and quality information. November, 2004. **http://www.kff.org/kaiserpolls/upload/National-Survey-on-Consumers-Experiences-With-Patient-Safety-and-Quality-Information-Survey-Summary-and-Chartpack.pdf** (accessed 27 March 2007).

8. Gallagher TH, Garbutt JM, Waterman AD, *et al*. Choosing your words carefully: how physicians would disclose harmful medical errors to patients. *Arch Intern Med* 2006; **166**(15): 1585–1593.

9. Gallagher TH, Waterman AD, Garbutt JM, *et al*. US and Canadian physicians' attitudes and experiences regarding disclosing errors to patients. *Arch Intern Med* 2006; **166**(15): 1605–1611.

10. Studdert DM, Mello MM, Gawande AA, *et al*. Disclosure of medical injury to patients: an improbable risk management strategy. *Health Aff (Millwood)* 2007; **26**(1): 215–226.

11. Institute of Medicine (US). Committee on Quality of Healthcare in America. *To Err is Human: Building a Safer Health System*. Washington, DC: National Academy Press; 2000.

12. Gallagher TH, Waterman AD, Ebers AG, *et al*. Patients' and physicians' attitudes regarding the disclosure of medical errors. *JAMA* 2003; **289**(8): 1001–1007.

13. Surbone A, Rowe M, Gallagher TH. Confronting medical errors in oncology and disclosing them to cancer patients. *J Clin Oncol* 2007; **25**(12): 1463–1467.

14. Kash KM, Holland JC, Breitbart W, *et al*. Stress and burnout in oncology. *Oncology (Williston Park)* 2000; **14**(11): 1621–1633; discussion 1633–1624, 1636–1627.

15. Physician Insurers Association of America. *Breast Cancer Study: Third Edition*. Washington, DC: Physician Insurers Association of America; 2002.

16. Lamb RM, Studdert DM, Bohmer RM, *et al*. Hospital disclosure practices: results of a national survey. *Health Aff (Millwood)* 2003; **22**(2): 73–83.

17. Gallagher T, Brundage G, Bommarito, KM, *et al*. Risk Managers' attitudes and experiences regarding patient safety and error disclosure: a national survey. *J Healthcare Risk Management* 2006; **26**: 11–16.

18. Mazor KM, Simon SR, Gurwitz JH. Communicating with patients about medical errors: a review of the literature. *Arch Intern Med* 2004; **164**: 1690–1697.

19. Chan DK, Gallagher TH, Reznick R, *et al*. How surgeons disclose medical errors to patients: a study using standardized patients. *Surgery* 2005; **138**(5): 851–858.

20. Hickson GB, Clayton EW, Githens PB, *et al*. Factors that prompted families to file medical malpractice claims following perinatal injuries. *JAMA* 1992; **267**(10): 1359–1363.

21. Levinson W, Roter DL, Mullooly JP, *et al*. Physician–patient communication. The relationship with malpractice claims among primary care physicians and surgeons. *JAMA* 1997; **277**(7): 553–559.

22. Vincent C, Young M, Phillips A. Why do people sue doctors? A study of patients and relatives taking legal action. *Lancet* 1994; **343**(8913): 1609–1613.

23. Kraman SS, Hamm G. Risk management: extreme honesty may be the best policy. *Ann Intern Med* 1999; **131**(12): 963–967.

24. Clinton HR, Obama B. Making patient safety the centerpiece of medical liability reform. *N Engl J Med* 2006; **354**(21): 2205–2208.

25. COPIC. COPIC's 3R Program. **http://www.callcopic.com/resources/custom/PDF/3rs-newsletter/vol-3-issue-1-jun-2006.pdf** (accessed 27 March 2007).

26. Hobgood C, Xie J, Weiner B, *et al.* Error identification, disclosure, and reporting: practice patterns of three emergency medicine provider types. *Acad Emerg Med* 2004; **11**(2): 196–199.

27. Crigger NJ. Always having to say you're sorry: an ethical response to making mistakes in professional practice. *Nurs Ethics* 2004; **11**(6): 568–576.

28. National Quality Forum: Safe Practices for Better Healthcare. **http://www.qualityforum.org/projects/completed/safe_practices/** (accessed 25 July 2007).

29. Gallagher TH, Studdert D, Levinson W. Disclosing harmful medical errors to patients. *N Engl J Med* 2007; **356**(26): 2713–2719.

30. Taft L. On bended knee (with fingers crossed). *Depaul Law Review* 2005; **55**: 601–616.

Chapter 29

Clinician perspectives on shared decision-making

Martin HN Tattersall

Introduction

Shared decision-making (SDM) between physician and patient is now widely considered to be a desirable goal in many healthcare contexts. However, little is known about current SDM practice in cancer care. Moreover there are few data about physician perceptions of SDM or about outcomes for patients.

Patients vary in the extent to which they wish to participate in decisions and in the decisions in which they wish to participate. Patients in the developed world are increasingly health consumers, and want to be active participants in medical decision-making. A survey of 8,119 European adults reported that over 50% preferred to share decisions with their healthcare provider (1), with the highest rates (74%) found in the younger age group (<35 years). In contrast, few patients report achieving the level of involvement in clinical decision-making that they would like (2). Patients tend to leave doctors who fail to involve them in decisions (3). Responding to the growing expectations of patients to participate in medical care decisions creates significant difficulties for healthcare providers in many countries (4).

Surveys of patients with advanced cancer have revealed that patients' desire for information and involvement in decision-making is high. Cancer patients' expectations for information and involvement in decision-making have changed rapidly, since only 50 years ago, most patients in the USA were not told their diagnosis, and the doctor's role was to participate in a conspiracy of silence or euphemism, and to decide treatment in the best interests of the patient. Now, most cancer patients are told the diagnosis, and expect to be informed about their disease and its management.

There are many reasons for the recent increased emphasis on patients' rights. As communities have become better educated and information about healthcare issues has become more accessible, a fundamental shift in society's expectations of the appropriate role for physicians has occurred. Calls for increased accountability have also emanated from within professional and government ranks, in efforts to standardize clinical practice according to best medical evidence, and to enhance healthcare outcomes. Moreover, consumer advocacy groups have added momentum to legitimizing information provision to patients and their participation in treatment decisions. As we enter the twenty-first century, there is a growing awareness of the importance of involving patients in making decisions about their care, because this can contribute to better quality decisions, and perhaps improve compliance and health outcomes.

If patients are to be active participants in decisions about their care, the information they are given must accord with available evidence and be presented in a form that is acceptable and useful. However, many patient information materials currently in use do not meet these standards (5). The growth and wider availability of the internet will greatly increase access to health information. There are well over 10,000 health-related websites, and over a third of internet users access the web to retrieve health and medical information. However, much of the information on the internet is inaccurate or misleading. The importance of paying attention to the quality of information obtained by patients has been highlighted. An over-optimistic view of medical investigations or treatment may enhance demand for inappropriate interventions, leading to iatrogenic harm, increased patient dissatisfaction and unnecessary costs. The provision of accurate information that patients find useful may enhance the quality of care.

Surveys of patients with advanced cancer have revealed not only that patients' desire for information and involvement in decision-making is high, but also that patients whose condition has recently worsened are more likely to want progressively less involvement in decision-making (6). In this chapter, literature pertaining to the potential relevance of the particular patient circumstance and the consequences for embracing shared decision-making are reviewed.

Shared decision-making

Shared decision-making (SDM) describes a partnership between health professional and patient, in which each contributes to decisions about treatment or care. Physicians in the developed world are increasingly urged to practice shared decision-making. When the aim is to include patients in decision-making, it is the process of involvement, rather than its outcome, that is relevant.

Shared decision-making can be evaluated in terms of information delivered on treatment options, checking of understanding and preferences, and making a shared decision (7). These steps can be monitored best using consultation audio-tapes. We have used audio-recordings of oncologist consultations to examine information discussed, the role of question-prompt lists and oncologist endorsement of patient participation (8–11).

Importance of the physician in facilitating SDM

A survey of oncologists involved in breast cancer care in Ontario, Canada (12) reported that patient involvement in decision-making was less than the oncologist would like. This finding suggests that patients need to be prepared for their potential role in decision-making. Other studies have suggested that physicians need to play a major role in this preparation. In one study, we aimed to determine whether a successful tailoring of patient participation conferred benefits to patients, and whether patients who jointly decided on treatment with their oncologist experienced better outcomes (13). A match between preferred and perceived roles in decision-making was found for just over one-third of patients, with 29% more active than preferred and 37% participating to a lesser degree than preferred. Patients whose level of participation was less than desired wanted more information about treatment options and side-effects, and expressed a greater need for assurance, as well as a chance to talk about their fears. Patients less active in decision-making than desired were also significantly less satisfied. Irrespective of preference, patients who reported a shared role in decision-making were most satisfied with their consultation, with their oncologist and with information about treatments and emotional support. Importantly, patient reports of their levels of participation in decision-making were correlated with oncologist, but not their own, behaviour. This finding suggests that the consultation itself, and the oncologist's behaviour in particular, may be pivotal in generating the discrepancy between preferred and actual roles in reaching treatment decisions. Physician training to promote increased compatibility between patient information needs and participation expectations may be useful.

Elit *et al.* (14) interviewed women with advanced ovarian cancer to identify the extent to which they perceived they had treatment options, understood treatment-related risks and benefits, and preferred to participate in treatment decision-making. Most women felt that they made their treatment decision, but most felt they did not have a treatment choice. Women reported trust and hope as describing the patient–doctor interaction, but with an absence of words describing doctor exploration of patient preference or values. They observed that women with advanced epithelial ovarian cancer did not describe the treatment decision-making as shared, but rather an interaction that was directed largely by the doctor. They conclude that the *onus is on the doctor to ensure that there is an environment for shared decision-making*, in the event that the patient is interested in such an interaction.

Assessment of physician SDM behaviours during consultations

Specific criteria for SDM have not been developed, although over-arching themes have begun to appear in the literature. Stewart (15) reported provision of clear information was one of four communication dimensions. The others were questions from the patient, willingness to share decisions, and willingness to share decisions and agreement between physician and patient about the problem and the management plan. Ford *et al.* (16) identified the elements and skills required for a successful evidence-based SDM consultation. Six themes were identified, namely: research evidence/medical information, the physician–patient relationship, patient perspectives, decision-making processes, time issues and establishing the patient problem.

We developed a list of physician behaviours and actions in cancer consultations encompassing the concepts presented by Gattellari *et al.* (9) and the six themes elucidated by Ford *et al.* (16). The coding scheme is shown in Table 29.1. The individual behaviours were scored as present = 1 or absent = 0. If the behaviour was non-applicable, it was scored as 1. A total score was calculated by summing the SDM scores. Sixty-three medical and radiation oncology consultations with patients with primary cancer involving consideration of adjuvant therapy after surgery were audio-recorded, transcribed and coded. Oncologists demonstrated, on average, a little under 12/20 SDM behaviours. Behaviours involving discussion of evidence and seeking the patient perspective were particularly uncommon, with few consultations containing interactions on these issues. SDM behaviours were more common in consultations involving female patients. Previous studies have found that female cancer patients are more likely to prefer shared decision-making than males, and perhaps oncologists are responding to these preferences. There was a strong trend for patients to feel their involvement preference was met, depending on the SDM score, a relationship providing preliminary evidence of the validity of the coding scheme. These results support our previous finding that physician intervention is an essential part of the means to enhance SDM.

When is SDM most important?

Shared decision-making is most appropriate in situations of uncertainty, in which two or more clinically reasonable alternatives exist (17). When there is only one realistic choice, patient and physician may gather and share information; however, the patient cannot be empowered to make choices that do not exist. Entwistle *et al.* (18) reported a qualitative study of how people interpret and respond to structured questions about decision-making about their healthcare. They note that attempts to assess patients' perceptions of the quality of decision-making in 'routine' practice face greater difficulties than evaluations of a particular decision aid. In the latter setting, the decision of interest is specified for patients, and is the same for each of them. However, in 'routine' practice, especially those consultations that consider more than one clinical problem, they propose that patient-based measures, such as the control preference scale, should not be assumed to

Table 29.1

Elements of shared decision making (9).
Information disclosure
Effect of treatment on tumor (action of treatment)
Told aim of treatment
Told disease if incurable
Drawbacks of treatment
Information about life expectancy
Presented with treatment alternative
Beneficial effect of treatment on quality of life
Doctor encouragement of patient participation
Acknowledges uncertainty that treatment will achieve aim
Elicitation of patient values
Acknowledges trade-offs
Offers treatment choice
Checks patient understanding

reflect models of decision-making described in the literature. They propose a structured set of questions to encourage people to describe the options considered and selected might facilitate attempts to examine attitudes to and achievement of decisions faced and made by patients.

Physicians' perspectives on shared decision-making

A UK study sought to identify the importance of patient-centred behaviour according to general practitioners (GPs) and patients (19). Sixty-four GPs and 410 patients completed questionnaires rating each element on a 5-point Likert scale, where 1 = not important and 5 = totally important. Overall, the GPs believed patient-centred behaviours were very important with mean scores >4 for all items, except for 'allowing the patient to make the final decision'. Involving the patient in treatment decisions recorded the highest mean score, 4.46.

Changing attitudes to involving patients in decision-making were documented in a study investigating the effect of training GPs in risk communication (20). Measures aimed to elicit attitudes to the importance of involving patients in decision-making, their frequency of involving patients in decisions and the GPs competence in this approach. The GPs reported involving their patients in decision-making prior to the training programme less often than they did post-training (mean score 2.2), but it is unknown as to how long this effect lasts.

A USA study using semi-structured interviews with 53 academic and private practice physicians from primary care and surgical specialties identified three justifications for involving patients in decision-making: respect for autonomy, beneficence and self-interest (21). The majority of doctors in this study preferred the role of the doctor as an expert who educates patients and directs the decision-making process. Some participants supported a collaborative relationship with their patients; however, many saw a reduced role for patients, where there is only one medically reasonable choice. Treatment decisions with no clear best answer or with moral dimensions were deemed particularly suitable for increased patient control.

Focus groups with six experienced GPs explored the appropriateness of involving patients in decision-making and the required skills and methods (22). The participants expressed positive attitudes to patient involvement; however, they were concerned that this involvement should not be forced and that the patient's right not to be involved should be respected. A recent study examining attitudes to SDM of 41 Norwegian GPs (23) reported high support of, and preference for, SDM.

A large study investigated the attitudes of German physicians to SDM and compared these to patients (24). Sixty-seven percent of physicians reported that decisions should be shared, 8% that patients should take the lead and 21% that doctors should make the decisions. Younger physicians (≤45 years) reported greater endorsement of SDM.

Oncologists' perspectives on shared decision-making

In some circumstances, where there is a clearly superior treatment, clinicians have indicated a belief that patient preferences can contribute little to clinical decision-making (25). In other situations, particularly where the benefit–cost ratio of a treatment option is small, where options produce similar survival but different quality-of-life outcomes, or where there are no clear data on outcomes, preference about treatments will vary substantially. In these cases—called preference-sensitive decisions—the preferences that drive decision-making must be those of the patient, because patient and clinician preferences may be in disagreement. Examples in cancer care are decisions about whether to have a mastectomy versus lumpectomy plus radiotherapy for early stage breast cancer, and whether to take hormone replacement therapy. A survey of 100 patients and 156 clinical specialists, regarding preferences for different surgical options for managing large bowel cancer, reported preferences differed significantly between them (26). Thus it is important to identify preference-sensitive decisions (in the opinion of both patients and physicians) and to target interventions to elicit these preferences effectively.

Few physicians beyond academic environments elicit their patients' preferences for involvement in decision-making. A recent audit of oncology consultations in Sydney, discussing seeking consent for a clinical trial, reported that the patient preferences and concerns were elicited in only 39% of the consultations and ongoing decisional support was offered in 34% (27).

One of the earliest studies investigating attitudes of health professionals to patient input in decision-making was undertaken in breast cancer care in the USA (28). Oncologists, nurses and patients were all asked to complete the 15-item Locus of Decisional Authority in Decision-making survey. For each item, three responses were possible: 0 = doctor should make the decision, 1 = doctor and patient should make the decision, 2 = patient should make the decisions. A score of 15 indicated that respondents felt all decisions should be shared. Total scores for the three groups were below 15, indicating they felt that physicians should have overall decisional authority. The mean score for the physicians' group was the lowest, 10.23 compared to 12.49 for the patients and 13.74 for the nurses. Attitudes of the different clinician disciplines represented in the sample were also reported: surgical oncologists showed increased support for patient involvement in decisions compared to medical and radiation oncologists. This study also explored differences in attitudes according to age and gender. No significant differences were found in attitude to patient involvement for patient age or physician's gender; however, increased age of clinicians, both nurses and doctors, was associated with reduced advocacy for increased patient involvement.

A Canadian cross-sectional survey has explored the views and understanding of surgeons and oncologists specializing in breast cancer (29). Participants were asked to report their use and comfort with SDM and their perception of the mechanics of SDM, as outlined in a framework published by the authors previously (30, 31). This framework was based on semi-structured interviews, conducted initially with breast cancer patients, to investigate their understanding and experience when making treatment decisions with their physicians (32). The results of these interviews were then adapted for use with physicians in the form of a questionnaire. Separate focus groups of medical and radiation oncologists and breast surgeons identified their perceptions of SDM and its meaning, their use and comfort with this consultation style and the existence of obstacles or aids to putting this approach into practice.

Eighty-seven medial and radiation oncologists and 203 breast surgeons answered the open-ended question concerning what SDM means. The majority of respondents provided responses congruent with SDM, as outlined in the framework. A minority described SDM as information transfer alone. Some physicians suggested that, if the patient's treatment preference and their own recommendation were not the same, further discussion would be warranted to reach a consensus. The survey included examples of decision-making styles designed to depict the four models of decision-making, namely: paternalistic, information-sharing only, shared and informed. The majority of surgeons (94%) and oncologists (87%) identified the example intended to describe SDM as the one most like their own definition of SDM. The example that described information-sharing but clear retention of decisional authority by the physician was selected by 28% of surgeons and 34% of oncologists as their interpretation of SDM, while a similar proportion of surgeons (26%) and oncologists (21%) regarded the informed decision-making example as the most like SDM. The essential ingredients of SDM were further explored by asking respondents to rate the importance of seven characteristics using a 5-point Likert Scale (1 = not important, 5 = extremely important). Items that were rated with either a 4 or 5 were grouped together. Surgeons reported discussion of pros and cons of an intervention (100%), giving information to the patient (99%) and agreeing on the treatment to be given (86%) as very/extremely important. Oncologists reported giving information to the patient (99%), discussion of pros and cons (96.9%) and agreeing on the treatment to be given (95%) as very/extremely important.

Examples of four decision-making styles (paternalistic, information-sharing only, shared and informed) were presented in the survey and participants selected the one most akin to their usual style. Over half (56%) of oncologists and two-thirds (69%) of surgeons stated that their approach to a decision-making consultation was most similar to the shared decision-making example and 27 and 17%, respectively, to the information-sharing style (29). Less than 3% of both groups reported using a paternalistic approach and 8% reported embracing an informed or patient-led approach. These self-reported use statistics were compared to the self-reported comfort with each of the four styles outlined above and a significant discrepancy was noted between the usual approach to reaching a treatment decision and the approach with which they stated they were very or extremely comfortable. Both surgeons (89%) and oncologists (87%) stated they were very or extremely comfortable with the shared decision-making approach, a difference of 20 and 31%, respectively, to their reported use of this style.

We surveyed cancer physicians across Australia to seek their views on SDM to discover whether their views differed systematically according to physician characteristics (33). We hypothesized that specialty training, practice setting and patient caseload would influence support of, and use of, SDM in practice. Altogether 630 surveys were returned from 1,062 eligible participants (response rate 59%). The majority (62%) reported that their usual approach to decision-making with cancer patients was most like the SDM approach; 23% used an information-sharing approach. A paternalistic approach and the informed decision-making approach were selected by 1 and 8%, respectively. In regard to comfort levels with each of the four decision-making approaches, the SDM approach was most favoured. The amount and type of information oncologists routinely give to newly diagnosed patients were significantly greater by physicians who reported using SDM, compared to those not using this approach. Medical oncologists (66%) and surgeons (66%) more commonly reported an SDM approach than radiation oncologists (52%), haematologists (78%)

or paediatric oncologists (33%). In multivariate regression analysis, physicians treating breast cancer and urological cancer were 2.5 times as likely to be very comfortable with SDM compared to colorectal, gynaecological oncologists or haematologists. Female physicians were 2.3 times more likely to be very comfortable with SDM compared to their male colleagues. There was a mismatch between usual practice of SDM compared to high comfort with this approach, and this was greatest for gynaecological oncologists (48%).

Our findings in regard to attitudes of physicians treating breast cancer, mirror almost exactly the reported decision-making practices in Canada. Shared decision-making was also strongly supported by urologists in our study. Conversely, support for SDM was lower among paediatric oncologists and haematologists. Paediatricians may feel that parents of seriously ill children need to be informed about treatment but led to the recommended treatment approach because of the extremely emotional context.

Physician-identified factors affecting patient participation in treatment decision-making

In our survey of cancer clinicians across Australia, we asked participants to rate, on a 4-point Likert scale, to what extent they experienced selected items as barriers or facilitators to decision-making (34). Physicians treating breast or urological cancer were also asked to report their support for a range of listed interventions to encourage patient involvement and reflect on treatment options during the decision-making process. The listed barriers and facilitators, and interventions are presented in Tables 29.2, and 29.3, respectively.

Perceived barriers to treatment decision-making

Experience of items perceived as barriers to treatment decision-making is presented in Table 29.2. Response categories were on a 4-point Likert scale: never, sometimes, often and almost always. The most frequently oncologist-identified difficulty items were: having insufficient information to make a decision at the first consultation (6.6%); and insufficient time to spend with the patient (5.5%). Difficulties related to patient factors reported 'often' or 'almost always' included patients having other health problems, having misconceptions about their disease or treatment, being indecisive, being too anxious and not understanding the information given.

Facilitators to treatment decision-making

The most important facilitators to shared treatment decision-making identified by oncologists were that the patient trusted them, the patient being accompanied in the consultation, the patient wanting to participate and providing written information (see Table 29.3)

Eliciting patient preference for involvement in decision-making

In spite of recommendations from many authors that physicians should elicit patient preferences for involvement in decision-making, it is not clear that this approach is in general use among family practitioners or among cancer physicians. Data from the Evidence-Based Medicine working group, a group of 45 clinicians highly skilled and committed to practicing evidence-based shared decision-making, are illustrative. Even in this atypical group of physicians, only 15 reported sometimes using a quantitative rating of patient's preferences, 8 sometimes used written scenarios to enhance patient understanding of outcome states and 11 used patient decision aids (23).

In Australia, a recent audit of oncologist consultations discussing consent for a clinical trial reported that patient preferences and concerns were elicited in only 39% of the consultations

Table 29.2 Potential Barriers to Shared Decision-making

Doctors factors
I have insufficient information to make a decision about treatment at the first consultation.
There is insufficient time to spend with the patient.
I experience difficulty knowing how to frame the treatment options for the patient.

Patient factors
The patient has other health problems. (E.g. heart disease)
The patient has difficulty accepting s/he has cancer.
The patient has misconceptions about the disease or treatment.
The patient does not understand the information I have given.
The patient is indecisive.
The patient is too anxious to listen to what I have to say.
The patient does not want to participate as much as I would like him/her to.
The patient wants to make a decision before receiving the information from me.
The patient wants to participate more than I would like him/her to.
The patient comes expecting a certain treatment rather than a consultation.
The patient brings too much information to dicuss.
The patient has received conflicting recommendations from various specialists.
The patient requests a treatment not known to be beneficial.
The patient refuses a treatment that may benefit him/her.
There are cultural differences between the patient and me.
The patient's family overrides the decision-making process.

and ongoing decisional support was offered in 34% (24). This demonstrates the low levels of preference elicitation in a situation (involving consent), where one would hope it would be high (if not 100%).

Little is known about variation in physician consultation behaviours according to patient preferences for involvement in decision-making. Almost all the audio-recordings of cancer consultations have been with patients with English language skills; the efficacy of communication with patients with low literacy and from different cultures is largely unexplored. Moreover, few studies have compared differences in physician attitudes and practice when communicating about health decisions across cultures.

Conclusions

Overall, the studies of family practitioners show broad support for involving patients in decisions about their treatment, but family physicians acknowledge that actual involvement of patients is not routine. Reasons for this disparity include physicians not feeling comfortable with patients being assertive, respecting the right of patients not wanting to be involved and asserting that the role of the patient is minimal, if only one medically reasonable treatment option exists.

Physicians treating cancer patients are also broadly supportive of SDM with a minority advocating a paternalist approach. In the large Canadian study of physicians managing breast

Table 29.3 Potential Facilitators to Shared Decision-making

Patient facilitators
The patient trusts the doctor.
The patient has someone with them at the consultation.
The patient wants to participate in making the treatment decision.
The patient is emotionally ready for decision-making.
The patient is prepared (knowledgeable about disease and treatment) for the consulation.

System facilitators
Access for medical practitioners to training to enhance skills in meeting patients' preferenes for SDM
Input from Cancer Nurse Coordinator/CNC prior to consultation
Preparing patient for a greater role in decision-making, by offering question prompt lists prior to the consultation.
Giving the patient a booklet explaining clinical decision-making.
Giving the patient a booklet about patient roles, explaining shared decision-making.
Having a third person in the room.
Audio-taping consultation.
Explaicitly negotiating shared decision-making.
Offering the patient written information about the treatment options available.
Input from Cancer Nurse Coordinator/CNC *post* consultation.
Encourage patient to talk to treatment team and general practitioner.
Worksheets for the patient to help him/her articulate what is important for him/her.
Telephone follow up to discuss treatment decision.
Follow up appointment to make a decision.

cancer, self-reported use of SDM was high, with almost two-thirds of surgeons claiming this to be most like their own approach. Similarly in Australia, physicians treating breast cancer or urological cancer are supportive of SDM, more so than physic1ans managing haematological cancer or children with cancer. The reason for this discrepancy could be linked to the existence of treatment options and the acknowledgement of a clear treatment choice with similar survival outcomes, e.g. mastectomy vs lumpectomy plus breast radiation in breast cancer. A number of studies report some differences between physician specialties and age, with younger doctors reporting greater support for SDM.

Physician-identified barriers to SDM highlight administrative obstacles, namely: insufficient information at the time of the initial consultation and insufficient time. Facilitators of SDM included patient trust in the physician, providing written information about treatment options and the presence of a third person during the consultation.

References

1. Coulter A, Jenkinson C. European patients' views on the responsiveness of health systems and healthcare providers. *Eur J Public Health* **15**: 355–360, 2005.
2. Gattellari M, Butow PN, Tattersall MHN. Sharing decisions in cancer care. *Soc Sci Med* **52**, 1865–1878, 2001.

3. Kaplan SH, Greenfield S, *et al.* Characteristics of physicians with participatory decision-making styles. *Ann Internal Med* **124**: 497–504, 1996.

4. Braddock III CH, Edwards KA, *et al.* Informed decision-making in outpatient practice: time to get back to basics. *JAMA* **282**: 2313–2320, 1999.

5. Coulter A, Entwistle V, Gilbert D. Sharing decisions with patients: is the information good enough? *BMJ* **318**: 318–22, 1999.

6. Butow PN, Maclean M, Dunn SM, *et al.* The dynamics of change: cancer patients' preferences for information, involvement and support. *Ann Oncol* **8**: 857–863, 1997.

7. Edwards A, Elwyn G, Covey J. Presenting risk information a review of the effects of framing and other manipulations on patient outcomes. *J Health Comm* **6**: 61–82, 2001.

8. Butow PN, Dunn SM, Tattersall MHN, *et al.* Patient participation in the cancer consultation: evaluation of a question prompt sheet. *Ann Oncology* **5**: 199–204, 1994.

9. Gattellari M, Voigt KJ, Butow PN, *et al.* When the treatment goal is not cure: are cancer patients equipped to make informed decisions? *J Clin Oncol* **20**: 503–513, 2002.

10. Leighl NB, Butow PN, Tattersall MHN. Treatment decision aids in advanced cancer: when the goal is not cure and the answer is not clear. *J Clin Oncol* **22**:1759–1762, 2004.

11. Brown RF, Butow PN, Ellis P, *et al.* Seeking informed consent to cancer clinical trials: describing current practice. *Soc Sci Med* **58**: 2445–57, 2004.

12. Charles C, Gafni A, Whelan T, *et al.* Self-reported use of shared decision-making among breast cancer specialists and perceived barriers and facilitators to implementing this approach. *Health Expect* **7**: 338–48, 2004.

13. Gattellari M, Butow PN, Tattersall MHN. Sharing decisions in cancer care. *Soc Sci Med* **52**: 1865–78, 2001.

14. Elit LM, Levine LM, Gafni A, *et al.* Patients' preferences for therapy in advanced epithelial ovarian cancer: development, testing, and application of a bedside decision instrument. *Gynec Oncol* **62**: 329–335, 2003

15. Stewart MA. Effective physician-patient communication and health outcomes: a review. *Can Med Assoc Journal* **152**: 1423–1433, 1995.

16. Ford S, Schofield T, *et al.* What are the ingredients for a successful evidence-based patient choice consultation? A qualitative study. *Soc Sci Med* **56**: 589–602, 2003.

17. Whitney, SN. A new model of medical decisions: exploring the limits of shared decision-making. medical decision-making. *Med Dec Making* **23**: 275–280, 2003

18. Entwistle VA, Watt IS, *et al.* Assessing patients' participation and quality of decision-making: insights from a study of routine practice in diverse settings1. *Pat Educ Counsel* **55**: 105–113, 2004.

19. Ogden J, Ambrose L, Khadra A, Manthri S, Symons L, Vass A, Williams M. A questionnaire study of GPs and patients beliefs about the different components of patient centredness. *Pat Educ Couns* **47**: 223–227, 2002.

20. Edwards A, Elwyn G. Involving patients in decision-making and communicating risk: a longitudinal evaluation of doctors' attitudes and confidence during a randomized trial. *J Eval Clin Prac* **10**: 431–437, 2004.

21. McGuire AL, McCullough LB, Weller J, *et al.* Missed expectations? Physicians' views of patients' participation in medical decision-making. *Med Care* **43**(5): 466–470, 2005.

22. Elwyn G, Edwards A, *et al.* Shared decision-making and the concept of equipoise: the competencies of involving patients in healthcare choices. *Brit J Gen Prac* **50**: 892–897, 2000)

23. Carlsen B, Aakvik A. Patient involvement in clinical decision-making: the effect of GP attitude on patient satisfaction. *Health Exp* **9**: 148–157, 2006.

24. Floer B, Schnee M, *et al.* Shared decision-making. The perspective of practicing physicians. *Med Klinik* **99**: 435–440, 2004.

25. Whitney SN, McGuire AL, McCullough LB. A typology of shared decision-making, informed consent, and simple consent. *Ann Intern Med* **140**, 54–59, 2004.

26. Solomon MJ, Pager CK, Rex J, *et al.* Randomized, controlled trial of biofeedback with anal manometry, transanal ultrasound, or pelvic floor retraining with digital guidance alone in the treatment of mild to moderate fecal incontinence. *Dis Colon Rectum* **46**, 703–710 2003.

27. Brown RF, Butow PN, Elli P, *et al.* Seeking informed consent to cancer clinical trials: describing current practice. *Soc Sci Med* **58**: 2445–2457, 2004.

28. Beisecker AE, Helmig L, Moore G. Attitudes of oncologists, oncology nurses, and patients from a women's clinic regarding medical decision-making for older and younger breast cancer patients. *Gerontologist* **34**: 505–512, 1994.

29. Charles C, Gafni A, Whelan T. Self-reported use of shared decision-making among breast cancer specialists and perceived barriers and facilitators to implementing this approach. *Health Exp* **7**: 338–348, 2004.

30. Charles C, Gafni A, Whelan T. Shared decision-making in the medical encounter: what does it mean? (or it takes at least two to tango). *Soc Sci Med* **44**: 681–92, 1997.

31. Charles C, Gafni A, Whelan T. Decision-making in the physician-patient encounter: revisiting the shared treatment decision-making model. *Soc Sci Med* **49**: 651–661, 1999.

32. Shepherd HL, Tattersall MHN, Butow PN. The context influences doctors' support of decision-making in cancer care. *Br J Cancer* **97**: 6–13, 2007.

33. Shepherd HL, Tattersall MHN, Butow PN. Physician-identified factors which affect patient participation in reaching treatment decisions. *J Clin Oncol* **26**: 1724–31, 2008.

Chapter 30

Audio-recording important consultations for patients and their families—putting evidence into practice

Thomas F Hack and Lesley F Degner

Introduction

The experience of cancer is one of the most challenging and potentially devastating events that can befall a person. Physical and psychosocial threats abound throughout the disease continuum; from the point in time when the presence of cancer in the body is suspected, through the diagnostic period and treatment phase(s), and further to palliation and the final breaths of life. From the patient and family perspective, the process of adjustment to cancer involves a myriad of coping responses, many of which involve processing information to inform treatment decisions relevant to patient care. Effective communication between the patient, family, and healthcare professional is pivotal to adequately informing the patient about disease and treatment options, promoting patient participation in medical decision-making, and fostering psychosocial adjustment in the patient. It is through patient–professional discourse that patients come to better understand the nature of their specific form of cancer, as well as their unique treatment needs. These professional consultations are the vehicle by which patients can participate knowledgeably in the treatment decision-making process, yet patients commonly enter the consultation room in a state of elevated anxiety and leave with a weak recollection of information provided to them. For this reason, health professionals frequently encourage patients to ask a family member to accompany them to important consultations. Family members can be a source of emotional support and provide assistance with decision-making but they, like patients, have poor memories for what is said during consultations. If the information that is imparted during any given consultation is essential for making informed decisions, then interventions are needed to enhance patient comprehension of this information, thereby enabling patient and family participation in medical care decisions. One intervention that holds empirical promise in this regard is that of furnishing patients and their families with audio-recordings of important consultations.

The purpose of this chapter is 3-fold:

(1) to briefly review the empirical literature on the value of consultation audio-recordings for patients and families;

(2) to conduct a theory-driven examination of the factors that limit practice uptake of this intervention; and

(3) to provide practical suggestions for how these factors might best be addressed to enhance clinical uptake of consultation audio-recording use.

Review of empirical evidence

It is important that patients understand their disease and treatment options sufficiently to enable them to be effective treatment consumers. While not all patients may express a wish to have greater control over the medical decisions that affect their well-being, research evidence suggests it is in their best interest to do so: Patients who adopt a passive role in decision-making have overall poorer adjustment to their cancer than patients who are actively involved. Many factors likely contribute to rendering patients quiet when they meet with health professionals: lack of disease knowledge, lack of general education, lack of ability to respond assertively, and fears of death, all serve to silence patients during consultations. If the values we espouse for communication during oncology consultations include patient–professional collaboration, fully informed patient consumers, and greater decision-making control by patients, then efforts are needed to enhance the processes involved in conveying information to patients.

One intervention that holds promise in addressing the unmet needs and concerns of newly diagnosed and follow-up cancer patients is the consultation recording (1–18). Reviews of the empirical evidence support the conclusion that audio-recordings of oncology consultations provide valuable benefits to patients (19–21). Consultation recordings allow for memories to be refreshed, for the learning of information not recalled from the consultation, for a clearer understanding of one's cancer treatment (1, 6, 11–13), for greater confidence that critical aspects of the disease and treatment have been discussed (7–9), and for greater information recall in comparison to non-tape controls (3–5, 15–16). Consultation recordings provide patients with a means by which to initiate disease and treatment discussions with family members (4, 11–15) and help patients assume a significantly more active role in subsequent consultations (6). Consultation recordings are well received by the majority of cancer patients; patient satisfaction with the intervention is high (1–2, 4–5, 8–9, 13, 15–16, 18). Practitioner support for this intervention has generally been implied by their study participation or indicated via follow-up interviews (22) but no detailed, prospective account of oncologist use of the consultation recording has been reported to date.

From the research conducted in this area we can conclude that consultation recordings improve information recall, reduce anxiety, enhance patient satisfaction with communication, and increase patients' perceptions that essential aspects of their disease and treatment have been addressed during the consultation (19–21). The Cochrane Collaborative Group, in its revised systematic review of the consultation recording research literature (20), concluded that 'the provision of recordings or summaries of key consultations may benefit most adults with cancer. Although more research is needed to improve our understanding of these interventions, most patients find them very useful. Practitioners should consider offering people tape recordings or written summaries of their consultations.' (p.1)

Theoretical considerations

Despite the empirical evidence supporting the provision of consultation recordings in oncology, the uptake of this intervention into practice has been limited. Knowledge translation theories are useful for understanding why the uptake of promising psychosocial interventions is slower than might be expected, given the supportive evidence base. These theories also suggest that efforts towards wide-scale dissemination should be delayed until the obstacles that impede uptake have been sufficiently identified and addressed.

While translation of healthcare knowledge is not successful if the knowledge itself is not relevant, unbiased, and based on all available evidence (23), translation is also not possible if the knowledge is not adequately transferred. Knowledge transfer is a component of knowledge translation and refers to the technical process that brings information from the empirical literature to practitioners and caregivers. One of the more common findings from health service research is a failure to routinely translate research findings into daily clinical practice (24). Simple diffusion and passive dissemination of research findings are largely ineffective at changing practice (25). Some practitioners have difficulty finding, assessing, interpreting, and applying the best evidence (26–28). This problem has arisen, in part, from empirical information overload and the complexity of research findings (23).

One useful theoretical framework to consider when moving empirically promising communication interventions into mainstream clinical practice is the Promoting Action on Research Implementation in Health Services (PARIHS) Framework (29). The PARIHS framework was conceived by colleagues at the Royal College of Nursing (RCN) Institute in the United Kingdom (30–32). They posited that knowledge translation can be explained as a function of the relationship between *evidence* (research, clinical experience, and patient preferences), *context* (culture, leadership, and measurement), and *facilitation* (characteristics, role, and style), with these three elements having a dynamic, simultaneous relationship. The most successful implementation occurs when evidence is robust, the context is receptive to change, and where the change process is appropriately facilitated (31). Without a thorough understanding of the contextual factors that serve to stimulate, support, and reinforce the use of audio-recordings in oncology, this practice is likely to fail. Given the inter-relationship between evidentiary, contextual, and facilitative factors, it is necessary to examine the complexities of these relationships if audio-recording use is to be successfully diffused and taken up into practice.

Evidence

Evidence (33) comes from four sources: research, clinical experience, patients, and the local context/environment. Research organizations have traditionally focused on the generation of research evidence demonstrating effectiveness. This is certainly the case for consultation audio-recordings.

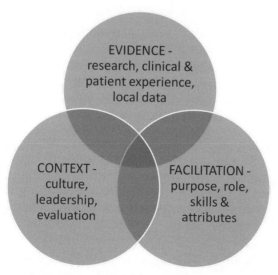

Fig. 30.1 PARIHS framework: Knowledge translation as interrelationship of evidence, context and facilitation.

Systematic reviews of the empirical literature, such as the Cochrane review of consultation recording studies, quicken the rate at which research findings are understood but provide no promise of integration of clinical practice and research findings. This lack of integration may be a function of well-intentioned clinicians trying their best to work in healthcare settings that are too busy and complicated (24). When research is successfully translated, this is often after considerable, unacceptable delay (28). Rycroft-Malone calls for an enhanced understanding of the ways in which research evidence interacts with the evidence of clinical practice, the needs and experiences of patients, and the feedback mechanisms of the social and professional networks that comprise the organizational history and culture. By this definition, evidence in support of consultation audio-recording use is broader than published empirical reports of effectiveness, and efforts to transfer consultation audio-recording knowledge become multi-faceted. For example, little research has been conducted to understand the behavioural propensity of oncologists towards consultation audio-recording use, or the attitudes held by oncologists with respect to their appreciation of the consultation recording literature. The latter is probably best explained by oncologists' lack of exposure to this body of research.

With respect to patient needs and experiences, while the empirical literature unequivocally demonstrates benefits associated with having a consultation audio-recording, we do not know the mechanism(s) by which these benefits are derived. While the benefit of recall is clearly associated with listening to the recorded consultation, it is not known why and how anxiety is reduced and why patients are satisfied with the intervention. While it may be inferentially argued that more informed patients are consequently more satisfied treatment consumers, little is known about how patients derive benefit from listening to the audio-recording. For example, what information on the audio-recording is most helpful to patients and families? Does the audio-recording inform treatment decision-making? Is there a more intangible benefit to having a recording, such as being more positively disposed towards the oncologist, or feeling more 'connected' to family members who listen to the audio-recording? The factors that contribute to the derivation of patient benefit need to be systematically identified. With this knowledge we can then facilitate uptake of consultation audio-recording use in a manner that maximizes benefit.

Context

Context (32) is characterized as having three themes: culture, leadership, and measurement or evaluation. Culture is defined as 'the way things are done around here', and includes 'the forces at work which give the physical environment feel'. The culture of a practice context needs to be understood if meaningful and lasting change is to be achieved. By examining the context of consultation audio-recording use in selected cancer centres, the cultural, leadership, and measurement factors that shape the uptake of consultation-recording use can be identified. With respect to organizational climate, to our knowledge there are no formal policies or even tacit rules governing consultation-recording use. Indeed, oncologists rarely speak of this intervention, and discussions of the merits of this intervention usually take place in the context of an existing consultation audio-recording study. These studies are infrequent and usually pioneered by a researcher with a professional designation other than that of oncologist. Without 'buy in' from oncologists, and in the absence of regular discourse on this topic, the transfer and uptake of consultation audio-recording use is stalled.

Although many important barriers to knowledge translation exist at the level of the healthcare professional (29), there are structural and organizational barriers to integrating research evidence into practice, which operate at levels beyond the control of the individual clinician. Structural barriers are those environmental factors that impede knowledge translation. In oncology settings, a frequently occurring structural barrier to adoption of psychosocial interventions is a lack of financial resources; consultation recording equipment must be purchased and staff resources may be necessary to enable implementation. A potential organizational barrier is the absence of institutional or collegial peer pressures to use this intervention. The likelihood of uptake of consultation recordings may be enhanced through the support of the Chief Executive Officer of the cancer centre or one or more oncologists who can serve as 'champions' in encouraging the use of consultation recordings.

Facilitation

Facilitation (30) refers to the process of enabling the implementation of evidence into practice; 'enabling others' rather than 'doing for others'. In the context of knowledge translation, 'enabling' may have a greater impact than 'doing' because practitioners need time to ponder and assimilate research findings. If oncologists tend to only use consultation recordings within the context of a research study, then we may be merely obtaining time-limited 'buy-in', 'doing for others' or, more precisely, 'guiding the hands of others' rather than enabling oncologists to become self-motivated and self-directed in using this intervention.

Motivation is a critical behaviour change factor that underlies the use of consultation audio-recordings by oncology professionals. Lack of exposure to the benefits of consultation audio-recordings may result in clinicians who believe there is a lack of positive, consensus evidence for their use. Where unfounded negative attitudes towards this intervention exist, these attitudes may serve as heavy barriers for implementation. For this reason, efforts to educate oncologists about the benefits of consultation audio-recordings may be a fundamental component of oncologist acceptance of the intervention and successful implementation. Where positive oncologist attitudes towards consultation audio-recording use exist, those who form an intention to do so may later forget or lose interest in doing so if they are not reminded or otherwise reinforced.

Social barriers to knowledge translation are often critical ones when groups of individuals are encouraged to adopt an intervention. The successful uptake of consultation audio-recording use relies on a substantial proportion or 'critical mass' of oncologists integrating the intervention into clinical practice. Social network theory is useful for examining ideas about the best ways to overcome the social barriers that impede the transfer and uptake of consultation audio-recording use. Social network theory predicts that an intervention is more likely to be adopted, the greater the number of individuals who use it and if an integrated social structure can be established to support adoption (34). By deliberate rewiring of the interactions between oncologists, nurses, patients, and families through the provision and explanation of evidence, support in the use of consultation audio-recordings, and by increasing health professionals' interactions with each other while using this intervention, we may potentially increase the density of the cancer patient–professional social network (35). West argued that a dense social network has advantages for knowledge translation: 'The multiplicity of ties gives members the opportunity to persuade, cajole, and monitor the performance of others' (p.635). An objective for promoting consultation audio-recording use is to utilize the professional hierarchy of oncology practice to provide for 'cascades' of consultation audio-recording evidence, increasing the density of the social context of consultation audio-recording use, and thereby facilitating uptake into clinical practice. Social network theory also suggests that those individuals with the most influence or power in using the intervention and promoting its use among others should be identified as change agents. Among oncologists, disease site leaders might be identified and approached, particularly if these oncologists can instruct other oncologists within their disease specialty to adopt consultation audio-recording use.

An implicit assumption in much of the writing on social barriers is that most knowledge translation activities should be directed toward the health professional. There are proportionately fewer studies that identify selected patient groups as the target for change. This is perhaps not surprising given that the goal of most knowledge-transfer activities is to change the practice style of treating clinicians. However, there may be evidence that is sufficiently compelling to cause a significant portion of cancer patients or the general public to mobilize in an effort to change clinical practice. The significance of cancer patients and their advocacy organizations in promoting interventions that may enhance their psychosocial well-being should not be under-estimated. Studies are needed to identify and address the role of cancer patients and their advocacy groups as change agents in the consultation audio-recording transfer process.

Case study: assessment of receptiveness to consultation audio-recordings

By way of example, we will use our consultation recording research programme to illustrate the application of the PARIHS framework to enhancing the transfer and uptake of the consultation audio-recording intervention. Consistent with the functions of knowledge 'brokering', if the translation goal is to see more clinicians using a new intervention, then the probability of success will be enhanced if clinicians are included as co-investigators of the research and if they are involved in an advisory capacity throughout the research process (36). We sought after oncologists who have used consultation audio-recordings in clinical practice and hold senior positions within their respective cancer disease sites. We identified health professionals who are well suited by their practice history and power status to serve as local champions for the use of consultation audio-recordings, and invited them to join the research team as co-investigators.

In the development phase of a recent project, the first author travelled to each participating centre to interview the oncologists and front-line staff about consultation recording use, asking them to share their opinions on the relative merits, perceived barriers, and facilitative facets of this intervention. Given that an understanding and acceptance of the best empirical evidence in support of consultation recording use is fundamental to successful uptake, the principal investigator arrived at each interview with evidence in hand: a copy of the Cochrane Collaboration systematic review of consultation recording use (20), copies of publications of the consultation recording studies conducted by the research team, and a copy of a recent newspaper article speaking to the value of consultation audio-recordings for newly diagnosed oncology patients. These materials were offered to the interviewee, depending on the direction of the interview. Nearing the end of each interview, the interviewer explained that a detailed proposal to examine the transfer and uptake of the consultation audio-recording intervention would be developed only if there was sufficient interest among the oncologists and nurses being interviewed. It was encouraging that all of the interviewees supported the idea and expressed their willingness to participate. The interview transcripts showed that the oncologists and nurses were able to identify several barriers and contextual factors that explain the current use of consultation audio-recording in their centre. The respondents frequently differed both in their assessment of the benefits to patients of receiving a consultation audio-recording, and in their identification of factors that are critical to enhancing the uptake of consultation audio-recording use. These considerations of evidence, context, and facilitation are presented in Box 30.1 as guidelines for use when designing a research study to examine the consultation audio-recording intervention within a knowledge translation framework.

Box 30.1 Evidence, context, and facilitation considerations for consultation audio-recording studies

Knowledge of consultation recording evidence. Are patients, families, and oncology staff aware of the evidence?

Perceived quality of evidence. How do patients, families, and oncology staff rate the quality of the evidence?

Perceived value and benefit. What is the perceived value and benefit of consultation recordings?

Relative value and benefit. How does this intervention compare against other ways of providing information?

Perceived impact of consultation recording on oncologist behaviour. Will oncologist involvement possibly reduce spontaneity during consultation; improve the quality of communication?

Leadership. Is there an individual to or group to champion the intervention?

Legal concerns. Who owns the recording—the patient, oncologist, or cancer centre? Can oncology staff or the cancer care organization be successfully sued for what is said on the recording? Is there a need to consult legal counsel?

Time constraints. Is there sufficient time for oncology staff to record consultations?

Privacy. What protective measures need to be taken to minimize patient risk?

Data storage. Where and how will recordings be stored?

Lack of infrastructure. Is there a sufficient number of recording devices and associated materials available in clinic?

Resource cost. What is the staff cost to implement *and* sustain the intervention?

Intervention cost. What is the ongoing cost to sustain the intervention indefinitely?

Motivation. Will oncology staff be compensated or reinforced for participating? Will oncology staff performance be evaluated?

Technology type. What options are available for recording the consultation—CD? USB key (memory stick)? Should the digital recording be converted to a text file? Should one type of technology be used for all patients or should options be available?

Availability of technology. Are all patients able to access the chosen technology? Do older patients have access to computers? Is there a need to accommodate different computer operating systems? Do patients need to own a computer to participate?

Delivery mode. Will the patient or cancer centre supply the recording equipment? Will the intervention patient or provider driven? Who will press the 'record' button? How will the recording be accessed by patients and family members?

Staff support. Who will identify eligible patients—ward clerks, nurses?

Message. Will the entire consultation be recorded or only a portion thereof? Will the medical history be recorded? Will the physical examination be recorded? Will only the oncologist be recorded, or the nurse and resident as well?

Looking forward

For oncology professionals who want to integrate audio-recording of key consultations into their practice, we offer the following basic suggestions:

◆ Secure the availability of audio-recording equipment in all clinic rooms.

◆ Assign responsibility for recording the consultation to a specific staff member or class of oncology professional.

◆ Introduce the topic of recording the consultation by saying something to the patient like: 'Today I will provide you with important information about your disease and treatment that you may want to remember. To make it easier to remember what we talk about, many patients find it helpful to receive an audio-taped recording of the discussion. I would like to offer you an audio-recording of our discussion. You can then take the recording home with you to listen to on your own or with family and friends.'

◆ Obtain, from the patient, informed written consent to be recorded. Consider including a disclaimer statement to protect the recorded professional from medico-legal liability associated with patient use of the recording.

◆ As an expression of respect for patient privacy, do not record the physical examination portion of the consultation.

◆ Retain a copy of the recorded consultation within the oncology department.

◆ Solicit patient feedback on the utility and value of the recorded consultation.

While recent reviews provide a compelling, evidence-based case for consultation audio-recording use, additional studies are warranted. Studies are needed to examine the process of implementing consultation audio-recording use into oncology practice. We need to address the factors that retard the transfer and uptake of consultation audio-recording use and test ideas about the best ways to transfer intervention knowledge and support intervention uptake. These studies should be guided by theoretical frameworks relevant to knowledge transfer and uptake, such as the PARIHS Framework and Social Network Theory. The field of knowledge translation is growing rapidly, and new theoretical frameworks are being developed, while existing ones are being adapted for use as knowledge translation frameworks. Further research is needed to examine the suitability or heuristic value of these theories to examinations of the transfer and uptake of the consultation audio-recording intervention.

Using prospective, longitudinal designs, we need to follow patients more closely during the first few days following receipt of the consultation audio-recording, i.e. the time at which the recording tends to be listened to, to document the patient's perspective with respect to the specific benefits that are realized. It is important that these benefits be measured systematically because benefit articulation is an essential component of successful uptake of psychosocial interventions by practitioners. Patients' stories of the benefits received from having the recording may be a powerful, reinforcing influence on consultation-recording use by oncologists and nurses. The use of patients as 'change agents' should therefore be explored by systematically documenting the benefits that patients derive from the recorded consultation and passing this benefit knowledge on to the oncologists and nurses as a means of facilitating patient–professional communication about this intervention. One possibility is to have patient and family feedback presented in a letter to the oncology staff that expresses patient and family appreciation for the consultation audio-recording.

While the empirical evidence-base demonstrates the value of furnishing patients with consultation audio-recordings, greater attention needs to be paid to the benefits that family members receive from listening to the audio-recording, the manner by which patients and families derive benefit and value, and the benefits to clinicians of having their consultations recorded for use by patients and family members. We need to identify and describe any subgroups of patients and families for whom consultation audio-recordings are most beneficial. Last, we need to document the types of consultations that are most valuable to patients and families. While most of the empirical literature has focused on the initial treatment consultation, there may be potential risks or unique benefits associated with providing patients with audio-recorded consultations during which discouraging news is provided, such as news of a relatively poor prognosis or indication of disease progression.

References

1. Ah-Fat FG, Sharma MC, Damato BE (1998). 'Taping outpatient consultations: a survey of attitudes and responses of adult patients with ocular malignancy'. *Eye*, **12**, 789–91.

2. Bowden JR, Brennan PA, Butler-Keating R, *et al.* (2003). 'Use of audiotaped patient consultations in a head and neck oncology clinic and survey of patient attitudes to this facility'. *J Laryngology Otology*, **117**, 879–82.

3. Bruera E, Pituskin E, Calder K, *et al.* (1999). The addition of an audiocassette recording of a consultation to written recommendations for patients with advanced cancer'. *Cancer*, **86**, 2420–5.

4. Deutsch G (1992). 'Improving communication with oncology patients: taping the consultation'. *J Clin Oncol*, **4**, 46–7.

5. Dunn SM, Butow PN, Tattersall MHN, *et al.* (1993). 'General information tapes inhibit recall of the cancer consultation'. *J Clin Oncol*, **11**, 2279–85.

6. Ford S, Fallowfield L, Hall A, *et al.* (1995). 'The influence of audiotapes on patient participation in the cancer consultation'. *Eur J Cancer*, **31A**, 2264–9.

7. Hack TF, Pickles T, Bultz BD, *et al.* (1999). 'Feasibility of an audiotape intervention for patients with cancer: a multicenter, randomized, controlled pilot study'. *J Psychosocial Oncol*, **17**, 1–15.

8. Hack TF, Pickles T, Bultz D, *et al.* (2003). 'Impact of providing audiotapes of primary treatment consultations to men with prostate cancer: a multi-site, randomized, controlled trial'. *Psycho-Oncology*, **16**, 543–52.

9. Hack TF, Pickles T, Bultz BD, *et al.* (2003). 'Impact of providing audiotapes of primary adjuvant treatment consultations to women with breast cancer: a multi-site, randomized, controlled trial'. *J Clin Oncol*, **21**, 4138–44.

10. Hack TF, Whelan TJ, Olivotto IA, *et al.* (2006). 'Standardized audiotape versus recorded consultation to enhance informed consent to a clinical trial in breast oncology: a feasibility study'. *Psycho-Oncology*, **16**, 371–6.

11. Hobgin B, Fallowfield L (1989). 'Getting it taped: the 'bad news' consultation with cancer patients'. *Br J Hosp Med*, **41**, 330–3.

12. Johnson AA, Adelstein DJ (1991). 'The use of recorded interviews to enhance physician-patient communication'. *J Cancer Educ*, **6**, 99–102.

13. Knox R, Butow PN, Devine R, *et al.* (2002). 'Audiotapes of oncology consultations: only for the first consultation?' *Annals Oncol*, **13**, 622–7.

14. McHugh P, Lewis S, Ford S, *et al.* (1995). 'The efficacy of audiotapes in promoting psychological well-being in cancer patients: a randomised, controlled trial'. *Br J Cancer*, **71**, 388–92.

15. North N, Cornbleet M A, Knowles G, *et al.* (1992). 'Information giving in oncology: a preliminary study of tape-recorder use'. *Br J Clin Psychol*, **31**, 357–9.

16. Ong LML, Visser MRM, Lammes FB, *et al.* (2000). 'Effect of providing cancer patients with the audiotaped initial consultation on satisfaction, recall, and quality of life: a randomized, double-blind study'. *J Clin Oncol*, **18**, 3052–60.

17. Reynolds PM, Sanson-Fisher RE, Poole AD, *et al.* (1981). 'Cancer and communication: information giving in an oncology clinic'. *Br Med J*, **282**, 1449–51.

18. Tattersall MHN, Butow PN, Griffin AM, *et al.* (1994). 'The take-home message: patients prefer consultation audiotapes to summary letters'. *J Clin Oncol*, **12**, 1305–11.

19. McClement SE, Hack TF (1999). 'Audio-taping the oncology treatment consultation: a literature review'. *Patient Educ Couns*, **36**, 229–38.

20. Scott JT, Harmsen M, Prictor MJ, *et al.* (2007). 'Recording or summaries of consultations for people with cancer (Review)'. *The Cochrane Collaboration*, Issue 2.

21. Tattersall MH, Butow PN (2002). 'Consultation audio tapes: an underused cancer patient information aid and clinical research tool'. *Lancet Oncol*, **3**, 431–7.

22. Stockler, M, Butow PN, Tattersall MHN (1993). 'The take-home message: Doctors' views on letters and tapes after a cancer consultation'. *Annals Oncol*, **4**, 549–52.

23. Boissel, JP, Amsallem E, Cucherat M, *et al.* (2004). 'Bridging the gap between therapeutic research results and physician prescribing decisions: knowledge transfer, a prerequisite to knowledge translation'. *Eur J Clin Pharmacol*, **60**, 609–16.

24. Grimshaw JM, Eccles M, Tetroe J (2004). 'Implementing clinical guidelines: current evidence and future implications'. *J Contin Educ Health Prof*, **24**(Suppl 1), S31–7.

25. Chilvers R, Harrison G, Sipos A, *et al.* Evidence into practice (2002). 'Application of psychological models of change in evidence-based implementation'. *Br J Psychiatry*, **181**, 99–101.

26. Ely JW, Osheroff JA, Ebell MH, *et al.* (2002). 'Obstacles to answering doctors' questions about patient care with evidence: qualitative study'. *BMJ*, **324**, 1–7.

27. Haynes B, Haines A (1998). 'Barriers and bridges to evidence based clinical practice'. *BMJ*, **317**, 273–6.

28. Pearcey PA (1995). 'Achieving research-based nursing practice'. *J Adv Nurs*, **22**, 33–9.

29. Rycroft-Malone J (2004). 'The PARIHS framework—a framework for guiding the implementation of evidence-based practice'. *J Nurs Care Qual*, **19**, 297–304.

30. Harvey G, Loftus-Hills A, Rycroft-Malone J, *et al.* (2002). 'Getting evidence into practice: the role and function of facilitation'. *J Adv Nurs*, **37**, 577–88.

31. Kitson A, Harvey G, McCormack, B (1998). 'Approaches to implementing research in practice'. *Qual in Healthcare.* **7**, 149–59.

32. McCormack B, Kitson A, Rycroft-Malone J, *et al.* (2002). 'Getting evidence into practice: the meaning of 'context''. *J Adv Nurs*, **38**, 94–104.

33. Rycroft-Malone J, Seers K, Titchen A, *et al.* (2004). 'What counts as evidence in evidence-based practice?' *J Adv Nurs*, **47**, 81–90.

34. West E, Barron DN, Dowsett J, *et al.* (1999). 'Hierarchies and cliques in the social networks of healthcare professionals: implications for the design of dissemination strategies'. *Soc Sci Med*, **48**, 633–46.

35. Buchanan, M (2002). *Nexus: small worlds and the groundbreaking theory of networks.* W.W. Norton & Company, New York.

36. Lomas J (2007). 'The in-between world of knowledge brokering'. *BMJ*, **334**, 129–32.

Chapter 31

Working with interpreters and achieving culturally competent communication

Steven Klimidis and Harry Minas

Introduction

Healthcare around the world is currently experimenting with the development of culturally and linguistically competent workforces and systems of care (e.g. 1). Fundamental to this enterprise is redressing the problems of language and cultural barriers between the community and service providers. Language interpreting is becoming an essential service. There remain issues of accessibility, coverage of languages in increasingly multilingual societies, the setting of standards for interpreting, and competing funding models for such services (e.g. 2–4). For the clinician, there is a need to develop the knowledge and skills for working with culturally and linguistically diverse patients and their families, including those relevant to working effectively with interpreters. In this chapter, we focus on the issues of interpreting: understanding interpreting as a process; its nature and limitations; and progress towards a guide for clinicians in working effectively with interpreters. We begin with a brief account of the current evidence for the effectiveness of interpreting.

Effectiveness of interpreters in medical settings

The question of whether interpreters are effective in improving clinical consultation and in fostering improved outcomes has been subject to a growing body of research, most of which is included in recent reviews (5, 6). Here we summarize the general findings, incorporating some newer research. The main results indicate that interpreted interviews return improvements in the clinical encounter and patient outcomes over non-interpreted interviews. This is the case especially when professional (rather than untrained) interpreters are engaged. However, interpreted interviews are inferior to interviews where clinicians are able to speak the patient's language. This suggests that there is scope for improvements to be made in interpreted interviews (7). This generally favourable picture, however, is based on merging results from different clinical settings, in none of which have interview process and patient outcomes been evaluated together. Limitation in space precludes detailed consideration of the many methodological issues and areas in need of further research.

A focus on communication

Communication is complex. It involves achieving consensus in meaning between communicators who may approach their encounter from different perspectives, different communicative styles and behaviour, and differences in representing meaning in words and actions. There are cultural and situational influences, variations in intimacy, trust and power in relationships, as well as many other factors that can influence communication. Basic aspects of communication are comprehension and production of speech, gestures, text and other communicative modes. At a psychological level, these involve processing of acoustic, phonological and morphemic information, syntactical forms, relationships between words, and so on. These tasks are generally accomplished without the need for awareness and attention to process. Language analysis decodes a sequential message by incorporating prior syntax and semantics into an evolving understanding. Language production assembles a vast network of associations into a meaningful, sequential, semantically and syntactically coherent form. The fact that human languages can differ substantially in structure and semantics (8) means that transfer of meaning across languages can be easily compromised, particularly in verbal communication.

Common meaning through shared culture has major implications for successful communication. Dysard-Gale (9) gives an example where the doctor is requesting an interpreter to ask a Moroccan male if the patient has a history of same-sex relationships. The interpreter asked if the patient had 'relations with a person other than the patient's wife'. Such miscommunication could be regarded as an error with potential clinical significance (e.g. 10). However, the interpreter was well aware that '[t]hat's a 100% impossible question in our religion. He [the patient] would kill me [had I asked him that]. You'd hear 'Code blue, Kamal [the interpreter] is dead!'… if I asked that.' (p.243, 9). One of the key issues in clinician– patient communication is the clinician's own awareness and cultural sensitivity in her communications with patients. What might be regarded, in the clinician's culture, as a relatively 'normal' question, could pose significant problems to the patient, to the clinical relationship and to the content of what is communicated by an interpreter. In a process that is influenced by factors from basic information processing through to social, cultural and situational, there is much opportunity for communication failure, i.e. a failure to transfer the intended meaning between communicators across two languages.

An example is the sociolinguistic analysis of doctor–patient communication by Marshall (11). Doctor–patient communication is not everyday conversation. Mishler (12), reflecting on the cultural gap between doctors and patients, suggests that the doctor and patient speak with discordant voices—the doctor's is the voice of medicine, while the patient's is the voice of lived experience (e.g. 13, 14). Translated into communications for the purpose of achieving a diagnosis, the doctor's voice is structured to elicit relevant history and presence or absence of symptoms, guided by her knowledge of biomedical syndromes and clinical experience. There are constraints on the doctor, including time pressure and institutional protocols to be followed, and other issues that influence communication. The patient often does not have the same understanding of the specific purpose of the communication or the methods used, and commonly does not share the same broader influences on the communication process. Nor is there, usually, the same underlying theory of illness (the main business of diagnostic communication), let alone any sharing of the language of medicine. In the patients' experience, pain, distress, mood variations, and so on—the whole-personal experience of illness—are embedded in the stories of their lives. Usually they are presented in rich narrative form, context- and situation-bound, and may not necessarily be brought together meaningfully in the patient's mind by any underlying disease concept. Even where the patient does have a clear illness concept that explains her predicament, it may differ significantly from the dominant conceptions of biomedicine (e.g. 13–19). Communication can sometimes be characterized by a lack of conversational cooperation between clinician and patient. Procedurally, as shown by Marshall (11), this is indicated by ambiguities between the patient's and the clinician's expressions going unresolved, clinician-led conversation, lack of appropriate conversational 'turn-taking', clinician interruptions that change the topic, inferred (but not actual) experiences read into the illness experience of the patient, and misinterpretation of the patient's condition. Such difficulties in communication can clearly compromise all aspects of the clinical process.

Erzinger (20) conducted an analysis of communication between Spanish-speaking patients in the USA and their doctors, highlighting the influence of ethno-cultural differences. In this work, cultural values, such as *sympatia* (expressions of personal warmth and concern) and *personalismo* ('formal friendliness')—both features of *respeto* (respect)—translate into specific styles of conversation, with particular rules guiding patient and doctor communications. When doctor and patient share a culture such rules are understood implicitly and their conversations are characterized by greater conversational cooperation. In other cases, where there is cultural mismatch, doctors, as Erzinger's (20) analysis shows, may fail to respond according to the patient's cultural expectations (as in Kamal's dilemma, above), leading to communication failures, deterioration of the clinical relationship and possible problems in treatment (for discussion of inter-cultural factors see: 19, 21, 22).

While focusing in this chapter on issues of interpreting, it is important for the reader to keep in mind that clinician–patient communication is inherently problematic, particularly when communication involves the meeting of two cultures. Gregg and Saha (7) point out that research (and resultant policies) in cross-language communication in medical settings has been guided by the unfounded assumptions that languages share a roughly common grammar and words, and that 'language barriers can be considered a problem of simple [word or] code-switching, in which individuals who speak different languages merely require a "code-breaker"' (p.368). Larsen's (8) textbook for translators lists over 150 qualities of world languages that influence comprehension and reproduction of text from one language to another. For communication to be meaningful, extra-linguistic factors and effects of context, such as who is communicating with whom, where, how and why, among other things, come into play. Hymes (23) referred to this as 'communicative competence'. Gregg and Saha (7) suggest that a focus on interpreted interactions as communicative competence may be where interpreted encounters could be improved, with optimal benefits to patients.

An issue of some importance is the diversity of views concerning whether medical interpreters should also assume the role of 'culture brokers' (e.g. 9, 24), acting beyond the inter-language code-switching and participating in cross-cultural information exchange, across the divide between biomedicine and patient cultures. This may include explaining biomedical terminology, diseases and processes of disease and treatment to patients in a manner likely to be understood by patients, and explaining to the clinician the possible cultural origins of the patient's illness perspective and illness behaviour, and broader cultural factors that may be influencing the patient and the patient's communication with the clinician (9, 24). There is a difference of opinion between clinicians and interpreters about what constitutes an appropriate role for interpreters in the clinical encounter. Abbe *et al.* (2006), for example, indicated that, while oncologists typically preferred word-for-word translation, interpreters' views were that clinicians often misunderstood the nature of inter-cultural communication and pointed to the need for interpreters to be able to act as cultural brokers. It should also be pointed out that there is considerable diversity of opinion among interpreters concerning whether it is appropriate in clinical settings for interpreters to assume this cultural brokerage role.

Interpreters and translators

An interpreter is an intermediary between two people who are communicating through speech. A translator is more strictly focused on rendering text from one form to another. While translators are important to the development of linguistic and culturally appropriate text-based medical communications (e.g. consent forms, patient information materials, etc.), there is greater urgency in multi-lingual and multi-cultural societies to ensure that there is access to professional interpreters in clinical settings (e.g. 5, 6). The interpreter is ideally bilingual *and* bicultural in the deepest sense. That is, they have a deep understanding of the two cultural groups in the communication encounter, in addition to an extensive and readily accessible knowledge of the two languages. Indeed, interpreters in settings dealing with immigrants need to have cultural and linguistic knowledge of the local community, given that immigrant cultural identity, practices and language can be subject to local variations. This is particularly so for long-term resident communities in the country of settlement. For interpreters, this notion extends to special settings such as the medical setting, where specific communication practices can be complex, involve particular terminologies, and an interpreter's ignorance of these cultural and linguistic aspects can severely impair communication, leading to significant errors (e.g. 5, 26, 27).

Communicative complexity

Because of convenience or patient preference it is common to conscript family members (often adolescent children), bilingual hospital staff and, sometimes, other patients into the medical interpreting role (28, 29). In Fagan *et al.* (30) over 50% of interpreted interviews occurred with family members or friends doing the interpreting (this not an unusual rate, e.g. 31). This practice reflects a serious under-estimation of the complexity of the medical interpreting task. Different types of clinical encounters cary greatly in communicative complexity. A typical example of a high-complexity situation is the communication of negative prognosis and end-of-life (EOL) issues in late-stage terminal illness. Clayton *et al.* (32) have developed practice guidelines for such situations, summarised in Box 31.1.

By comparison with Marshall's (11) diagnostic process, the EOL interview highlights many highly sensitive interpersonal strategies, in addition to information exchange, which make it considerably more complex to negotiate. In EOL discussions an interpreter is required to join

---

Box 31.1 Summary of end-of-life communication process

- Preparation for the communication before meeting with the patient and family.
- Heightened sensitivity and empathy towards the emotional safety of the patient and family.
- Delicacy in how clinicians relate 'bad news'.
- Respects and negotiates decisions about disclosure to the patient taking time to understand people's motivations to, and not to, disclose.
- Gives appropriate time and space for patients and family members to understand, pursue or not pursue information given their emotional readiness for it.
- Expects and respects emotional outpourings or 'shock'.
- Deals with patient and family emotions strategically by clinicians remaining open, available and responsive to their immediate needs.
- Engages sensitively into issues to be considered, as they will emerge in the course of time (cautiously condensing into the reality of what is ahead for the patient and the family).
- Incorporates cultural understandings and expectations.

(32, 33)

a more complex process, where interpersonal strategies, perhaps more than technical medicine, are important in the exchange between communicators. The interpreter will need to be able to personally cope with the content and process of what is being communicated and will need to sensitively maintain fidelity to the methodology of clinical tasks pursued by the clinicians (tasks that are inherently unpalatable and demanding of the clinicians themselves). Further, in such situations, interpreters will need to be experienced enough to be able to handle the connotative, nuanced, euphemistic aspects of the language involved (34), as clinicians, patients and family members commonly 'soften' the emotional impact of topics of death and dying (e.g. 35). It should be obvious that the interpreter must adhere strictly to their role, lest the delicate dynamic between clinicians and the patient and family be disturbed and give rise to misunderstandings.

Issues in the use of untrained interpreters

Other than inaccuracy and the potential for errors of clinical significance (e.g. 10, 36), the practice of engaging untrained interpreters, particularly the general public and family members, is highly problematic. The interpreting process requires an intimate, extensive, readily accessible and symmetrical knowledge of the two languages and of the rich cultural connotations or senses of meaning encapsulated in words or larger units of speech. Although informal interpreters may be thought to be bilingual and bicultural, in the main they may not meet the requirements for effective interpreting. This is particularly so in situations of high complexity where specialist terminology is used or abstract concepts, such as emotions, pain type and severity, probabilities of cure, medication side-effects, decline in health, etc., are discussed. Moreover, the fact of acculturation, and individual variations in this process, questions the validity of engaging untrained interpreters who may not be able to represent the cultural features of the patient. To some extent, it can also be argued that interpreters who have not specialized in their training in medical interpreting, or have little experience in such settings (or even in specialized tasks such as EOL communications), may lack the requirements to effectively interpret.

Using members of the general public as interpreters also presents particular issues as to how their relationships with the patient might influence communication. Children of patients as interpreters, for example, may not be able to communicate freely on topics that may be embarrassing and inappropriate for their age, given their cultural background, such as issues related to libido or sexual behaviour as affected by illness or medication side-effects or issues of sexuality, as in the personal and conjugal implications for women with breast removal (e.g. 37). Topics such as disclosure of diagnosis or poor prognosis may be uncomfortable for a family member and may be subject to censorship in contexts where there are cultural preferences for non-disclosure. Often non-disclosure is construed as a means of protecting the emotional wellbeing of the patient, in the belief that such disclosure will lead to loss of hope in the patient and contribute to a decline in wellness or preclude recovery (e.g. 38, 39). Using strangers who are members of the ethno-cultural group of the patient has its own problems, including confidentiality issues. Patients, particularly those from a small local community, may be inhibited in communication given the perceived threat of having their condition known to others in their community. This may be especially important in communities where illnesses such as cancer may carry shame and stigma (e.g. 16).

There is evidence suggesting that health workers untrained in interpreting, under some circumstances, may be able to provide sufficient interpreting quality for medical communications. Moreno *et al.* (40), for example, tested bilingual skills in 840 'dual-role' staff. It was found that 77% of the sample scored at the level sufficient for medical interpreting. This group was typified by those with some formal education in their language other than English. The remainder had basic conversational knowledge of English or their other language, often making errors in translation and in oral interpreting, including errors considered to be of clinical significance. Therefore, some dual-role staff could be a valuable resource within a healthcare system where professional interpreter access is an issue. In deciding on the use of untrained interpreters, one approach is to consider the task itself. 'Bilingual' family members may be useful in assessing need for a trained interpreter, to identify the patient's preferred language, dialect, preferred interpreter gender and so on. In more complex negotiations, such as consent for medical procedures (e.g. 41), untrained family members may not be able to interpret effectively. With dual-role staff it may be necessary to know their capability for the interpreting role (40), but also for the organization to consider the costs of taking staff away from their primary role (42). Generally, it may be useful for services to identify clinically critical communicative situations where professional interpreters should always be engaged and other situations of lower complexity where available skills can be matched to communicative situations and balanced against their potential adverse impact on the overall care process and clinical outcomes. This is a matter of setting policy to guide clinicians' decisions at the point of practice.

Professional interpreting and the nature of interpreting

There are various forms of professional interpretation. The interpreter may be present in the room with the healthcare provider and the patient, present via audiovisual relay, or remotely linked via an audio system (e.g. telephone, intercom). Needless to say, in remote interpreting, all involved in the communication should have access to the utterances of the interpreter. Cases have been noted where this has not occurred, with poor outcomes for the patient and service provider alike (27). Types of interpretation may be either simultaneous, involving (nearly) word-for-word interpretation of the speaker's utterance, or consecutive, where the interpreter listens to a sample of speech in one language and then relates this to the listener in the other.

An important difference between the two is the greater opportunity in consecutive interpreting for the interpreter to take responsibility for the conveyance of meaning between the speaker and the listener, compared with the simultaneous method, where achieving an appropriate interpretation of the speaker's message, in its fullest cultural nuance, is the responsibility of the listener. The cognitive demands differ too. In simultaneous interpreting, the interpreter engages in three tasks at broadly the same time, with delays averaging three to four words between input and translated reproduction (43): monitoring the speaker's input, 'code-switching', and production and monitoring of their own output. Experienced simultaneous interpreters are able to do this task effectively because they have more symmetrical bilingual vocabulary and syntactical access competencies than other bilinguals. Through training, experienced interpreters have developed superior skills in storing and manipulating information in 'working memory' (roughly, the memory system holding a telephone number while dialling). They may also be better able to inhibit interference between the two languages, an established phenomenon in bilinguals (44). Thus experience and practice are important determinants of successful simultaneous interpretation. Situational factors, such as rate of speech delivered by communicators, combined with the length of the message, can hamper the interpreter's performance, particularly where the interpreter is less experienced with simultaneous interpreting. Unfamiliarity with specialist terminology and the constructs discussed, lack of equivalency in structure between languages (e.g. different subject–verb–object arrangements, differences in pronominal structure, morpheme ambiguity differences, lack of vocabulary correspondences among other variations) may also contribute to lowering performance in simultaneous interpretation.

In consecutive interpreting, it may be expected that message length by the speaker, especially when a correctly sequenced reproduction is required, will influence interpretation accuracy. Thus in either simultaneous or consecutive interpreting, speakers should be wary of the cognitive demands of their utterances on interpreters and should make relevant adjustments by segmenting their speech sequence so that key single ideas are the usual basis of the segments. Patients cannot be expected to follow such rules, particularly in emotionally charged situations, but clinicians could be mindful of the need to support interpreters in their task. If correct sequencing is not an issue and a main idea needs to be communicated, then memory demands will not be as high, as the focus will be on the interpreter understanding the main point to be conveyed to the patient in broadly the same manner. Consecutive interpreting allows more flexibility for idea transmission under conditions of prior agreement between the interpreter and the clinician that the inter- preter's role may be allowed to extend beyond language 'code-switching'.

There are also differences between audio-only remote versus in-person (in the room or by audio-visual link) interpreting situations. Typically simultaneous interpreting is not reasonable in in-person interpreting due to acoustic interference and patient confusion about who to focus on during the communication. Both consecutive and simultaneous can be done remotely, while consecutive is more typical of in-person situations. An important difference between in-person and remote methods is in the availability to the interpreter of the non-verbal behaviour of the speaker, which may be important in being able to relay emotional displays, interest or disengage- ment, non-verbal emphases of particular phrases and other aspects that serve as context for the verbal message. At its best, in-person interpretation can allow some level of mimicry by the inter- preter of non-verbal behaviour, transmitting not only words but also emotional and gestured punctuations of the speech act. Conversely, on occasion, an inexperienced interpreter may show disparities between verbal and non-verbal communicative acts, e.g. smiling when the patient is relating information in a serious manner, because of personal embarrassment or other reasons. On such occasions, the interpreter may be overstepping her role as facilitator and becoming an active participant, communicating non-verbally her personal judgements of the patient's experi- ence. This could act to alienate the patient.

Another important difference is in the relationships between interpreter and each of the two people communicating, as these may potentially impact on the relationship between the two primary communicators (e.g. doctor–patient). Alliances between communicators and the inter- preter are more likely to form in in-person interpreting. Remote interpreting is more impersonal and, because of this, some patients may feel more comfortable with issues of confidentiality (e.g. 45). Alliances between interpreters and patients may be beneficial. Interpreters often play a wider role in the patient care or broader social support process of the patient (e.g. 24), as patients invite them into this role. Patient–interpreter alliances may emerge from the need for language minority patients to negotiate a complex system of care, including the exigencies that constrain clinicians as these are transferred into their communications with patients in busy medical care settings (e.g. 11, 28). However, issues of divided loyalties may arise for the interpreter. Dohan and Levintova (46) give the example where a family member admonishes the interpreter for following the doctor's insistence to disclose the patient's diagnosis of cancer to the patient, in a culture where it was expected that the interpreter should comply with the cultural demand for non-disclosure (see also, 47–49). Excessive alliance between patients and interpreters may lead clinicians to feel left out of the communicative process and to question the adequacy of the interpretation process (e.g. 24). The clinician's intention is usually to fortify a clinical relationship with the patient in order to develop trust that is important in ensuring treatment negotiation and consequent therapeutic outcomes (50). Sideline conversations between patient and interpreter, the interpreter acting as advocate or taking over the patient's role as an active communicator (e.g. answering for the patient), may be signs of such an alliance.

Another circumstance is where there is strong alliance between the clinician and interpreter. In this case, the interpreter may be seen by patients to be representing the interests of the clinician or the service. In cases of disagreement between patients and clinician (e.g. 39), the interpreter is likely to be construed as an agent for the clinician and the service, leading potentially to patient disengagement. Lastly, in certain situations, interpreters may be seen as disinterested or disengaged with the care process (e.g. 51). There may be good reasons for such behaviour, such as the interpreter's personal security or emotional safety, other than a lack of experience. All potentially damaging alliances should be discussed and redressed between clinicians and interpreters.

Whichever variation of interpreting is used, professional interpreters will communicate in the first person when this is appropriate to the conversation between the primary communicators (which is most of the time). This is in keeping with their role as the *facilitator* of communication rather than an *actor*. Also in keeping with this role, and with the aim of supporting the clinician–patient relationship, it is important for clinicians and patients to be talking directly with each other, in both verbal and non-verbal communicative acts. Exceptions to this are when there is prior agreement between clinician and interpreter for the interpreter to be able to interject and help repair the communication between the clinician and the patient. Kamal's dilemma, above, could have been resolved without his distorting the message to the patient if Kamal was, by agreement, able to stop the interaction and act as cultural broker clarifying the culturally problematic nature of the doctor's request for information.

Sometimes there will be significant differences between the length of the patient's or clinician's verbal productions and those of the interpreter. Often this is thought as reflecting interpreter incompetence, and clinicians may mistrust the interpreting process (e.g. 24). Interpreter incompetence may or may not be the cause. Here there is a need for clinicians and interpreters to converse about the situation, and often for the clinician to take responsibility and control of the communication content and process. On occasion, words like cancer, allergy, psychosis, depression, etc., may not have direct translations in the language of the patient, requiring explanation of the construct itself. Patient education is the responsibility of the clinician and there may be a need to step back from the conversation to incorporate clinician-guided explanation of the construct being addressed.

As mentioned, an interpreter's role, as cultural broker, is to communicate professional constructs and terminology to the patient in the form that is most likely to be understood. However, it remains important for clinicians to be at the centre of what is to be communicated to patients, given that the clinician's medical expertise will not be matched by the interpreter. Conversely, clinicians cannot entirely rely on interpreters to inform them about the cultural predilections and behaviour of patients. Cultural stereotypes as expressed by interpreters, acting as cultural brokers, may not apply to a particular patient due to the patient's possible acculturation and individual variation in cultural identity and participation with the culture of origin, especially with respect to illness behaviour and clinical process issues (e.g. 21, 52). Second, often it is not clear that the interpreter is an infallible informant about cultural features of the patient. Stereotyped views (developed through consultation with an interpreter or otherwise by reference to published accounts, e.g. 38, 39) should hold a position of expanding the clinician's range of possibilities (clinical hypotheses) for understanding the patient's behaviour, but they must always be qualified by direct clinical evidence for their relevance to any particular patient.

Another important issue for consideration, affecting repeated consultations with patients, is whether or not it is advantageous to have the same interpreter each time. There are many advantages to communication in having the same interpreter, including less need for briefing the interpreter about the patient's history, greater development of collaboration between clinicians and interpreters, familiarity in having negotiated together difficult issues of communication in the past and the establishment of rules and patterns of communication to resolve emergent difficulties, patient comfort in identifying with a single interpreter as part of the treatment process, and lessening of patient concerns about confidentiality issues by demonstrated confidentiality adherence, among other advantages. Disadvantages include the potential for counter-productive alliances developing between the interpreter and the patient.

Lastly, much of the literature on interpreting, on errors of communication, for example, attributes miscommunication to the (in) competence of interpreters. As indicated, it is important also to recognize the contribution of clinicians to communication difficulties. Aranguiri *et al.* (53) analysed communication between primary care physicians and patients as interpreted, primarily, by dual-role staff. In one example of the doctor's message to the patient, we counted 84 words, packing in some 40 concepts or ideas, and littered with 21 instances of technical medical terms. The interpreter's relay contained 28 words and a vast omission of the details, including blurring of the main message that the doctor intended to convey. As indicated earlier in the discussion of cognitive demands on interpreters, clearly one aspect of improved communication has to be clarity and succinctness on the part of clinicians.

Working effectively with interpreters

There is some consensus (e.g. 54, 55) that structuring the interpreted consultation into three stages, preparation, interview and post-interview review, may facilitate communication, particularly for higher complexity communications. Space precludes a fuller account; however, we give several recommendations for useful strategies within a three-stage model. First, preparation is just as important as the clinical interview itself. In the preparation stage, even before meeting with an interpreter, the clinician should have organizd the meeting with the interpreter based on a clear understanding of the patient's language and dialect, and any particular preferences for the gender and age of the interpreter. When meeting the interpreter, the clinician will need to know the experience of the interpreter in relation to the communication task ahead. The clinician's own needs for support to conduct the interview may be useful to discuss if the clinician is inexperienced with an interpreted interview. The interpreter will need to be briefed on the patient and the nature and purpose of the interview. A description of the methods to be used by clinicians would be useful to interpreters, including any that may involve intentional interpersonal strategies (as in the EOL example earlier). If technical medical terms will be related, it would be useful for the clinician to discuss these, with alternative means of communication agreed upon where direct translation is impossible or constructs might be unknown. If it is probable that the interview will be emotionally charged, this should be discussed with the interpreter, examining the latter's confidence that the situation can be handled effectively with respect to both the interpreter's emotional comfort and safety, and with respect to the communication process itself. In relation to the interview, the clinician may confirm its confidential nature and set out the ground rules with the interpreter for dealing with emergent ambiguities or difficulties (e.g. will the interpreter be allowed to interrupt the interview to clarify issues of communication). It may be useful for the clinician to discuss seating arrangements, forms of address, interpersonal distance, eye-contact and touching, effects of clinician–patient gender or age differences, and any other related topics that may be subject to cultural influences or taboo, especially if this is an unfamiliar patient for the clinician. Expectations of a post-interview briefing should be raised at this point and any issues resolved about this prior to the interview. The interpreter should be given an opportunity to ask any questions to resolve any uncertainties about what is ahead.

During the interview, the clinician should inform the patient regarding the ground rules that will operate regarding the interpreted discussion, giving the patient permission to interrupt to clarify ambiguities. Confidentiality should be discussed, particularly in relation to the interpreter's presence. The clinician should talk directly with the patient and encourage the patient to talk directly to the clinician. The interpreted interview should afford the clinician time to think about their communications and to 'package' them into effective, non-verbose messages. This will allow the clinician to be able to monitor the overall communication but also ensure that messages are as succinct as they can appropriately be, to support the interpreter in the communication process. The clinician should monitor indicators that may signal difficulties in the communication or that there is a need for review or conversational repair. Such indicators include disproportionate lengths of messages, disparities between verbal and non-verbal behaviours, discontinuities in verbal content and emotional reactions, etc., in the exchanges between clinician, interpreter and patient. Discomfort with any of these may indicate the need for communication repair, particularly through a discussion with the interpreter. The clinician should also take note of any less urgent issues that may need to be followed up with the interpreter after the interview.

During the post-interview review the interview may be skeletally reconstructed and reviewed. Any issues of miscommunication should be raised and discussed. As continuous learning, it may be useful for the clinician to ask the interpreter to reflect on the clinician's style and performance. The interview should be reviewed with respect to whether its purpose has been achieved and to assess what additional issues need follow-up because of communication failures. Just as significant, in situations that have been emotionally difficult, the clinician should enquire about the emotional state of the interpreter. It is not unusual for interpreters to have experienced similar circumstances as the patient (cancer in the family, refugee trauma, etc.). If significant distress is indicated and there is no facility for appropriate debriefing, the clinician may wish to advise the interpreter of relevant professional services.

Concluding comment

There is a need for greater appreciation among clinicians of the complexity and difficulty of the communicative task in patient–clinician communication, particularly when patient and clinician do not share a common language and must rely on the assistance of an interpreter. Cultural differences between clinician and patient add to the difficulty of achieving effective communication. The common practice of relying on untrained interpreters is not acceptable and frequently leads to avoidable error in communication, with sometimes serious clinical consequences. There is a need also for clinicians to learn the methods that are required for working effectively with an interpreter.

References

1. Anderson, L. M., Scrimshaw, S. C., Fullilove, M. T., *et al.* and The Task Force on Community Preventive Services (2003). Culturally competent healthcare systems: asystematic review. *American Journal of Preventive Medicine*, **24**, 68–79.

2. Bowen, S. (2001). *Language Barriers in Access to Care*. Ottawa: Health Canada.

3. Miletic, T., Minas, I. H., Stolk, Y., *et al.* (2006). *Improving the Quality of Mental Health Interpreting in Victoria*. Melbourne: Victorian Transcultural Psychiatry Unit.

4. Regenstein, M. (2007). Measuring and improving the quality of hospital language services: Insights from the *Speaking together* collaborative. *Journal of General Internal Medicine*, **22**(Suppl 2), 356–359.

5. Flores, G. (2005). The impact of medical interpreter services on the quality of health care: a systematic review. *Medical Care Research & Review*, **62**, 255–299.

6. Karliner, L. S., Jacobs, E. A., Chen, A. H., *et al.* (2006). Do professional interpreters improve clinical care for patients with limited English proficiency? A systematic review of the literature. *Health Services Research*, **42**, 727–754.

7. Gregg, J., Saha, S. (2007). Communicative competence: A framework for understanding language barriers in health care. *Journal of General Internal Medicine*, **22**(Suppl 2), 368–370.

8. Larsen, M. (1984). *Meaning-based Translation: A Guide to Cross-Language Equivalence.* New York & London: University Press of America.

9. Dysard-Gale, D. (2007). Interpreters. Negotiating culturally appropriate care for patients with limited English ability. *Family & Community Health*, **30**, 237–246.

10. Flores, G., Laws, M. B., Mayo, S. J., *et al.* (2003). Errors in medical interpretation and their potential clinical consequences in pediatric encounters. *Pediatrics*, **111**, 6–14.

11. Marshall, R. S. (1988). Interpretation in doctor-patient interviews: a socio-linguistic analysis. *Culture, Medicine & Psychiatry*, **12**, 201–208.

12. Misher, E. G. (1984). *The Discourse of Medicine: Dialectics of Medical Interviews.* Norwood, NJ: Ablex Publishing Corp.

13. Snow, L. F. (1983). Traditional health beliefs and practices among lower class black Americans. *The Western Journal of Medicine*, **139**, 820–128.

14. Yeo, S. S., Meiser, B., Barlow-Stewart, K., *et al.* (2005). Understanding community beliefs of Chinese-Australians about cancer: Initial insights using an ethnographic approach. *Psycho-oncology*, **14**, 174–186.

15. Dein, S. (2004). Explanatory models of and attitudes towards cancer in different cultures. *The Lancet Oncology*, **5**, 119–124.

16. Goldstein, D., Thewes, B., Butow, P. (2002). Communicating in a multicultural society II: Greek community attitudes towards cancer in Australia. *Internal Medicine Journal*, **32**, 289–296.

17. Hubbell, F. A., Chavez, L. R., Mishra, S. I., *et al.* (1996). Differing beliefs about breast cancer among Latinas and Anglo women. *The Western Journal of Medicine*, **164**, 405–409.

18. Landrine, H., Klonoff, E. A. (1992). Culture and health-related schemas: a review and proposal for interdisciplinary integration. *Health Psychology*, **11**, 267–276.

19. Ong, K. J., Back, M. F., Lu, J. J., *et al.* (2002). Cultural attitudes to cancer management in traditional South-East Asian patients. *Australian Radiology*, **46**, 370–374.

20. Erzinger, S. (1991). Communication between Spanish-speaking patients and their doctors in medical encounters. *Culture, Medicine & Psychiatry*, **15**, 91–115.

21. Huang, X., Butow, P., Meiser., B., *et al.* (1999). Attitudes and information needs of Chinese migrant cancer patients and their relatives. *Australian and New Zealand Journal of Medicine*, **29**, 207–213.

22. Schouten, B. C., Meeuwesen, L. (2006). Cultural differences in medical communication. A review of the literature. *Patient Education and Counselling*, **64**, 21–34.

23. Hymes, D. (1962). The ethnography of speaking. In T. Gladwin & W. C. Sturtevant (eds.), *Anthropology and Human Behaviour*, pp.13–53. Washington: The Anthropology Society of Washington.

24. Kaufert, J. M., Koolage, W. W. (1984). Role conflict among 'culture brokers': the experience of Native Canadian medical interpreters. *Social Science and Medicine*, **18**, 283–286.

25. Abbe, M., Simon, C., Angiolillo, A., *et al.* (2006). A survey of language barriers from the perspective of pediatric oncologists, interpreters. *Pediatric Blood Cancer*, **47**, 819–824.

26. Divi, C., Koss, R. G., Schmaltz, S. P., *et al.* (2007). Language proficiency and adverse events in US hospitals: a pilot study. *International Journal for Quality in Health Care*, **19**, 60–67.

27. Johnstone, M.-J., Kanitsaki, O. (2006). Culture, language, and patient safety: making the link. *International Journal for Quality in Health Care*, **18**, 385–388.

28. Davidson, B. (2001). Questions in cross-linguistic medical encounters: te role of the hospital interpreter. *Anthropological Quarterly*, **74**, 170–178.

29. Richter, R., Daly, S., Clarke, J. (1979). Overcoming language difficulties with migrant patients. *The Medical Journal of Australia*, **1**, 275–276.

30. Fagan, M. J., Diaz., J. A., Reiner, S. E., *et al.* (2003). Impact of interpretation method on clinic visit length. *Journal of General Internal Medicine*, **18**, 634–638.

31. Andrulis, D., Goodman, N., Pryor, C. (2002). *What a Difference an Interpreter Can Make. Health Care Experiences of Uninsured with Limited English Proficiency*. Boston: The Access Project.

32. Clayton, J. M., Hancock, K. M., Butow, P. N., *et al.* (2007). Clinical practice guidelines for communicating prognosis and end-of-life issues with adults in the advaced stages of a life-limiting illness, and their caregivers. *Medical Journal of Australia*, **186**(12) (Supp), s77-s108.

33. Back, A. L., Curtis, J. R. (2002). Communicating bad news. *The Western Journal of Medicine*, **176**, 177–180.

34. Westermeyer, J., Janca, A. (1997). Language, culture and psychopathology: conceptual and methodological issues. *Transcultural Psychiatry*, **34**, 291–311.

35. Rodriguez, K. L., Gambino, F. J., Butow, P., *et al.* (2007). Pushing up daisies: implicit and explicit language in oncologist-patient communication about death. *Support Care Cancer*, **15**, 153–161.

36. Sabin, J. E. (1975). Translating despair. *American Journal of Psychiatry*, **132**, 197–199.

37. Ashing-Giwa, K. T., Padilla, G., Tejero, J., *et al.* (2004). Understanding the breast cancer experience of women: a qualitative study of African American, Asian American, Latina and Caucasian cancer survivors. *Psychooncology*, **13**, 408–428.

38. Lipson, J. G., Meleis, A. I. (1983). Issues in health care of Middle Eastern patients. *The Western Journal of Medicine*, **139**, 854–861.

39. Muller, J. H., Desmond, B. (1992). Ethical dilemmas in a cross-cultural context: a Chinese example. *The Western Journal of Medicine*, **157**, 323–327.

40. Moreno, M. R., Otero-Sabogal, R., Newman, J. (2007). Assessing dual-role staff-interpreter linguistic competency in an integrated health care system. *Journal of General Internal Medicine*, **22**(Suppl 2), 331–225.

41. Hunt, L. M., de Voogd, K. B. (2007). Are good intentions good enough? Informed consent without trained interpreters. *Journal of General Internal Medicine*, **22**, 598–605.

42. Timmins, C. L. (2002). The impact of language barriers on the health care of Latinos in the United States: a review of the literature and guidelines for practice. *Journal of Midwifery & Women's Health*, **47**, 80–96.

43. Treisman, A. M. (1965). The effects of redundancy and familiarity on translating and repeating back a foreign and a native language. *British Journal of Psychology*, **56**, 369–379.

44. Christoffels, I. K., de Groot, A. M. B., Kroll, J. F. (2006). Memory and language skills in simultaneous interpreters: The role of expertise and language proficiency. *Journal of Memory and Language*, **54**, 324–345.

45. Gany, F., Leng, J., Shapiro, E., *et al.* (2007). Patient satisfaction with different interpreting methods: a randomised controlled trial. *Journal of General Internal Medicine*, **22**(Suppl 2) 312–318.

46. Dohan, D. L., M. (2007). Barriers beyond words: Cancer, culture, and translation in a community of Russian speakers. *Journal of General Internal Medicine*, **22**(Suppl 2), 300–305.

47. Mystakidou, K., Tsilika, E., Parpa, E., *et al.* (2005). Patterns and barriers in information disclosure between health care professionals and relatives with cancer patients in Greek society. *European Journal of Cancer Care*, **14**, 175–181.

48. Papadopoulos, I., Lees, S. (2004). Cancer and communication: similarities and differences of men with cancer from six different ethnic groups. *European Journal of Cancer Care*, **13**, 154–162.

49. Turner, L. (2005). From the local to the global. Bioethics and the concept of culture. *Journal of Medicine and Philosophy*, **30**, 305–320.

50. Mechanic, D., Meyer, S. (2000). Concepts of trust among patients with serious illness. *Social Science & Medicine*, **51**, 657–668.

51. Nailon, R. E. (2006). Nurse's concerns and practices with using interpreters in the care of Latino patients in the emergency department. *Journal of Transcultural Nursing*, **17**, 119–128.
52. O'Malley, A. S., Kerner, J., Johnson, A. E., *et al.* (1999). Acculturation and breast cancer screening among Hispanic women in New York City. *American Journal of Public Health*, **89**, 219–327.
53. Aranguri, C., Davidson, B., Remirez, R. (2005). Patterns of communication through interpreters: a detailed sociolinguistic analysis. *Journal of General Internal Medicine*, **21**, 623–629.
54. Farooq, S., & Fear, C. (2003). Working through interpreters. *Advances in Psychiatric Treatment*, **9**, 104–109.
55. Miletic, T., Piu, M., Minas, I. H., *et al.* (2006). *Guidelines for Working Effectively with Interpreters in Mental Health Settings*. Melbourne: Victorian Transcultural Psychiatry Unit.

Chapter 32

Challenges in communicating with ethnically diverse populations

Bejoy C Thomas, Joshua J Lounsberry, and
Linda E Carlson

Introduction

In the United States, visible minorities currently constitute 29% of the total population, and by the year 2050, estimates suggest that nearly 50% of Americans will be people of colour (1). In Canada, average immigration rates recorded over a 5-year span increased by 15% from 1986–1991 to 1996–2001 (2). In addition, between 2001 and 2006, Canada's foreign-born population increased by 13.6%, while the Canadian-born population increased by only 3.3%. Currently, foreign-born Canadians represent almost one in five of the total population. Worldwide, the highest proportion of foreign-born population is in Australia (22.2 %), followed by Canada (19.8%) and the USA (12.5%) (3).

Incidence of cancer amongst these ethnic minorities is generally comparable to that of the host population (4–6). Research also suggests that access to healthcare amongst visible minority populations is comparable to host populations in tax-dollar facilitated healthcare systems, such as Canada (7). However, creating universal access to healthcare may not imply comparable utilization amongst different groups. Indeed, differences in the use of hospital and screening services by visible minorities have been identified. This discordancy in utilization of services may contribute to the creation of health-status disparities for visible minorities.

Health-status disparities are complex and often poorly understood. Some research suggests that these disparities may largely reflect socio-economic differences, which in turn may influence health-related risk factors (8, 9). However, research has shown that ethnic differences persist even when variables such as socio-economic status and education do not differ or are statistically controlled (10–12). Interestingly, this disadvantage appears to occur only for the patient when they are a minority in the host society. Research has shown that the psychosocial impact of cancer on patients seems to be globally consistent and comparable across nations. For example, quality-of-life (QOL) scores in cancer populations in India (13–15), China (16) and Japan (17) are comparable to findings seen in similar non-Hispanic White cancer patient populations in the United States (13–15, 18). Migration seems to change the dynamics of QOL, satisfaction, and biomedical and psychosocial outcomes.

The Institute of Medicine 2002 report entitled 'Unequal treatment: Confronting racial and ethnic disparities in heath care' (9) stated that ethnic minorities in the USA are often at a later stage of cancer when diagnosed and are less likely to receive appropriate treatment. Studies have also noted that racial and ethnic minorities are less likely to possess health insurance (19), are more likely to rely of publicly funded health insurance (20) and, even when insured, are likely to face additional barriers to care due to other socio-economic factors, such as higher co-payments or insufficient transportation (9). Minorities are also more likely to report higher levels of dissatisfaction and distrust with treatment and care (21).

Communication: the role of the patient and the care provider

In general terms, communication difficulties can be described with reference to problems of diagnosis, a lack of patient involvement in discussions around diagnosis and treatment options, or the inadequate provision of information to the patient (22). Studies have shown that across patient groups: nearly 50% of psychosocial and psychiatric problems are missed by general practitioners (23); patients are interrupted an average of 18 seconds into the description of the presenting problem (24); about 50% of patient problems and concerns are never mentioned by either the patient or the physician (25); patient and physician agree on the presenting problem in less than 50% of visits (26); and patients are often dissatisfied with the information provided to them by physicians (27). Clearly then, communication between the physician and patient can be tenuous; when language issues, cultural diversity, and prejudice are added to the mix, communication may become even more problematic.

In the early 90s, Sondra Thiederman authored the book *Profiting in America's multicultural marketplace* (28). While this book deals with economics in the multicultural business world, some of the concepts mesh nicely with the difficulties faced in multicultural cancer care. There may be reluctance on the part of caregivers to notice, or act upon, cultural differences in patients for several reasons, such as:

◆ the fear of being construed as being racist;

◆ the fear that if we focus on how patients differ, we will fail to see how they are similar;

◆ the fear of perpetuating stereotypes;

◆ the fear of making it complex;

◆ facing the uncomfortable truth that there may be multiple and equally valid approaches to life.

How communication unfolds in medical encounters depends on a number of factors, such as doctors' and patients' beliefs and goals, styles of communicating, perceptions of each other and how each adapts to, and accommodates, the communication style of the other (27) (see Box 32.1). There are two common reasons for disparities in doctor–patient communication. First,

Box 32.1 The six basic requirements of successful service, discussion, and treatment in a multicultural hospital setting

◆ You must build trust with the patient.

◆ You must build rapport and be liked by the patient.

◆ You need to be able to communicate.

◆ You need to know and satisfy the patient's needs and expectations.

◆ You need to make the patient feel comfortable.

◆ You must make it easy for the patient to choose and adhere to treatment.

Adapted from the six requirements of sales, service, and negotiation (28).

doctors may believe that some patients (e.g. middle-aged, more educated, white) are more interested in, more capable of understanding, or in greater need of information than are other patients (29). Second, when doctors are passive in either providing or eliciting information, patients are less likely to gain adequate understanding of their health condition and treatment options (30), are less likely to adhere to the doctor's recommendations (31), and may experience poorer health after the consultation (22). Moreover, when patients assume a passive role in the interaction, doctors may not get sufficient information to make appropriate treatment recommendations (32) and patients may be less committed to, and less satisfied with, those recommendations (33, 34).

Research has indicated that visible minorities and patients in ethnically discordant consultations (patient and physician are of different ethnicity) tend to be less communicative with physicians and typically elicit less information from physicians (35, 36). However, this disparity cannot be wholly attributed to poor communication, as cultural differences are likely to play a role as well. For example, in several cultures (e.g. Middle Eastern and South Asian cultures) the physician is akin to a demigod. In these cultures, patients rarely disagree with physicians, and when they do, a great deal of guilt and anguish is experienced. Thus, the biases brought into the mix by both parties can be quite influential in producing unsatisfactory communication (35, 36).

Language issues

In recent years, several studies have identified language problems as one of the biggest challenges facing immigrant populations. Language barriers can impede healthcare access (37, 38), lower quality of care (39, 40) and result in dissatisfaction with care (41, 42). However, Ponce *et al.* (43) noted that there is a scarcity of studies that address how the gradations of English proficiency might affect health status and healthcare access.

Host language proficiency has been shown to be a dominant component of acculturation to the host society (44), and may bring about socio-economic stability and improved healthcare navigation skills (43). However, Berry *et al.* (45) have hypothesized that acculturation may lead to acculturative stress—feelings of marginalization and alienation—which often results in the reduction of health status of individuals in the form of distress. Ponce *et al.* (43) postulated that, if being English proficient could enable the individual to gain better healthcare access and better health status, then the outcomes of the English-proficient population (those who are fluent in English but speak a different language as their mother tongue) would be comparable to those of the English-only population (host population). In their study testing this hypothesis, English-proficient individuals were not found to differ from English-only individuals on healthcare access or health status. However, limited-English-proficient individuals (those not fully fluent in English) were found to have significantly worse access to care and health status compared to the English-only individuals. Interestingly, both limited-English-proficient and English-proficient individuals had a statistically higher risk of reporting poorer emotional health when compared to the English-only individuals (43). Some suggest that this represents a shift from the somatization of stressors—which is normal in some cultures—to a more Westernized emotional recognition of stress (46, 47). Others have attributed it to the unique emotional difficulties that may be faced when attempting to straddle two disparate cultures (48). Another possible distinguishing characteristic of English-proficient individuals is the likelihood of possessing higher socio-economic status (SES) in the country of origin, potentially followed by a decline in social class and occupational status after immigrating to the host nation, be it the United States, Canada or Australia (43). Hence, the immigration experience may have deflated their individual self-worth, resulting in an increase in depressive symptoms (49–51).

Potential interventions for communication problems

Use of translators

Although the cost of interpretational services seems prohibitory, research has shown that, if services are offered in multiple languages, cancer screening rates and access to cancer care are likely to increase among ethnically diverse populations (52–55). A case-control evaluation study by Jacobs *et al.* (56), found that patients who used interpreter services had a greater uptake of recommended preventive services. They felt that, given the improvement in quality and uptake of services amongst immigrant groups, the estimated $279 per person for interpreter services is justifiable.

Professional interpreters are trained not just to promote accuracy of communication by translating both physician and patient statements verbatim, but also by becoming as 'invisible' as possible in the doctor–patient relationship (57). Unfortunately, limited resources or uncommon languages can hinder this process. When using untrained interpreters, such as family members or staff, errors in interpretation can occur, such as omission (message completely or partially deleted by the interpreter), addition (information not expressed by the patient), condensation (response is simplified and paraphrased), and substitution (replacement of one concept with another) (58, 59) (see Box 32.2). Although not an ideal choice, the ability to 'professionalize' an *ad hoc* interpreter becomes an essential skill of the physician (57). In these situations, physicians can emphasize the importance of accuracy (no adding, omitting, or substituting), position (behind the patient), eye contact (with the doctor, not the patient), and employing clarification or back translation, when needed (60). Despite this suggestion in the literature, such training is not a common feature of medical programmes, and there are few standardized methods to evaluate this competency (61, 61).

Box 32.2 The importance of good patient–physician communication: a case example

Mohammad Kochi is a 59-year-old man living in Fremont, California. Mr Kochi and his family emigrated from Kabul in war-torn Afghanistan eighteen years ago. Many of his family members were lost in the war, and most of his family's possessions were left behind. Even though Mr Kochi has lived in North America for quite some time, he still lives as would a traditional Afghani. His family is highly patriarchal and his home is replete with the trappings of the society from which he came. As a devout follower of Islam, Mr Kochi prays five times a day, fasts during Ramadan, and has done the pilgrimage to Mecca (Haj) seven times in his life. Mr Kochi is often seen wearing traditional garments, a white cylindrical hat, and slippers. Most of Mr Kochi's time is spent within his Afghani/Muslim community, resulting in Mr Kochi still lacking a working knowledge of English. While Mr Kochi does like watching baseball and football on television, he has not become acculturated into the North American way of life. His strong religious and cultural beliefs still inform all aspects of his life.

Mr Kochi began experiencing stomach pains and was referred to a specialist by his family doctor. Following diagnostic testing, the specialist determined that Mr Kochi had gastric cancer. At the time, Mr Kochi's daughter, Habiba, was translating for him and, on the advice of her brother-in-law, told Mr Kochi that it was a bacteria rather than cancer. As is traditional within the Afghani culture, they thought to save him the trauma of thoughts surrounding a terminal illness. Unbeknownst to his daughter, Mr Kochi did hear the word 'cancer' and understood its meaning; however, he chose to keep this knowledge to himself in

> **Box 32.2 (continued) The importance of good patient–physician communication: a case example**
>
> order to not upset his family. After a lengthy discussion with his family, Mr Kochi decided to go ahead with the suggested surgery to remove his stomach. During this successful procedure, the surgeon notice enlarged lymph nodes in the area and Mr Kochi was sent to an oncologist, Dr Fisher, for further treatment.
>
> At this initial appointment with Dr Fisher, it was determined that Mr Kochi would benefit from adjuvant chemotherapy. The most effective method for administering the chemotherapy was to use an intravenous line and a pump to be worn on the belt. However, Mr Kochi refused the chemotherapy for what was at the time assumed by Dr Fisher to be religious reasons. This belief held by Dr Fisher was supported by Mr Kochi's use of phrases such as 'It is in Allah's hands'.
>
> Mr Kochi's cancer continued to worsen and at each follow-up appointment he was encouraged to accept the chemotherapy treatment. Then almost a year after his surgery, one of Mr Kochi's other daughters, Noozria, accompanied him on his appointment as translator. It is at this point that the tragic miscommunication became clear. The language barrier—perhaps in conjunction with the family's attempts to keep Mr Kochi unaware of his condition—resulted in Mr Kochi understanding that the only treatment option was the chemotherapy dispensed by the pump and permanent central line. All along when Dr Fisher was referring to chemotherapy, Mr Kochi was thinking about the pump. He remained unaware that there were many different options for receiving chemotherapy.
>
> As it turned out, Mr Kochi's reluctance to undergo chemotherapy was based more in misunderstanding than religious objections. Muslim religious doctrines dictated that Mr Kochi be clean and pure before prayer. Normally, this includes the performance of ritualistic ablutions, but also includes a prescription against bleeding or having anything injected while praying. Mr Kochi could easily have received chemotherapy via an intravenous line at the hospital in, between times of prayer. Indeed, once the misunderstanding had been resolved, Mr Kochi did receive chemotherapy in this manner.
>
> Unfortunately, the chemotherapy was ineffective because the cancer had been left untreated for almost a year. Shortly thereafter, Mr Kochi succumbed to the disease at his home surrounded by his grieving family.
>
> Synopsis of the film *Hold Your Breath*, Directed by Maren Grainger-Monsen. For more details please visit Fanlight Productions at **www.fanlight.com**

Other interventions

Healthcare navigators may help to overcome the patient's lack of familiarity with the healthcare system and educate their lack of perception of risk or awareness. An agreed-upon management plan may facilitate the communication process and provide benefit to both the physician and the patient (22). This type of engagement is based on communication skills that can be taught. Patients' communication with their physicians can be improved by introducing some rudimentary training to increase participation in medical encounters (62). Communication interventions using printed material to prompt patients to write down questions before a visit (63) or using patient education video-tapes to role-model active behaviours (64), have been shown to increase patients' participation in medical consultations. Patients can also be encouraged to bring a companion to important consultations, such as the discussion of potential cancer diagnosis and treatment (36).

Likewise, training medical students and healthcare professionals on ethnic differences may improve communication (61, 65). Effective communication benefits not only the emotional health of the patient, but also leads to greater symptom relief, functional and physiologic status, and pain control (22). In order to create effective communication, it has been suggested that physicians ask a wide range of questions, not only about the physical aspects of the patient's problem, but also about the patient's feelings and concerns, understanding of the problem, expectations of therapy, and perceptions of how the problem affects function. Stewart (22) recommended that patients:

- Need to feel that they are active participants in care and that their problem has been discussed fully.
- Should share in decision-making when a plan for management is formulated.
- Should be encouraged to ask questions and given clear verbal information supplemented by emotional support and written informational packages.

The need for the physician to attend to the patient's expectations, feelings and ideas, as well as to provide clear information during discussion of the management plan, has been well-established (66–68). Authors have described attending to patient feelings as exploring the 'illness experience' during history-taking (69) and providing clear information as 'finding common ground' (70) (see Box 32.3).

Box 32.3 Communication tips for healthcare providers (71)

Non-verbal communication

While there are many non-verbal signals that may seem familiar, it is important to remain mindful that these signals may not always mean the same thing to all people. Clarifying these non-verbal signals will reduce misunderstandings caused by cultural differences in their use.

Facial expressions

Many facial expressions are universally recognizable including: anger, disgust, fear, happiness, sadness, and surprise. However, individuals from similar cultural backgrounds are better at interpreting facial expressions of their peers. This may be due to cultural norms in expressivity and intensity of expression (15).

Eye contact

In many cultures, eye contact indicates respect, while in others mainataining eye contact with an authority figure is seen as a sign of disrespect. Females in many cultures may also keep their eyes downcast as a sign of respect to a healthcare provider. Remaining aware that there are cultural differences in the acceptability of eye contact will forestall any misunderstandings.

Gestures

In many Latin American cultures, head-nodding is a sign of respect; however, this can easily be misinterpreted as an assentive behaviour. In India, it would be usual to specifically seek a 'yes' or 'no' at the end of an explanation and perhaps have the patient reiterate the conversation in their own words.

Box 32.3 (continued) Communication tips for healthcare providers (71)

Personal space

The personal space that a person requires around them is very much culturally influenced. Sitting close and leaning forward is expected by Hispanic patients. Patients in the Indian subcontinent and the Middle East would judge a doctor poorly if he/she did not come close or pat their shoulder. Other cultures perceive touching by a healthcare provider as an invasion of personal space—providers should take their cues from patient behaviour and knowledge of the patient's cultural background.

Verbal communication

Various cultures may use intonation, cadence and volume differently to enhance the meaning of the spoken word. For example, individuals from the Middle East may speak loudly to demonstrate the importance of the content matter and this should not be interpreted as anger.

Forms of address

In several different cultures it is considered disrespectful for an individual's given name to be used by casual acquaintances. Addressing patients from these cultures as Mrs or Mr may convey more respect than using first names. Addressing caregivers will vary from first name interaction in the West, to formal titles such as 'Doctor' with the last name or just 'Sir' and 'Nurse' or 'Sister' or 'Madam' in places like India.

Gender influences

Having a doctor of the opposite sex can be problematic for some patients, especially if the concern involves sensitive issues. Conversely, some cultures respect only males as physicians and would not be comfortable with a female doctor. Patient preferences for, and comfort with, doctor gender should be addressed at the outset.

Religious influences

In some cultures illness is thought to be a natural phenomenon—phrases like 'its in God's hands, let His will be done' can be common (see Box 32.2 as an example). However, it should not be assumed that the individual may not seek medical care. In some cultures, treating illness without considering the spiritual side amounts to incomplete care.

Redefining the problem

Most researchers agree that the biggest stumbling block in ethnicity or minority population research is categorizing the population. There is a lot of variance in the 15–20% that comes under the 'other' ethnic category. This results because individuals have emigrated from very different and divergent nations (see Box 32.4).

When cancer patients are in their native cultural environments, they ask more or less similar questions regarding the logistics involved with a diagnosis and treatment of a cancer. They also voice very similar concerns in regards to family, employment, and outcomes. In addition to

> ### Box 32.4 Race vs. Ethnicity
>
> #### Race
>
> Historically, the term 'race' has been used to define a group of people classified together on the basis of common physical characteristics (e.g. skin colour, height, facial features, etc.). However, this term has been discredited because it denotes superficial biological differences that have been used to imply socially constructed similarities.
>
> #### Ethnicity
>
> Ethnicity implies a shared cultural identity reflected in values, beliefs, and traditions. Identifying with a particular ethnicity usually implies a common cultural heritage, religion, language, place of birth, or ancestry.

difficulties with communication due to language barriers, there are other problems and challenges faced in communication with immigrant populations. The host country's healthcare system is typically designed and maintained to meet the needs of the host country population—the visible majority. Visible minorities are generally expected to use one of two methods to navigate the system:

(1) rely on external sources, such as navigation systems or coordinators instituted by health administrations, or

(2) rely on internal resources by adapting or acculturating one's self to the system and attempting to navigate the system for themselves.

Not speaking English as a primary language often signals a distinct set of patient attitudes, experiences and beliefs that could be critical in understanding what informs and influences cancer care behavior (72, 73). For the healthcare provider, the stimulus of a racially discordant interaction may also trigger a distinct set of attitudes, experiences, and meanings assumed from the patient's apparent ethnicity/race.

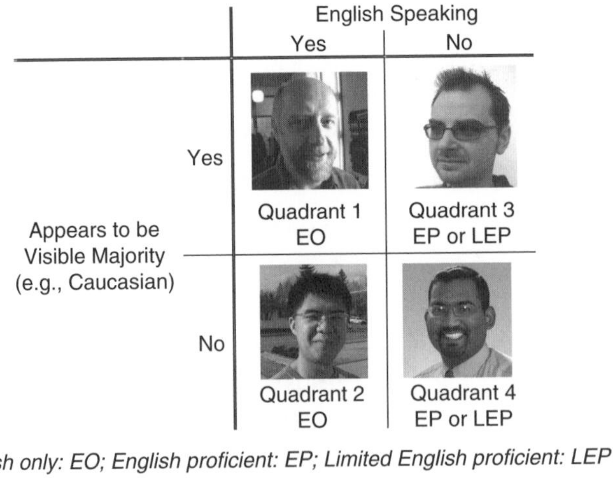

English only: EO; English proficient: EP; Limited English proficient: LEP

Fig. 32.1 The multicultural patient population.

The two most tangible and easily assessable potential 'markers' of patients' access to the healthcare system are proficiency in the host language and physical resemblance to host population. Figure 32.1 is a hypothesized representation of the population served in a multi-cultural nation (74).

There are two points of interest in Fig. 32.1. Just because someone looks more similar to a non-host ethnicity/race (quadrant 2) does not preclude them from considering themselves to be part of the host population (e.g. a person with an Asian background defining/categorizing themselves as Canadian or Australian, despite the obvious non-Canadian or non-Australian features). Also, individuals in quadrant 3 may look the part in regards to physical features compatible with the host population; however, they may consider themselves of a different race/ethnicity (e.g. a cancer patient originally from Italy who speaks fluent English may consider themselves Italian first and Canadian second). Potential patient-related outcomes for the four quadrants may be as follows.

Quadrant 1—English-speaking and appears to be visible majority: optimal access, navigation, and physical and emotional health status

As representatives of the host population, patients in this quadrant are expected to posssess the requisite understanding of access and navigation of the healthcare system. Researchers generally utilize this population as the baseline comparison in studying health status and outcomes.

Quadrant 2—English-speaking and visible minority: optimal access, navigation and physical health status, but sub-optimal emotional health status

Patients in this quadrant would also consider themselves as members of the host population; however, their physical features may cause the health system to view them as a visible minority. Clinical experience has shown that these patients are often asked inappropriate questions (e.g. How long have you been in Canada? Do you require a translation services). This marginalization by the healthcare system may lead to increased emotional distress.

Quadrant 3—non-English speaking and appears visible majority: sub-optimal access, navigation, and physical and emotional health status

While language issues would be of concern for navigation of the healthcare system, these first-generation immigrants would have lesser concerns of marginalization or exclusion in the host system due to their physical apperance.

Quadrant 4—non-English speaking and visible minority: sub-optimal access, navigation, and physical and emotional health status

Patients in this quadrant would generally be first-generation immigrants from predominantly non-English speaking countries. A subset of them may be English-Proficient, yet their physical appearance, perhaps combined with an accent, would likely result in a high degree of marginalization. Difficulties in navigating in a new healthcare system would be compounded by this marginalization and possible language barriers. Significant psychological concerns may result fron this stereotyping and marginalization.

Conclusions

People from ethnically diverse backgrounds with cancer are at risk for poor outcomes when they are immigrants to a new country. This disparity takes many forms and can impact both access to care and use of available treatment services, ultimately resulting in poorer physical and psychological outcomes. Communication difficulties between patients and healthcare providers may be a significant cause of these less-than-optimal outcomes for people new to the system. Both language and cultural barriers can contribute to this problem. Some solutions to overcome language differences are to have trained translators present, and follow several simple rules to facilitate accurate translation. Healthcare providers can also improve communication through awareness of different cultural styles of communication, including expectations and cultural effects on non-verbal communication. Different styles of decision-making across cultures also need to be taken into account by healthcare providers. Optimally, healthcare providers need to acknowledge and examine their beliefs, stereotypes and prejudices around different cultures, and question how these affect their behaviour with patients. Developing sensitivity to the impact of patient appearance and language ability on how patients are treated is essential. Research efforts in these areas need to determine the critical characteristics that influence how patients are treated in medical settings, ultimately leading to the development of further changes to the overall healthcare system that will optimize patient care for the diverse range of people who require care. In the meantime, openness on the part of healthcare providers and willingness to examine our own prejudices and assumptions are keys to ultimately improving the cancer care provided to all patients, regardless of their appearance, background, or ability to communicate.

References

1. US Census Bureau. *US interim projections by age, sex, race, and Hispanic origin.* 2004. Available at: **http://www.census.gov/ipc/www/usinterimproj/**. Accessed 28 November 2007.

2. Statistics Canada. *Immigration from 1851 to 2001.* 2005. Available at: **http://www40.statcan.ca/101/cst01/demo03.htm?sdi=immigration**. Accessed 27 November 2007.

3. Statistics Canada. *Immigration in Canada: a portrait of the foreign-born population, 2006 census.* 2007: 97–557-XIE.

4. Jain RV, Mills PK, Parikh-Patel A. Cancer incidence in the south Asian population of California, 1988–2000. *J Carcinog* 2005; **4**: 21.

5. Luo W, Birkett NJ, Ugnat AM, *et al.* Cancer incidence patterns among Chinese immigrant populations in Alberta. *J Immigr Health* 2004; **6**(1): 41–48.

6. Singh GK, Hiatt RA. Trends and disparities in socioeconomic and behavioural characteristics, life expectancy, and cause-specific mortality of native-born and foreign-born populations in the United States, 1979–2003. *Int J Epidemiol* 2006; **35**(4): 903–919.

7. Quan H, Fong A, De Coster C, *et al.* Variation in health services utilization among ethnic populations. *CMAJ* 2006; **174**(6): 787–791.

8. Williams DR Race, socioeconomic status, and health. The added effects of racism and discrimination. *Ann NY Acad.Sci* 1999; **896**: 173–188.

9. Smedley BD, Stith AY, Nelson AR. *Unequal treatment: confronting racial and ethnic disparities in health care.* Washington DC: The National Academies Press; 2002.

10. Lannin DR, Mathews HF, Mitchell J, *et al.* Influence of socioeconomic and cultural factors on racial differences in late-stage presentation of breast cancer. *JAMA* 1998; **279**(22): 1801–1807.

11. Pearlman DN, Rakowski W, Ehrich B, *et al.* Breast cancer screening practices among black, Hispanic, and white women: reassessing differences. *Am J Prev Med* 1996; **12**(5): 327–337.

12. Williams DR. The concept of race in Health Services Research: 1966 to 1990. *Health Serv Res* 1994; **29**(3): 261–274.

13. Pandey M, Sebastian P, Ahamed IM, *et al.* A case-control study into the quality of life of women with breast cancer. *Cancer Strat* 2000; **2**: 61–68.

14. Thomas BC, Pandey M, Ramdas K, *et al.* FACT-G: reliability and validity of the Malayalam translation. *Qual Life Res* 2004; **13**(1): 263–269.

15. Pandey M, Thomas BC, Ramdas K, *et al.* Quality of life in breast cancer patients: validation of a FACT-B Malayalam version. *Qual Life Res* 2002; **11**(2): 87–90.

16. Alagaratnam TT, Kung NY. Psychosocial effects of mastectomy: is it due to mastectomy or to the diagnosis of malignancy? *Br J Psychiatry* 1986; **149**: 296–299.

17. Bando M. Experiences of breast reconstruction following mastectomy in cases of cancer and evaluation of psychological aspects of the patients. *Gan To Kagaku Ryoho* 1990; **17**(4 Pt 2): 804–810.

18. Meyerowitz BE, Richardson J, Hudson S, *et al.* Ethnicity and cancer outcomes: behavioral and psychosocial considerations. *Psychol Bull* 1998; **123**(1): 47–70.

19. Collins KS, Hall A, Neujaus C. *US minority health: a chartbook.* 1999.

20. The Henry J. Kaiser Family Foundation. *Health Insurance Coverage in America—1999 data update;* 2000.

21. Thomas BC, Groff S, Tsang K, Carlson LE. *Patient ethnicity: a key predictor of cancer care satisfaction.* Ethn Health, Mar 2006 [E pubahead of print].

22. Stewart MA. Effective physician–patient communication and health outcomes: a review. *CMAJ* 1995; **152**(9): 1423–1433.

23. Davenport S, Goldberg D, Millar T. How psychiatric disorders are missed during medical consultations. *Lancet* 1987; **2**(8556): 439–441.

24. Frankel R, Beckman H. Evaluating the patient's primary problem(s). In: Stewart M, Roter D, eds. *Communicating with medical patients.* Newbury Park, California: Sage Publications; 1989, pp.86–98.

25. Stewart MA, McWhinney IR, Buck CW. The doctor/patient relationship and its effect upon outcome. *J R Coll Gen Pract* 1979; **29**(199): 77–81.

26. Starfield B, Wray C, Hess K, *et al.* The influence of patient-practitioner agreement on outcome of care. *Am J Public Health* 1981; **71**(2): 127–131.

27. Street RL. Communicative styles and adaptations in physician-parent consultations. *Soc Sci Med* 1992; **34**(10): 1155–1163.

28. Thiederman S. *Profiting in America's multi-cultural marketplace: how to do buisness across cultural lines.* NY: Lexington Books; 1991.

29. Waitzkin H. Information giving in medical care. *J Health Soc Behav* 1985; **26**(2): 81–101.

30. Hall JA, Roter DL, Katz NR. Meta-analysis of correlates of provider behavior in medical encounters. *Med Care* 1988; **26**(7): 657–675.

31. Bultman DC, Svarstad BL. Effects of physician communication style on client medication beliefs and adherence with antidepressant treatment. *Patient Educ Couns* 2000; **40**(2): 173–185.

32. Henbest RJ, Stewart M. Patient-centredness in the consultation. 2: Does it really make a difference? *Fam Pract* 1990; **7**(1): 28–33.

33. Young M, Klingle RS. Silent partners in medical care: a cross-cultural study of patient participation. *Health Commun* 1996; **8**(1): 29–53.

34. Rost K, Carter W, Inui T. Introduction of information during the initial medical visit: consequences for patient follow-through with physician recommendations for medication. *Soc Sci Med* 1989; **28**(4): 315–321.

35. Johnson RL, Roter D, Powe NR, *et al.* Patient race/ethnicity and quality of patient-physician communication during medical visits. *Am J Public Health* 2004; **94**(12): 2084–2090.

36. Gordon HS, Street RL,Jr, Sharf BF, *et al.* Racial differences in doctors' information-giving and patients' participation. *Cancer* 2006; **107**(6): 1313–1320.

37. Woloshin S, Schwartz LM, Katz SJ, *et al.* Is language a barrier to the use of preventive services? *J Gen Intern Med* 1997; **12**(8): 472–477.

38. Jacobs EA, Karavolos K, Rathouz PJ, *et al.* Limited English proficiency and breast and cervical cancer screening in a multiethnic population. *Am J Public Health* 2005; **95**(8): 1410–1416.

39. Ngo-Metzger Q, Massagli MP, Clarridge BR, *et al.* Linguistic and cultural barriers to care. *J Gen Intern Med* 2003; **18**(1): 44–52.

40. Seid M, Stevens GD, Varni JW. Parents' perceptions of pediatric primary care quality: effects of race/ethnicity, language, and access. *Health Serv Res* 2003; **38**(4): 1009–1031.

41. Weech-Maldonado R, Morales LS, Elliott M, *et al.* Race/ethnicity, language, and patients' assessments of care in Medicaid managed care. *Health Serv Res* 2003; **38**(3): 789–808.

42. Carrasquillo O, Orav EJ, Brennan TA, *et al.* Impact of language barriers on patient satisfaction in an emergency department. *J Gen Intern Med* 1999; **14**(2): 82–87.

43. Ponce NA, Hays RD, Cunningham WE. Linguistic disparities in health care access and health status among older adults. *J Gen Intern Med* 2006; **21**(7): 786–791.

44. Lara M, Gamboa C, Kahramanian MI, *et al.* Acculturation and Latino health in the United States: a review of the literature and its sociopolitical context. *Annu Rev Public Health* 2005; **26**: 367–397.

45. Berry JW, Kim U, Minde T, *et al.* Comparative studies of acculturative stress. *Intern Migr Rev* 1987; **21**: 491–511.

46. Chen H, Guarnaccia PJ, Chung H. Self-attention as a mediator of cultural influences on depression. *Int J Soc Psychiatry* 2003; **49**(3): 192–203.

47. Uppaluri CR, Schumm LP, Lauderdale DS. Self-reports of stress in Asian immigrants: effects of ethnicity and acculturation. *Ethn Dis* 2001; **11**(1): 107–114.

48. Burr JA, Mutchler JE. English language skills, ethnic concentration, and household composition: older Mexican immigrants. *J Gerontol B Psychol Sci Soc Sci* 2003; **58**(2): S83–92.

49. Vega WA, Kolody B, Aguilar-Gaxiola S, *et al.* Lifetime prevalence of DSM-III-R psychiatric disorders among urban and rural Mexican Americans in California. *Arch Gen Psychiatry* 1998; **55**(9): 771–778.

50. Takeuchi DT, Chung RC, Lin KM, *et al.* Lifetime and twelve-month prevalence rates of major depressive episodes and dysthymia among Chinese Americans in Los Angeles. *Am J Psychiatry* 1998; **155**(10): 1407–1414.

51. Yeung A, Chan R, Mischoulon D, *et al.* Prevalence of major depressive disorder among Chinese-Americans in primary care. *Gen Hosp Psychiatry* 2004; **26**(1): 24–30.

52. Fernandez-Esquer ME, Espinoza P, Ramirez AG, *et al.* Repeated Pap smear screening among Mexican-American women. *Health Educ Res* 2003; **18**(4): 477–487.

53. Peek ME, Han JH. Disparities in screening mammography. Current status, interventions and implications. *J Gen Intern Med* 2004; **19**(2): 184–194.

54. Karliner LS, Perez-Stable EJ, Gildengorin G. The language divide. The importance of training in the use of interpreters for outpatient practice. *J Gen Intern Med* 2004; **19**(2): 175–183.

55. Brach C, Fraser I, Paez K. Crossing the language chasm. *Health Aff* (Millwood) 2005; **24**(2): 424–434.

56. Jacobs EA, Shepard DS, Suaya JA, *et al.* Overcoming language barriers in health care: costs and benefits of interpreter services. *Am J Public Health* 2004; **94**(5): 866–869.

57. Zabar S, Hanley K, Kachur E, *et al.* 'Oh! She doesn't speak English!' Assessing resident competence in managing linguistic and cultural barriers. *J Gen Intern Med* 2006; **21**(5): 510–513.

58. Marcos LR. Effects of interpreters on the evaluation of psychopathology in non-English-speaking patients. *Am J Psychiatry* 1979; **136**(2): 171–174.

59. Putsch RW,3rd. Cross-cultural communication. The special case of interpreters in health care. *JAMA* 1985; **254**(23): 3344–3348.

60. Baker DW, Hayes R, Fortier JP. Interpreter use and satisfaction with interpersonal aspects of care for Spanish-speaking patients. *Med Care* 1998; **36**(10): 1461–1470.

61. Carrillo JE, Green AR, Betancourt JR. Cross-cultural primary care: a patient-based approach. *Ann Intern Med* 1999; **130**(10): 829–834.

62. Greenfield S, Kaplan S, Ware JE,Jr. Expanding patient involvement in care. Effects on patient outcomes. *Ann Intern Med* 1985; **102**(4): 520–528.

63. Cegala DJ, McClure L, Marinelli TM, *et al.* The effects of communication skills training on patients' participation during medical interviews. *Patient Educ Couns* 2000; **41**(2): 209–222.

64. Anderson LA, DeVellis BM, DeVellis RF. Effects of modeling on patient communication, satisfaction, and knowledge. *Med Care* 1987; **25**(11): 1044–1056.

65. Culhane-Pera KA, Reif C, Egli E, *et al.* A curriculum for multi-cultural education in family medicine. *Fam Med* 1997; **29**(10): 719–723.

66. Pendleton D. *The consultation: an approach to learning and teaching.* Oxford, Oxfordshire; New York: Oxford University Press; 1984.

67. Levenstein JH, McCracken EC, McWhinney IR, *et al.* The patient-centred clinical method. 1. A model for the doctor-patient interaction in family medicine. *Fam Pract* 1986; **3**(1): 24–30.

68. Riccardi VM, Kurtz SM. *Communication and counseling in health care.* Springfield, Ill.: C.C. Thomas; 1983.

69. Weston WW, Brown JB, Stewart MA. Patient-centered interviewing. Part 1: Understanding patients' experiences. *Can Fam Physician* 1989; **35**: 147–151.

70. Brown JB, Weston WW, Stewart M. Patient-centered interviewing. Part II: Finding common ground. *Can Fam Physician* 1989; **35**: 151–158.

71. MacLeod-Glover N. *Communication in a multi-cultural society.* Communications Centre,CE; 2006.

72. Lee T. *Language-of-Interview effects and Latino mass opinion.* 2001; RWP01–041: 1–31.

73. Ponce NA, Chawla N, Babey SH, *et al.* Is there a language divide in pap test use? *Med Care* 2006; **44**(11): 998–1004.

74. Thomas BC, Carlson LE, Bultz BD. *Cancer patient ethnicity and associations with emotional distress–the 6th vital sign: A new look at defining patient ethnicity in a multicultural context.* J. Immigr, Minor, Health 2008 Seps. [E pub ahead of print].

Chapter 33

Intercultural communication in palliative care

James Hallenbeck and Vyjeyanthi S Periyakoil

Since technology deprives me of the intimacy of my illness,
makes it not mine but something that belongs to science, I wish
my doctor could somehow restore it to me and make it personal
again. Just as he orders blood tests and bone scans of my body,
I'd like my doctor to scan me, to grope for my spirit as well as
my prostate. While he inevitably feels superior to me because he
is the doctor and I am the patient, I'd like him to know that I
feel superior to him too, that he is my patient also and I have my
diagnosis of him. There should be a place where our respective
superiorities could meet and frolic together.
Anatole Broyard in Doctor, talk to me

Introduction

Communication occurs in cultural contexts, which are in turn determined by a host of variables—
ethnicity, religion, geographic origin, gender, sexual orientation, social role, and age, among others.
Anthropologist Edward Hall noted that social interactions and associated communication can be
broadly classified as being relatively high or low in their cultural context (1–5).

◆ Low-context communication is task-oriented, emphasizing straightforward, unambiguous
   spoken or written communication. Asking and receiving street directions is an example of
   low-context communication.

◆ High-context communication embeds large amounts of meaning within the actual situation
   (or context). within which communication is occurring and tends to compress meanings in
   spoken, written, and non-verbal communication. In high-context situations, where people are
   communicating (public or private, formal or informal space). who is present and how they
   position themselves relative to one anotherr, are all parts of the episode of communication.
   High-context communication is relational. That is, establishment or clarification of relationships is itself a goal of communication, beyond any more concrete tasks to be accomplished.

Serious illness and dying are experienced as a complex web of low- and high-context interactions
(6, 7). Current medical training tends to focus almost exclusively on low-context aspects of communication. This chapter will provide an introduction to high-context communication,

as it applies to palliative care, and will discuss educational strategies for improving related communication skills.

Relevance of high-context communication to palliative care

As a broad generalization, Northern European and related cultures tend to use lower contextual styles of communication. Asian, Southern European, Arab, African—indeed most other cultures, tend to use higher contextual styles (8). However, in all cultures certain types of interactions are intrinsically high context, such as situations in which some degree of dependence exists among people. High-context situations tend to blur private and public aspects of people's lives and to entail both risk, if the relationship goes badly, and reward, if it goes well. Courtship behaviour, such as dating, and gang activity are non-medical examples of high-context interactions. While no validated scales exists in judging how high in context particular activities are, situations involving serious illness and dying exhibit all the features typical of high-context interactions. Very sick people are highly dependent upon others for a variety of needs. Sickness is both a very private and a public experience, requiring collaboration among patients, families, and clinicians and entailing potentially great risk and reward.

The culture of biomedicine

Biomedicine, the particular medical system evolving out of Northern Europe over the last few hundred years, often called, simply 'modern medicine', is a culture unto itself (9–12). This culture has been adapted by the myriad countries within which biomedicine is practiced, but a certain cultural identity is retained. As a cultural system, biomedicine is low context and extremely task-oriented. Anthropologists have noted that biomedicine is reductionist in its approach to sickness and healing; espousing a belief system that focuses on progressively microscopic aspects of the human body (10). The belief and hope is that by fixing on more elemental problems, the sick body can be 're-built' into a healthy one from the ground up (11, 13).

Psychiatrist and anthropologist, Arthur Kleinman, has noted that the culture of biomedicine differs in certain ways from other cultures of medicine (9). Such differences are of relevance to palliative care. He notes that suffering is not a primary concern of biomedical practice. The dominant belief is that suffering will disappear if a healthy body is properly reconstructed and thus the primary goal of medicine should be bodily cure (14). Of course, such a belief system becomes extremely problematic when cure is not possible, as is usually the case for patients receiving palliative care. In contrast, most other world medical systems stress the concept of a balancing of life forces, as in the Chinese concept of *yin* and *yang* (15). The goal of medical care in most other systems is not the attainment of some idealized state of bodily perfection, but of optimized balance, regardless of the overall state of health. Finally, Kleinman notes that biomedicine is unusual in its emphasis on illness occurring in individual bodies. Other systems tend to view illness as arising from complex interactions of forces, natural and human, that result in imbalance. Medical systems that philosophically recognize the primacy of suffering, the importance of balance, and the inter-relatedness of physical, psychological, social, and spiritual dimensions of illness, would seem much closer to tenets of palliative care as originally espoused by hospice founder, Cicely Saunders, in her writings on 'total pain' (16, 17).

In keeping with its overtly low-context cultural framing, communication in biomedicine tends to stress efficiency, clarity, and task completion. For certain problems this works quite well. However, in high-context situations, as commonly occur in the practice of palliative care, such a low-context approach often fails, just as overly direct communication styles tend to fail in other high-context situations, such as dating. Neglect of relational aspects of communication often results in miscommunication. Worse, offence may be taken, hindering future relationship-building and subsequent problem-solving. By analogy, in low-context communication the shortest distance between two points (quickest route to goal completion) is a straight line. However, in high-context situations an alternate 'physics' is a work; the shortest distance between two points is usually a curve. That is, an excessively direct approach to problem-solving in the name of efficiency often backfires, paradoxically resulting in it taking longer to reach one's goal (18). If offence is taken, it will take even more time to undo the damage, repair the relationship, and proceed to problem resolution. While investment in relationship-building (the curve) may be viewed as a 'waste of time' in terms of low-context values, in high-context situations such an investment may result in more rapid and successful problem resolution and goal attainment.

Communication training in palliative care and high-context content

In palliative care, most communication training, as elsewhere in medicine, is task-oriented. Common examples include training in how to deliver bad news or address goals of care. Such training often includes an outline of suggested steps. Delivery of bad news offers perhaps the clearest example—preparation, setting, advanced alert, delivery, of news, pause and so on (19–21). The advantages of such an approach are clarity in educational presentation and ease of recall for the learner. However, some risk is also entailed. A complex, intrinsically high-context interaction, as we would argue this is, may be reduced to a low-context task. Good curricula and texts on communication in palliative care clearly recognize this risk (22–24). While reference is not generally made explicitly to intercultural communication theory, attention to certain contextual concerns, such as setting, non-verbal communication, relationships, and demonstration of respect, among others, are consistent with such theory. Below, we will outline in more detail concepts and suggested exercises that may be of help in improving intercultural communication skills in palliative care. While discrete high-context training and exercises may be developed, we would suggest that more overt incorporation of related skills into more traditional communication training might enhance their educational effectiveness as well.

Most cross-cultural healthcare education in general and in palliative care has revolved around issues of ethnicity (25–27). Conversely, most communication training in palliative care has not stressed cross-cultural issues. While intercultural communication training is relatively new in healthcare, such is not the case elsewhere. An extensive literature exists on both the theory and practice of such training (28–34). The discussion that follows can be understood as an extrapolation from this literature, adapted to the world of palliative care.

Relational communication skill development

Core concepts: in high-context situations, work on the nature of participants' relationships is often central to the episode of communication. Effective use of intercultural communication skills facilitates this task. Such work may include:

♦ Establishing new, positive relationships among participants.

♦ Fostering mutual respect and trust within relationships.

♦ Clarifying relationships, where uncertainty or ambiguity exists about respective roles exists.

♦ Addressing problems that may arise in the evolution of relationships such as:

  • Distrust.

- Conflicts regarding relative power.
- Role conflict.
- Cross-cultural miscommunication.

Palliative care practitioners usually first meet patients and families during times of great stress. Most lay people have not previously heard of palliative care. What they may have heard, positive or negative, may be quite inaccurate. While patients and families are usually hopeful, they may also be doubtful. Given the intensely personal nature of the crises commonly faced, patients and families may be concerned as to how well clinicians will honour and respect their ways. Will they understand and honour the often complex, unspoken rules in the family network regarding roles and customs? If so, then perhaps they can be of great assistance. If not, then involvement will only add to the burden. Such questions, we believe, are often the unspoken subtexts to initial palliative care encounters. Fostering of positive relationships is a key goal in working with patients and families.

Disagreements and damage repair

Sometimes the major problem to be addressed in a palliative care encounter is damage already done to relationships. When arguments break out, is the primary issue that participants really disagree on a care plan or could it be that the relationship has become so damaged that participants are unable to consider the positions of others? If the issue is a damaged relationship, what is the cause—disrespect or neglect, bad intent, or perhaps a misunderstanding? Somewhat different skills are required for successful repair, if possible, of such relationships (35).

Relationships can go awry in a number of ways. People may feel disrespected or neglected if they believe they have not been heard or their interests have not been taken seriously. As disagreements progress, participants may resort to progressively strong statements and behaviours intended to represent power and dominance over the other. More subtly, damage can result when participants' roles are threatened. Family roles, such as patriarch, maternal nurturer, caregiver, decision-maker, may come under threat simply through the process of illness. For example, family roles may be thrown into conflict when a family patriarch is incapacitated by illness and others in the family are forced into roles contrary to their usual familial roles, a form of role conflict. A daughter might feel forced into a position of relative dominance by way of being a translator for a non-English speaking elder or forced to provide personal hygiene care for a father, which is perceived as being shameful by both father and daughter. Clinicians, similarly, may experience role conflict. When clinicians believe they are being forced to provide ill-advised medical care out of respect for patient/proxy autonomy, they may experience a conflict with their self-perceived role of medical expert and healer.

Damage can easily result from cross-cultural miscommunication. Such miscommunication can be as simple as a 'cultural miss'—one party not doing or saying something expected by the other. For example, in one study, Hispanic mothers of paediatric patients took some offence when non-Hispanic paediatricians moved too quickly (low-context approach) to the business at hand, without a proper compliment of the child by way of introduction—*Que linda*! [How beautiful, your child is] (36). A more serious error can result from a cultural *faux pas* (37). In a cultural *faux pas*, the meaning intended by one person is misinterpreted by another, when the cultural framing of the communication differs between the two. For example, a non-Hispanic individual might send marigolds to a Mexican with a 'get well' intent, unaware that these flowers are used during the Mexican Day of the Dead festival. A hint to such misunderstandings is when the recipient responds to the communicated message in a manner very different or opposite to that expected.

Ambiguity, compression of meaning, and subtexts

Ambiguity

While ambiguity tends to be scorned in low-context communication, ambiguity is often purposely used in high-context communication when discussing difficult or dangerous topics (38). Ambiguity, skillfully used, can enable participants to choose whether or not to pursue a particular topic or discuss it in greater depth. For example, a question such as, 'What do you make of your situation?' may be a good, 'open-ended' (albeit ambiguous) question. The patient's response, 'You mean about my dying?' or, 'Not great, but I always hope for the best', may give the clinician a good idea how explicitly he or she may discuss topics related to dying. However, ambiguous speech is prone to misunderstanding. Thus, a related skill is recognition of possible misunderstanding and needed clarification (39). For example, a patient might ask a clinician, 'Will you be there for me, when the time comes?'. This question might simply be asking for support or it might be an intentionally ambiguous request for assisted suicide. Clarification is necessary. Related communications skills that can be practiced include sharing common examples of skilled use of ambiguity in palliative care and highlighting examples of where clarification of ambiguity is indicated.

Compression of meaning

High-context verbal communication often 'compresses' meaning, much like a compression software program compresses computer files (39). Compressed communication, e.g. metaphor or jokes, is highly efficient in data transmission, but is prone to serious misunderstanding if the recipient does not share the implied meaning. Expressions like 'passed away' and 'kicked the bucket' are simple examples of nuanced meanings of dying (40). Non-native speakers of English may misunderstand such nuances, resulting in cross-cultural miscommunication. Related communication skills include, first, recognition of compressed meaning and then the skilled use of compressed meaning, such as metaphor, in enabling participants to discuss and explore complex and difficult topics (41–45). A superb example of such skill use is included in an article by Hutchings (46). In the presented case a dying patient introduces a metaphoric thread, which is picked up by the nurse. 'I thought now with my kids raised, I was out of the woods'. The nurse then skillfully continued the metaphor, 'Till this cloud on the horizon'. The cloud continues the metaphor, but is intentionally ambiguous. Will the cloud blow away or will the skies darken? 'Till this big, black cloud on the horizon', replied the patient. Through this metaphor the patient and the nurse discuss her dying without ever using the 'd' word.

Subtexts

High-context communication is usually heavily laden with subtexts—beliefs, affect, hopes, and fears that are usually not verbalized directly. Subtexts are discussed in more traditional communication training, often with an emphasis on identifying cognitive and affective components of communication (39, 47). Here, as an example, we will briefly discuss relative trust or mistrust as a subtext. Trust or lack thereof, is often suggested through non-verbal communication and implied, but less commonly stated (intentionally ambiguous) in verbal communication. The first skill in dealing with subtexts is recognition of their existence.[1] The clinician may then consciously determine whether to deal with the subtext as a subtext (e.g. by working to build trust) or to raise

---

[1] See Pedersen's discussion of triad models of counselling for analogous concepts. In triad cross-cultural counselling an individual familiar with the culture of the client/patient, verbalizes unstated 'subtexts', which the counsellor may not recognize, to assist in developing awareness of such subtexts (29).

the subtext to the 'text' of the conversation. No easy guidelines can be given as to which strategy is correct in particular situations, but flexibility and skill in 'raising the subtext' is a high-context communication skill. For example, if mistrust is suspected or present, the clinician may say something like, 'From what you are saying, it sounds like you may be distrustful. If possible, I would like to work toward building trust. Could you tell me more about your concerns?'. Raising subtexts is a form of naming or mirroring, as commonly taught in communication training in dealing with affect (48). A risk in raising subtexts is escalation in any conflict. Thus, positive and sympathetic framing with a clearly stated intent to resolve the problem is suggested.

Cultural awareness exercises

High-context aspects of communication normally function out of consciousness or at its periphery. Thus, bringing into consciousness high-context issues is the critical first step in skill improvement (29, pp.19–37, 31, pp.258–280). In terms of relations, one might start with a question, 'What relational issues are at work here?'.[2] Categorization of common relational issues may help flesh-out this answer, as outlined above in the section on relational skill development. For initial training in high-context skills, we encourage trainers to start with clear instructions to learners *not* to do anything different from their usual patterns, but just work to increase their awareness of underlying issues. Learners may first be asked to watch others (film, role plays, or real interaction observation) and be given the task of noting relational issues that arise along the lines discussed above. Learners may then be encouraged to observe themselves in episodes of communication, attending to relational issues as they arise, practicing a form of 'mindfulness'. Only later should learners be encouraged to change their behaviours.

Behavioural instruction and exercises

Non-verbal communication exercises: culturally-specific behaviours (primarily in terms of ethnicity) can first be reviewed to highlight different ways non-verbal communication can be used to communicate one's intended relationship to the other. Common gestures, such as smiling, looking at a person (or looking down), can serve as examples of non-verbal communication working to communicate very different things in different cultures (33, pp.124–145, 49). Given that the relational goal for the clinician is to establish, strengthen or repair damaged relationships, particular attention should be given to gestures that will be viewed as trust-enhancing and respect-building. Such instruction should be adapted to ethnic populations with whom the learner group frequently interacts. Cultural guides knowledgeable about such groups should be consulted in curriculum development.

Relationship enhancing verbal communication and related exercises

Perhaps the most basic verbal communication skill in relationship building is to increase the proportion of time spent listening relative to talking (47). The simplest exercise in this regard is

---

[2] Koester and Olebe have developed similar criteria for evaluating intercultural skills, called the BASICs (behavioral assessment scale for intercultural competence scale). While a detailed discussion of this scale is beyond the scope of this work, major dimensions of the scale include: display of respect, orientation to knowledge, empathy, interaction management, task-role behaviour, relational role behaviour, tolerance for ambiguity, and interaction posture (34).

to first practice awareness of the amount of time spent speaking relative to listening and then set a goal of increasing time spent listening by some degree (39). Another simple exercise is to practice avoiding interruptions and prolonging pauses following another speaking.

Certain types of speech are particularly useful for enhancing relationships. Positively framed role-related speech, is an example. Role-related speech addresses the social roles of participants—patients, families, and clinicians. Positive framing of such speech accentuates good aspects of individuals in their social roles. For example, in meeting a mother with a sick child, attention might be brought not only to the daughter (*Que linda*! how beautiful), but to the mother's role relative to the daughter, '*Que linda*! What a beautiful daughter you have'. The clinician might also praise the mother more directly, 'Your daughter is lucky to have such a fine mother, who takes such good care of her!'.

Role-obligation speech: when disagreements with patients or families arise, the clinician may wish to offer an opinion based on his or her understanding of perceived benefits and burdens, as typically taught (a low-context, rational approach). However, particularly where patients or families are advocating for a particular course of action via the ethical principle of role obligation (50) (a belief that the greatest good will occur if one is true to one's role, such as that of a father or wife), then a more appropriate response may be to incorporate clinician role-obligation speech into one's opinion. For example, the clinician might say, 'I respect that as a wife you feel a strong obligation to ask that we do all we can to keep your husband alive. As your husband's physician, I too feel a strong obligation to him. I must do all I can to ensure the best possible care. I am concerned that if we do [whatever], he will not likely have his life prolonged, but he may have a more difficult time. As his physician, this would be hard for me.' For another example, if asked not to disclose a terminal diagnosis to a patient (request for non-disclosure), the clinician may demonstrate respect that family members feel obligated to make such a request, while also asking that they respect that he or she has an obligation not to lie, if directly asked a question by the patient (51).

The patient as a person: respect and trust can also be engendered by asking questions about a person and their life outside those questions typically associated with one's clinical role. For example, in meeting a family of a patient with advanced dementia, the family may fear that clinicians will not appreciate what a special person their father is, given his or her debilitated state. For a physician to go beyond standard history and physical questions in talking with family members can be reassuring and engender trust. For example, the physician might say, 'I wish I had the opportunity to know your father before he became ill. I know he was not always like this. If he could speak, what do you think he would say was his greatest accomplishment in life?' or, 'I will never know your Dad the way that you do. But tell me, what would you like me to know about your father, as a person?'.

Following concept introduction and awareness exercises, relationship enhancing speech can be practiced first in role plays and later in clinical practice (52).

Personal disclosure

Patients and families encountered in palliative care often need to establish more personal relationships with clinicians beyond those arising from narrowly defined clinical roles (53).[3] Can the clinician as a person relate to the struggles of the patient and family? Is the clinician personally trustworthy? We see in this need a blurring of public and private selves typical to high-context

---

3   Indeed, it would not be a stretch to say that Dame Cicely Saunders inspiration for the hospice movement evolved out certain key relationships with patients in which professional and personal boundaries were blurred (54).

Table 33.1 Examples of personal disclosure-related speech

Patient	Clinician
I don't know how you do this work.	It can be difficult. Sometimes, it makes me very sad. But I find it personally rewarding.
What do you think happens after death?	That's a question I struggle with too. If you would like, I can share my thoughts, but I'd first like to hear what you think.

relationships (7). Personal disclosure is a teachable and learnable skill. Attention is first drawn to patient/family cues that personal disclosure might be welcomed. Cues may be indirect in their invitation for disclosure, 'I don't know how you people do this kind of work,' or more direct, 'If it were your father, what would you do?'. Before providing disclosure, the clinician should pause and reflect deeply regarding whom the disclosure is serving—the patient, family, or the clinician. A good check for the appropriateness of disclosure is that it must first and foremost serve the needs of the patient or family (54). Finally, disclosure, when provided, usually should emphasize the clinician's humanity outside the clinical role. Often, disclosure is used to establish some common ground in wrestling with difficult issues related to mortality or spirituality. Educational exercises related to disclosure may establish guidelines, as above, provide examples of situations and speech in which disclosure is useful, and discuss boundaries. Examples of disclosure-related speech are included in Table 33.1.

Summary

The above discussion serves as an introduction to the topic of intercultural communication in palliative care. Suggestions are made for developing educational exercises dealing with these topics. While the authors have personally tried the various suggested educational strategies, as is too often the case in the communication education literature, the evidence base behind these strategies is weak. To the best of our knowledge, well-evaluated or reviewed curricula in palliative care education along these lines do not exist. We would certainly welcome such evaluation.

References

1. Hall E. *The Hidden Dimension*. Garden City: Doubleday; 1966.
2. Hall E. *Beyond Culture*. Garden City: Anchor Press; 1976.
3. Hall E. *The Dance of Life*. NY: Anchor; 1983.
4. Hall E. *The Silent Language*. NY: Anchor; 1990.
5. Hall E. Context and meaning. In: Samovar L, Porter R, eds. *Intercultural Communication*, 8th edn. Belmont: Wadsworth; 1997, pp.45–54.
6. Hallenbeck J. Intercultural differences and communication at the end of life. *Primary Care: Clinics in Office Practice* 2001; 28(2): 401–413.
7. Hallenbeck J. High context illness and dying in a low context medical world. *Am J Hosp Palliat Care* 2006; **23**(2): 113–118.
8. Samovar L, Porter R, eds. *Intercultural Communication*, 8 edn. Belmont: Wadsworth; 1997.
9. Kleinman A. *Writing in the Margin: discourse between Anthropology and Medicine*. Berkeley: University of California Press; 1995.
10. Hahn R. *Sickness and Healing—An Anthropological Perspective*. New London: Yale University Press; 1995.

11. Fabrega H. *Evolution of Sickness and Healing*. Berkeley: University of California Press; 1997.

12. Starr P. *The Social Transformation of American Medicine*. NY: Basic Books; 1982.

13. Frank A. *The Wounded Storyteller—Body, Illness, and Ethics*. Chicago: University of Chicago Press; 1995.

14. Hallenbeck J. Cross-cultural issues in end-of-life care. In: Berger A, Shuster J, Von Roenn J, eds. *Palliative Care and Supportive Oncology*, 3rd edn. Phildelphia: Lippincott; 2007, pp.517–525.

15. Brady E, ed. *Healing Logics—Culture and Medicine in Modern Health Belief Systems*. Logan: Utah State University Press; 2001.

16. Saunders C, Baines M. *Living with Dying—The Management of Terminal Disease*. Oxford: Oxford University Press; 1983.

17. Clark D. 'Total pain', disciplinary power and the body in the work of Cicely Saunders, 1958–1967. *Soc Sci Med* 1999; **49**(6): 727–736.

18. Levinson W, Gorawara-Bhat R, Lamb J. A study of patient clues and physician responses in primary care and surgical settings. *JAMA* 2000; **284**(8): 1021–1027.

19. Buckman R. *How to Break Bad News*. Baltimore: Johns Hopkins University Press; 1992.

20. Ptacek JT, Eberhardt TL. Breaking bad news. A review of the literature [see comments]. *JAMA* 1996; **276**(6): 496–502.

21. Baile WF, Buckman R, Lenzi R, *et al*. SPIKES-A six-step protocol for delivering bad news: application to the patient with cancer. *Oncologist* 2000; **5**(4): 302–311.

22. von Gunten CF, Ferris FD, Emmanuel L. Ensuring competency in end-of-life care—communcation and relational skills. *JAMA* 2000; **284**(23): 3051–3057.

23. Quill TE. *Caring for Patients at the End of Life*. New York: Oxford University Press; 2001.

24. Back AL, Arnold RM, Baile WF, *et al*. Efficacy of communication skills training for giving bad news and discussing transitions to palliative care. *Arch Intern Med* 2007; **167**(5): 453–60.

25. Purnell L, Paulanka B. *Transcultural Health Care—a Culturally Competent Approach*. Philadelphia: FA Davis; 1998.

26. Lipson JG, Minarik PA, Dibble SL. *University of California San Francisco. School of Nursing. Culture & Nursing Care: a Pocket Guide*. San Francisco, CA: UCSF Nursing Press; 1996.

27. Braun K, Pietsch J, Blanchette P. *Cultural Issues in End-of-Life Decision Making*. Thousand Oaks: Sage; 2000.

28. Hoopes D, Ventura P, eds. *Intercultural Sourcebook—Cross-Cultural Training Methodologies*. Washington: Intercultural Press; 1979.

29. Pedersen P. *A Handbook for Developing Multicultural Awareness*. Alexandria: American Association for Counseling and Development; 1988.

30. Brislin R, Yoshida T. *Intercultural Communication Training: an Introduction*. Thousand Oaks: Sage; 1994.

31. Chen G, Starosta W. *Foundations of Intercultural Communication*. Boston: Allyn and Bacon; 1998.

32. Fowler S, Mumfort M, eds. *Intercultural Sourcebook: Cross-Cultural Training Methodologies*. Boston: Intercultural Press; 1999.

33. Martin J, Nakayama T. *Experiencing Intercultural Communication*. Mountain View: Mayfield; 2001.

34. Lustig M, Koester J. *Intercultural Competence—Interpersonal Communication Across Cultures*. Boston: Allyn and Bacon; 2003.

35. Chen G, Starosta W. Intercultural conflict management. In: *Foundations of Intercultural Communication*. Boston: Allyn and Bacon; 1998, pp.140–162.

36. Contro N, Larson J, Scofield S, *et al*. Family perspectives on the quality of pediatric palliative care. *Arch Pediatr Adolesc Med* 2002; **156**(1): 14–19.

37. Hallenbeck J, Goldstein MK, Mebane EW. Cultural considerations of death and dying in the United States. *Clin Geriatr Med* 1996; **12**(2): 393–406.

38. Rodning CB. Coping with ambiguity and uncertainty in patient-physician relationships: III. Negotiation. *J Med Humanit* 1992; **13**(4): 211–222.

39. Hallenbeck J, Stratos G, Katz S. Stanford End of Life (ELC). Curriculum, Module 3: *Communicating with patients and families*. Available at: **http://www.mywhatever.com/cifwriter/library/stanford/modules.html**; 2003.

40. Wen-Shu L. That's Greek to me: between a rock and a hard place in intercultural encounters. In: Samovar L, Porter R, eds. *Intercultural Communication*. Belmont: Wadsworth; 1997, pp.213–220.

41. Froggatt K. The place of metaphor and language in exploring nurses' emotional work. *J Adv Nurs* 1998; **28**(2): 332–338.

42. Mattingly C. *Healing Dramas and Clinical Plots—the Narrative Structure of Experience*. Cambridge: Cambridge University Press; 1998.

43. Kirmayer L. Broken narratives—clinical encounters and the poetics of illness experience. In: Mattingly C, Garro L, eds. *Narrative and the Cultural Construction of Ilness and Healing*. Berkeley: University of California Press; 2000, pp.153–180.

44. Reisfield GM, Wilson GR. Use of metaphor in the discourse on cancer. *J Clin Oncol* 2004; **22**(19): 4024–4027.

45. Rallison L, Limacher LH, Clinton M. Future echoes in pediatric palliative care: becoming sensitive to language. *J Palliat Care* 2006; **22**(2): 99–104.

46. Hutchings D. Communicating with metaphor: a dance with many veils. *The American Journal of Hospice & Palliative Care* 1998; **15**(5): 282–284.

47. Suchman AL, Markakis K, Beckman HB, *et al*. A model of empathic communication in the medical interview. *JAMA* 1997; **277**(8): 678–682.

48. Wagner PJ, Lentz L, Heslop SD. Teaching communication skills: a skills-based approach. *Acad Med* 2002; **77**(11): 1164.

49. Devito J, Hecht M, eds. *The Nonverbal Reader*. Prospect Heights: Waveland Press; 1990.

50. Hallenbeck J, Goldstein MK. Decisions at the end-of-life: cultural considerations beyond medical ethics. GENERATIONS/Care at the End-of-Life: Restoring a balance 1999 (Spring, 1999): 24–29.

51. Hallenbeck J, Arnold RM. A request for nondisclosure: don't tell mother. *Journal of Clinical Oncology* 2007; **26**(31): 5030–5034.

52. McCaffery J. The role play: a powerful but difficult training tool. In: Fowler S, Mumfort M, eds. *Intercultural Sourcebook: Cross-Cultural Training Methods*. Boston: Intercultural Press; 1995, pp.17–25.

53. Yedidia MJ. Transforming doctor–patient relationships to promote patient-centered care: lessons from palliative care. *J Pain Symptom Manage* 2007; **33**(1): 40–57.

54. Hallenbeck J. A dying patient, like me. *Am Fam Physician* 2000; **62**: 888–890.

Chapter 34

Communicating about infertility risks

Zeev Rosberger, Jeanne Carter, Marie Achille,
Barry D Bultz, and Peter Chan

Background and evidence from literature about communication strategies and skills

Infertility is a consequence of many cancer diagnoses and/or treatments for both male and female patients (1). This is particularly true for those who require cancer treatment comprised of high-dose chemotherapy (2, 3), combination chemotherapy (4, 5), radiation therapy to the pelvis (6, 7) and/or surgical removal of the reproductive organs as part of their cancer treatment (8).

While the issues of prognosis, survival and treatment regimen decisions initially generally assume prime importance, the communication of risk information regarding fertility is usually presented in the context of other potential cancer treatment side-effects. In this context, patients must assimilate much complex information having both immediate and potentially long-term consequences. Ideally, the potential for cancer treatment to negatively impact a patient's fertility should be addressed during the treatment planning process. However, current research suggests that the dialogue between physician and patient occurs neither uniformly nor routinely (9–12).

Recent research indicates that, while fertility issues may not be viewed as paramount at the time of diagnosis, they can become increasingly important over time in cancer survivorship (12, 13). Parenthood for many cancer patients is a fundamental goal of cancer survivorship. Studies documenting the attitudes of young cancer survivors have revealed that parenthood is viewed as a positive experience. Survivors have also expressed that their experience with cancer would make them better parents (14). Additionally, 60% of young cancer survivors reported they would attempt to achieve the role of being a parent as an important life goal, even if they were to die young (15).

The limited data available to provide guidance to physicians initiating this conversation contribute to this challenge. Additionally, the existing long-term studies have limitations due to altered standards of care with medical advancement over time, reducing the applicability of the findings to current treatment regimes (7). Low levels of accurate knowledge, comfort with communication, timing and other factors have been found to contribute to poor fertility-risk communication (15). Nevertheless, existing research provides a helpful framework in which to start discussions and to prepare patients and their loved ones for possible reproductive health consequences of treatment.

Male fertility

For young males with cancer who either have or have not yet considered fatherhood, potential risks of infertility due to surgery (e.g. orchiectomy), radiation (e.g. to the pelvis) or gonadotoxic chemotherapy regimens are clearly important considerations.

The most prevalent cancers in young men include testicular cancer, lymphoma (Hodgkin and non-Hodgkin) and leukaemia. While 5-year survival rates have improved significantly in recent years (95% for testicular and approximately 80% for the lymphomas; 16, 17) resulting in long-term survival, fertility presents as an important issue for these men. It has been fairly well-established that the systemic effects of the disease process prior to diagnosis may already compromise spermatogenesis significantly, resulting in subnormal semen parameters and hormonal profiles. Current treatment regimens for testicular cancer include surgical removal of the affected testis. For advanced and metastatic diseases, additional surgery (retroperineal lymph node dissection) may be necessary for diagnostic and therapeutic considerations. This procedure often results in additional sexual side-effects, including dry ejaculation (anejaculation) and erectile dysfunction. Adjuvant chemotherapy and radiation may affect sperm production and quality (e.g. motility, DNA integrity), further limiting future fertility (18). Current data suggest that these cancer therapies will result in impaired fertility in virtually all men, either temporarily (with recovery in up to two years) or perhaps permanently for 15–30% of men.

Reproductive options

Modern assisted reproduction techniques (ART), such as intra-cytoplasmic sperm injection (ICSI) in which only a single living sperm is required to inject directly into an oocyte to achieve fertilization, make it feasible for cancer survivors who have significant impairment in semen profile post-treatment to father genetic children. Even for cancer survivors who have no spermatozoa found in semen (azoospermia), micro-surgical retrieval of sperm within the testes is feasible in about half of these patients to have sperm usable for procreation (19). These techniques are highly technical and may not be widely available. Given the availability of these and other modern ART and cryopreservation technologies, sperm-banking prior to treatment in cancer patients is currently the most important fertility-preservation approach. Gonadal stem cell retrieval and testis tissue preservation are currently in experimental stages of research and have not yet demonstrated efficacy in fertility preservation.

Communication

Young men with cancer are interested in understanding their infertility risk and related management issues. Most are interested in fatherhood, whether they are in a significant relationship currently or not; do not remember being informed about their risk; and, of about 50% who were offered sperm banking, only half of those complied. Some patients, especially younger adolescents, may be embarrassed to discuss infertility and sperm-banking methods in the presence of their parents. In addition, survivors feel that their cancer experience will make them better parents and feel healthy enough to have the energy to be good parents (14, 15, 20).

Female fertility

For the female cancer patient undergoing treatment with obvious direct effect (i.e. surgery) to the reproductive organs, discussions about fertility issues may be more readily addressed, but still many remain surprised by unexpected premature menopause (11). One recent study demonstrates that childhood cancer survivors who experience spontaneous menstruation five years or greater after their cancer diagnosis, are at 13-fold increased risk of non-surgical premature menopause in comparison to siblings (7). Young breast cancer survivors also have been found to be at increased risk of premature menopause. Many factors have been shown to be associated with chemotherapy induced premature menopause including an individual's age at the time of treatment, the type of chemotherapy regime and the number of months since completion of treatment (4).

Loss of fertility as the result of their cancer treatment has been shown to cause persistent feelings of sadness and grief lasting more than a year post-treatment in female cancer survivors (21). Qualitative research suggests that fertility and menopause are important for young cancer survivors. Chemotherapy places women at risk of premature menopause and infertility. Oestrogen deprivation can cause other side-effects (i.e. hot flashes, sexual dysfunction) (9, 12). Premature menopause or loss of reproductive function has been shown to be associated with poorer emotional functioning and greater risk for sexual difficulties (22). Following stem cell transplant, concerns about fertility have been reported by some even ten years post-treatment, and especially among younger women and survivors without children (23). Wenzel and colleagues also evaluated the relationship between infertility and long-term quality of life in female cancer survivors and found reproductive concerns of great importance and centrally linked to psychosocial outcomes (24). Interestingly, even those individuals who undergo fertility preserving surgery have been noted to experience persistent distress and reproductive concerns over time post-operatively (25).

Reproductive options

As medical technology advances, childhood and young cancer patients diagnosed with, and treated for, cancer not only have an improved likelihood of survival, but also the availability of emerging assisted-reproductive techniques. In some cases, individuals may be eligible for conservative fertility-preserving surgical treatment, as is the case for specific types of early stage gynaecologic (8, 26) and testicular cancers. For other types of cancers, such as breast cancer, leukaemia and lymphoma, cryopreservation of gametes (ooycte or sperm) and/or embryos (27) can be a viable option for biological offspring, when concerns exist about premature menopause and sterility. However, upon completion of treatment, this option would require a functional uterus and no contra-indications to pregnancy, which can be a complex issue in individuals with hormone-receptive cancers. Otherwise, family building may require the assistance of another individual or third party.

Third-party parenting (i.e. the involvement of a third person beyond the parenting couple or single parent) in order to create a baby is possible in the case of individuals where treatment causes gonadal toxicity. Techniques can include egg (oocyte) donation, sperm donation, embryo donation, *in vitro* fertilization (IVF), with or without a gestational carrier (surrogacy), and/or adoption. When possible, preservation of the ovaries offers the possibility of a biological child through assisted reproduction with egg retrieval.

Many young cancer patients will be faced with treatment options that may require surgical removal of some or all reproductive organs. For these individuals, family-building options will require the assistance of another individual or third-party reproduction. Adoption is another alternative for family building in cancer survivorship. It should be noted that, for some individuals, this process presents both difficult and emotional challenges. Some survivors not only confront their loss of reproductive function, but question the possibility of a hostile legal environment towards being a parent and a cancer survivor. A recent study found that adoption agencies may be reluctant to consider cancer survivors as potential parents (28). Growing concern over the late health risks after cancer treatment may also present barriers to the adoption process (11, 28).

Communication issues

Despite the risk of cancer-related infertility, current research demonstrates a lack of communication on this topic. This is problematic for the young cancer survivor. Zebrack and colleagues (28) examined a cohort of young adult survivors of childhood cancer and found that nearly 60% reported uncertainty about their fertility status, and only half recalled a healthcare provider discussing potential reproductive problems associated with treatment (29). Many women report having unmet informational needs about reproductive health, either prior to, or during, treatment. In recent studies with young cancer survivors, women indicated that the information received on fertility and the sequelae of treatment (i.e. menopause, sexuality and mood) prior to treatment was either insufficient or unavailable (10, 29). For example, in a study with young female breast cancer survivors, 72% noted a discussion occurred about the topic of fertility with their doctor, with only 51% reporting satisfaction that their concerns were adequately addressed (10). Of note, this study was conducted with a sample of women from a high SES. In comparison, Duffy *et al.* (9) surveyed a diverse sample of 170 newly diagnosed breast cancer patients under the age of 45 years, about fertility counselling. Within this sample, only 34% reported a discussion with a doctor about fertility, but 68% recalled a discussion about possible premature menopause (9).

These findings suggest that communication regarding reproductive concerns is not universally performed and that a physician's comfort level may vary by the topic of treatment sequelae. Some medical professionals may feel more completely trained to discuss menopause versus issues of reproductive health, which includes sexual function. In a recent qualitative study exploring cancer survivors and their health professionals' communication about changes to their body secondary to cancer treatment, two major themes were noted. Cancer survivors had concerns about the idea of not having their informational needs being met, as well as noting mismatched expectations on the part of patient and physician. Cancer survivors indicated that they would want negotiated time to discuss with their health professional the topic of intimate and sexual changes as a consequence of treatment (30). Delivery of adequate information to prepare patients for treatment has been noted to reduce anxiety/distress, to improve coping with treatment and to enhance quality of life (31). The theme of mismatched expectations between patients and physicians reveals that healthcare professionals may not discuss issues of reproduction health based on stereotypical assumptions of age, gender, cancer diagnosis, culture and/or partner status (30). Corney and colleagues (32) found that women experiencing infertility following treatment for gynecological malignancies felt deprived of choice, and that medical professionals tended to minimize the sense of loss experienced by older women (32). Additionally, lack of time or privacy in which to broach these sensitive issues, and/or discomfort with the topic, can also be a barrier to doctor–patient communication (30). The current literature describes urgency of treatment, a lack of information regarding reproductive options and limited resources, both geographically and economically, to reproductive medicine specialists or services, as additional barriers to efficient reproductive health communication.

As noted previously, some cancer survivors may be overwhelmed by their cancer diagnosis and unable to process or retain information initially outlined by the oncologist regarding possible side-effects of treatment. As a result, many patients may be caught unaware or surprised by their loss of fertility (14). Some researchers suggest that the period of diagnosis and treatment tends to focus on the cure and symptom management, and, as a result, quality-of-life issues may be ignored (33).

Goal of clinical encounter and guidelines

Clinical goals for both the patient and healthcare provider should include discussions of reproductive health issues, not only prior to treatment, but also throughout the continuum of their care, to ensure the assimilation of information and address evolving questions regarding fertility. The American Society of Clinical Oncology formally released guidelines on fertility preservation (34) and called attention to issues of reproductive knowledge and access. Fertility preservation is possible in people undergoing cancer treatment. ASCO recently published guidelines that should be incorporated into medical practice (34).

ASCO Recommendations include:

(1) Oncologists discuss risk of infertility as early as possible.

(2) Referral to reproductive specialist as early as possible.

(3) Encourage patients to enrol in clinical trials to advance knowledge in the field.

It is also important to address potential barriers to fertility preservation, which include:

(1) Lack of knowledge about infertility risk and possible alternatives for future fertility (i.e. cryo-preservation, third-party parenting and/or adoption).

(2) Failure to discuss/consider options with the patient prior to treatment.

(3) Limited discussion due to concerns about insurance coverage and high cost.

(4) Investigational status of many of the techniques available, in particular for women.

Oncologists and other healthcare professionals (e.g. reproductive specialists) should be well-informed of the available evidence for risk of infertility (both short- and long-term), depending tumour type, staging, and treatment options and duration (13, 34). Discussions concerning fertility risks must take place *prior* to the initiation of systemic therapies, as even one chemo-therapy infusion may significantly affect sperm production and quality. Patients have indicated in numerous studies that open discussion and dialogue between the oncologist and patient will enhance trust and facilitate communication (13, 35). Sperm-preservation methods and cost should be discussed with sperm banking (cryopreservation) encouraged and insisted upon by the physician for possible later use in ART, if necessary. Safety of preserved sperm (e.g. transmission for increased risk of cancer and/or teratogenic effects in offspring) should be discussed. Age and relationship status of the patient are critical. Patients should be encouraged to involve partners/spouses in decision-making, as data suggest that their involvement facilitates sperm-banking agreement. Younger patients (of age for personal health decision-making) may wish parents to be either involved or uninvolved, while those below age of consent will require parental consent to produce and bank sperm. Desire for fatherhood and/or current fatherhood status is variable (and age-dependent) but should be explored as should future oriented thinking around fatherhood, even if the patient is currently not in a relationship. This discussion will also improve adherence to banking, even if morbidity and especially mortality, are of current primary concern to the patient. Reassurance should be given regarding concerns about damaged sperm or transmission of increased cancer risk to progeny, for which there is no current evidence. Referral to a fertility specialist should be encouraged (13, 35).

Educational resources are available to assist the medical professional in educating themselves, as well as their patients, about available reproductive health issues. Excellent information is avail-able through multiple non-profit organizations about family-building options (Fertile Hope: **www.fertilehope.org**), cancer and intimacy (American Cancer Society: **http://www.cancer.gov/**) and survivorship (Lance Armstrong Foundation: **http://www.laf.org/**), to name just a few. Fertile Hope also offers a national referral list of reproductive specialists, which can be extremely helpful in addressing the survivorship issues of cancer patients.

Key communication skills

+ Clear concise factual information provided, both verbally and written, regarding fertility risk and preservation methods in the context of diagnosis and treatment prior to initiation of treatment.

+ Including significant others in discussions, as appropriate, including consultation with spiritual leaders, where appropriate and necessary.

+ Direct, firm directions on cryopreservation, where clearly indicated (e.g. sperm banking for men)

+ Ongoing continuous discussion of fertility issues through treatment and survivorship stages

Model statements

'I know you are most concerned with just getting through your treatment and 'surviving', but it is important for you to know that one of the potential side-effects of your treatment is infertility and there are a number of things you can do about it, because if you don't do it now, you may regret it later.'

'Sperm banking will give you a chance to have children in the future, even if you are not planning to now or in the near future.'

'Any sexual dysfunction side-effects you may experience are not related to whether you can preserve your fertility in the future.'

Practical checklist

+ Assure a private setting for conversation regarding infertility.

+ Refer to a qualified reproductive specialist, if available locally.

+ In the case of males, make certain that referral is made to a reputable sperm-banking facility.

+ Provide written information pamphlets outlining procedures, cost, and so on.

+ Provide access for patients to address emerging questions (e.g. telephone hotline, reliable, evidence-based websites, such as: **www.livestrong.org**; **www.fertilehope.org**; **www.asrm. org/Patients/FactSheets/cancer**).

Clinical scenarios

Males

Testicular cancer patient

A 21-year-old male university student, living with his girlfriend, is diagnosed with a testicular cancer after experiencing a swollen testicle for several weeks and feeling listless for a number of weeks. He was initially reassured by his GP that this was likely just an infection, but finally was referred for a urology consultation after the symptoms failed to remit after antibiotic treatment. Additional evaluation, including testicular sonography and serum markers, confirmed the diagnosis of testis cancer for which he underwent an orchiectomy. Additional surgery with retroperineal lymph node dissection was required. He experienced anenjaculation post-operatively. He was referred to oncology for adjuvant chemotherapy. While discussing his need for chemotherapy, his oncologist informed him that there was a significant risk that he would become either temporarily or even permanently infertile, and recommended a referral to a fertility specialist. The patient stated that he was not really concerned about fertility as his major fixation was on his survival. The oncologist informed the patient that while his prognosis was excellent with chemotherapy treatment (approximately 90% 10-year survival), he insisted that the patient provide a sample of sperm for banking (cryopreservation) prior to the initiation of further treatment for future use in assisted reproductive therapy. The student balked at the fees charged by a private sperm-banking facility. The doctor encouraged the young man to discuss this issue with his family to see if financial help could be found. Since he was unable to produce a sample through masturbation, electro-ejaculation procedure (stimulation of ejaculation by applying electrical stimulation to the prostate) was used. At subsequent follow-up visits, the healthcare team again brought up the patient's evolving plans for fatherhood. As recovery progressed and the patient returned to normal activities, his interest in ultimately fathering his own children became more salient.

Lymphoma patient

A 29-year-old male construction worker, married for three years with one child (aged 2 years), was diagnosed with non-Hodgkin lymphoma. He had been experiencing unexplained fevers for several months, increasing weakness and fatigue, until he noticed a lump in his neck that was biopsied to confirm the final diagnosis. A combination of chemotherapy and radiation therapy was proposed. In discussing the potential side-effects of the treatments with the patient and his wife, the oncologist mentioned the potential for permanent or temporary infertility. While sperm banking was recommended, the patient felt that, since he already had one child, he was not that concerned. However, his wife felt that since his prognosis was very good, she was optimistic and insisted that he bank sperm, as they had talked about having several children and she did not wish to overlook an opportunity in case his fertility did not return. After completing chemotherapy and radiation treatments, he returned to work and regular activities, though fatigue was a significant problem during the first year. His sexual function returned to the pre-diagnosis state. Two years post-treatment, his semen profile reviewed normal levels of sperm concentration and motility. In discussion with his physician, he was assured that fertility had returned and that he could attempt to have another child.

Females

Early stage cervical cancer patient

A 31-year-old woman was found to have an abnormal pap smear and underwent cone biopsy, which revealed stage 1B1 cervical cancer. The standard of care for early stage cervical cancer is a radical hysterectomy, resulting in cancer-related infertility. The patient voiced a strong desire for fertility and for information about options for fertility preservation and alternative family building methods.

The fertility-preserving surgical treatment option of radical trachelectomy has been established in the field of gynaecologic oncology for almost two decades. This procedure provides adequate tumour control, while allowing for the preservation of the uterus with promising gynaecologic and obstetrical outcomes (25, 36, 37). Surgical criteria are specific, and this procedure is only offered to women with a strong desire to preserve fertility. It has been estimated that 48% of young women diagnosed with early-stage cervical cancer would meet the criteria for a trachelectomy (38).

However, if the patient does not choose, or meet, the criteria for radical trachelectomy, alternate methods for family building can be addressed. Since radical hysterectomy requires the removal of the uterus, a third party will be necessary to carry a pregnancy for the patient, such as surrogate or gestation carrier. Patients choosing this option will have to undergo ovarian stimulation for oocyte (egg) retrieval, which then can be fertilized with a partner's sperm or donor sperm. The embryo or fertilized egg would then be transplanted in the surrogate/gestation carrier or cyropreserved for later implantation.

In some cases, women who have undergone radical trachelectomy or radical hysterectomy, may be recommended to undergo adjuvant treatment (chemotherapy and /or radiation therapy) based on final pathology review of the surgical specimen. In this particular circumstance, patients may choose the option of oocyte and/or embryo cryopreservation, based on preference and partner status, prior to initiating post-operative treatment. Additionally, adoption is always a viable option for the individual who may not be in favour of current reproductive medicine techniques.

Premenopausal breast cancer patient

A 36-year-old woman was found to have a lump in her right breast and underwent breast scans to evaluate extent of disease. The patient was diagnosed with an early stage breast cancer and was recommended to undergo surgical resection and sentinel lymph node mapping and sampling. The patient was advised to receive adjuvant chemotherapy post-operatively.

Based on the current literature (4), it is unclear whether the patient will have return of menses. Therefore, options for fertility preservation should be explored as soon as possible to minimize delays in treatment. Since the patient is at risk for premature menopause, due to her age and possible chemotherapy regime, it should be suggested that the patient be advised of the risk of premature menopause and provided with information about the available reproductive options, prior to the initiation of chemotherapy.

Even if a patient returns to a premenopausal state after adjuvant treatment, the window of fertility may be shortened (39). Many patients choose to undergo ovarian stimulation in order to retrieve ooyctes (egg) for cryopreservation or for fertilization with partner's sperm or sperm donation for cryopreservation of embryos. Some have suggested using letrozole as part of ovarian stimulation protocol to lower peak levels of oestradiol (40). Another available option which is still considered 'experimental' is the option of ovarian tissue cryopreservation, with the goal of re-implantation for ooycte retrieval post-treatment (41, 42).

Concerns about pregnancy after breast cancer is also an issue of debate, especially since a paucity of data exist on fertility and pregnancy outcomes in breast cancer survivors. Women are commonly recommended to wait 2 years from treatment completion prior to conception. This 2-year period appears to be the time of greatest risk for aggressive breast cancer recurrence (5). In women with hormone-receptive cancer, the waiting period prior to attempted conception may be as long as 5 years, due to standard duration of hormonal therapy (5). This time delay can be an issue of concern for breast cancer survivors of more advanced years and declining reproductive function wishing fertility options, if they were fortunate enough to have return of menses post-treatment.

Summary of outcomes for patients and families resulting from communication

Many survivors report that they are satisfied that their health care professionals insisted that they engage in discussions and act proactively on fertility-preservation options. Discussions with parents (in younger adolescents) and significant others (e.g. spouses, girl/boy friends) leads to better mutual adjustment and satisfaction, even when fertility return ultimately results in natural progeny outcomes.

References

1. Bahadur G. Fertility Issues for cancer patients. *Mol Cell Endocrinol* 2000; **169**: 117–122.

2. Sanders JE, Buckner CD, Amos D, *et al*. Ovarian function following marrow transplantation for aplastic anemia or leukemia. *J Clin Onc* 1988; **6**: 813–818.

3. Schechter T, Finkelstein Y, Doyle J, *et al*. Pregnancy after stem cell transplantation. *Can Fam Physician* 2005; **51**: 817–818.

4. Petrek JA, *et al*. Incidence, time course, and determinants of menstrual bleeding after breast cancer treatment: a prospective study. *J Clin Oncol* 2006; **24**: 1045–1051.

5. Partridge A, Gelber S, Gelber RD *et al*. Age of menopause among women who remain premenopausal following treatment for early breast cancer: long-term results from International Breast Cancer Study Group Trials V and VI. *Eur J Cancer* 2007; **43**: 1646–1653.

6. Meirow D, Nugent D. The effects of radiotherapy and chemotherapy on female reproduction. *Human Reprod Update* 2001; **7**: 535–543.

7. Sklar *et al*. Premature menopause in survivors of childhood cancer: a report from the childhood Cancer Survivor Study. *J National Cancer Instit* 2006; **98**(13): 890–896.

8. Gershenson DM. Fertility-sparing surgery for malignancies in women. *J Natl Cancer Inst Monogr* 2005; **34**: 43–47.

9. Duffy CM, Allen S M, Clark MA. Discussions regarding reproductive health for young women with breast cancer undergoing chemotherapy. *J Clin Oncol* 2005; **23**(4), 766–773.

10. Partridge AH, Gelber S, Peppercorn J, *et al*. Web-based survey of fertility issues in young women with breast cancer. *J Clin Onco* 2004; **22**(20), 4174–4183.

11. Schover LR. Psychosocial aspects of infertility and decisions about reproduction in young cancer survivors: a review. *Medical and Pediatric Onc* 1999; **33**: 53–59.

12. Thewes B, Meiser B, Rickard J, *et al*. (2003). The fertility- and menopause-related information needs of younger women with a diagnosis of breast cancer: a qualitative study. *Psycho-Oncology* 2003; **12**(5), 500–511.

13. Achille MA, Rosberger Z, Robitaille R, *et al*. Facilitators and obstacles to sperm banking in young men receiving gonadotoxic chemotherapy for cancer: the perspective of survivors and health care professionals. *Hum Reprod* 2006; **21**(12), 3206–3216.

14. Schover LR, Rybicki LA, Martin BA, *et al*. Having children after cancer. A pilot survey of survivors' attitudes and experiences [original article]. *Cancer* 1999; **86**(4), 697–709.

15. Schover LR, Brey K, Lichtin A, *et al*. Knowledge and experience regarding cancer, infertility, and sperm banking in younger male survivors. *Journal of Clinical Oncology* 2002; **20**(7), 1880–1889.

16. Sonneveld DJ *et al*. Improved long term survival of patients with metastatic nonseminomatous testicular germ cell carcinoma in relation to prognostic classification systems during the cisplatin era. *Cancer* 2001; **91**(7), 1304–1315.

17. Jemal A *et al*. Annual report to the nation on the status of cancer, 1975–2001, with a special feature regarding survival. *Cancer* 2004; **101**(1), 3–27.

18. O'Flaherty C, Hales BF, Chan P, Robaire B, Impact of chemotherapeutics and advanced testicular cancer of Hodgkins lymphoma on sperm deoxyribonucleic acid integrity Fertil Steril, 2009 Jul 8 (epub ahead of print) PMID: 19591994

19. Chan PTK, Palermo GD, Veeck LL, *et al*. Testicular sperm extraction combined with intracytoplasmic sperm injection in the treatment of men with persistent azoospermia postchemotherapy. *Cancer* 2001; **92**(6), 1632–1637.

20. Robitaille R, Rosberger Z, Achille M, *et al*. Infertility concerns in young male cancer survivors: a qualitative study. unpublished manuscript

21. Carter J, Rowland K, Chi D, *et al*. Gynecologic cancer treatment and the impact of cancer-related infertility. *Gynecologic Oncology* 2005; **97**(1), 90–95.

22. Ganz *et al*. Health status and quality of life in patients with early-stage Hodgkin's disease treated on Southwest Oncology Group Study 9133. *J Clin Oncol* 2003; **21**(18), 3512–3519.

23. Hammond C, Abrams JR, Syrjala KL. Fertility and risk factors for elevated infertility concern in 10-year hematopoietic cell transplant survivors and case-matched controls. *J Clin Oncol* 2007; **25**(23), 3511–3517.

24. Carter J, Sonoda Y, Abu-Rustum N. Reproductive concerns of women treated with radical trachelectomy for cervical cancer. *Gyn Onc* 2007; **105**(1): 13–16.

25. Wenzel L, Berkowitz RS, Newlands E, *et al*.: Quality of life after gestational trophoblastic disease. *J Reprod Med* 2002; **47**: 387–394.

26. Plante M, Renaud MC, Francois H, *et al*. Vaginal radical trachelectomy: an oncologically safe fertility-preserving surgery. An updated series of 72 cases and review of the literature. *Gynecol Oncol* 2004; **94**: 614–623.

27. Sonmezer M, Oktay K. Fertility preservation in female patients. *Hum Reprod Update* 2004; **10**: 251–66.

28. Rosen A. Third-party reproduction and adoption in cancer patients. *J Natl Cancer Inst Monogr* 2005; **34**: 91–93.

29. Zebrack BJ, Casillas J, Nohr L, *et al.* Fertility issues for young adult survivors of childhood cancer. *Psycho-oncology* 2004; **13**(10), 689–699.

30. Hordern AJ, Street AF. Communicating about patient sexuality and intimacy after cancer: mismatched expectations and unmet needs. *MJA* 2007; **186**(5): 224–227.

31. Toubassi D, *et al.* The informational needs of newly diagnosed cervical cancer patients who will be receiving combined chemoradiation treatment. *J Cancer Educ* 2006; **21**: 263–268.

32. Corney R, Everett H, Howells A, *et al.* The care of patients undergoing surgery for gynaecological cancer: the need for information, emotional support and counselling. *J Adv Nurs* 1992; **17**: 667–671.

33. Katz A. The sounds of silence: sexuality information for cancer patients. *J Clin Onc* 2005; **23**(1), 238–241.

34. Lee SJ, Schover LR, Partridge AH, *et al.* American Society of Clinical Oncology Recommendations on Fertility Preservation in Cancer Patients. [ASCO special article]. *J Clin Onc* 2006; **24**(18), 2917–2931.

35. Chapple A, Salinas M, Ziebland S, *et al.* Fertility issues: the perceptions and experiences of young men recently diagnosed and treated for cancer [original article]. *J Adolesc Health* 2007; **40**(1), 69–75.

36. Plante M, Renavd MC, Hoskins IA, Roy M. Vaginal radical tracelectomy: a valuable fertility-preserving option in the management of early stage cervical cancer. A series of 50 pregnancies and review of the literature. *Gynecol Oncol* 2005; **98**: 3–10.

37. Sonoda Y, *et al.* Initial experience with Dargent's operation: The radical vaginal trachelectomy. *Gynecol Oncol* 2008; **108**(1): 214–219

38. Sonoda Y, Abu-Rustum NR, Gemignani ML, *et al.* A fertility-sparing alternative to radical hysterectomy: how many patients may be eligible? *Gynecol Oncol* 2004; **95**: 534–538.

39. Partridge AH, Rubby KJ, Fertility and adjuvant treatment in young women with breast cancer. *The Breast* 2007; **16**(Suppl): S11–S12.

40. Oktay K, *et al.* Fertility preservation in breast cancer patients: a prospective controlled comparison of ovarian stimulation with Tamoxifen and letrozole for embryo cryopreservation. *J Clin Oncol* 2005; **23**: 4347–53.

41. Demeestere I, *et al.* Options to preserve fertility before oncological treatment: cryopreservation of ovarian and its clinical application. *Acta Clin Belg* 2006; **61**: 259–263.

42. Oktay K, *et al.* Embryo development after heterotopic transplantation of cryopreserved ovarian tissue. *Lancet* 2004; **363**: 837–840.

Chapter 35

Communicating about sexuality in cancer care

John W Robinson and Joshua J Lounsberry

Extensive research has shown that cancer, and the treatment thereof, can interfere with healthy sexual functioning. Indeed, sexual dysfunction is frequently cited as one of the top adverse effects of cancer treatment (1). However, while healthcare professionals routinely discuss quality-of-life issues with cancer patients, the literature suggest that too often this does not include an assessment of sexual concerns. One study reported that 96% of healthcare professionals stated that discussing sexuality was part of their job, while only 2% said that they regularly spoke to patients about sexuality (2). When questions incorporating sexual functioning were included in routine patient assessments, approximately 41% of patients indicated problems with sex (3). However, if patients are not asked specifically about sexual functioning, less than 10% will raise sexual concerns (4). Clearly, the responsibility to initiate discussion on sexuality rests with the healthcare professional.

Establishing the sexuality information needs of the cancer patient can sometimes be difficult and it becomes more so when healthcare professionals make erroneous assumptions concerning sexuality. Healthcare professionals often hold the belief that cancer patients are, and should be, most concerned with treating the cancer and that other considerations are tangential (5). In fact, some patients are willing to trade years of life to maintain sexual function (6). Further, healthcare professionals often believe that the responsibility for discussing sexuality lies with someone else, which often results in no one assuming the responsibility (7, 8). Even when the healthcare professional does accept the responsibility, there are a host of commonly stated reasons for not initiating the conversation, including: limited time; a lack of education; embarrassment; the feeling that it is not a part of the presenting problem; a preference for same-gender consultation; the sexual orientation of the patient; the assumption that sexuality is not a concern for either the very young or the older patient; and possible religious or language barriers (8–10). However, patients often express a desire to receive information regarding sexuality, and irrespective of patient age, sex, partnership status, culture, or site of cancer, patients have stated that their needs in this area often go unmet (5).

Unresolved sexual problems can have devastating effects on the lives of both the patient and their partner. These effects can range from mild embarrassment, unhappiness, and frustration to profound humiliation, loss of self-esteem, erosion of the relationship bond, and complicated mental health issues. Indeed, patients need information detailing how to stay sexually active for as long as they wish, in spite of their illness. Thus, whether or not to assess sexuality is no longer an issue; it must be a routine part of cancer care.

The PLISSIT model

While there are several different models of intervention for patients suffering from sexual difficulties, the model known by the acronym PLISSIT is frequently used in cancer centres and can easily be adapted to various types of practice (11, 12). The model describes four progressive levels that can be used to guide assessment and intervention (13).

- PERMISSION. Raise the topic of sexuality so that patients feel that they have permission to talk about sexual concerns.

- LIMITED INFORMATION. Provide information to address the sexuality concerns of the patient, including sexual sequelae common to their situation.

- SPECIFIC SUGGESTIONS. Taking into consideration their sexual history and relationship, provide specific strategies for dealing with problems and maintaining sexuality.

- INTENSIVE THERAPY. Refer to a specialist those patients who have premorbid sexual concerns, mental health problems, or those with more complex problems.

While the model is designed with a hierarchical structure, practically, it is not a tool to be used in a strictly linear fashion. There are many areas of overlap between each of the levels and, as different issues develop, the healthcare professional may be required to move back and forth between levels. The PLISSIT model should be used fluidly as a guideline to inform practice.

PERMISSION

Raising the subject of sex during the first meeting grants the patient permission to talk about their concerns and serves to legitimize the existence of sexual thoughts, feelings, and desires. Thus, granting permission should be implemented with all patients regardless of demographic variables or disease status, so that the choice of pursuing this topic is left to the patient.

The importance of addressing sexuality early is highlighted by findings that ignoring sexual dysfunction after cancer treatment can lead to erosion in the marital bond (14), self-concept, and social relationships (15). On the other hand, early intervention can lead to the resumption of sexual activity, which has been shown to enhance quality of life (16) and to increase the chances of optimal recovery of sexual function (17). Incorporating a generic question about sex into an initial history or follow-up visit can be an effective first step. These openings provide patients with an opportunity to ask questions and to indicate their level of sexual functioning. While the therapeutic benefit of the mere disclosure of personal information to a trusted healthcare professional has long been recognized (18), patients/couples may not want further discussion, so the issue should not be forced. The patient may wish to concentrate on their primary treatment or may not yet have concerns regarding sexuality. However, by granting permission the healthcare professional has let the patient know that it is a valid concern.

Questions to initiate discussion:

- What impact has cancer had on your sex life?

- Are you experiencing any loss of sexual function?

- Do you feel any different about yourself as a man/woman as a result of your cancer?

- Many people are concerned about how their illness will affect their sexuality. What concerns do you have?

Patient sexuality is more often overlooked when the sexual organs are not directly involved; however, there are a number of sexual side-effects to treatment that are common to most cancers (5). Patients often struggle with incontinence, hygiene, fatigue, pain, dependency on others, and loss of earning power; all of which can adversely affect the patient's sense of sexual appeal. Following cancer treatment, most patients are also affected by changes in their perceived body image. In some cases the changes are intuitive such as alopecia, breast loss, ostomy, or laryngectomy. In other cases the loss is less obvious but nonetheless heartfelt: loss of body hair, uterus, rectum, physical strength, or stamina. Few patients are unaffected by such challenges, and thus the majority require information on sexuality regardless of the cancer site or type of treatment.

Some patients may be too young at the point of diagnosis or treatment to be engaged in sexual activity; however, given the ever increasing survival rates for cancer, the patient will likely become sexually active at some point in their lives. Thus, provisions must be made to ensure that the patient is informed of the likely effects of cancer/cancer treatment on both sexuality and fertility. On the other end of the spectrum are those who may be 'too old' or 'too sick' to be sexually active. The healthcare professional must remain aware of the fact that couples in their 60s to 70s still want to be sexually active (19) and that even palliative patients find comfort in sexual intimacy (20).

Relationship status is another important consideration when discussing sexuality. Whether or not the patient is currently engaged in a romantic relationship has bearing on the types of concerns that they are likely to have. Also, it is incumbent upon the healthcare professional to determine the sexual orientation of the patient, rather than assuming them to be heterosexual. This can be easily accomplished by asking the patient's relationship situation.

Finally, ethnic or religious diversity can become a factor. The healthcare professional should always remain aware of the part played by the cultural/religious assumptions of both themselves and the patient with regard to sexuality. That being said, while there are likely to be many differences in the desired method of communication, the types of sexual dysfunction after cancer are common to patients from all ethnic or religious groups.

Box 35.1 Clinical example

Chris and Patti, a Canadian couple in their late-forties, had been married for 25 years and had become caught up in their busy life. Then, Patti was diagnosed with cancer and underwent an allogeneic stem cell transplant.

Everything was going well with regard to Patti's physical recovery at a 9-month follow-up, but there had been some changes in the couple's relationship. Both Chris and Patti reported having felt closer than ever during the crisis of initial diagnosis and primary treatment. However, now that Patti was out of the hospital and was doing well, things had begun to deteriorate. They had become frustrated with one another and had begun bickering over minutia.

I informed the couple that it is common for issues to arise once the threat of cancer subsides. Sometimes this uprising of issues can be related to the disruption in the level of sexual intimacy in the relationship and the uncertainty about resuming sexual relations. As it turned out, Patti was having concerns that Chris was no longer attracted to her, while Chris was patiently waiting for Patti to let him know when she was ready to resume their sexual relationship.

As we talked, the couple began to realize that the tension they had been feeling in the relationship was coming from the pent-up feelings they both had about this issue. The couple expressed relief and gratitude about finally breaking the silence around sexuality.

LIMITED INFORMATION

The next level of intervention is the provision of information pertinent to patient concerns. Although the healthcare professional may need to warn the patient that cancer treatment can impair sexual functioning, it is crucial to convey the message that sexual activity is not at an end. Patients may wonder if they can continue sexual relations during treatment, they may have concerns about changes in their body following treatment, or they may have concerns about satisfying their partner. Failure to provide information may lead the patient to expend needless emotional energy worrying about concerns that could easily have been allayed. It is also important to remember that the patient will likely feel overwhelmed when initially diagnosed with cancer and may forget much of the sexual information provided. Therefore, during follow-up visits, patients will benefit from being asked again about their sexual concerns and having them addressed.

Following primary treatment, the patient should be provided with resources outlining the lasting effects of cancer treatment in general, as well as specifics for their particular situation. Written information can be particularly helpful because it allows the patient to work with the material on their own time (21). Numerous reliable sources of written information are available for patients.

- Schover L (1998). *Sexuality and cancer: for the woman with cancer and her partner.* New York, NY: American Cancer Society.

- Schover L (1998). *Sexuality and cancer: for the man with cancer and his partner.* New York, NY: American Cancer Society.

- Cancer Council of Victoria (2004). *Sexuality and cancer: a guide for people with cancer.* Carlton, Australia: Cancer Council of Victoria.

- Canadian Cancer Society (2006). *Sexuality and cancer: a guide for people with cancer.* Toronto, Canada: Canadian Cancer Society.

- Schover L (1997). *Sexuality and fertility after cancer.* Toronto, Canada: John Wiley & Sons, Inc.

Sexual response cycle

The sexual response cycle is a helpful model for explaining both sexual functioning and the ways in which various treatments will likely affect sexual functioning (22, 23). In addition to the diagram outlining the sexual response cycle (Fig. 35.1), patients often find 3-D models of pelvic

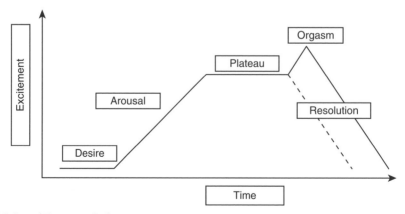

Fig. 35.1 Sexual Response Cycle

anatomy helpful when trying to understand the changes that are taking place at the various stages of the cycle.

The sexual response cycle is usually presented as a linear series of phases beginning with Desire. Desire is commonly experienced as sexual thoughts/fantasies or spontaneous sexual urges. When a person acts upon their desire they move to the Arousal phase. Lingering in a state of sexual arousal is referred to as Plateau, from which the sexual tension that is built up in the arousal phase can, with further stimulation, be released in what is called an Orgasm. There is, however, no imperative for a sexual encounter to culminate with an orgasm. The tension that builds during sexual play can be allowed to dissipate on its own without harm, and arousal can be enjoyed in its own right. The Resolution phase refers to the period during which the body returns to physiological norms. If the sexual experience has gone well, this is the phase where many couples experience the greatest emotional closeness.

Revised sexual response cycle

Loss of sexual desire is one of the most common sexual effects of cancer treatment. Basson's (24) refinement of the sexual response cycle can be particularly useful in helping patients understand the changes that they are experiencing (Fig. 35.2). While in the past the revised model has been applied specifically to females, clinically it appears to have applicability to both female and male cancer patients. This model differentiates between spontaneous/innate sexual desire and receptive/responsive sexual desire. Spontaneous desire corresponds to the aforementioned conceptualization of the sexual response cycle beginning with Desire. Basson theorizes that desire often follows arousal, rather than precedes it. Thus, if the patient is motivated to engage in potentially arousing sexual activity, and if they begin to feel sexually aroused, desire will be triggered. The importance of enhancing motivation and understanding the patient's fears about engaging in sexual activity are highlighted in this revised conceptualization.

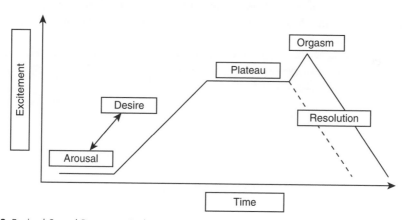

Fig. 35.2 Revised Sexual Response Cycle

Many cancer patients find that the French axiom, 'L'appetit vient en manegeant' or 'Appetite comes while we eat' is one that captures this concept and resonates with their experience. Just as cancer patients commonly lose their spontaneous appetite for food, so too do they often lose their appetite for sexual relations. When the appetite is weak, the mere idea of being expected to eat an entire four-course meal is sure to stifle any willingness to taste the first course. However, if patients are gently encouraged to taste some food knowing that they can just nibble the bits that they find appealing, there will often be an enjoyment and a concomitant awakening of appetite. Similarly, many patients are more willing to engage in sexual touching when there is no pressure to reach climax or to engage in sexual activity that is not appealing.

Resuming sexual intercourse

The sexual response cycle can be used to help the patient understand that the impairment of one aspect of sexual functioning does not preclude satisfying experiences in other aspects. For example, when a female patient has been instructed to refrain from sexual intercourse, she and her partner may be unaware that other sexual activity is a possibility. Similarly, after radical prostatectomy, sexual desire, pleasurable genital sensation resulting in arousal, and the ability to have an orgasm often are not impaired, even though the patient may experience erectile difficulties. For a man, arousal is usually palpable and there is often a direct association between the sight/sensation of an erection and a report of subjective arousal (24). Thus, when there is a loss of erectile function the man often overlooks the remaining subtle and less familiar sensations, making the erroneous conclusion that arousal is unattainable. This concept of orgasm without erection seems counterintuitive to most patients. Men will often find it helpful to have information on the physiology of orgasm, particularly with regard to the fact that the nerves that are involved in erectile function are different from those involved in sensation and orgasm. Analogies, such as those described in Box 35.2, can be an effective way of simplifying complicated concepts.

Box 35.2 Helpful analogies

Christmas light analogy

The Christmas light analogy can be helpful in explaining the phenomenon of orgasm without erection. Many men believe that they are wired like an old string of Christmas lights where, if one bulb burns out (the ability to have an erection), the whole sting goes out. Further, there is the belief that if you cannot replace that bulb and regain the ability for erection, you may as well throw out the whole string because none of the bulbs will light. However, we know that men can, in fact, experience orgasm without an erection, so all the Christmas lights do not go out when one bulb burns out.

Orgasm/sneeze analogy

It is sometimes instructive for patients to think of orgasms as pelvic sneezes. The tension in the face and the tickle in the nasal passages indicate that a sneeze is building. Likewise, for orgasm there is a build-up of muscle tension and congestion, in other words arousal. Sneezes can be stifled and the tension allowed to dissipate on its own, just as arousal can be allowed to dissipate without orgasm. While sneezes release the tension in the face, orgasm releases sexual tension.

To carry the metaphor further, we can have a wet sneeze if there is mucus in the nasal passages and dry sneezes if there is none. Similarly, men have wet orgasms—ejaculate—if they have a functioning prostate that produces seminal fluid and dry orgasm if they don't. Wet and dry sneezes feel different and yet they are both unmistakably sneezes.

Issues of fertility

Although fertility issues are most pressing for patients who still wish to have children, the ability to procreate can be an important part of a positive sexual image, independent of the wish to reproduce (25). The loss of fertility can exacerbate the struggle to maintain a positive body image after cancer and can result in the feeling of being damaged goods. Given that chemotherapy and broad irradiation are likely to affect fertility, it is incumbent upon the healthcare professional to provide the patient with options for preserving fertility. Research suggests that, unless the healthcare professional takes the initiative to refer patients to a fertility specialist, it is unlikely that patients will go of their own accord (26, 27). For more information on this issue see Chapter 34.

Box 35.3 Clinical example

Chris and Patti did have questions and concerns about resuming sexual intimacy, so the conversation continued on to these topics. Patti brought up the common concern of changes in how her body responds sexually. I informed the couple that these changes are quite common and that the loss of spontaneous desire is particularly common. When the idea of 'our appetite develops as we eat' was presented to the couple, they both found that it applied well to their situation. I also informed the couple that while women do have an awareness of the physiological sensations of arousal, it is the thoughts and emotions that she experiences that determine subjective arousal. If Patti were to embrace her perceptions of sexual feelings and thoughts, her arousal might be reinforced. Normalizing the situation reduced the couple's anxiety and allowed Patti to look for solutions, rather than concentrate on the bodily changes. I also provided the couple with a booklet that contained an explanation of the changes that were likely following cancer treatment, so that they might review things on their own. While the couple was provided with the tools to resolve their issues, the door was left open to take the conversation further, if the couple so desired.

SPECIFIC SUGGESTIONS

Attention to patient context is always important, but it is even more so when providing specific suggestions. While people across cultures, religions, and sexual orientations are more alike than they are different, it is important to remain aware that there may be issues specific to particular groups. Resources are available to help healthcare professionals become more sensitive to diversity issues (28–35). However, patients themselves are often more than willing to explain how their background and upbringing informs their sexuality and they often appreciate the healthcare professional taking the time to ask. The key is not to make an assumption about your patient because there are likely factors involved of which you are unaware. For example, the adoption of Euro-Canadian sexual attitudes and beliefs is often not related to length of residency but rather to acculturation into Western culture (36). That being said, many of the suggestions that healthcare professionals offer apply across cultures and sexual affiliations.

It is important to include partners in the conversation when providing specific suggestions. Partners often have concerns of their own, but can also play a vital role in helping the patient overcome any difficulties. It will be helpful to obtain a brief sexual history in order to understand the dynamics of the couple's intimate relations (Box 35.4). The sexual history will also help to reveal the true source of the sexuality problem. If the patient states that they have lost desire, but the healthcare professional is unaware that they are experiencing dyspareunia, the root cause will have been missed and any suggestions to improve desire will likely fail.

Box 35.4 Sexual function assessment questions

Desire phase

Are there times when you spontaneously experience desire for sexual activity? If so, how frequently?

If your partner approaches you sexually, how do you usually respond?

Arousal phase

How easy or difficult is it for you to become sexually aroused or excited?

Men: Do you ever experience difficulties obtaining or maintaining an erection?

Women: Do you experience a sense of pelvic fullness and find that your labia become engorged? Do you find that you lubricate or become wet?

Do you ever experience pain with sexual activity?

Orgasm phase

On most occasions, when you wish to are you able to reach orgasm?

Do you sometimes find that you reach orgasm faster than you want or that it takes longer than you would like?

Everybody is different in the types of stimulation that best help them reach orgasm. What types of stimulation work best in helping you reach orgasm?

Resolution

When you reflect back on your recent sexual experiences, how do you usually feel?

Are you concerned with any aspect of how your body responds sexually, with your sexual relationship, or you ability to be a good lover?

Another important contextual factor is the use of medications that interfere with sexual functioning. For example, depression is strongly associated with sexual dysfunction and the use of antidepressants often exacerbates the problem (37). More than half of those who take antidepressant medications, especially selective serotonin reuptake inhibitors, experience decreased desire, difficulties becoming aroused, and problems reaching orgasm (37). However, there are antidepressants (Mirtazapine, Moclobemide, Nefazodone, Reboxetine) that have been found to have limited negative effects on sexual functioning (37, 38) and Bupropion is reported to have actually improved sexual function for women treated for breast cancer (39). Switching to Bupropion has also been shown to be effective for men who are experiencing erectile dysfunction or delayed ejaculation (40). Clearly then, it is important for the healthcare professional to remain aware of the medications that the patient is taking and to intervene on their behalf if a change in medication would improve sexual functioning.

In order to become effective in the provision of specific suggestions, the healthcare professional will need to acquaint themselves with the sexual sequelae for the patient population in question. Describing the approaches to treating the sexual difficulties for all of the specific cancer sites is beyond the scope of this chapter; however, there are sequelae that are common to most cancers. It is important to remember that it is rarely cancer itself that directly interferes with sexual functioning; rather it is the treatment that most often causes the problems. An understanding of the important advances in our knowledge of the mechanisms of sexual functioning and the effects of cancer treatments will be required for skilled intervention at this level. At the very least, healthcare professionals should be knowledgeable concerning the most common sexual sequelae; vaginal dryness and dyspareunia (painful intercourse), loss of desire, and erectile dysfunction.

Vaginal dryness and dyspareunia

Vaginal dryness and female dyspareunia are common after chemotherapy and pelvic radiotherapy (41, 42). Oestrogen-replacement therapy (ERT) can be an effective treatment—possibly even for hormonally sensitive patients (43). Some findings suggest that localized forms of ERT, such as virginal creams, pessary, or ring, can be effective in reducing vaginal dryness without significantly increasing serum levels of oestrogen in hormonally sensitive cancer survivors (43). However, combining pelvic floor muscle relaxation with water-based lubricants, vaginal moisturizers (t.i.w.), and vitamine E (100-600 IU/day orally or localy) is perhaps more effective in treating dyspareunia than hormonal treatment (42, 44-46). Non-hormonal polycarbophil moisturizing gel (Replens) has been shown to improve vaginal health and sexual functioning for women with a history of breast cancer (47) who are unable or reluctant to use hormone replacement therapy (48).

Loss of desire

Another common problem is the loss of desire. Androgen replacement is often cited as the only real 'cure' for women who experience a loss in sexual desire after losing ovarian function (49). Improvements in sexual response have been shown with the supplementation of testosterone to high physiologic levels (50, 51). While androgen replacement has been considered safe by some, even in women with hormone sensitive tumours (52), many caution against its use (53). Men too, commonly experience a loss of sexual desire following certain cancer treatments. Androgen-deprivation therapy, a treatment for prostate cancer, often results in a physical inability of experiencing a sexual response because of the castrate levels of testosterone.

Psychosocial variables are equally, if not more, important than hormonal variables in the subjective experience of desire (54). For example, there does appear to be some evidence that men are capable of a full sexual response despite castrate levels of testosterone (55, 56). Similarly, contextual and relationship factors were found to be more important than hormonal ones in a study of women who underwent surgical menopause (57, 58). Behavioural interventions, especially those addressing motivational issues, have shown promise, even for women with low androgen levels (24).

Erectile dysfunction

Erectile dysfunction is the most common sexual problem for which men seek treatment (59). The majority of men treated for prostate cancer will lose the ability to obtain an erection sufficient for intercourse (15). Men having pelvic surgeries, such as cystectomy or anterior–posterior resection, and those receiving pelvic radiotherapy may experience erectile dysfunction as well. Health care professionals should be aware of the most effective interventions for helping couples maintain sexual intimacy despite erectile dysfunction (60). These high rates of dysfunction may decline in the future with the increased awareness of the benefits of early intervention. It has been shown that men who start the use of an erectile aid, such as a vacuum erection device or phosphodiesterase-5 inhibitor medication, soon after radical prostatectomy or cryoablation improve their chances of recovering erectile function (61–64). Early use of erectile aids has also been shown to preserve penile length after primary treatment (62).

Sensate focus

Sensate focus exercises provide a safe and comfortable framework through which couples can begin to explore sexuality with sensual touch. Couples learn to focus on the feelings that arise as they are pleasuring their partner and are being pleasured, without the expectation or pressure to become aroused or engage in activities that are anxiety provoking. Special consideration must be given to the cancer patient because they are sometimes self-conscious about their body due to weight loss, scarring, or an ostomy. The patient is encouraged to start with what is comfortable for them, and to proceed at their own pace. There are materials available to help healthcare professionals to implement this strategy (65, 66). Brotto and colleagues (36) have found that training in mindfulness also helps women stay focused on sensual feelings and improves their sexual function.

Box 35.5 Clinical example

The tone of the conversation suggested that both Chris and Patti would be open to moving beyond limited information into the provision of specific suggestions. I provided the couple with instructions on the use of sensate focus techniques and encouraged them to try. If they started slow, with no intention of sexual intercourse, Patti's appetite might slowly start to develop. Both Patti and Chris agreed that this would be a good solution. The couple was also provided with a water-based lubricant, and were told that following a stem cell transplant many women do experience labial and virginal dryness. I also asked the couple to report any vaginal stenosis—which is common after a stem cell transplant—because there are effective treatments available (67)

When I next saw the couple I could immediately see the difference in how they were relating to one another. When I commented on the change, they explained that the sensate focus exercises had provided them with a comfortable way of reconnecting physically and emotionally. They had come to the realization that while sexuality is not the glue that holds them together, it is the lubricant that helps smooth out the rough patches.

Intensive Therapy

Research has shown that 80% of cancer patients' sexual concerns can be managed by intervention at the first three levels of the PLISSIT model (68). Nonetheless, the healthcare professional should be able to recognize the point at which the patient/couple should be referred to a specialist. Intensive Therapy is needed for patients with more complex medical problems or if there are relationship or attitudinal factors that impede their ability to use the information or suggestions. A history of poor psychological coping, sexual or physical abuse, chemical dependency, or previous sexual dysfunction are also associated with an increased propensity for major sexual difficulties (11).

The healthcare professional may also be faced with compliance issues following the provision of specific suggestions. It has been repeatedly shown that merely recommending that women use vaginal dilators to prevent virginal stenosis after pelvic radiotherapy results in very low compliance rates (69, 70). Likewise, the advent of phosphodiesterase-5 inhibitor medications have led some to believe that erectile dysfunction is now easily treated. However, a recent review of the literature (15) found that 50% of men stop using the aid within a year. Most concerning are the patients who, when medical treatments do not seem to work, withdraw from all intimate contact and become despondent. A more intensive intervention may be required to ensure optimal recovery of sexual functioning through compliance with treatment. In the previous example of the use of vaginal dilators, the information motivation behaviour model has been proven more effective than simply providing information (69). Biopsychosocial interventions also seem to increase the likelihood of remaining sexually active (71). However, these types of interventions are best left to those who have been professionally trained in their use.

Box 35.6 Clinical example

Although it was unlikely that the couple needed intensive therapy, I made sure that they were aware that seeing a specialist was possible and not out of the ordinary. I pointed out that, if left to their own devices, couples often avoid talking about sensitive issues because they are afraid of making matters worse. Couples who do seek professional counselling improve their chances of maintaining or improving sexual intimacy because it can help couples to have meaningful discussions about difficult issues and to express pent up feelings.

Reflecting on practice

Just as patients have a right to know if treatments will result in hair loss or nausea, so too do they have a right to know the ramifications of treatment on their sexuality. Rather than perpetuating the culture of silence around sexuality, healthcare professionals can work to improve or maintain sexual health. Most patients' needs are easily met through the normalization of thoughts and feelings, the presentation of accurate information, and the provision of appropriate suggestions. For more complex issues, the healthcare professional simply refers the patient to a specialist. Proficiency in communicating about sexuality with the cancer patient requires little more than knowledge of sexual sequelae of the cancer in question and a willingness to initiate the conversation.

Clearly, healthcare professionals endeavour to provide the best possible care. Thus, as conscientious healthcare professionals, we must ask why sexuality is so often overlooked when its importance has been repeatedly demonstrated. Our intent in these pages was to provide a tool to facilitate communication, while inviting a critical appraisal of the healthcare professional's beliefs, assumptions, and stereotypes. The hope being that healthcare professionals will reflect on the manner in which their context affects practice; that is, to base practice on evidence rather than assumption and to assign priority to the patient's wellbeing.

References

1. Hampton T. Cancer survivors need better care: new report makes recommendations. *JAMA* 2005 Dec 21; **294**(23): 2959–2960.
2. Hautamaki K, Miettinen M, Kellokumpu-Lehtinen PL, *et al.* Opening communication with cancer patients about sexuality-related issues. *Cancer Nurs* 2007 Sep–Oct; **30**(5): 399–404.
3. Baker F, Denniston M, Smith T, *et al.* Adult cancer survivors: how are they faring?. *Cancer* 2005 Dec 1; **104**(11 Suppl): 2565–2576.
4. Driscoll CE, Garner EG, House JD. The effect of taking a sexual history on the notation of sexually related diagnoses. *Fam Med* 1986 Sep–Oct; **18**(5): 293–295.
5. Hordern AJ, Street AF. Communicating about patient sexuality and intimacy after cancer: mismatched expectations and unmet needs. *Med J Aust* 2007 Mar 5; **186**(5): 224–227.

6. Singer PA, Tasch ES, Stocking C, *et al.* Sex or survival: trade-offs between quality and quantity of life. *J Clin Oncol* 1991 Feb; **9**(2): 328–334.

7. Dixon K, Dixon P. The PLISSIT model: care and management of patients' psychosexual needs following radical surgery. *Lippincotts Case Manag.* 2006 March/April; **11**(2): 101–106.

8. Stead ML, Brown JM, Fallowfield L, *et al.* Lack of communication between healthcare professionals and women with ovarian cancer about sexual issues. *Br J Cancer* 2003 Mar 10; 88(5): 666–671.

9. Gott M, Galena E, Hinchliff S, *et al.* 'Opening a can of worms': GP and practice nurse barriers to talking about sexual health in primary care. *Fam Pract* 2004 Oct; **21**(5): 528–536.

10. Katz A. The sounds of silence: sexuality information for cancer patients. *J Clin Oncol* 2005 Jan 1; **23**(1): 238–241.

11. Schover LR, Jensen SB. *Sexuality and chronic illness: a comprehensive approach.* New York, NY, US: Guilford Press; 1988.

12. Robinson JW. Sexuality and cancer. Breaking the silence. *Aust Fam Physician* 1998 Jan–Feb; **27**(1–2): 45–47.

13. Annon JS. *Behavioral treatment of sexual problems: brief therapy.* Oxford, England: Harper & Row; 1976.

14. Navon L, Morag A. Advanced prostate cancer patients' ways of coping with the hormonal therapy's effect on body, sexuality, and spousal ties. *Qual Health Res* 2003 Dec; **13**(10): 1378–1392.

15. Matthew AG, Goldman A, Trachtenberg J, *et al.* Sexual dysfunction after radical prostatectomy: prevalence, treatments, restricted use of treatments and distress. *J Urol* 2005 Dec; **174**(6): 2105–2110.

16. Fialka-Moser V, Crevenna R, Korpan M, *et al.* Cancer rehabilitation: particularly with aspects on physical impairments. *J Rehabil Med* 2003 Jul; **35**(4): 153–162.

17. Mulhall J, Land S, Parker M, *et al.* The use of an erectogenic pharmacotherapy regimen following radical prostatectomy improves recovery of spontaneous erectile function. *J Sex Med* 2005 Jul; **2**(4): 532–540.

18. Balint M. *The doctor, his patient and the illness,* 2nd rev. and enl edn. London, Pitman Paperbacks; 1968.

19. Adler NE, Page AE (Eds.) *Cancer care and the whole person: meeting psychosocial health needs.* Washinton, DC: Institute of Medicine; 2007.

20. Lemieux L, Kaiser S, Pereira J, *et al.* Sexuality in palliative care: patient perspectives. *Palliat Med* 2004 Oct; **18**(7): 630–637.

21. Hewitt ME, Greenfield S, Stovall E, National Cancer Policy Board, Committee on Cancer Survivorship: Improving Care and Quality of Life. *From cancer patient to cancer survivor: lost in transition.* Washington, DC: The National Academies Press; 2006.

22. Singer Kaplan H. *Disorders of sexual desire and other new concepts and techniques in sex therapy.* New York: Simon & Schuster; 1979.

23. Masters WH, Johnson VE. *Human sexual response.* Boston: Little, Brown; 1966.

24. Basson R. Women's sexual dysfunction: revised and expanded definitions. *CMAJ* 2005 May 10; **172**(10): 1327–1333.

25. Rieker PP, Fitzgerald EM, Kalish LA. Adaptive behavioral responses to potential infertility among survivors of testis cancer. *J Clin Oncol* 1990 Feb; **8**(2): 347–355.

26. Achille MA, Rosberger Z, Robitaille R, *et al.* Facilitators and obstacles to sperm banking in young men receiving gonadotoxic chemotherapy for cancer: the perspective of survivors and health care professionals. *Hum Reprod* 2006 Dec; **21**(12): 3206–3216.

27. Schover LR, Brey K, Lichtin A, *et al.* Knowledge and experience regarding cancer, infertility, and sperm banking in younger male survivors. *J Clin Oncol* 2002 Apr 1; **20**(7): 1880–1889.

28. Blank TO. Gay men and prostate cancer: invisible diversity. *J Clinl Oncol* 2005 Apr 20; **23**(12): 2593–2596.

29. Boehmer U, Case P. Physicians don't ask, sometimes patients tell: disclosure of sexual orientation among women with breast carcinoma. *Cancer* 2004 Oct 15; **101**(8): 1882–1889.

30. Boehmer U, Linde R, Freund KM. Breast reconstruction following mastectomy for breast cancer: the decisions of sexual minority women. *Plast Reconstr Surg* 2007 Feb; **119**(2): 464–472.

31. McGoldrick M, Giordano J, Garcia-Preto N. *Ethnicity & family therapy*, 3rd edn. New York: Guilford Press; 2005.

32. Nagel J. *Race, ethnicity, and sexuality: intimate intersections, forbidden frontiers.* New York: Oxford University Press; 2003.

33. Perlman G, Drescher J. *A gay man's guide to prostate cancer.* New York, NY, US: Haworth Press; 2005.

34. Sinding C, Grassau P, Barnoff L. Community support, community values: the experiences of lesbians diagnosed with cancer. *Women Health* 2007; **44**(2): 59–79.

35. Mautner Project—Home Page. Available at: **http: //www.mautnerproject.org/home/**. Accessed 11/26/2007, 2007.

36. Brotto LA, Krychman M, Jacobson P. Eastern approaches for enhancing women's sexuality: mindfulness, acupuncture, and yoga (CME). *J Sex Med* 2008 Dec; **5**(12): 2741-2748.

37. Balon R. Depression, antidepressants, and human sexuality. *Primary Psychiatry* 2007 Feb; **14**(2): 42–44, 47–50.

38. Balon R. The effects of antidepressants on human sexuality: diagnosis and management update 2004. *Primary Psychiatry* 2004 Mar; **11**(3): 58–66.

39. Mathias C, Cardeal Mendes CM, Ponde de Sena E, *et al.* An open-label, fixed-dose study of bupropion effect on sexual function scores in women treated for breast cancer. *Ann Oncol* 2006 Dec; **17**(12): 1792–1796.

40. Clayton DO, Shen WW. Psychotropic drug-induced sexual function disorders: diagnosis, incidence and management. *Drug Safety* 1998 Oct; **19**(4): 299–312.

41. Bergmark K, Avall-Lundqvist E, Dickman PW, *et al.* Vaginal changes and sexuality in women with a history of cervical cancer. *N Engl J Med* 1999 May 6; **340**(18): 1383–1389.

42. Ganz PA, Rowland JH, Meyerowitz BE, *et al.* Impact of different adjuvant therapy strategies on quality of life in breast cancer survivors. *Recent Results Cancer Res* 1998; **152**: 396–411.

43. Ponzone R, Biglia N, Jacomuzzi ME, *et al.* Vaginal oestrogen therapy after breast cancer: is it safe? *Eur J Cancer* 2005 Nov; **41**(17): 2673–2681.

44. Schover LR, Jenkins R, Sui D, *et al.* Randomized trial of peer counseling on reproductive health in African American breast cancer survivors. *J Clin Oncol* 2006 Apr 1; **24**(10): 1620–1626.

45. SOGC Clinical Practice Guidelines. The detection and management of vaginal atrophy. *Int J Gynaecol Obstet.* 2005; 88: 222–228.

46. Derzko C, Elliott S, Lam W. Management of sexual dysfunction in postmenopausal breast cancer patients taking adjuvant aromatase inhibitor therapy. *Curr. Oncol.* 2007 Dec; Suppl 1: S20-40.

47. Gelfand MM, Wendman E. Treating vaginal dryness in breast cancer patients: results of applying a polycarbophil moisturizing gel. *J Womens Health* 199; **3**(6): 427–434.

48. Ganz PA, Greendale GA, Petersen L, *et al.* Managing menopausal symptoms in breast cancer survivors: results of a randomized controlled trial.see comment. *J Natl Cancer Inst* 2000 Jul 5; **92**(13): 1054–1064.

49. Schover LR. Is the fault in our steroids or in our selves?. *J Clin Oncol* 2006 Aug 1; **24**(22): 3519–3521.

50. Buster JE, Kingsberg SA, Aguirre O, *et al.* Testosterone patch for low sexual desire in surgically menopausal women: a randomized trial. *ObstetGynecol* 2005 May; **105**(5 Pt 1): 944–952.

51. Shifren JL, Braunstein GD, Simon JA, *et al.* Transdermal testosterone treatment in women with impaired sexual function after oophorectomy. *N Engl J Med* 2000 Sep 7; **343**(10): 682–688.

52. Dimitrakakis C, Jones RA, Liu A, *et al.* Breast cancer incidence in postmenopausal women using testosterone in addition to usual hormone therapy. *Menopause* 2004 Sep –Oct; **11**(5): 531–535.

53. Stahlberg C, Pedersen AT, Lynge E, *et al.* Increased risk of breast cancer following different regimens of hormone replacement therapy frequently used in Europe. *Int J Cancer* 2004 May 1; **109**(5): 721–727.

54. Walker L, Robinson J. Androgen deprivation therapy for prostate cancer: Unique needs of couples. *J Sex Marital Ther.* 2009; In press.

55. Warkentin KM, Gray RE, Wassersug RJ. Restoration of satisfying sex for a castrated cancer patient with complete impotence: a case study. *J Sex Marital Ther* 2006 Oct–Dec; **32**(5): 389–399.

56. Wassersug RJ. Mastering Emasculation. *J Clin Oncol* 2009 Feb; 27(4): 634-636

57. Dennerstein L, Lehert P, Burger H. The relative effects of hormones and relationship factors on sexual function of women through the natural menopausal transition. *Fertil Steril* 2005 Jul; **84**(1): 174–180.

58. Kotz K, Alexander JL, Dennerstein L. Estrogen and androgen hormone therapy and well-being in surgically postmenopausal women [see comment]. *J Womens Health* 2006 Oct; **15**(8): 898–908.

59. McKee AL, Jr, Schover LR. Sexuality rehabilitation. *Cancer* 2001 Aug 15; **92**(4 Suppl): 1008–1012.

60. Beck AM, Robinson JW, Carlson LE. Sexual intimacy in heterosexual couples after prostate cancer treatment: What we know and what we still need to learn. *Urol. Oncol.* 2009; 137-143.

61. Ellis DS, Manny TB, Jr, Rewcastle JC. Cryoablation as primary treatment for localized prostate cancer followed by penile rehabilitation. *Urology* 2007 Feb; **69**(2): 306–310.

62. Köhler TS, Pedro R, Hendlin K, *et al.* A pilot study on the early use of the vacuum erection device after radical retropubic prostatectomy. *BJU Int* 2007; **100**(4): 858–862.

63. Raina, R. Pahlajani, G. Agarwai, A. *et al.* Early penile rehabilitation following radical prostatectomy: Cleveland clinic experience. *Int J Impot Res* 2007 Mar-Apr; 20(2): 121-126.

64. Zippe CD, Pahlajani G. Penile rehabilitation following radical prostatectomy: role of early intervention and chronic therapy. *Urol Clin North Am* 2007; **34**(4): 601–618.

65. Singer Kaplan H. *The illustrated manual of sex therapy.* New York: Quadrangle/New York Times Book Co.; 1975.

66. Schover LR. *Sexuality and fertility after cancer.* New York: Wiley; 1997.

67. Spiryda LB, Laufer MR, Soiffer RJ, *et al.* Graft-versus-host disease of the vulva and/or vagina: diagnosis and treatment. *Biol Blood Marrow Transplant* 2003 Dec; **9**(12): 760–765.

68. Schover LR, Evans RB, von Eschenbach AC. Sexual rehabilitation in a cancer center: diagnosis and outcome in 384 consultations. *Arch Sex Behav* 1987 Dec; **16**(6): 445–461.

69. Jeffries SA, Robinson JW, Craighead PS, *et al.* An effective group psychoeducational intervention for improving compliance with vaginal dilation: a randomized controlled trial. International *Int J Radiat Oncol Biol Phys* 2006; **65**(2): 404–411.

70. Robinson JW, Faris PD, Scott CB. Psychoeducational group increases vaginal dilation for younger women and reduces sexual fears for women of all ages with gynecological carcinoma treated with radiotherapy. *Int J Radiat Oncol Biol Phys* 1999; **44**(3): 497–506.

71. Canada AL, Neese LE, Sui D, *et al.* Pilot intervention to enhance sexual rehabilitation for couples after treatment for localized prostate carcinoma. *Cancer* 2005 Dec 15; **104**(12): 2689–2700.

Section D

Communication issues across the disciplines

Section editor: Ilora Finlay

This section covers the perspective of particular disciplines and pertinent issues that are specific to the needs of each group. The emphasis is not on repeating the basics that are common to all disciplines, but identifying matters unique to each discipline that nonetheless impact on care delivery by the whole healthcare team. The very young and very elderly are included here. Use of the humanities enriches any approach to teaching medicine across all of its disciplines.

Chapter 36

The challenges and rewards of communication skills training for oncology and palliative care nurses in the United Kingdom

Sandra Winterburn and Susie Wilkinson

Introduction and background

In this chapter the authors describe a number of key communication challenges for nurses working in a modern cancer and palliative care setting. An overview of the growing evidence base for communication skills training is given, and these findings are related to experiences of developing and delivering training as part of the English National Advanced Communication Skills Training Programme. Finally, recommendations are made for the future provision of post-registration nurse training by outlining a core curriculum for communication skills.

The past three decades have witnessed a considerable growth in the amount of research directed at examining communication skills in healthcare. Earlier efforts set out to describe the problems in communication between patients and providers, whilst later studies focussed on the skills to be taught and the training techniques to be used. Whilst much of this early work concentrated on the primary care setting [1], subsequent work developed from within the field of oncology. The efforts of Wilkinson (1991) [2], Maguire et al (1996) [3], Fallowfield et al (1998) [4], Heaven (1998) [5] and Razavi et al (1993) [6] are of particular relevance to this chapter, as they focus explicitly on the experiences and training needs of nurses. Development of this knowledge base has meant that the ability to communicate effectively with patients has gained increasing attention, resulting in an acceptance of communication as a core skill for all professions.

The challenges of communicating with oncology and palliative care patients within contemporary healthcare

The patient's perspective

It is recognised that cancer patients, particularly those with advanced disease, have complex needs of a physical, psychological and social nature. Optimum communication with these patients is essential in order both to maximise quality of life and reduce the incidence of psychological morbidity, which is estimated to occur in approximately 23% to 40% of all cancer patients [7, 8].

Studies eliciting patient's views demonstrate that people with serious illness have special expectations of their nurses [9]. They expect understanding, empathy and support and often consider the nurse to be the primary communication link to the medical system and as a result, their future treatment and chances of survival [10].

It has been argued that effective communication should be viewed as central, rather than peripheral, to the actual outcome of cancer treatment [11, 12]. Being the patients advocate, and providing information and emotional support may well result in significant stress reduction and the adoption of adaptive coping strategies, which in turn may lead to improved functioning of the immune system and ultimately affect the course of the disease itself [13–15]. There is a correlation between the extent to which patients feel that they were treated with dignity and respect and their overall perception/satisfaction with the professionals delivering their care [16]. Inadequate communication in itself may be the source of distress for patients and ultimately inhibit psychological adjustment to the cancer or other life threatening illnesses [17]; it has also been linked to adverse effects on patient's compliance with recommended treatment regimes [18].

The changing role of the patient

Within present-day healthcare the expectations of patients and their carers are heightened, with many wanting more detailed information about their cancer diagnosis, prognosis, and treatment options. This has been accompanied by a reduction in the practice of paternalistic medicine and an increased emphasis in involving patients in the decision making process [19, 20].

The last decade has seen an increase of online information regarding cancer and the development of cancer information centres. Whilst studies demonstrate that newly diagnosed cancer patients perceive the Internet as a powerful tool, both for acquiring information and for enhancing confidence to make informed decisions, healthcare professionals do not always share this view [21].

Nurses themselves have been shown to find communication with "expert patients" a particular challenge [22]. This may lead to reluctance to engage in giving any information at all or answering patients' questions, for fear of getting it wrong and being subject to litigation. It is impossible with the complexities of modern cancer care to have a system free from complaints, but at the same time it must be acknowledged that good communication can do much to minimise many of the misunderstandings that currently arise and as a result can reduce complaints [23].

Although many patients within the UK report positively on their experience of cancer care, there are many who claim that they did not receive the information and support that they needed [24]. Patient complaints frequently highlight a perceived failure in communication (an inability to adequately convey a sense of care) rather than a lack of clinical competence as their main concern [25, 26].

These findings are echoed in the most recent UK national cancer survey [16] which found that 21% of UK hospital patients said that they had not received enough information about their condition or treatment and 28% said that doctors sometimes or often talked in front of them as if they weren't there.

The changing role of the nurse

Nurses and midwives comprise the largest staff group in the UK National Health Service (NHS), delivering an estimated 80% of all care. Multiple NHS reorganisations over the past 30 years have aimed to improve the efficiency and quality of the services provided. Within these changes there has been considerable development of the role of the oncology/ palliative care nurse which has impacted greatly on communication with patients [27].

With many of the traditional nursing roles now being performed by health care assistants, it could be argued that there is less time spent at the "bedside" by registered nurses, where an opportunity to build relationships and communicate with patients arise.

Reduction in junior doctor's hours has led to a blurring of roles between nurses and doctors [28]. The extended role of the nurse, which often lends itself to more technical tasks, puts pressure on the nurse in terms of the time to talk, but can also be a source of confusion for patients who feel unfamiliar with the roles and responsibilities of professionals in the "new health service". The more recent growth of clinical nurse specialists, nurse consultants and nurse prescribing has contributed to this confusion for both nurses and patients alike.

Following the recommendations of the 1995 Calman-Hine report [29], tumour site-specific nurses were introduced into UK cancer services, particularly within hospitals. Whilst these nurses were, on the whole, seen as a welcome addition to the multi-disciplinary team, there is a recognised tension between how they may wish to operate and the demands of an overstretched NHS. Increased burden on an already limited number of ward staff, has led to the practice of routinely referring patients to specialist nurses, instead of undertaking regular communication tasks themselves. Such reliance on specialist services has the effect of eventually deskilling/devaluing general nurses, who no longer recognise communication as part of their role or feel that they have the necessary skills to undertake it. Feeling de-skilled in communication has been shown to lead to increased stress, lack of job satisfaction and emotional burnout amongst health care professionals [30, 31].

Nurse training in communication skills

Where health professionals lack communication skills, the solutions lie with undergraduate and continuing education.

(Audit commission) [25]

Pre-registration education

Although considerable emphasis has been placed on teaching communication skills as part of doctors training [32], with 60% of medical schools adopting a systematic approach to communication skills based on models such as the Calgary-Cambridge Guide [33, 34], the same is not true for pre-registration nurse training.

Nurses continue to learn vital communication skills on the job and are dependent on finding good role models to teach them. The ward environment and associated ideology, together with the "atmosphere" created by the ward sister have been shown to be influential on how, and even if, student nurses feel able communicate with patients [2, 35]. Examination of the literature relating to pre-registration nurse training highlights a fundamental problem with teaching communication skills with a tendency to deliver training in a problem focussed and mechanistic way [36]. The now familiar model of large group pedagogic training neither reflects individual learning styles nor the evidence base which support small group experiential approaches to acquiring skills.

Although there are specific standards of proficiency relating to communication laid out by the Nursing and Midwifery Council [37], they are very broad and not mapped against expected competencies at different stages of training or against branche of nursing. As such these are open to interpretation by those designing and delivering the pre-registration curriculum, leading to inconsistencies in teaching across the UK.

Post-registration training

For a number of years we have had clear evidence that specific communication skills training can lead to an improvement in the behaviour of experienced doctors and nurses working in cancer care [6, 38, 39, 40]. Two systematic reviews undertaken [41, 42] also offer support to this argument. A recent multi-centre randomised controlled trial [43] makes a significant contribution to this body of evidence. One hundred and seventy two post-registration nurses were randomly allocated to undertake a three-day course or to a control group (no course). The intervention group improved in all areas of the assessment compared to the control group. Most progress in the intervention group was made in the emotionally-laden areas of the assessment, aided by the use of more facilitating behaviours and less blocking behaviours compared with the control group.

Gratifyingly more than just short term gains have been demonstrated. Skills such as open questions, clarification and picking up verbal cues had been maintained, and improved upon, five years post training[44]. Wilkinson et al [45] evaluated a communication skills training programme delivered to 110 post-registration oncology and palliative care nurses as part of ongoing further education. The mean time since completing training was 2.5 years although some nurses had undertaken training five years previously. It was noted that overall the level of competence when assessing patients was maintained over time, with a significant improvement in the ability to explore in-depth psychological issues.

Development of a National training programme for communication skills training

In response to the views of the public and professionals alike, and influenced by the growing evidence base which indicates communication skills can be taught and maintained over time, there has been a significant national drive and investment on the part of the English Government to develop a national training programme to systematically improve the communication skills of senior health care professionals working within the field of oncology [46, 24, 47]. The Advanced Communication Skills Training (ACST) Programme was initiated in response to the recommendations of the NHS Cancer Plan [46] which stated:

> "there will be new joint training across professions in communication skills.....it will be a precondition of qualification that they (oncology staff) are able to demonstrate competence in communication with patients. Advanced communication skills training will form part of continuing professional development programmes".

(7.11)

Table 36.1 Template for National Model

Template for the national ACST model

Programme aimed at senior health care professionals working in oncology. Consultants, Registrars, Nurses and Allied Health Professions e.g. Occupational Therapist (band 6 and above).

Each workshop/course is

- three days in duration
- delivered in a safe environment away from the workplace
- a maximum of 12 participants
- bound by agreed ground rules
- based on a learner centred agenda
- experiential in its approach
- delivered by a pair of facilitators, at least one of whom is a Department of Health recognised facilitator

Table 36.2 Learning outcomes

The course enables learners to:

♦ Reflect upon and critically appraise own and others communication skills

♦ Demonstrate the skills required to facilitate a structured patient focused, assessment/consultation

♦ Utilise specific strategies required to handle difficult communication scenarios

Table 36.3 Quality Assurance Measures

Monitoring and Quality Assurance Measures

♦ **Learners**
Pre and post course confidence questionnaire
Course evaluation
Verbal feedback

♦ **Facilitators**
Competency based assessment
Evaluation questionnaire

♦ **Actors**
Evaluation form

This commitment was reinforced by the National Institute for Clinical Evidence (NICE) guidance on supportive and palliative care [24], which emphasised that commissioners should ensure that accredited training courses are available for all health and social care staff working with cancer patients.

To make these commitments a reality, the ACST programme has been developed for the NHS by leaders in the field by Cancer Research UK and Marie Curie Cancer Care. The programme is based on evidence showing the effectiveness of three-day workshops that are learner–centred and involve role-play and feedback. It has been piloted and validated and a cadre of facilitators have been trained to deliver these courses to senior health professionals across the country.

Identifying the basic components for an experiential workshop

It has been established that the evidence base strongly supports the development of communication skills training which employs an experiential rather than didactic approach to teaching.

"Knowledge does not translate directly to performance, a further step of specific experiential work is required to acquire new skills and change learner's behaviour"

Kurtz (p63) [34].

With this in mind, what follows is a description of the agreed core components of the national ACST programme. The teaching methods incorporated into the workshops have been based on what we have learnt from the literature as well as being aimed at offering enough variety in teaching techniques to appeal to a broad range of learning styles [48].

Table 36.4 Core components of the ACST programme

Core components and teaching methods for the national ACST workshops

Didactic Components—Two presentations delivered on first day

◆ Evidence Base and rationale for training

◆ The Micro-Skills of communication

Facilitating skills and blocking behaviours. Structure of a patient assessment. Experiential methods

◆ Agenda setting

Learner group sets own agenda for workshop by identifying challenging situations with patients, carers or colleagues. This process aims to make workshop both learner-centered and responsive to specific individual training needs.

◆ Ground rules

Group-generated ground rules to ensure safety and equal participation.

◆ Critique of Trigger Tapes

Group evaluation of the strengths and weaknesses of the communication skills demonstrated in pre-recorded video tapes known to be representative of issues that oncology nurses have identified as difficult, e.g. handling anger.

◆ Interactive demonstration

Agreed clinical scenario role-played by one facilitator and an actor (Patient role). The specific skills and strategies to be tried are suggested by the learner group.

◆ Group exercises

Interactive exercises used to demonstrate specific learning points such as how to give complex information.

◆ Discussion

Debate encouraged around key communication issues.

◆ Role play

Largest component of workshop is video recorded learner centered role-plays based on the communication issue delegate has identified as challenging during the agenda setting process.

Actors playing the role of patient/carer/colleague are seen as fundamental in terms of offering **standardisation** (reproducibility of same issue/content a number of times) and **customisation** (pitching role play to learners individual needs and level of experience).The group is encouraged to imagine how the patient may be feeling. **Patient prediction** is aimed at increasing understanding of patient perspective and encouraging use of empathy.

Experiences of delivering the workshops. What do nurses see as the challenges?

Each of the three day workshops provides nurses with the opportunity to describe, explore and practice what they believe to be the major challenges in communication. A number of core themes repeatedly emerge. These themes are discussed in detail below and are accompanied by recommendations for a core curriculum if nurses are to address these issues in clinical practice.

The challenge of time

Often the primary concern expressed by nurses is a perceived lack of time and space to spend with patients. This raises an important question as to whether the issue is actually time, or rather a lack of communication skills which would enable nurses to engage and disengage confidently with patients in a therapeutic way.

Core content for teaching- Using time more effectively

Although nurses often state that they feel uncomfortable in agreeing a time limit with patients, it is argued that time boundaries can be negotiated in such a way that is inclusive to the patient and enables shared responsibility for time keeping.

Consider the examples below

"We've got about 10 minutes to talk about your pain today – how does that sound to you?"
"As you are new to the unit I would like to undertake a nursing assessment which usually takes about 20 minutes. Would that be O.K?

In using time boundaries in this way nurses are encouraged to rethink the following commonly held beliefs;

◆ **Patients will only tell me their concerns if I spend a long time putting them at their ease.**
Establishing rapport and building relationships is an important task but there is evidence to show that this need not be a lengthy process. [49, 50]

◆ **There are certain issues that it is not appropriate to address in the first meeting with a patient.**
Nurses report that personal issues such as sexual functioning are not appropriate to address in an initial assessment and as a result these issues frequently get overlooked altogether. An ability to provide opportunities for patients to describe what is an issue for them can be taught by increasing nurses awareness of the different questioning styles and the context within which they can be used, e.g. broad open questions such as; **"How is the illness affecting the relationship with your husband?"**

◆ **The longer I spend with the patient the more helpful it is likely to be.**
It depends entirely upon the skills used by the nurse and whether the patients concerns have been addressed and. [5] Short focussed interviews can be just as effective as marathon consultations, particularly for ill patients who tire easily.

◆ **I need to cover everything in this one interview or the patient may not open up again.**
Research indicates that patients hold realistic beliefs about the roles of health care professionals and are on the whole capable of prioritising their concerns and dealing with a few at a time[34].

The challenge of assessment

The workshops have demonstrated a marked lack of structure in undertaking patient assessment concurring with the results of a recent randomised controlled trial examining the communication skills of senior nurses [43]. Nurses consistently reveal a tendency to take refuge in the realms of information-giving and problem-solving, with very little time being spent on eliciting the patient's actual concerns. Transition to problem-solving so early in the interview can be fraught with problems, as we know from the work of Beckman and Frankel [49] which states that patients do not reliably disclose their greatest concern first.

There is also a dilemma around the extent to which the interview should be directed by the nurse, and how much should be patient led. This is particularly true in treatment areas where there is a large amount of information to impart.

Core content for teaching—The importance of assessment

The importance of a regular and rigorous assessment cannot be under estimated. Assessment is an integral part of nursing practice and needs to be taught in a systematic way, paying attention not only to content but also to the manner in which it is structured. Only by assessing the patient's key problems and establishing which of these problems are a concern to the patient, can we hope to deliver care that tailored to meet individuals needs. [51]

Health professionals need to show patients that they are as interested in their psychological, social and spiritual concerns as they are in physical problems.

"They need to interview in a proactive way that makes it clear to patients that it is legitimate to disclose any concerns rather than only those of a physical nature"

Heaven & Maguire [52]

Developing a logical flow in assessments

"If you don't know where you are going you might end up in the wrong place"

Old adage

Nurses need to be taught a systematic approach to structuring their assessments. Recognised frameworks such as the Calgary Cambridge guide [33] have much to offer in this area. An adapted version of the guide is described below.

Introduction

- ♦ Preparation—Ensure enough time and necessary information to undertake assessment.
- ♦ Establish initial rapport by introducing self, state name and role and ask for patient's preferred form of address.
- ♦ Negotiate length of time required for assessment. Briefly outline of the purpose of this task.
- ♦ Attend to "patient's agenda" and ascertain if they have anything in particular that they wish to discuss.

Information Gathering

- ♦ Undertake exploration of the patient's main problems to discover any physical, social, spiritual or psychological concerns.
- ♦ Demonstrate an interest in both the **disease process**- bio-mechanical description of the signs and symptoms- as well as the **illness perspective** (individual description of ill health which is based on personal experience).
- ♦ Check if anything has been missed by asking a **screening** question such as;

"is there something else that you want to tell me about before we move on to looking at how we might help?"

- ♦ Ask patient to prioritise their concerns, so that the most important ones are addressed first.

Information Giving

Information giving and problem solving should occur only when key concerns have been elicited.

- ♦ Give correct type and amount of information in small bite-size pieces, using the patient's language.
- ♦ Check out the patient understanding of the information given;

"Can you tell me in your own words what you have understood from our conversation today".

- ♦ Together with the patient agree a shared plan of action.

+ Closing the session.
+ Thank patient for time.
+ Inform patient of how and who to contact for help if it is required.

The challenge of strong emotions

Nurses frequently describe uneasiness around patients and relatives expressing strong emotions, saying that they feel ill equipped to deal with these situations. Often the fear is that rather than making it better, they will make the situation much worse. A degree of self-protection is also acknowledged as to enquire about the patient's feelings may mean that that the individual nurse has to open themself up to the pain that another person is experiencing.

Core content for teaching—Handling strong emotions

Psychological distress is common among people affected by cancer and is an understandable and natural response to a traumatic and threatening situation.

NICE 5.1 p74. [24]

NICE proposes a four tier model which encompasses the range of psychological skills and expertise upon which patients may draw. It is recommended that senior nurses working in oncology and palliative care should undertake training which would enable them to work at least at the level of being able to screen for Psychological distress and apply psychological techniques such as problem solving.

In addition nurses need to:

+ Be familiar with and suitably skilled in using a range of strategies which will assist them in the task of assessing and managing strong emotions, such as managing anger and the distressed patient.
+ Become familiar with the range of tools available to measure the presence and severity of anxiety and depression.
+ Proactively explore and develop reliable support structures within the clinical setting, such as clinical supervision, peer review, debriefing and critical incident reporting.

The challenge of breaking bad news

Responsibility for breaking bad news at diagnosis continues to sit largely with the medical team. However, the recent growth of tumour site specific nurses and those in diagnostic roles has contributed to a noticeable change in this practice.

Kaye, [53] defines bad news as:

"any information that drastically alters a patient's view of their future for the worse."

It is apparent from this definition that breaking bad news can be considered in a much wider context than the task of informing the patient about the initial diagnosis. Telling patents that discharge home is no longer possible, telling families of imminent or recent death or handling difficult questions such as "is it cancer?" are all examples of nurses breaking bad news in everyday clinical practice.

Nurses consider breaking bad news as one of the greatest communication challenges, knowing that the way that this situation is handled will have a lasting effect on how the news is received and dealt with.

If we get it right the patient will never forget us; if we get it wrong, they will never forgive us.

Buckman [54]

Core content of teaching—Breaking Bad news

A number of authors have proposed frameworks for breaking bad news [53, 55, 57] and nurses need to become familiar with these principles which are as follows:

- Preparation
  Provide a suitable physical environment. Attend to patient comfort and ask if they would like anyone present

- Find out how much the patient already knows

  "Had you had any thought on what it might be?"

- Find out how much the patient wants to know

  "Are you the sort of person who likes to have all the information?"

- Give a warning shot

  "I'm afraid it could be more serious than we thought."

- Deliver the news at the patients pace, in manageable chunks avoiding jargon
- Check out what they have understood and how they are feeling
- Respond to their feelings and invite questions
- Agree a plan of action and arrange follow up

The challenge of denial

A wealth of studies offer mixed opinions as to the adaptive and maladaptive properties of denial, [57–59] which adds to the dilemma of teaching nurses in terms of when and if denial should be supported or tackled. Although denial is often described by them as being functional in the immediate phase of coping, it is often implied that denial is seen as maladaptive when it persists over time. However, what is considered as a "reasonable" time-frame remains unclear.

Core content of teaching—Working with denial

Nurses attending workshops are encouraged to think about denial in terms of whether the patient needs to know. Does the patient have important treatment decisions to make or do they seem distressed by not knowing all the facts? Having considered these issues then the following framework is proposed as a way of exploring the strength of denial;
Looking for a window on denial:

- Present

  "how do you feel things are going at the moment?"

- Past

  "has there ever been a moment when you thought things may not work out?"

- Future

  "how do you see your illness affecting your future?"

- If it appears that the patient does not wish to discuss their illness, leave it there, but assure follow up and further opportunities to talk should the patient want to in the future.

The challenge of collusion

"Patients are not protected by their ignorance, only isolated"

Litcher [60]

A review of the literature by Wilkinson et al [61] highlighted strong evidence to suggest that patients prefer full and open disclosure about their diagnosis with non-informed patients experiencing a greater incidence of psychological distress. Ambiguous or conflicting information was also shown to increase anxiety.

Despite this knowledge there are still individuals who seek to protect other family members from information that they perceive to be harmful. Collusion may also be initiated by professionals who aim to shield patients from the "whole truth" by withholding certain aspects of information.

Core content—Dealing with collusion

The following is a framework for managing collusion:

♦ Recognise that requests for collusion are usually related to high levels of anxiety and a strong need to protect

♦ Focus on the person asking professionals to collude

♦ Arrange a time to meet and explore how they are feeling about the situation

♦ Establish the emotional cost to both family and patient of keeping up the collusion i.e. not being able to openly discuss feelings or plans for the future

♦ Assess what questions the patient has been asking about their illness and pick up on any which suggest the patient may already know what is happening

♦ Inform of plans to interview the patient and assure that information about the disease will only be given if the patient asks or if they are "ready to hear the truth"

The challenge of working with colleagues

There are many occasions in healthcare when differences of opinion arise; some can lead to difficulties in working relationships between staff, either from the same or from differing disciplines. Conflicts may occur when areas of expertise or roles overlap, leading to disagreements about the way forward with care. An example of this is when continuing a treatment is considered inappropriate for certain patients.

Core content—working with colleagues

In these very difficult situations it is considered appropriate to use the breaking bad news strategy outlined in section 5.4.

Conclusion and the way forward

This chapter has addressed a number of key challenges faced by oncology and palliative care nurses when communicating with patients. Using examples from the National ACST programme it has offered suggestions for a core curriculum when undertaking training with nurses. There is however, still much work to be done. The introduction of frameworks such as the Liverpool Care Pathway and Gold Standards Framework [62, 63] have brought with them a new set of challenges for nurses as they encourage proactive communication much earlier in the disease trajectory. It has become clear with the emerging Department of Health End of Life Strategy, that programmes such as the one described here need to be extended to areas other than cancer in order to meet the needs of the wider NHS population.

Courses aimed at testing the feasibility of extending the national programme to conditions other than cancer have already taken place with nurses working with children and young people or heart failure patients. Both courses evaluated well in terms of the teaching methods and the core content described in this chapter and demonstrating noticeable changes between the pre-course and the post-course confidence scales. Ongoing work with work with the British Heart Foundation nurses [64] has led to plans to roll out the programme to all 250 heart failure nurses across the UK.

In considering the future it seems vital that communication skills training for pre-registration nurses, healthcare assistants and nursing home staff need to take place as a matter of some urgency if long-term across the board change is to be achieved.

References

1. Levinson W, Roter D (1993) The effects of two continuing medical education programmes on communication skills of practicing primary care physicians. *J Gen Intern Med*, **8**:318–324

2. Wilkinson S (1991) Factors which influence how nurses communicate with cancer patients. *J Adv Nurs*, **16**, 677–68

3. Maguire P, Boot K, Elliot C (1996) Helping health professionals involved in cancer care acquire key interviewing skills: the impact of workshops. *Eur J Cancer*, **32A**:1486–1489

4. Fallowfield L, Lipkin M, Hall A (1998) Teaching senior oncologists communication skills: results from phase I of a comprehensive longitudinal program in the United Kingdom. *J Clin Oncol*, **16**(5): 1961–1968

5. Heaven C M Maguire P (1998) Relationship between patient's concerns and psychological distress in a hospice setting. *Psychooncology*, **7**: 502–507

6. Razavi D, Devlaux N, Marchal S (1993) The effects of 24–hour psychological training program on attitude, communication skills and occupational stress in oncology: a randomized study. *Eur J Cancer*, **29A**:1858–1863

7. Greer S, Moorey S, Braunch JDR *et al* (1992) Adjuvant psychological therapy for patients with cancer: A prospective randomised trial. *BMJ*, **304**(6828): 675–680

8. Stark D, Kiely M, Smith A, Velikova G, House A, Selby P (2002) Anxiety disorders in cancer patients: Their nature, associations and relation to quality of life. *J Clin Oncol*, **20**(14) 3137–3148

9. Verhallen W.C,Timmermans L, Van Dulmen S (2004) Observation of nurse–patient interaction in oncology: review of assessment instruments. *Patient Education and Counseling*, **54**:307–320.

10. The BAM (1999) Palliatieve behandeling en communicatie: een onderzoek naar optimisme op herstel van longkankerpatienten (palliative treatment and communication: a study into optimism about recovery in lung cancer patients) Houten Bohn Staffleu Van Longhum.

11. Thorne S.E (1999) Communication in cancer care: what science can and cannot teach us. *Cancer Nurs*, **22**:370–378

12. Spiegel D, Sephton S.E (2001) Psychoneuroimmune and endocrine pathways in cancer: effects of stress and support. *Semin Clin Neuropsychiatry*, **6**:252–256

13. Spiegel D, Bloom J.R, Kraemer H.C, Gottheil E (1989) Effect of psychosocial treatment on survival of patients with Metastatic breast cancer. *Lancet*, **8668**:888–891

14. Anderson B (1994) Quality of life in progressive ovarian cancer. *Gynecol Oncol*, **55**: 151–155.

15. Spiegel D (2001) Mind Matters: coping and cancer progression. *J Psychosom Res*, **50**: 287–290.

16. Department of Health (2002) National surveys of NHS patients: cancer national overview 1999–2000. London, DoH

17. Kruijver I, Kerkstra A, Bensing J, Van der Wiel H (2000) Nurse/patient communication in cancer care. A review of the literature. *Cancer Nurs*, **23**(1):20–31

18. Turnberg L (1997) Improving communication between doctors and patients. A report of a working party. Royal Collge of Physicians, London.

19. Degner LF, Kristjanson LJ Bowman D et al (1997) Information needs and decisional making preferences in women with breast cancer. JAMA, **277**:1485–1492

20. Gatterlari M, Buttow P, Tattersall MHN (2001) Sharing decisions in cancer care. Soc Sci Med, **51**: 1865–1878

21. Bass SB, Ruzek SB, Gordon TF, Fleisher L, Mckeown-Conn N, Moore D (2006) Relationship of Internet health information use with patient behavior and self-efficacy: experiences of newly diagnosed cancer patients who contact the National Cancer Institute's Cancer Information Service. J Health Commun, **11**(2):219–236

22. Wilson PM, Kendall S, Brooks F (2006) Nurses responses to expert patients: The rhetoric and reality of self management in long term conditions: A grounded theory study. Int J Nurs Stud, **43**: 803–818

23. Brown RF, Buttow P, Henman MA et al (2002) Responding to the active and passive patient: flexibility is the key. Health Expectations, **5** (3):236–245

24. National Institute for Clinical Excellence (2004) Guidance on Cancer services: Improving Supportive and Palliative Care for Adults with Cancer. The manual NICE, London.

25. Audit Commission (1993) What seems to be the matter? Communication between Hospitals and Patients. HMSO, London

26. Healthcare Commission (2006) The views of hospital patients in England. Healthcare Commission, London.

27. Seymour J, Clark D, Hughes P et al (2002) Clinical nurse specialists in palliative care. Part 3. Issues for the Macmillan Nurse role. Palliat Med, **16**: 386–394

28. Dowling S, Martin, Skidmore P, Doyal L, Cameron A, Lloyd S (1996) Nurses taking on doctors work: a confusion of accountability. BMJ, **312**:1211–1214

29. Calman K, Hine D (1995) A Policy framework for commissioning cancer services: A report by the expert advisory group on cancer to the chief medical officers of England and Wales. Department of Health, London.

30. Wilkinson S.M (1994). Stress in cancer nursing-does it really exist? J Adv Nurs, 20:1079–1084.

31. Ramirez A.J, Graham J, Richards M.A et al (1995) Burnout and psychiatric disorder among cancer clinicians. Br J Cancer, **71**, 1263–1269.

32. General Medical Council (2003) Tomorrows doctors. General Medical Council Publications, London

33. Silverman J, Kurtz S, Draper J (1998) Skills for communicating with patients, second edition. Radcliffe Publishing, Oxford

34. Kurtz S, Silverman J, Draper J (1998) Teaching and learning communication skills in medicine, second edition. Radcliffe Publishing, Oxford

35. Wilkinson S (1992) Good communication in cancer nursing. Nurs standard 7(9) 35–39

36. Chant S, Jenkinson T, Randle J, Rush G (2002) Communication skills: some problems in nursing education and practice. J Clin Nurs, 11:12–21

37. Nursing and Midwifery Council (2004) Standards of proficiency for pre-registration nursing education. NMC publications, London

38. Razavi D, Devlaux N, Marchal S et al (2002) Does training increase the use of more emotionally laden words by nurses when talking to cancer patients? A randomised study. Br J Cancer, **87**:1–7

39. Wilkinson SM, Roberts A, Aldrdge J (1998) Nurse-Patient Communication in Palliative Care: An Evaluation of Communication Skills Programme. Palliat Med,12:13–22

40. Fallowfield L, Jenkins V, Farewell V, Saul J, Duffy A, Eaves R (2002) Efficacy of a Cancer Research UK communication skills training model for oncologists: a randomised controlled trial. Lancet, **359**: 650–656

41. Aspergen K (1999) Teaching and learning communication skills in medicine: a review with quality grading of articles. Med teacher, **21**:563–570

42. Fellowes D, Wilkinson S, Moore P (2004) Communication skills training for health professionals working with cancer patients, their families and/or carers. Cochrane Database of Systematic Reviews

43. Wilkinson S, Linsell L, Perry R, Blanchard K (2008) Effectiveness of a three-day communication skills course in changing nurses' communication skills with cancer/palliative care patients: A randomised controlled trial. *Palliat Med*, **22**: 365–375

44. Maguire P, Fairburn S, Fletcher C (1986) Consultation skills of young doctors. Benefits of feedback training in interviewing as students persist. *BMJ*, **292**:1573–1576

45. Wilkinson S, Bailey K, Aldridge J, Roberts A (1999) A Longitudinal evaluation of a communication skills programme. *Palliat Med*, **13**(4): 341–348

46. Department of Health (2000) The NHS Cancer Plan: A plan for investment, a plan for reform. The Stationary office, London.

47. Department of Health (2007) Cancer Reform Strategy. Crown, Department of Health, London

48. Honey P, Mumford A (2000) The Learning style Questionaire: 80-item version. Peter Honey Publications Ltd, Berks, UK

49. Beckman HB Frankel RM (1984) The effects of Physician behaviour on the collection of data. *Ann Intern Med*, 101:692–696

50. Rowe MB (1986) Wait time: Slowing down may be a way of speeding up. *J Teacher Educ*, **37**:43–50

51. Richrdson A (2007) Holistic Common Assessment of Supportive and Palliative Care Needs for adults with Cancer. Report to the National Cancer Action Team. Kings College, London.

52. Heaven C, Maguire P (1997) Disclosure of concerns by Hospice patients and their identification by Nurses. *Palliat Med*, **11**:283–290

53. Kaye P (1996) Breaking Bad News: A 10 Step Approach. EPL Publications, Northampton

54. Buckman R (1996) Talking to patients about cancer: no excuse for not doing it now. *BMJ*, **313**: 699–700

55. Buckman R(1992)How to break bad news: a guide for health care professionals. Papermac, Basingstoke

56. Faulkner A (1998) When the news is bad: a guide for health professionals. Stanley Thones Ltd, Cheltenham

57. Kubler-Ross E (1969) On death and dying. Macmillan, New York

58. Claxton J W (1993) Paving the way to acceptance. Psychological adaptation to death and dying in cancer. Professional Nurse **8**(4) 206–211

59. Burgess D (1994) Denial and terminal illness Am J Hospice and Palliative Care

60. Litchner I (1978) Communication in cancer care. Churcill Livingsrone, Edinburgh

61. Wilkinson SM, Fellowes D, Leliopoulou C (2002) does truth telling improve psychological distress of palliative care patients? A systematic review. The University of York NHS Centre for Review & Dissemination, Database of Abstracts of Reviews of Effectiveness:*http://nhscrd.york.ac.uk/online/dare/20028114.htm*

62. Ellershaw J, Wilkinson S- Editors (2003) Care of the dying: A pathway to excellence. Oxford University Press, Oxford

63. Thomas K (2003) The Gold Standards Framework in Community Palliative care. *Eur J Palliat Care*, 10:113–115 *www.goldstandardsframework.nhs.uk*

64. Wilkinson SM, Linsell L, Perry R, Blanchard K (2007) A feasibility project to test the transferability of the advanced communication skills training course in cancer and palliative care for senior healthcare professionals working with patients with heart disease. Awaiting publication

Chapter 37

Ambulatory care nurses responding to depression

Anthony De La Cruz, Richard Brown, and Steve Passik

A significant percentage of patients with cancer develop concomitant psychiatric disorders, such as adjustment disorders, demoralization, and depression; and those with advanced disease are a particularly vulnerable group (1). Or not infrequently oncology nurses in the ambulatory setting may develop long and enduring relationships with their patients. They often spend more time with their patients than other health professionals do, so they may be better able to identify problems and provide specific interventions (2). Because nurses are in a key position to identify and respond to a patient's emotional distress, their ability to establish a dialogue about emerging symptoms is invaluable. In this chapter we will present a model of core communication components consisting of strategies, skills, and process tasks. This model will enable nurses to gain an understanding of the patient's experience and assist in the recognition and treatment of depression.

Nature of depression

In a comprehensive review of more than 100 studies of patients with cancer, Massie found a wide range (0–58%) in the reported prevalence of depression spectrum syndromes. Cancer, irrespective of site, is associated with a higher rate of depression than in the general population (3). In spite of the high prevalence, health professionals fail to recognize depression about half of the time (4). Surveys of oncology nurses reveal similar statistics (5). Fincannon found that, although oncology nurses may not always be able to identify specific psychiatric diagnoses, they are skillful in the recognition of psychological distress in patients (6). Patients faced with a diagnosis of cancer experience a broad spectrum of emotions, including depressive symptoms that range from normal unhappiness, to adjustment disorder with depressed mood, to major depression.

Clinical depression is distinguished by its intensity, duration, and the extent to which an individual's functioning is compromised (7). The National Institute of Mental Health, a division of the United States National Institutes of Health, describes a depressive disorder as an illness that involves the body, mood, and thoughts. It affects how a person behaves (e.g. loss of appetite, insomnia), feels about himself or herself (e.g. hopeless, worthless, guilty), and thinks (e.g. inability to concentrate; thoughts about death). These changes are pervasive and affect every aspect of the patient's being.

In diagnosing depression, mental health professionals often use criteria set out in the American Psychiatric Association's Diagnostic and Statistical Manual of Mental Disorders (DSM-IV-TR). Specific criteria help distinguish between major depression, dysthymic disorder, minor depression, and adjustment disorder with depressed mood.

The perplexing symptoms a patient exhibits may leave nurses feeling ill-equipped to differentiate sadness from depression that needs treatment (8). Although the ambulatory care nurse is not

Box 37.1 Criteria for diagnosis of a major depressive episode

Five (or more) of the following symptoms must have been present for a 2-week period and represent a change from previous functioning. At least one of the symptoms is depressed mood (#1) or loss of interest or pleasure (#2).

1. Depressed mood most of the day.

OR

2. Markedly diminished interest or pleasure in almost all activities.
AND at least 4 additional symptoms:

3. Increase or decrease of appetite.

4. Insomnia or hypersomnia.

5. Psychomotor agitation or retardation.

6. Fatigue or loss of energy.

7. Feelings of worthlessness or excessive guilt.

8. Diminished ability to think or concentrate.

9. Recurrent thoughts of death or suicidal ideation.

Adapted with permission from American Psychiatric Association[10]

expected to diagnose a depressive disorder, an understanding of the diagnostic criteria is important in recognizing a patient's symptoms. Box 37.1, adapted from the DSM-IV-TR, summarizes the criteria for a major depressive episode. Depressive disorders have been associated with an increased symptom burden, poorer medical outcomes, and overall decreased quality of life (9).

Risk factors

Numerous physiological and psychological factors increase a patient's likelihood of developing a depressive disorder. These fall into four broad categories (listed in Table 37.1): the cancer and its treatment, the patient's psychiatric history, and social factors (1).

Uncontrolled pain is the most common cause of a depressive episode in patients (11). Many of the medications used to treat cancer can also trigger symptoms—corticosteroids in particular may cause the patient to be emotionally labile, becoming tearful easily, euphoric or irritable, and can lead to a depressive episode. In addition, there are a number of metabolic and endocrine abnormalities—such as calcium, potassium particularly may cause the patient to be euphoric, irritable or emotionally labile, becoming tearful easily, which can lead to a depressive episode or sodium imbalances, and thyroid dysfunction—that are associated with depression.

Barriers to recognizing depression

Patients, family, and even healthcare providers can have a number of misconceptions about the recognition and treatment of depression. One common presumption is that all people with cancer must be depressed. This can minimize caregivers' perception, not only of the degree of suffering associated with depression but also its impact on a person's quality of life, and it frequently leads to the undertreatment of depression (12). Another misconception is that eliciting strong emotions will harm rather than help the patient. Nurses report feeling reluctant to ask

Table 37.1 Factors influencing the risk of depression in patients with cancer

Related to cancer	Related to cancer treatment
Advanced stage of disease	Chemotherapy agents
Tumor type and site	Interferon-alpha
Endocrine abnormalities	Corticosteroids
Metabolic abnormalities	Interleukin-2
Physical symptoms	Barbiturates
Pain	
Increased physical impairment	
Neurologic/paraneoplastic syndrome	
Psychiatric history	**Social factors**
History of depression	Concurrent life stressors
Bereavement experience	Absence of social support
Substance abuse	Family history of cancer
Anxiety disorders	Family history of depression
Psychotic disorders	

Adapted with permission from Springer Science and Business Media (1).

about depressive symptoms for fear of upsetting the patient (13), especially if their training has not equipped them to deal with the patient's psychosocial concerns (14).

In the ambulatory setting, nurses often focus on physical aspects of treatment and the management of side-effects, and avoid emotional issues, possibly because of an unfounded belief that they must 'remedy' distress. Many patients are reluctant to express their sadness or depression for fear that they may burden the treatment team or may even be stigmatized (15). Understanding these factors will assist nurses in identifying and effectively assessing patients at risk of developing depression, and will allow them to be more confident in their ability to discuss these sensitive issues with the patient.

Symptoms associated with depression

Fatigue, weight loss, insomnia, and lack of appetite are somatic symptoms that are often cited as criteria used in establishing a diagnosis of depression in the physically healthy individual. But in patients with cancer, the symptoms of depression, the side-effects of treatment and the symptoms of the cancer are often very difficult to distinguish. Fatigue and lack of appetite may be associated with a chemotherapy regimen or with the cancer itself. Insomnia may be the result of pain or other symptoms related to the cancer.

Inquiring about psychological as well as physical symptoms is crucial to distinguishing between the two and enhancing the recognition of depression. Feelings of worthlessness, hopelessness, excessive guilt, and diminished interest in usual activities are common and reliable diagnostic pointers to depression. A patient who is not depressed may lose hope for a cure but still maintain hope that pain or other distress can be controlled. Hopelessness that is pervasive and is accompanied by a sense of despair and guilt is more likely to represent clinical depression (12). Asking about these feelings is a way to open up a dialogue with patients who might otherwise be reluctant to discuss them.

Patients with depression may be at increased risk of suicide. Asking a patient about thoughts of, or plans for, suicide does not initiate such ideas. On the contrary, they may be relieved if they are asked directly about their thoughts and feel that you are interested in their situation (16). If suicidal ideation is present, the patient should be referred urgently for psychiatric evaluation and, very occasionally, the patient may even need compulsory treatment.

Strategies for responding to depression

Nurses who lack either communication skills or confidence in their skills are more likely to use distancing behaviours, instead of actively participating in helping patients cope with psychological distress (17). Maguire *et al.* conducted a communication skills training workshop with 206 health professionals, predominantly nurses (65%), which involved practice in assessing patient concerns (18). Participants first identified the areas that were most problematic for them (e.g. breaking bad news and eliciting and discussing patients' feelings about their disease), then watched a video comparing assessment behaviours that either promote disclosure or inhibit it, and then role-played specific communication techniques. Before the workshop, each participant interviewed a simulated patient in order to elicit the patient's current problems; after training, each participant conducted a similar assessment with a different simulated patient. Maguire *et al.* reported a significant increase in participants' use of facilitative behaviour (i.e. they engaged in more behaviour that elicited their patient's concerns) and a significant reduction in the use of questions that focused solely on physical issues.

In another study, 61 clinical nurse specialists took part in a three-day communication skills training workshop, after which 29 of them were randomized to receive follow-up clinical supervision for four weeks. Simulated patient assessments conducted before and after the workshop indicated that the training programme was effective in increasing nurses' ability to use key skills, respond to patient cues, and identify patient concerns. Furthermore, the nurses who received clinical supervision were better able to transfer their skills to the clinical setting (19).

Wilkinson and colleagues (20) demonstrated the efficacy of a 26-hour communication skills training programme for nurses in a palliative context. Over a period of six months, 110 nurses participated in the programme, which focused on skills acquisition, knowledge improvement, and attitude change. Overall, when pre-course and post-course audio-taped interactions with patients were compared, these nurses demonstrated a statistically significant improvement in skills in assessing patient's concerns. In a long-term follow-up on this cohort two and a half years later, the nurses responding to the follow-up assessment continued to demonstrate those skills (21). In some areas, notably psychological assessment, long-term improvement was found. In another study, Wilkinson et a1. (22) evaluated a communication skills programme delivered to 308 oncology nurses. After the course, the nurses displayed statistically significant improvements in nine areas of assessment. The most significant improvements were in areas with high emotional content.

Key communication skills and process tasks

Well-developed communication that includes supportive and empathetic responses serves to comfort and inspire patients, and becomes a useful therapeutic intervention (23). Using an evidence-based approach, we developed six core communication strategies to assist ambulatory care nurses in recognizing and responding to a patient's depression. The six strategies were developed in collaboration with groups of ambulatory care nurses and make use of established communication techniques. Skills and process tasks have been identified for each strategy, and

Strategy #1 Make a transition to a discussion about emotional issues

Process tasks:

Ensure that the setting is appropriate:
- seating arrangement;
- be at eye level with the patient;
- avoid interruptions;
- have tissues on hand.

Skill	Description	Example
Make a 'take stock' statement.	Creates a pause in the dialogue to review the prior discussion and seek the patient's permission to move on.	'Now, we have talked about your physical symptoms. But it seems to me that you look sad today. Would it be all right to talk about this?'
Ask open-ended questions.	Questions that allow the patient to respond in any manner they choose.	'So, can you tell me more about how you are feeling?'
Normalize.	Respond with a comparative statement asserting that a particular emotional response is not out of the ordinary.	'It is not uncommon to feel this way a time like this.'

examples of how nurses may approach or respond to a patient are provided. The goal is to gain an understanding of the patient's experience and to assist the patient in seeking treatment. These strategies may also be incorporated into role-playing scenarios or practiced independently as a way to improve communication skills.

These strategies are not meant to be used sequentially; in fact they may be repeated and occur over multiple encounters.

Strategy #1 enables the nurse to initiate a dialogue and will shift the assessment from physiological symptoms to emotional concerns. It allows the nurse to assess the patient's needs and provides an opportunity to educate the patient on issues related to depression. By using open-ended questions, the nurse may be able to elicit information, and even when the concerns cannot be directly resolved, the opportunity to discuss them can be beneficial (14).

Even when patients give cues, healthcare professionals often fail to ask questions that would reveal symptoms of anxiety and/or depression (24). Nurses are in a strategic position to detect psychological distress because most nurse–patient interactions require establishing some kind of dialogue. This allows nurses to assess patients' needs and also provides important information.

Strategy #2 Discuss patient's emotional experience

Process tasks:

- Discuss patient's preference for who is present for the discussion.
- Ask direct questions.

Skill	Description	Example
Encourage expression of feelings.	Express to the patient that you would like to know how he or she is feeling.	'It is important to me to understand how you are dealing with all of this emotionally.'
Ask open-ended questions.	Questions that allow the patient to respond in any manner they choose.	'So, can you tell me more about how you are feeling?'

Strategy #3 Discuss patient's symptoms and risk factors

Process tasks:

– Review patient's experience.
– Explore patient's previous coping mechanism and support.

Skill	Description	Example
Clarify.	Ask a question to better understand what the patient is saying.	'I am not sure I understand what you mean. Can you explain a little more?'
Restate.	State in your own words what you think the patient is saying.	'It sounds like you do not enjoy things that you used to love to do.'
Check patient's medical knowledge.	Ask the patient about his understanding of the medical terminology.	'What do you understand depression to?

Nurses should be direct in pursuing information when patients provide cues that indicate psychological distress. If nurses address sensitive patient concerns with self-confidence, patients may be more likely to reveal their distress (16).

Strategy #3 addresses the overlap between depressive and physical symptoms which complicates the recognition and diagnosis of depression. Many of the classic symptoms of depression may be due to physical illness or depression or both. In discussing symptoms and risk factors, the nurse will be able to identify the patient's needs and respond. It is important to be able to pick up, acknowledge, and explore cues patients have given, particularly about experiences of key symptoms or psychological reactions (25).

Strategy #4 Empathize with patient's emotional distress

Process tasks:

– Provide hope and reassurance.
– Allow patient time to process feelings.

Skill	Description	Example
Acknowledge.	Make a statement that indicates recognition of the patient's emotion or experience.	'It sounds as if you have found all this very distressing?
Validate.	Make a statement expressing that a patient's emotional response to an event or an experience is appropriate and reasonable.	'You have been through a difficult time; it is certainly understandable to feel the way you do.'
Normalize.	Respond with a comparative statement asserting that a particular emotional response is not out of the ordinary.	'Many people feel the way you do in this type of situation.'
Praise patient's efforts.	Make a statement that validates a patient's attempts to cope with his emotional issues.	'It sounds like you have been trying hard to keep things as normal as you can.'

The use of empathy in Strategy #4 is very important in establishing a patient's true feelings (26). Asking questions about the impact of events—and how these events have affected aspects of the patient's life—is crucial in allowing the nurse to empathize with the patient.

Didactic training in the recognition of depression has been found to be effective in increasing nurses' awareness of symptoms (27). A better understanding of depression gives healthcare providers a sense of confidence in their ability to discuss the disorder with the patient. Patients may feel confused and embarrassed and reluctant to discuss emotional difficulties. It is important to try to dispel negative perceptions by explaining the causes and risk factors, as well as the many treatment options available. Providing information about treatment options and their effectiveness may ease the patient's anxiety.

Therapies for depression include a variety of pharmacological and non-pharmacological approaches. Five categories of pharmacotherapy typically used in the cancer setting are selective serotonin reuptake inhibitors (SSRIs), atypical antidepressants, tricyclic antidepressants, psychostimulants, and, rarely, monoamine oxidase inhibitors (MAOIs) (11). Nurses should familiarize themselves with these general categories and the associated side-effects. SSRIs have become the first line of treatment for depression. They are effective and well-tolerated in many patients, and are not as toxic in high doses as the older tricyclic antidepressants (28).

Psychotherapy is also frequently used in combination with pharmacological intervention. Several psychotherapeutic techniques have been successful in treating patients with cancer. Two commonly used modalities are supportive psychotherapy and cognitive-behavioural therapy (28).

Offer the patient a variety of alternatives when discussing referrals. A psychologist, psychiatrist, or social worker can be a source of support. Depending on institutional practice, a counselling service may be available. In addition, numerous community resources may be available and accessible to the patient.

Strategy #5 Educate the patient about depression

Process tasks:

- Provide vocabulary and avoid jargon.
- Explain sources of information.
- Allow the patient time to integrate the information.

Skill	Description	Example
Preview information.	Give an overview of the main points that you are about to cover.	'I would like to discuss some aspects of depression that you may not be aware of.'
Summarize.	Recap the main details conveyed.	'So, let me summarize what we have said -, there are many different approaches to treating depression.'
Check patient understanding.	Ask the patient about his understanding or previously conveyed information or the current situation.	'We spoke about a lot of different risk factors. Can you tell me which ones you may have?'
Invite patient's questions.	Make it clear to the patient that you are willing to answer questions and address concerns.	'Please feel free to call me from home if you have any questions.'

Strategy #6: Discuss whether a referral would be appropriate

Process tasks:

 - Explore the patient's attitude about treatment for depression.
 - Maintain eye contact.

Skill	Description	Example
Express a willingness to help.	Make a specific offer to help or a general statement about being available for future help with a decision.	'If there is anything I can do to help you with a decision, please let me know.'
Review next steps.	Go over with the patient the possible next steps and make sure the patient is clear on them.	'I just want to go over the next steps that we discussed to make sure we both understand the plan.'
Invite patient's questions.	Make it clear to the patient that you are willing to answer questions and address concerns.	'What questions do you have?'
Make a partnership statement.	Convey an alliance with the patient.	'Let's figure out when would be the best time to continue our discussion.'
Offer time to delay a decision.	Reinforce the idea that the patient has time to make a decision about treatment.	'There is no rush. You can decide in your own time whether you want to speak with someone or not.'
Summarize.	Recap the main ideas conveyed.	'Let's summarize the next steps.'

Key questions to ask

In one small study, simply asking the patient if she or he is depressed was shown to be highly correlated with the presence of depression (29). Table 2.3 lists some additional questions that may be used to guide the nurse's assessment and assist in determining if a referral is needed (30).

Table 37.2 Key questions to ask

Question	Symptoms/factors being assessed
How well are you coping?	Mood
How are your spirits? Do you feel down, sad, depressed? Are you crying a lot?	Mood/emotions
Are there things you still enjoy doing, or have you lost pleasure in the things you used to do?	Anhedonia; loss of interest
Are there things that you are looking forward to?	Hopelessness
Do you feel that things are out of your control?	Helplessness
How are your memory and concentration?	Concentration
Do you ever feel so bad that you feel it is not worth going on, maybe wishing you could go to sleep and not wake up again?	Suicidal ideation
Do you ever have thoughts about suicide?	Suicidal ideation
Do you feel exhausted or weak? Do you feel rested after sleeping?	Energy/fatigue
How are you sleeping at night? Do you have trouble falling asleep?	Sleep
How is your appetite? Have you gained or lost weight recently?	Appetite

Conclusion

Establishing and maintaining a dialogue is critical in assessing and responding to a patient's depression. Understanding the illness, its symptoms, and its impact enables nurses to support and promote referrals not only for patients exhibiting signs of depression but also for those at risk. Developing key communication skills is essential to meeting the needs of our patients. Mastering these techniques will enable nurses to relinquish inhibitory behaviours and help their patients explore their feelings, no matter where on the continuum of depression they lie or how distressing they seem. Depression is treatable. Recognizing and responding to a patient's depression can greatly improve their quality of life.

References

1. Breitbart W (1995). 'Identifying patients at risk for, and treatment of major psychiatric complications of cancer'. *Support Care Cancer*, **3**(1), 45–60

2. Lovejoy NC, Matteis M (1997). 'Cognitive-behavioural interventions to manage depression in patients with cancer: research and theoretical initiatives'. *Cancer Nurs*, **20**(3), 155–167

3. Massie MJ (2004). 'Prevalence of depression in patients with cancer'. *J Natl Cancer Inst Monogr*, **2004**(32), 57–71

4. Katon W (1987). 'The epidemiology of depression in medical care'. *Int J Psychiatry Med*, **17**(1), 93–112

5. McDonald MV, Passik SD, Dugan W, *et al.* (1999). 'Nurses' recognition of depression in their patients with cancer.' *Oncol Nurs Forum*, **26**(3), 593–599

6. Fincannon JL (1995). 'Analysis of psychiatric referrals and interventions in an oncology population.' *Oncol Nurs Forum*, **22**(1), 87–92

7. Bowers L, Boyle DA (2003). 'Depression in patients with advanced cancer.' *Clin J Oncol Nurs*, **7**(3), 281–288

8. Block SD (2000). 'Assessing and managing depression in the terminally ill patient. ACP-ASIM End-of-Life Care Consensus Panel. American College of Physicians–American Society of Internal Medicine.' *Ann Intern Med*, **132**(3), 209–218

9. Katon W (1996). 'The impact of major depression on chronic medical illness.' *Gen Hosp Psychiatry*, **18**(4), 215–219

10. American Psychiatric Association (2000). *Diagnostic and statistical manual of mental disorders (DSM-IV-TR)*, 4th edn, text revision. American Psychiatric Association, Washington, DC

11. Pirl WF, Roth AJ (1999). 'Diagnosis and treatment of depression in cancer patients.' *Oncology (Williston Park)*, **13**(9), 1293–1301; discussion 1301–1302, 1305–1306

12. Passik SD, McDonald MV, Dugan WM, *et al.* (1997). 'Depression in cancer patients: recognition and treatment.' *Medscape Psychiatry & Mental Health eJournal* **2**(3), October 17, 2007

13. Valente SM, Saunders JM, Cohen MZ (1994). 'Evaluating depression among patients with cancer.' *Cancer Pract*, **2**(1), 65–71

14. Parle M, Maguire P, Heaven C (1997). 'The development of a training model to improve health professionals' skills, self-efficacy and outcome expectancies when communicating with cancer patients.' *Soc Sci Med*, **44**(2), 231–240

15. Lloyd Williams M, Payne S (2003). 'A qualitative study of clinical nurse specialists' views on depression in palliative care patients.' *Palliat Med*, **17**(4), 334–338

16. 'Practice guidelines for the assessment and treatment of patients with suicidal behaviours.' (2003). *Am J Psychiatry*, **160**, 1–60

17. Sivesind D, Baile WF (2001). 'The psychologic distress in patients with cancer.' *Nurs Clin North Am*, **36**(4), 809–25, viii

18. Maguire P, Booth K, Elliott C, *et al.* (1996). 'Helping health professionals involved in cancer care acquire key interviewing skills—the impact of workshops.' *Eur J Cancer*, **32A**(9), 1486–1489

19. Heaven C, Clegg J, Maguire P (2006). 'Transfer of communication skills training from workshop to workplace: the impact of clinical supervision.' *Patient Educ Couns*, **60**(3), 313–325

20. Wilkinson S, Roberts A, Aldridge J (1998). 'Nurse-patient communication in palliative care: an evaluation of a communication skills programme.' *Palliat Med*, **12**(1), 13–22

21. Wilkinson S, Bailey K, Aldridge J, *et al*. (1999). 'A longitudinal evaluation of a communication skills programme.' *Palliat Med*, **13**(4), 341–348

22. Wilkinson SM, Gambles M, Roberts A (2002). 'The essence of cancer care: the impact of training on nurses' ability to communicate effectively.' *J Adv Nurs*, **40**(6), 731–738

23. Kennedy Sheldon L (2005). 'Communication in oncology care: the effectiveness of skills training workshops for healthcare providers.' *Clin J Oncol Nurs*, **9**(3), 305–312

24. Butow PN, Brown RF, Cogar S, *et al*. (2002). 'Oncologists' reactions to cancer patients' verbal cues.' *Psychooncology*, **11**(1), 47–58

25. Maguire P, Pitceathly C (2003). 'Improving the psychological care of cancer patients and their relatives. The role of specialist nurses.' *J Psychosom Res*, **55**(5), 469–474

26. Maguire P, Faulkner A, Booth K, *et al*. (1996). 'Helping cancer patients disclose their concerns.' *Eur J Cancer*, **32A**(1), 78–81

27. Passik SD, Donaghy KB, Theobald DE, *et al*. (2000). 'Oncology staff recognition of depressive symptoms on videotaped interviews of depressed cancer patients: implications for designing a training program.' *J Pain Symptom Manage*, **19**(5), 329–338

28. Winell J, Roth AJ (2004). 'Depression in cancer patients.' *Oncology (Williston Park)*, **18**(12), 1554–60; discussion 1561–2

29. Chochinov HM, Wilson KG, Enns M, *et al*. (1997). ''Are you depressed?' Screening for depression in the terminally ill.' *Am J Psychiatry*, **154**(5), 674–676

30. Roth AJ, Holland JC (1994). 'Treatment of depression in cancer patients.' *Primary Care and Cancer*, **14**, 23–29

Chapter 38

Social work support in settings of crisis

Carrie Lethborg and Grace Christ

A diagnosis of cancer as a lived experience, is universally stressful. Improvements in anti-cancer treatments and early detection programmes have meant that, cancer is a chronic illness for many. But the initial expectation for most patients is that cancer is life threatening. As a result, this disease provokes fear in many areas of patient's lives, such as fear of uncontrolled pain, isolation, loss of control and loss of self. Indeed, a significant proportion (15–40%) of people living with a cancer diagnosis experience clinical levels of distress (1). The prevalence of such distress can fluctuate throughout each experience as treatments, support and physical factors change.

Social work has a long history of providing support to people living with cancer and their families. The overall objective of the social worker in this setting is to support and equip the patient and those close to them to navigate and adjust to the impact of the disease on their lives (2). However, the very nature of social work as a profession makes it somewhat complex to describe operationally. The International Federation of Social Workers characterizes the profession thus:

- The social work profession promotes social change, problem-solving in human relationships and the empowerment and liberation of people to enhance well-being.

- Utilizing theories of human behaviour and social systems, social work intervenes at the points where people interact with their environments.

- Principles of human rights and social justice are fundamental to social work.

This definition highlights the breadth of the social work focus, whereby the conceptualization of a problem may involve a political and policy perspective, a gender perspective, understanding of life stage and roles, and the client-described lived experience. In addition, the profession aims to focus on the strengths and resources a person brings to their life experiences. Interventions may involve the mobilizing of resources, family counselling, teaching problem-solving skills and multi-disciplinary team consultation. This multi-system and multi-modal focus is, in many ways, unique to social work (3).

The focus of this chapter will be on the social work role during the crisis periods of the cancer experience.

The importance of context, situation and meaning model

The social work perspective views living with cancer as an experience accompanied by a series of challenges as treatment decisions are made, side-effects are endured and relationships strained. For most patients, these challenges are managed with support from loved ones and their healthcare team. However, any one of these difficulties can develop into a crisis or a situation where customary methods of coping do not work and the person living with the disease feels overwhelmed (4).

The starting point, when working with a person experiencing a crisis, is to understand what is happening for this individual. While a crisis by its very nature requires efficient action, it is also important to clarify the issue(s) that have brought about the crisis; sometimes they differ from the presenting problem (5, 6). Acute responses to crisis include helplessness, confusion, anxiety, shock, anger, sadness and panic (7, 8). These responses can occur due to the difficulty exceeding the person's current resources and coping mechanism (9).

The model used here considers three broad aspects of a case: context, situation and meaning. Here, the context includes the specific factors that make up the individual and their life experience, the situation is the reason or trigger for the crisis and the meaning is how the individual experiences the situation. This model can be used in both assessment and intervention in the clinical setting.

The context, situation and meaning model in assessment

Context

The social work assessment considers cancer in relation to the many factors that make up each individual patient's life. It is acknowledged that a person brings to their cancer experience a number of factors that make this experience uniquely theirs such as:

- their age and the particular challenges of their life stage;
- their gender;
- the roles they play in their social and working lives;
- the relationships they have and how supportive or burdensome they are;
- their assumptive-world (10), including general world views and beliefs and cancer specific beliefs;
- the amount and efficacy of their social support;
- their psychosocial history, including past losses, trauma and other significant experiences;
- their cultural background, including beliefs, customs, roles;
- their socio-economic background, including the resources and choices available to them and their political and power status in their community.

The patient is also viewed from within their family context (where family is defined by the client themselves) with a family-centred approach being crucial to comprehensive care (11–13). Indeed, cancer is viewed as a 'family experience', whereby family members are reciprocally affected by illness in each other (14).

Situation

In any assessment, the situation that has brought about the crisis is an obvious concern. However, the presenting problem is not always the actual cause of the crisis and thus assessing the underlying problem(s) is important. Crises in the setting of cancer are seen by the social worker as fluid and ongoing throughout each individual experience of living with the disease. More recently, illness stages or crisis points have been conceptualized as transition points that present the patient and family with new coping tasks. Typically these stages relate to diagnosis, treatment induction and side-effects, treatment completion, recurrence/metastasis, advanced illness, terminal illness and family bereavement.

Particular stresses can be predicted during transitions from one phase of illness/treatment to another. Some of these transitions and their demands are obvious, (e.g. diagnosis, terminal illness) but others are less expected, such as the stresses associated with the successful completion of a treatment process:

As medical advances alter the course of the illness/treatment trajectory, the illness stages also change in intensity, duration and expected outcome. Thus the psychosocial challenge to the patient and family is altered. For example, the ability to control some disease metastases for many months or even years creates more hope for extended life, but also more treatment, side-effects, late effects; this requires that patients learn to live with greater ambiguity of outcome.

In the cancer setting, the presenting situation causing a crisis for the patient and/or their family is often triggered by a transition point. A patient who feels they 'coped well' with their initial diagnosis may struggle greatly with a recurrence, for example. However, the stress of the cancer experience may also trigger relational issues or concerns about finances or work situations that have been a problem for some time. Assessing the situation it thus central to focusing on an intervention.

Meaning

The stress of living with cancer becomes a crisis when the experience is intolerable to the person living with the disease. An important aspect of this experience is the meaning that it has for the individual. Crisis can thus be self-defined, whereby what is a crisis for one person may not be a crisis for another.

Within the assessment, understanding the meaning given to the event enhances the appreciation of why the situation has caused distress and assists in the development of the intervention. This is not to say that the patient is the cause of the distress, but it acknowledges that the way they view the situation is key to understanding their crisis. To give an example, one person might see their diagnosis as a battle they are going to fight with hope and much support around them; they may see themselves as lucky that they have the love and care that they have. Another person, with the same diagnosis and the same resources, might see this as yet another bad thing that has happened to them, a challenge they could never face and feel quite 'beaten' down by their cancer. The difference is partly due to the meaning they give to their cancer diagnosis.

The context, situation and meaning model in the clinical encounter

In the setting of cancer the following clinical goals are important (15):

- ◆ To understand the individual's unique lived-experience of the illness and treatment process.
- ◆ To identify the strengths embodied by the client.
- ◆ To identify the resources available to the client.
- ◆ To identify the specific concerns of the client at this stage.
- ◆ To prioritize concerns with the client into manageable components, so that the most distressing aspects can be dealt with quickly.
- ◆ To identify an agreed upon outcome goal(s).
- ◆ To develop a strategy or strategies to achieve this goal(s).

These goals are achieved using the following processes that are informed by the situation, context and meaning model:

- ◆ Developing a therapeutic relationship.
- ◆ Problem identification and the development.
- ◆ The implementation of strategies to manage concerns.

Each process will be described separately.

Developing a therapeutic relationship

The first of these processes is the same for any clinical encounter. A therapeutic intervention cannot occur without the development of a relationship of understanding between the clinician and the client. Such a relationship, often formed in times of stress and with short time-lines, requires the use of effective and empathic communication and relational skills.

Communication is a two-way process, whereby both parties hear and understand what each other is trying to say. This requires active listening, with the social worker asking the client to describe their perception of the situation and noting their verbal and non-verbal responses. In order to check that they have actually heard this information as the client stated, the social worker feeds back their understanding throughout the encounter. In addition to understanding what the client is saying, the social worker aims to understand the meaning that situation has for each individual.

In order for communication to occur most effectively, it is important that the setting is as comfortable as possible. In general, this requires that there are few distractions, is private, comfortable and that the discussion occurs at a time most conducive to open communication. Clearly, within the hospital or the outpatient setting these factors can be difficult to achieve, but they should remain an aim for each encounter.

Use of self is another communication skill important in joining with the client. The clinician monitors verbal and non-verbal cues and is cognizant of their 'tone'. If the client is angry and loud, for example, the social worker needs to reflect this energy whilst maintaining a sense of calm. If the client is tearful and withdrawn, then a more subdued response is required. The client's reactions and behaviours are not judged as pathological or wrong, but understood as efforts to cope with a highly stressful situation until proven otherwise.

Problem identification

Within the therapeutic relationship the clinician is able to discuss the specific source of the client's concerns. However, this can be a complex process. In the setting of cancer it is often assumed that the client is anxious because they have cancer and, indeed, this is often the case. However, identifying what it is about the cancer that is upsetting, how this is impacting on their life and what specific factors are contributing to their distress, is more involved. This is where the therapeutic relationship moves into a counselling relationship. The aim of counselling is to move a person from a state of unease (such as distress, sadness, anger and so on) to a state of coping (16). This requires, first, understanding the problem at hand and interpreting it to the client in a way that permits the provision of strategies to address this/these problems. The context, situation, meaning matrix is crucial at this stage.

The development and implementation of strategies

In the setting of a crisis it is important to ensure the safety of the client first and then to define the priority issues to focus on in an intervention. The model below offers three broad steps useful in this process:

- ◆ Step1. Ascertain safety of client. Rule out any safety issues for the client or others (e.g. clinical depression, domestic violence, medical concerns).
- ◆ Step 2. Assessment. The assessment process aims to understand, not only the presenting problem but also the wider aspects of the crisis. One of the most powerful skills available to the social worker in assessment is that of questioning. During the clinical encounter there are three kinds of questioning that can be helpful (with examples to illustrate):

Questions to gain information:

> Can you tell me more about that?

> Can you tell me what happened?

Questions to check understanding:

> So, what you're saying is you feel...?

> Can I just check with you, did you say your mother accompanied you to the doctor?

Questions to encourage further understanding of the situation or to test a theory about the situation:

> You mentioned that you have been the carer for everyone in your family and you are not used to needing help. I wonder how this impacts on the way you and your husband have interacted?

> It is interesting to me that you describe yourself as 'not coping' when you have just told me the things you accomplish in a week. Do you see a discrepancy between these two things?

◆ Step3. Intervention development.

Break down the crisis into smaller issues that can be addressed separately.

Work with client to develop strategies to address the issues identified.

Identify barriers and strengths to carry out these strategies.

These steps offer a framework for the clinical encounter that can be used in a crisis. An example of such a crisis in the setting of cancer is that of treatment completion; this framework will be illustrated below using a case example of this particular transition in the cancer experience.

The context, situation and meaning model—a clinical example

Treatment completion is a phase of common distress in the cancer experience. While there is often a sense of relief when anti-cancer treatment is completed, a crisis at the completion of treatment is not uncommon. The assessment of the cancer patient who is in crisis at the treatment-completion phase requires an understanding of their unique context and the meaning they give to treatment completion. However, the situation of treatment completion can differ from patient to patient also. Thus, it is important to begin with an understanding of treatment completion and the range of issues involved with this transition.

The patient's reaction to the end of treatment can vary depending on the reason for completion. It may have been a successful course of treatment, or it may have induced toxic reactions that had meant they had been unable to continue. Even when treatment has clearly been successful, patients may report feeling apprehensive about the decreased contact with medical staff and returning to normal living. Because they expect to feel more positive emotions, patients often think this anxiety is abnormal (17).

Families and partners also may expect the patient to return to normal life quickly following treatment, not realizing that psychosocial recovery often takes much longer than physical recovery. Finally, the healthcare system itself at times has unknowingly contributed to this anxiety by not clearly defining a patient care plan that specifies the terms of follow-up and ongoing access to knowledgeable medical and psychosocial care.

At treatment completion the client may need to:

◆ recognize the fear of having less medical surveillance and develop ways to cope with ambiguity and uncertainty, e.g. by creating a specific care plan with clear access to experts;

Box 38.1 Case study

Marcie is a 45-year-old woman. She is the mother of two teenage children, a daughter aged 15 and a son aged 17. She has been married to Steve for 20 years. Prior to her cancer diagnosis, Marcie worked as a writer for a women's magazine. Steve is an arts accountant.

Marcie completed treatment for early stage breast cancer five weeks ago. She was diagnosed almost twelve months ago and has undergone surgery and chemotherapy.

Aside from a two-week period, when her treatment had to be delayed due to a chest infection, Marcie describes her experience of diagnosis and treatment as 'hard but manageable'.

However, she has recently been having trouble sleeping, having headaches and feeling tearful. She has been fighting with Steve more and more, and wanting to retreat and be on her own. She believes she is not coping. She has asked to see the social worker urgently as she is concerned that her marriage is going to end.

- recognize the need to re-negotiate expectations of support from family and friends;
- normalize the stressful process of redefining self and family following confrontation with a life threatening condition.

The case study in Box 38.1 is from a real clinical situation, using different names and some details to maintain the client's anonymity. Having said this, the crisis situation being presented is not uncommon for people living with cancer.

Using the steps described previously, working with Marcie would begin in the following way.

Step 1: ascertain safety in crisis situation

In the first instance, it was important to ascertain if this situation puts her at risk at all. If she describes an inability to get to sleep and early waking, feelings of hopelessness and helplessness, and a loss of appetite over a 4-week period, for example, then the possibility of depression requiring treatment must be considered. However, if Marcie is still managing most aspects of her life, then the clinician can pursue the context/situation/meaning aspects of this referral.

Step 2: assessment

In talking with Marcie the social worker asked about her life experiences in general, her family, the support people in her life and so on. She also asked some general questions about Marcie's cancer experience, how she felt, what she thought, what she did in response to her diagnosis and treatment. The assessment then focused on the specific issue, of 'marital distress' and her feelings, thoughts and actions in relation to this. Using various kinds of questioning, the information from Marcie's assessment is summarized in Table 38.1.

Thus, Marcie's situation can be described in the following way:

The context of her crisis involves the setting of a cancer diagnosis 12 months ago and the completion of treatment within the past five weeks. In addition, the period of mid-life for a professional woman, mother, wife and friend. Marcie has a history of mild anxiety.

In relation to the situation of this case, Marcie's identified problem relates to marital discontent. The broader assessment of this situation includes post-traumatic stress following treatment completion, role confusion, managing uncertainty, withdrawal from social supports. Marcie also described a number of psychological and physical manifestations of distress. However, she did not have clinical levels of depression or anxiety.

Table 38.1 Information from Marcie's assessment

Context		Situation	Meaning
Gender	Female	Voiced concerns about loss of femininity due to cancer and challenges to her self- image.	'I don't know how to be around others right now, I feel anxious and unattractive.'
Roles	Mother	Reduction of energy, need to discuss role changes within family	
	Wife	Tension within marriage in relation to life threat and role change	'I was always able to manage the juggle of all these roles in the past, and I was proud of it'.
	Friend	Some friends have been there for Marcie but some have not.	
	Professional	Re-integrating back to work is causing anxiety.	
Life stage	Mid-life	Teenage children becoming independent Identity restructuring after confrontation with life threat	'I am not sure who I am right now, I don't know this 'me' and I don't know what is around the corner'
Health	Cancer diagnosis 12 months ago	Treatment completed, but full recovery takes more time for patient and family This was not what Marcie expected she is surprised that she is still experiencing stress related to her cancer.	'I thought it (the stress of cancer) would be over when treatment was over'
Psychological State	History of mild anxiety	Tearfulness, insomnia, worry about the future, describes withdrawing from family and friends. However, clinical depression ruled out at this point.	'Breaking down now means I am a failure, cancer has finally beaten me.'
		Fear of the unknown	'I don't know what my future holds – I feel like I have lost control.'
Client identified problem	Fighting with husband		'We seem further apart than ever – he has no idea what I am going through.'

For Marcie, the meaning of this crisis is that cancer has 'beaten her'. She described this crisis as a 'failure' and stated that she has never failed before. Pre-cancer, Marcie states that she always succeeded in whatever she took on and, though being a working mother at times took its toll, she had enjoyed the challenge and felt she did it well. She also described common feelings relating to living with uncertainty, feeling that her husband doesn't understand the ongoing nature of her cancer experience and not being sure about her life direction.

Marcie is still managing most aspects of her life but describes difficulty in knowing how to live with uncertainty, feeling that her husband doesn't understand the ongoing nature of her cancer experience, not being sure about her life direction and the need to re-define self and family after her traumatic confrontation with mortality.

Step 3: intervention development

Marcie's assessment illustrates how a presenting problem can reveal a range of concerns and issues. It is important to break down these into smaller issues and to work with the client to identify what are the most pressing and urgent concerns at that time. This is necessary both for practical reasons (most social workers have high case loads) and so that the action taken can be done in a manageable way with the client as a partner in the process.

When these issues were separated for the development of an intervention plan, the following points were agreed between Marcie and the social worker:

◆ Marcie is in no immediate danger to herself or others.

◆ Marcie describes feeling anxious about the future and doesn't know how to 'stop worrying'.

◆ Marcie feels that her husband is impatient for her to 'get back on with life' and that he doesn't understand her.

◆ Marcie is re-thinking her vocation as the time for her to resume work draws closer.

Prioritizing these issues, the problems, along with the identified barriers and strengths brought to this case, were identified in planning this intervention (see Table 38.2).

While couple therapy could have been offered to Marcie as an initial intervention, given the wider context and meaning it becomes clear that a range of interventions would be beneficial. It was likely that an effective intervention could involve counselling that focuses on cognitive, psychological and social aspects of managing uncertainty and post-traumatic response, as well as some couple counselling.

In fact, the intervention with Marcie took four sessions in total, although she rated a drop in her level of distress by half after session one. Marcie attributed her reduced distress to being able to better understand the process both she and her husband had been through since diagnosis and feeling that her current stress was normal and did not mean she had 'failed'. The sessions with Marcie are shown in Table 38.3.

It is important to point out that, while each step in the social work clinical encounter has been described here in detail, the process itself can occur quite quickly. The social worker aims to develop a realistic time-line to manage the identified problems that take into account both social

Table 38.2 Issues considered in planning intervention

Identified Issues	Focus of intervention
Anxiety about uncertainty.	Normalizing reaction to uncertainty. Cognitive skills to challenge automatic negative thoughts.
Marital tension.	Couple counselling to enable a sharing of the experience of living with cancer and of caring for someone with cancer.
Life review.	Goal-setting/meaning based intervention to review life goals and begin to plan for future goals.
Barriers to action plan.	Marcie describes herself as a 'worrier' for as long as she can remember and as having to have control over her life. She feels it will be hard to learn to 'let go' of these tendencies.
Strengths that will impact on action plan.	Marcie describes her marriage as being 'strong' in the past and that this is a surprise to her that they would be fighting now. She is sure her husband will come to counselling. She has been a successful woman in all roles in her life and is willing to learn how to overcome the current difficulties she is having.

Table 38.3 Intervention provided

Session One	Aimed to develop the therapeutic relationship, whereby Marcie felt safe enough to share her concerns and to identify the situation that had caused the crisis and the severity of her experience. It also aimed to assist Marcie to make sense of her situation in order to 'normalise' her distress.
Session Two	Aimed to work with the specific issues identified and in this case included teaching some cognitive skills, such as challenging automatic negative thoughts, problem-solving and relaxation techniques.
Session Three	Aimed to work on goal-setting for the future, including identifying life goals and purpose and to review the use of skills developed to date.
Session Four	A joint session with Marcie and her husband to discuss both their 'journeys' through cancer and for each other to hear the differences in their experiences and perceptions. This session resulted in a better understanding of each other's experiences and a joining together to begin to re-consider goals and future plans.

work resources and extent of the crisis. In Marcie's case, she was seen on the same day as her concerns were raised during a routine follow-up medical consultation.

This clinical encounter has been illustrated in this chapter as proceeding from the development of a therapeutic relationship to problem identification and intervention development. Of course this process is not always linear and the skills used to join with the client are required throughout the clinical encounter. However, the model presented illustrates the need for a comprehensive assessment before intervention development can begin. Interventions that are clinician-led and do not adequately take into account the client's perspective are going to be less effective than those that include the client as a 'partner' in the therapeutic relationship. Equally limiting are interventions that focus on the client as separate to their context (i.e. family, cultural background, gender, life stage, etc.).

The social work intervention in the setting of a crisis brought about by the cancer experience aims to fully understand the client and their specific concerns and to tailor interventions accordingly. Such an approach requires ongoing communication throughout the clinical encounter and an understanding of the complexity involved with living with this disease.

References

1. Zabora, J., BrintzenhofeSzoc, K., Jacobsen, P., *et al.* (2001). A new psychosocial screening instrument for use with cancer patients. *Psychosomatics*, **42**(3), 241–246.
2. Christ, G. (1991) Principles of oncology social work In A. Holleb, D. Fink, G. Murphy (eds.), *American Cancer Society Textbook of Clinical Oncology* (pp. 594–605). Atlanta, GA: American Cancer Society.
3. Hepworth, D., Rooney, R., Larson, J. (2002). *Direct Social Work Practice: Theory and Skills*, 6th edition. Pacific Grove, CA: Books/Cole.
4. Roberts, A. (2000). An overview of crisis theory and crisis intervention. In: Roberts, A (ed.). *Crisis Intervention Handbook: Assessment, Treatment, Research*. New York: Oxford University Press.
5. Parad, H. (1971). Crisis intervention. In R. Morris (ed), *Encyclopedia of Social Work*, 16th edition (pp 196–202. 202). New York: National Association of Social Workers.
6. Scheyett, A. M. (2002). Approaching complex cases with a crisis intervention model and teamwork: a commentary. *Journal of Genetic Counseling*, 11 (5), 377–382.
7. Golan, N. (1978) *Treatment in Crisis Situations*. New York: Free Press.
8. Lillibridge, E. M., Klukken, P. G.(1978) *Crisis Intervention Training*. Tulsa, OK: Affective House.

9. James, K. J., Gilliland, B. E. (2001) *Crisis Intervention Strategies.* Pacific Grove, PA: Brook/Cole.

10. Janoff-Bulman, R.(1989) Assumptive worlds and the stress of traumatic events: applications of the schema construct. *Social Cognition. Special Issue: Stress, coping, and social cognition.,* **7**(2), 113–136.

11. Quinn, W. H., Herndon, A. (1986). The family ecology of breast cancer. *Journal of Psychosocial Oncology,* **4**, 95–118.

12. Pederson, L. M., Valanis, B. G. (1988). The effects of breast cancer on the family: a review of the literature. *Journal of Psychosocial Oncology,* **6**, 95–118.

13. Zabora, J. R., Smith-Wilson, R., Fetting, J. H., Enterline, J. P. (1990). An efficient method for psychosocial screening of cancer patients. *Psychosomatics,* **31**(2),192–196.

14. Northouse, L. (1984). The impact of cancer on the family. *International Journal of Psychiatry in Medicine,* **14**, 215–242.

15. Christ, G. (1993) Psychosocial tasks throughout the cancer experience In N. Stearns, J. Herman, M. Lauria, P. Fogelberg (eds.), *Oncology Social Work: A Clinician's Guide* (pp. 79–99). Atlanta, GA: American Cancer Society.

16. Ragg, D. (2001). *Building Effective Helping Skills: The Building Effective Helping Skills: The Foundation of Generalist Practice.* Boston, MA: Allyn and Bacon.

17. Lethborg C, Kissane D (2003), 'It doesn't end on the last day of treatment': a psycho-educational intervention for women who have completed adjuvant treatment for early stage breast cancer. *Journal of Psychosocial Oncology,* **21**(3), 25–41.

Chapter 39

Communication in cancer radiology

Kimberly Feigin and Laura Liberman

Introduction

Diagnostic radiologists are often the first to know of a patient's medical abnormality, diagnosis, disease progression, or response to treatment. Traditionally, radiologists have been primarily consultants to referring physicians, reporting results of radiologic examinations to ordering physicians, who then relayed the information to patients. In recent years, radiology has evolved to include more procedures that bring radiologists into direct contact with patients. This is particularly true in certain subspecialties of radiology, such as interventional radiology and breast imaging. This chapter will explore current concepts in communication in radiology, often using the subspecialty of breast imaging as a model.

Communicating results of screening and diagnostic radiologic examinations

Communication with referring physicians

Communication with referring physicians is the most common type of communication a radiologist undertakes, usually in the form of an official written report. In the age of PACS (picture archiving and communication systems), wherein diagnostic images are readily available to all caregivers, a radiologist's interpretive report must be accurate, meaningful, and timely in order maximize the radiologist's contribution to patient care. Descriptions of radiologic findings must be accompanied by the radiologist's opinion of their significance, such as a specific diagnosis or differential diagnosis, so that the implications for patient management are clear to the referring physician. A purely descriptive, vague, or non-committal report is not only of little clinical value, it may lead to delay in diagnosis or treatment and leave the radiologist vulnerable to medical malpractice litigation (1, 2). Uniformity in radiology reporting is also necessary to convey a clear meaning to the recipient (3, 4). While the American College of Radiology (ACR), in its practice guideline for communication in diagnostic radiology, recommends that a radiology report should suggest 'follow-up or additional diagnostic studies to clarify or confirm the impression…when appropriate'(1), such a suggestion must be carefully worded in order to prompt appropriate patient management without unnecessarily constraining the referring physician (5).

In breast imaging, the need for uniformity and clarity in radiology reporting, along with the need for consistency of management recommendations, has resulted in the creation of the ACR's Breast Imaging Reporting and Database System (BI-RADS). BI-RADS is a lexicon and reporting format created to 'standardize (breast imaging) reporting, reduce confusion in breast-imaging interpretations and facilitate outcome monitoring' (6). All BI-RADS reports conclude with an overall assessment that assigns a precisely defined numerical classification to any abnormality and recommends the most appropriate course of action (see Table 39.1). Studies have shown

Table 39.1 Breast imaging reporting and data system (BI-RADS) assessment categories

Category	Definition	Recommendation
0	Incomplete	Needs additional imaging studies (as specified by radiologist)
1	Normal	Routine annual follow-up
2	Benign finding	Routine annual follow-up
3	Probably benign finding	Short-term follow-up (6 months)
4	Suspicions; biopsy should be considered	Biopsy
5	Highly suggestive of malignancy; appropriate action should be taken	Biopsy
6	Proven cancer	Management as clinically appropriate

Categories as defined in reference (6).

significant improvement in interpretive skills (7) and inter-observer agreement (8) among radiologists following training in the proper use of BI-RADS, suggesting that other radiology subspecialties might benefit from similar standardization of reporting.

In addition to routine reporting of imaging findings, the *ACR practice guideline for communication of diagnostic imaging findings* outlines steps that a radiologist must take when an imaging finding suggests a need for urgent intervention, when he or she discovers a significant and/or unexpected imaging finding, or when there is a discrepancy between a preliminary and final report. In such cases, in addition to a routine written report, the radiologist must directly communicate these findings to the referring clinician or his or her representative 'in a manner most likely to reach the attention of the treating or referring physician in time to provide the most benefit to the patient', such as in person or by telephone (1, 9). Documentation of this type of direct communication is also required (1). The European Association of Radiologists and the United Kingdom's Royal College of Radiologists have adopted similar guidelines (10), emphasizing their global importance.

Communication errors in radiology reporting result in substantial morbidity and mortality (11). For example, the Physician Insurers Association of America (PIAA) 1997 and 2002 claims studies revealed hundreds of claims and lawsuits with adverse patient outcomes that were the result of miscommunications in radiology (12, 13). Indeed, communication errors or delays are among the top five reasons radiologists are sued for medical malpractice (12, 14, 15); these errors are costly (13). In an analysis of medical liability cases in the United States from 1999 to 2003, radiologist defendants were held responsible for communication failures in 25 cases, over which the average indemnification (shared by co-defendants) was US $1.9 million (12).

Occasionally, clinicians will request an informal verbal 'curbside' radiology consultation. These types of consultations may expedite patient care, however the radiologist should engage with prudence. These consultations are frequently requested in an environment in which prior studies and reports are not available, patient history is incomplete, and viewing conditions are suboptimal. They require additional skills on the part of the radiologist, such as effective time management, a professional and collegial manner, and the ability to summarize pertinent findings instantly (16, 17), and the time and effort to perform these types of consultations are not financially compensated. Verbal consultations should be documented whenever possible to protect the radiologist from any potential inaccuracies recorded by the recipient (1, 12).

Communication with patients

Partially in response to malpractice lawsuits alleging failure to communicate urgent or significant radiographic abnormalities, a trend has recently emerged for radiologists to communicate results directly to patients. In several legal cases since in the 1990s, courts ruled that, occasionally, a radiologist has a duty to communicate abnormal findings directly to the patient (14, 15, 18). The *ACR practice guideline for communication of diagnostic imaging findings* states that, 'in certain circumstances, the radiologist may feel it is appropriate to communicate the findings directly to the patient' (1). The ACR's practice guideline suggests that this is particularly true when a patient is self-referred or is referred by a third party, such as an insurance company, employer, or federal benefit programme, and unexpected or serious findings result (1).

This trend of direct radiologist–patient communication has dovetailed with patients' increasing desire to participate in their own healthcare decision-making processes. Most patients prefer to hear radiology results from their radiologists upon completion of the imaging procedures, rather than waiting to hear their results at another time or from their own referring physicians, whether the results are normal or abnormal (19–23).

Additional advantages of the practice of communicating radiology results directly to patients include timelier reporting and the presence of a safeguard, should the referring physician fail to receive or respond to the written report. A radiologist is the physician in the best position to understand the meaning of the radiology test result in the context of the test's limitations and to suggest alternate imaging tests, if warranted. Furthermore, radiologists' direct communication with patients may improve radiologists' relationships with patients and 'enhance the visibility, status, and role of radiologists in the healthcare system' (24–26).

Disadvantages of direct radiologist–patient communication are also numerous. Radiology departments are typically not ideal places for delivering bad news, providing few supports for patients in such circumstances. In fact, the radiologist is often physically isolated from the patient in a reading room or at a clinical workstation. The extreme example of this is in transcontinental teleradiology. Also, time spent in consultation with patients and families detracts from time available to interpret radiology exams, and is, therefore, expensive (25, 27); yet patients are not willing to pay additional fees for this service (27).

Patients are only temporarily in the care of radiologists, who may not know relevant parts of the patient's history or other clinical findings. Radiologists are not usually responsible for clinical management and may not even know what should, or can, be done to treat a given patient, but patients often expect immediate therapeutic recommendations (28, 29). Referring physicians may not be adequately forewarned of the results and disclosure of them to the patient, and therefore may not be prepared to receive an urgent call from a distressed patient. Most referring physicians, therefore, want to know of a disclosed abnormal result as soon as possible and many prefer to tell the patient themselves (28, 30, 31). Studies have shown that patients' understanding of radiology results is suboptimal (32–34) and that wording of such discussions is important (35). For all of these reasons, some patients prefer to hear results from their own physician, with whom they generally have an established relationship (28).

Reporting of mammography results is a model for direct radiologist–patient communication. Many patients are self-referred for screening mammography, so that the radiologist must assume responsibility for communicating results to patients and for arranging for appropriate follow-up. In 1999, the United States Congress enacted the Mammography Quality Standards Act (36), which mandated written notification of mammography results directly to patients within 30 days of the examination. Since its implementation, this practice has virtually eliminated US medical malpractice lawsuits alleging failure of communication of mammographic findings (14, 15).

Radiologists who interpret mammograms, and patients themselves, generally prefer direct reporting of mammography results (25, 32, 37), and most patients prefer immediate in-person reporting of results of screening mammography to mailed written reports (27, 38, 39). Most patients (78%) are willing to wait an additional 30–60 minutes at the time of screening mammography for an immediate result, but the majority (89%) are not willing to pay extra for this service (27). Most women are willing to accept delayed reporting for screening mammograms if double interpretation is to be performed (40), suggesting that if patients understand that there is an advantage to be gained in waiting for results, they will better tolerate a delay.

In any case, when radiologists give results directly to patients, they must do so in a compassionate, yet unequivocal, way (41). Physician affect is important and should accurately reflect the seriousness of the situation, while remaining as encouraging and optimistic as possible. In one study, when ambiguous mammography results were the same, women receiving results from a perceptibly worried physician recalled less information, perceived the clinical situation as more severe, and were more anxious (by self-report and higher pulse rates) than when their physician did not seem worried (42). Radiologists should use plain terms in place of medical jargon and disclose information at a pace commensurate with the patient's ability to absorb it. Clarity of reporting is crucial for patient satisfaction, to guarantee patient understanding, and to ensure appropriate follow-up (34, 39, 43–45). Studies have shown that patient-reported results are least likely to agree with radiologist-documented results when results are abnormal (32, 33, 46).

Communicating with patients about image-guided percutaneous interventional procedures

Radiology has evolved to encompass minimally invasive image-guided diagnostic and therapeutic interventional procedures that bring radiologists into direct contact with patients in a dynamic similar to that of surgeons and their patients. Interventional oncology, in particular, is an arena in which the use of sophisticated cross-sectional imaging techniques, such as computed tomography (CT) and magnetic resonance (MR) imaging, has revolutionized image-guided tumour ablation, and molecular/functional imaging techniques promise even better tools for the future (24, 47). In breast imaging, percutaneous image-guided large-core breast biopsy performed by radiologists has become a mainstay of breast diagnosis (48). Radiologists who perform interventional procedures must be prepared to obtain informed consent for diagnostic and therapeutic image-guided procedures, to discuss their potential complications, and to discuss results of biopsies with patients.

Obtaining informed consent for an interventional radiology procedure entails discussing details of the proposed treatment, possible additional interventions that might be required during the course of the planned procedure, common and serious side-effects, the probability of success, and alternative treatment options (49). Additionally, patients are interested specifically in what to expect in terms of pain and potential disfigurement, and they want to know when they can expect to receive the results of the procedure (50). It is helpful if the patient is properly prepared, perhaps even given written information, about the procedure in advance (49, 51); also, whenever feasible, the radiologist performing the procedure should personally obtain the patient's informed consent (49). Clinic nurses and/or patient navigators can be very helpful in providing information, scheduling appointments, and giving emotional support to patients prior to their undergoing interventional radiology procedures (50, 52)

Principles for discussing biopsy results with patients are similar to principles for discussing complications or suboptimal outcomes of image-guided procedures. The Health Insurance Portability and Accountability Act (HIPAA) requires that results must be discussed directly and privately with patients, unless a patient has explicitly requested that results be given to a designated representative (53). Delivering biopsy results to patients is ideally done in person, but logistical considerations often prevent this, as patients may live far from their medical facilities, and scheduling return appointments routinely for all biopsy patients may be unduly burdensome for both patients and radiology facilities. In breast imaging, telephoning results of percutaneous core biopsies is often more expeditious and has been shown to be well-tolerated by patients, whether results are positive or negative (54). Telephoning results is preferable to mailing written results, as it is faster, women are more likely to understand the results (33), and women have an immediate opportunity to ask questions. Also, the patient can absorb results in private and prepare additional questions for subsequent appointments. Disadvantages of telephoning results are that the call may come at an unexpected or inconvenient time, particularly among mobile phone users, and that non-verbal communication cues are not available to either the patient or the radiologist. When radiologists discuss news with patients over the phone, therefore, they must first confirm that the patient is receiving the call at a time and place in which he or she can speak freely. As patients' emotional reactions may be difficult to discern without the benefit of non-verbal cues, radiologists must also ask patients to verbalize their responses and must be aware of emotional cues provided via paralanguage, such as tone, speech pattern, pauses, and pitch (55).

Whether or not a biopsy result is positive for cancer, the patient's understanding of the results must be optimized. First, radiologists should give results in the patient's preferred language. Medical interpreters are invaluable for this purpose (56). Second, radiologists must use unambiguous lay terms. For example, patients may confuse the meaning of 'positive' (abnormal) and 'negative' (normal) findings, since in medicine the meanings of these words are the opposite of their colloquial connotations (39). Third, radiologists should establish the patient's expectation of the result before giving information. Fourth, they must ask patients to verbalize their understanding of results to confirm their comprehension, and continue to present information to patients in alternate ways until the process of checking back confirms that adequate understanding is achieved (44).

When a biopsy yields cancer, clear and supportive communication is particularly important. Among breast cancer patients, for example, this diagnostic consultation is a highly memorable event (57). In one study of breast cancer patients, patients' perceptions of a physician's emotional supportiveness during the diagnostic consultation correlated with better later psychological adjustment to their illness, as measured by fewer cancer-related post-traumatic stress disorder symptoms, less depression, and less general distress (57). In another study of breast cancer patients, a variety of quality-of-life measures were significantly lower, even four years following diagnosis, among women over age 50 who reported receiving unclear or incomplete information at the time of diagnosis (58). Patients perceive radiologists to be supportive when their manner is unhurried, they invite and attend to patients' comments and questions, affirm patients' feelings, respect patients as individuals, focus on the positive, and are available to patients (41, 52, 59–61). Radiologists must offer hope, but avoid false reassurances. Specifically, they should mention any good prognostic features of a given lesion, such as small size, low histologic grade, or unifocality, but should not mislead the patient, as this may ultimately undermine trust (56, 59). The radiologist should give the patient an idea of what to expect in the future and an immediate concrete plan, such as a referral to a surgeon with a phone number to call to schedule an appointment. The radiologist should conclude the consultation by providing his or her own contact information and, if possible, contact information for an additional support staff member in case questions or problems arise (41, 52).

When a biopsy yields benign results, the radiologist should convey the good news first to relieve anxiety, so that patients will be better able to concentrate, and then explain results in more detail (60). One study found that patients undergoing breast biopsies that yielded benign results commonly sought information about three topics in particular, namely; the nature of their benign breast disease, e.g. 'what is fibrocystic [change]?'; the risk of breast cancer associated with benign breast disease, e.g. 'am I more prone to breast cancer now that I have [fibrocystic change]?'; and tests required to diagnose and treat benign breast disease. e.g. 'do I need follow-up tests if the biopsy is negative [for cancer]?' (50).

Special considerations in communicating radiology results

Cultural and sociodemographic factors

Physician–patient communication in radiology must be tailored to meet the needs of the individual patient, and cultural and sociodemographic factors must be considered. For example, many Navajo Native Americans perceive discussion of negative information to predict a bad outcome, so discussions with these patients must be adapted to respect their wishes (56, 61). Radiologists should familiarize themselves with cultural beliefs among patients in their practices and with findings in the literature that may help guide communications. Relatively less well-educated women, for example, have been found to experience greater levels of anxiety prior to breast biopsy (62) and to demonstrate persistent anxiety and lack of reassurance following benign diagnosis of breast symptoms, suggesting that these women may benefit from more detailed consultations or additional support services (63). It is unclear why certain minority populations have been shown to demonstrate relatively poor understanding of radiology results. In breast imaging, studies have shown a trend that African-Americans, Latinos, and Asians are more likely than white referents to report receipt of confusing or conflicting information at mammographic screening, even when language barriers and socioeconomic factors are taken into account (33, 46, 64). African-American women, whose breast cancers are diagnosed at a later stage on average than their white counterparts' breast cancers and who, therefore, have relatively high breast cancer mortality rates (65–67), were found to be more than 2.5 times more likely to complete timely and appropriate follow-up of abnormal mammograms when they reported that clinic staff informed them of what was to happen after the mammogram (45), confirming that clear communication with patients is crucial for screening efficacy. Younger women are also less likely to report a complete understanding of mammography results than older women (64) and are more likely to report experiencing significant stress upon receipt of an abnormal mammography result (68–70). Special care must be taken to consider patients' specific needs, to ensure their understanding of results, and to eliminate barriers to compliance, in order to improve healthcare outcomes (61, 71, 72).

Uncertainty in radiology

An issue that arises frequently in physician–patient communication, but is particularly relevant in radiology, is the discussion of uncertainty. Often, patients value their physicians' expertise above other characteristics and skills (59), so a great challenge for physicians is to explain what they do not know, while still inspiring their patients' trust. Uncertainty abounds in radiology, in that imaging examinations often have limited specificity and sensitivity.

The discovery of imaging findings of questionable clinical significance is common in radiology, particularly on screening examinations. Non-specific radiology results often lead to the performance of additional diagnostic tests, potentially fostering patient anxiety and/or confusion (15, 64). An empathetic explanation of the limitations of a given radiology examination is often required.

In breast imaging in particular, false-positive screening mammograms may lead to elevated levels of distress and anxiety that may even persist long-term (73), and they lead to increased utilization of healthcare resources, both for breast-related and non-breast-related reasons (74). Such false-positive examinations may breed less anxiety for patients undergoing mammographic screening when patients have been forewarned of the possibility of a recall or false-positive result (39), when radiologists use false-positive examination encounters with patients as 'teachable moments' to personally educate patients (60, 75), and when follow-up examinations can be performed promptly (41, 69, 76). Some authors suggest that this anxiety reduction in turn may lead to improved future compliance with follow-up recommendations (45, 75, 77, 78).

Not infrequently, limited radiological specificity results in the need for delayed follow-up imaging to assess for change over time in a relatively benign-appearing lesion. For example, renal cysts imaged on CT may receive a Bosniak IIF classification for a mild degree of complexity. Bosniak IIF lesions are likely to be benign, but require follow-up CT imaging to assess for stability over time (79). Similarly, a breast lesion on imaging may receive a BI-RADS assessment category of '3: probably benign' when a radiologist judges it to have a less than approximately 2% probability of malignancy. According to BI-RADS guidelines, the radiologist may recommend imaging surveillance of such a lesion over time instead of an immediate biopsy in an attempt to avoid performing a biopsy that is likely to be benign, thereby limiting attendant morbidity and cost (80). Patients may suffer adverse psychological consequences from waiting for follow-up (81); however, at least one study suggests that stress levels are lower among women undergoing short-interval follow-up mammography, than among women undergoing immediate core biopsy for such breast lesions that are probably benign (68). One study showed that women whose mammograms receive a classification of probably benign are less likely to understand their results than women with suspicious results requiring biopsy (33). Radiologists may clarify patients' results and allay patients' anxiety by explaining how their imaging findings fit known criteria for categorizing lesions as probably benign and by emphasizing the safety and effectiveness of radiologic surveillance as an alternative to core biopsy or other interventions for such lesions (80).

Imaging examinations also often have limited sensitivity, and radiologists must convey this concept to patients, lest patients be inappropriately reassured by a falsely negative test. For example, current estimates of the sensitivity of screening mammography are approximately 63–96% (82, 83), so that if a patient has a palpable breast mass or other salient sign or symptom suggestive of breast cancer, and a mammogram is negative, the radiologist must stress to both the patient and her referring physician the need to pursue a diagnosis.

Even percutaneous core biopsy results may not be definitive. For example, occasionally histopathologic results of a core biopsy are discordant, i.e. do not provide a sufficient explanation for the imaging features. Discordant lesions must be re-biopsied, usually by surgical excision, to avoid a delay in the diagnosis of breast cancer. Similarly, the presence of certain high-risk histologies at core breast biopsy, such as atypical ductal hyperplasia, may be associated with upgrades to carcinoma at surgery. Therefore, when a high-risk lesion is found at core biopsy, surgical excision is indicated (84). Discussing these possible outcomes during the process of obtaining informed consent, before performing the core biopsy, may help the patient understand, and emotionally prepare for, the possibility that despite a benign result at core biopsy, she may still require surgery.

Recent initiatives and future directions in radiology communication

Technology-based distribution of radiology results

Improving communication in radiology requires increasing efficiency in the distribution of results to referring physicians and patients. Recently, the adoption of speech-recognition software that provides contemporaneous computer-generated transcription has improved timeliness in report turnaround in many radiology facilities (4). In the future, PACS and related technology may also help facilitate efficient routine and non-routine reporting by automating two-way communication between radiologists and referring physicians. Thus electronically, a significant imaging finding may be directly linked with relevant report text, the referrer promptly alerted, receipt verified, and the communication archived (85). Findings of different levels of severity may be variously tracked, with different physicians notified at specified intervals, in order to optimize patients' safety and outcomes. Some authors advocate the use of secure HIPAA-compliant internet-based access of radiology reports for both referring physicians and patients in order to expedite and ensure their availability (26). The University of Pennsylvania radiology department sends letters to patients acknowledging that their radiology exams have been read by a radiologist and informing patients how to obtain copies of their reports (24).

Standardization of reporting

Improving communication in radiology also requires increasing accuracy and consistency of reporting. Some propose a move from the currently prevalent free-text (prose) radiology reports to a structured report format with a standardized language and content, much like the BI-RADS lexicon but for use throughout all imaging modalities (86). The Radiological Society of North America is in the process of developing such a unified imaging terminology resource called the RadLex project (4). Ideally, such an instrument would not only improve uniformity in reporting and thereby limit report ambiguity, but it would allow for automated data tracking and clinical outcomes analysis, by linking to other clinical data in a patient's electronic medical record and tracking compliance with follow-up recommendations

Promoting improvement in radiologists' communication skills

Finally, improving communication in radiology requires refining radiologists' competence in interpersonal and communication skills. The Accreditation Council for Graduate Medical Education (ACGME) mandated in 2002 that residents must demonstrate competency in interpersonal and communication skills. In radiology, this is defined as the ability to 'communicate effectively with patients, colleagues, referring physicians and other members of the healthcare team concerning imaging appropriateness, informed consent, safety issues, and results of imaging tests or procedures'. This type of training involves didactic instruction, supervised practice, and skills evaluations (86, 87). Performance measures include evaluations of residents' written reports and written evaluations by residents' superiors, peers, and subordinates (88). The Radiological Society of North America (RSNA) created a task force in 2006 to help develop effective communications curricula in radiology training programs (15, 24).

After training, radiologists must continue to demonstrate maintenance of their communication skills. In 2007, in order to align their goals with those of the ACGME and the American Board of Medical Subspecialties, the Joint Commission on the Accreditation of Healthcare Organizations published new guidelines for medical credentialing and privileging that require ongoing practitioner-specific data collection in several 'general competencies', one of which is practitioners' interpersonal and communication skills (89). Certain university radiology departments, such as Cincinnati Children's Hospital, have instituted initiatives to promote professionalism and effective communication and to document compliance with the Joint Commission standards (89, 90), such as eliciting patient input and educating radiologists in standards of customer service. Further adoption of such initiatives will likely foster widespread quality improvement in radiology communications.

Conclusion

Radiologists' communications with referring physicians must be accurate, meaningful, and timely, and therefore measures that improve uniformity and consistency of radiology reporting and prompt distribution of results are of paramount importance. The recent evolution of radiology to include more procedures that bring radiologists into direct patient contact has prompted the need for direct radiologist–patient communication that is likely to increase with continuing advances in radiology. It is essential that patients perceive these interactions as compassionate and comprehensible, and this is optimally achieved when radiologists tailor their communications to the needs of individual patients. For radiologists, improved communication with referring physicians and patients alike will ultimately result in timelier diagnoses, enhanced professional relationships, and superior healthcare outcomes.

References

1. American College of Radiology. *ACR practice guideline for communication of diagnostic imaging findings*. Reston, VA: American College of Radiology; 2005.
2. Berlin L (2000). Pitfalls of the vague radiology report. *AJR Am J Roentgenol* **174**, 1511–8.
3. Coakley FV, Liberman L, Panicek DM (2003). Style guidelines for radiology reporting: a manner of speaking. *AJR Am J Roentgenol* **180**, 327–8.
4. Reiner BI, Knight N, Siegel EL (2007). Radiology reporting, past, present, and future: the radiologist's perspective. *J Am Coll Radiol* **4**, 313–9.
5. Hricak H. *Oncologic imaging: essentials of reporting common cancers*. Philadelphia: Saunders Elsevier; 2007.
6. American College of Radiology. *BI-RADS Committee. ACR BI-RADS breast imaging and reporting data system: breast imaging atlas*, 4th edn. Reston, VA: American College of Radiology; 2003.
7. Lehman CD, Miller L, Rutter CM, *et al.* (2001). Effect of training with the american college of radiology breast imaging reporting and data system lexicon on mammographic interpretation skills in developing countries. *Acad Radiol* **8**, 647–50.
8. Berg WA, D'Orsi CJ, Jackson VP, *et al.* (2002). Does training in the Breast Imaging Reporting and Data System (BI-RADS) improve biopsy recommendations or feature analysis agreement with experienced breast imagers at mammography? *Radiology* **224**, 871–80.
9. Berlin L (2003). Duty to directly communicate radiologic abnormalities: has the pendulum swung too far? *AJR Am J Roentgenol* **181**, 375–81.
10. Garvey CJ, Connolly S (2006). Radiology reporting–where does the radiologist's duty end? *Lancet* **367**, 443–5.
11. Williamson KB, Steele JL, Gunderman RB, *et al.* (2002). Assessing radiology resident reporting skills. *Radiology* **225**, 719–22.
12. Kushner DC, Lucey LL (2005). Diagnostic radiology reporting and communication: the ACR guideline. *J Am Coll Radiol* **2**, 15–21.
13. Brenner RJ, Bartholomew L (2005). Communication errors in radiology: a liability cost analysis. *J Am Coll Radiol* **2**, 428–31.
14. Berlin L (2002). Communicating findings of radiologic examinations: whither goest the radiologist's duty? *AJR Am J Roentgenol* **178**, 809–15.
15. Berlin L (2007). Communicating results of all radiologic examinations directly to patients: has the time come? *AJR Am J Roentgenol* **189**, 1275–82.
16. Ouellette H, Kassarjian A, McLoud TC (2006). Teaching the art of verbal consultation. *J Am Coll Radiol* **3**, 9–10.
17. Gunderman RB (2001). A vital skill for radiologic education. *Acad Radiol* **8**, 651–5.

18. Berlin L (2006). Communicating radiology results. *Lancet* **367**, 373–5.

19. Ragavendra N, Laifer-Narin SL, Melany ML, *et al.* (1998). Disclosure of results of sonographic examinations to patients by sonologists. *Am J Roentgenol* **170**, 1423–5.

20. Vallely SR, Mills JO (1990). Should radiologists talk to patients? *BMJ (Clinical research ed)* **300**, 305–6.

21. Song (1993). Radiologists' responses to patients' inquiries about imaging results: a pilot study on opinions of various groups. *Investigative radiology* **28**, 1043–8.

22. Schreiber MH, Leonard M, Jr., Rieniets CY (1995). Disclosure of imaging findings to patients directly by radiologists: survey of patients' preferences. *AJR Am J Roentgenol* **165**, 467–9.

23. Peteet JR, Stomper PC, Ross DM, *et al.* (1992). Emotional support for patients with cancer who are undergoing CT: semistructured interviews of patients at a cancer institute. *Radiology* **182**, 99–102.

24. Ruiz JA, Glazer GM (2006). The state of radiology in 2006: very high spatial resolution but no visibility. *Radiology* **241**, 11–6.

25. Braeuning MP, Earp JL, O'Brien SM, *et al.* (2000). Informing patients of diagnostic mammography results: mammographer's opinions. *Acad Radiol* **7**, 335–40.

26. Johnson AJ, Hawkins H, Applegate KE (2005). Web-based results distribution: new channels of communication from radiologists to patients. *J Am Coll Radiol* **2**, 168–73.

27. Raza S, Rosen MP, Chorny K, *et al.* (2001). Patient expectations and costs of immediate reporting of screening mammography: talk isn't cheap. *AJR Am J Roentgenol* **177**, 579–83.

28. Lorch H, Scherer P (2007). Disclosure of diagnosis in ambulatory radiology practice: expectations of patients and referring physicians. *Rofo* **179**, 1043–7.

29. Zardawi IM (2002). Should radiologists and pathologists talk to patients? *Med J Aust* **177**, 222.

30. Storby G (1996). Disclosure of X-ray results by the radiologist? Yes, say the patients. May be, say the physicians. *Lakartidningen* **93**, 927–30.

31. Levitsky DB, Frank MS, Richardson ML, *et al.* (1993). How should radiologists reply when patients ask about their diagnoses? A survey of radiologists' and clinicians' preferences. *AJR Am J Roentgenol* **161**, 433–6.

32. Priyanath A, Feinglass J, Dolan NC, *et al.* (2002). Patient satisfaction with the communication of mammographic results before and after the Mammography Quality Standards Reauthorization Act of 1998. *AJR Am J Roentgenol* **178**, 451–6.

33. Karliner LS, Patricia Kaplan C, Juarbe T, *et al.* (2005). Poor patient comprehension of abnormal mammography results. *J Gen Intern Med* **20**, 432–7.

34. Poon EG, Haas JS, Louise Puopolo A, *et al.* (2004). Communication factors in the follow-up of abnormal mammograms. *J Gen Intern Med* **19**, 316–23.

35. Davey HM, Lim J, Butow PN, *et al.* (2003). Consumer information materials for diagnostic breast tests: women's views on information and their understanding of test results. *Health Expect* **6**, 298–311.

36. United States. Congress. House. Committee on Commerce. Subcommittee on Health and the Environment. Reauthorization of the Mammography Quality Standards Act hearing before the Subcommittee on Health and Environment of the Committee on Commerce, House of Representatives, One Hundred Fifth Congress, second session, 8 May 1998 (microform). Washington: US GPO: for sale by the US GPO, Supt. of Docs., Congressional Sales Office; 1998.

37. Levin KS, Braeuning MP, O'Malley MS, *et al.* (2000). Communicating results of diagnostic mammography: what do patients think? *Acad Radiol* **7**, 1069–76.

38. Wilson TE, Wallace C, Roubidoux MA, *et al.* (1998). Patient satisfaction with screening mammography: online vs off-line interpretation. *Acad Radiol* **5**, 771–8.

39. Padgett DK, Yedidia MJ, Kerner J, *et al.* (2001). The emotional consequences of false positive mammography: African-American women's reactions in their own words. *Women & Health* **33**, 1–14.

40. Hulka CA, Slanetz PJ, Halpern EF, *et al.* (1997). Patients' opinion of mammography screening services: immediate results versus delayed results due to interpretation by two observers. *AJR Am J Roentgenol* **168**, 1085–9.

41. Thorne SE, Harris SR, Hislop TG, Vestrup JA (1999). The experience of waiting for diagnosis after an abnormal mammogram. *Breast J* **5**, 42–51.

42. Shapiro DE, Boggs SR, Melamed BG, *et al.* (1992). The effect of varied physician affect on recall, anxiety, and perceptions in women at risk for breast cancer: an analogue study. *Health Psychol* **11**, 61–6.

43. Dolan NC, Feinglass J, Priyanath A, *et al.* (2001). Measuring satisfaction with mammography results reporting. *J Gen Intern Med* **16**, 157–62.

44. Lobb EA, Butow PN, Kenny DT, *et al.* (1999). Communicating prognosis in early breast cancer: do women understand the language used? *Med J Aust* **171**, 290–4.

45. Kerner JF, Yedidia M, Padgett D, *et al.* (2003). Realizing the promise of breast cancer screening: clinical follow-up after abnormal screening among Black women. *Prev Med* **37**, 92–101.

46. Jones BA, Reams K, Calvocoressi L, *et al.* (2007). Adequacy of communicating results from screening mammograms to African American and White women. *Am J Public Health* **97**, 531–8.

47. van den Bosch MA (2007). Re: interventional radiology: veni, vidi, vanished? *J Vasc Interv Radiol* **18**, 165; author reply, 6.

48. Fajardo LL, Pisano ED, Caudry DJ, *et al.* (2004). Stereotactic and sonographic large-core biopsy of nonpalpable breast lesions: results of the Radiologic Diagnostic Oncology Group V study. *Acad Radiol* **11**, 293–308.

49. O'Dwyer HM, Lyon SM, Fotheringham T, *et al.* (2003). Informed consent for interventional radiology procedures: a survey detailing current European practice. *Cardiovasc Intervent Radiol* **26**, 428–33.

50. Deane KA, Degner LF (1997). Determining the information needs of women after breast biopsy procedures. *AORN J* **65**, 767–72, 75–6.

51. Phatouros CC, Blake MP (1995). How much now to tell? Patients' attitudes to an information sheet prior to angiography and angioplasty. *Australasian Radiology* **39**, 135–9.

52. Northouse LL, Tocco KM, West P (1997). Coping with a breast biopsy: how healthcare professionals can help women and their husbands. *Oncol Nurs Forum* **24**, 473–80.

53. United States Department of Health and Human Services. *OCR guidance explaining significant aspects of the privacy rule 2003* (updated 2003; cited December 17, 2007); Available from: http://www.hhs.gov/ocr/hipaa/guidelines/personalrepresentatives.rtf.

54. Campbell L, Watkins RM, Teasdale C (1997). Communicating the result of breast biopsy by telephone or in person. *The British Journal of Surgery* **84**, 1381.

55. Reisman AB, Brown KE (2005). Preventing communication errors in telephone medicine. *J Gen Intern Med* **20**, 959–63.

56. Harvey JA, Cohen MA, Brenin DR, *et al.* (2007). Breaking bad news: a primer for radiologists in breast imaging. *J Am Coll Radiol* **4**, 800–8.

57. Mager WM, Andrykowski MA (2002). Communication in the cancer 'bad news' consultation: patient perceptions and psychological adjustment. *Psycho-oncology* **11**, 35–46.

58. Kerr J, Engel J, Schlesinger-Raab A, *et al.* (2003). Communication, quality of life and age: results of a 5-year prospective study in breast cancer patients. *Ann Oncol* **14**, 421–7.

59. Wright EB, Holcombe C, Salmon P (2004). Doctors' communication of trust, care, and respect in breast cancer: qualitative study. *BMJ (Clinical research ed* **328**, 864.

60. Ong G, Austoker J (1997). Recalling women for further investigation of breast screening: women's experiences at the clinic and afterwards. *J Public Health Med* **19**, 29–36.

61. Carrese JA, Rhodes LA (2000). Bridging cultural differences in medical practice. The case of discussing negative information with Navajo patients. *J Gen Intern Med* **15**, 92–6.

62. Northouse LL, Jeffs M, Cracchiolo-Caraway A, *et al.* (1995). Emotional distress reported by women and husbands prior to a breast biopsy. *Nurs Res* **44**, 196–201.

63. Meechan GT, Collins JP, Moss-Morris RE, *et al.* (2005). Who is not reassured following benign diagnosis of breast symptoms? *Psycho-oncology* **14**, 239–46.

64. Zapka JG, Puleo E, Taplin SH, *et al.* (2004). Processes of care in cervical and breast cancer screening and follow-up–the importance of communication. *Prev Med* **39**, 81–90.

65. Jemal A, Siegel R, Ward E, *et al.* (2007). Cancer statistics, 2007. *CA Cancer J Clin* **57**, 43–66.

66. Li CI, Malone KE, Daling JR (2003). Differences in breast cancer stage, treatment, and survival by race and ethnicity. *Arch Intern Med* **163**, 49–56.

67. Smith-Bindman R, Miglioretti DL, Lurie N, *et al.* (2006). Does utilization of screening mammography explain racial and ethnic differences in breast cancer? *Ann Intern Med* **144**, 541–53.

68. Lindfors KK, O'Connor J, Acredolo CR, *et al.* (1998). Short-interval follow-up mammography versus immediate core biopsy of benign breast lesions: assessment of patient stress. *AJR Am J Roentgenol* **171**, 55–8.

69. Lindfors KK, O'Connor J, Parker RA (2001). False-positive screening mammograms: effect of immediate versus later work-up on patient stress. *Radiology* **218**, 247–53.

70. Jatoi I, Zhu K, Shah M, Lawrence W (2006). Psychological distress in U.S. women who have experienced false-positive mammograms. *Breast Cancer Res Treat* **100**, 191–200.

71. Witt D, Brawer R, Plumb J (2002). Cultural factors in preventive care: African-Americans. *Prim Care* **29**, 487–93.

72. Wu TY, West B, Chen YW, *et al.* (2006). Health beliefs and practices related to breast cancer screening in Filipino, Chinese and Asian-Indian women. *Cancer Detect Prev* **30**, 58–66.

73. Brewer NT, Salz T, Lillie SE (2007). Systematic review: the long-term effects of false-positive mammograms. *Annals of Internal Medicine* **146**, 502–10.

74. Barton MB, Moore S, Polk S, *et al.* (2001). Increased patient concern after false-positive mammograms: clinician documentation and subsequent ambulatory visits. *J Gen Intern Med* **16**, 150–6.

75. Pisano ED, Earp J, Schell M, *et al.* (1998). Screening behavior of women after a false-positive mammogram. *Radiology* **208**, 245–9.

76. Barton MB, Morley DS, Moore S, *et al.* (2004). Decreasing women's anxieties after abnormal mammograms: a controlled trial. *J Nat Cancer Inst* **96**, 529–38.

77. Brett J, Austoker J (2001). Women who are recalled for further investigation for breast screening: psychological consequences 3 years after recall and factors affecting re-attendance. *J Public Health Med* **23**, 292–300.

78. McCann J, Stockton D, Godward S (2002). Impact of false-positive mammography on subsequent screening attendance and risk of cancer. *Breast Cancer Res* **4**, R11.

79. Israel GM, Bosniak MA (2005). An update of the Bosniak renal cyst classification system. *Urology* **66**, 484–8.

80. Sickles EA (1995). Management of probably benign breast lesions. *Radiol Clin North Am* **33**, 1123–30.

81. Ong G, Austoker J, Brett J (1997). Breast screening: adverse psychological consequences one month after placing women on early recall because of a diagnostic uncertainty. A multicentre study. *J Med Screen* **4**, 158–68.

82. Elmore JG, Armstrong K, Lehman CD, *et al.* (2005). Screening for breast cancer. *JAMA* **293**, 1245–56.

83. Humphrey LL, Helfand M, Chan BKS, *et al.* (2002). Breast cancer screening: a summary of the evidence for the U.S. Preventive Services Task Force. *Ann Intern Med* **137**, 347–60.

84. Berg WA (2004). Image-guided breast biopsy and management of high-risk lesions. *Radiol Clin North Am* **42**, 935–46, vii.

85. Brenner RJ (2006). To err is human, to correct divine: the emergence of technology-based communication systems. *J Am Coll Radiol* **3**, 340–5.

86. Sistrom CL, Langlotz CP (2005). A framework for improving radiology reporting. *J Am Coll Radiol* **2**, 159–67.

87. Sistrom C, Lanier L, Mancuso A (2004). Reporting instruction for radiology residents. *Acad Radiol* **11**, 76–84.

88. ACGME. Competency definitions (cited 17 January 2008). Available from: http://www.apdr.org/directors/pdffiles/competency_definitions.pdf.

89. Donnelly LF (2007). Performance-based assessment of radiology practitioners: promoting improvement in accordance with the 2007 joint commission standards. *J Am Coll Radiol* **4**, 699–703.

90. Donnelly LF, Strife JL (2006). Establishing a program to promote professionalism and effective communication in radiology. *Radiology* **238**, 773–9.

Chapter 40

Communication in surgical oncology

Alexandra Heerdt, Bernard Park, and Patrick Boland

Introduction

As in every field of oncology, the importance of communication for the surgical oncologist cannot be overstated. The surgeon may become involved with the cancer patient at almost any point in the disease process. In many instances, the surgeon performs the biopsy that diagnoses the cancer and needs to be able to appropriately convey, not only the diagnosis but also its implications. In other instances, surgery itself is the main treatment for the disease and the surgeon becomes the primary caregiver for these patients. Finally, the surgeon may become involved at a time when palliation is the main objective. In this situation, clarifying the role of surgery and its limitations in a manner which still provides some hope is of significant importance.

Several studies have indicated that patient satisfaction and trust in the treating physician are based on perceptions of appropriate communication (1–5). In each study, a patient-centred approach with excellent communication of information was found to be important (6). While there are some situations unique to each surgical subspecialty in surgical oncology, there are aspects of the surgeon's daily life that are common to all subspecialties. In order to properly address the patient's needs and to communicate effectively, it is helpful to have a framework to approach the common situations that arise.

The first appointment

As with any oncology specialty, the first meeting with a surgical oncologist is of paramount importance. In this consultation, the patient will look to the surgeon for information, not only about the surgical procedure itself but also about the cancer. It is helpful to provide the patient with a short synopsis of what one hopes to accomplish during this first appointment. Additionally, assuring the patient that there will be an opportunity to ask questions and voice concerns is always welcome. Be especially attuned to the fact that patients have varying degrees of understanding of the disease process and may require more or less explanation of any given aspect of your discussion.

A possible framework for the consultation would be as follows:

- Give an overview of the information that is already known regarding this patient's cancer.
- Be clear about what is not yet known about this cancer.
- Indicate your (the surgeon's) role in the treatment of the cancer.
- Describe the surgical procedure(s), including possible consequences of the procedure and variations in approach that could be considered.
- Indicate other healthcare providers who may be involved in the care of the patient, either now or at a later date.
- Establish lines of communication for the patient and review the next steps to be followed.

At the time of this initial meeting with a patient, various amounts of information may be available regarding the cancer with which they have been diagnosed. For instance, while a biopsy may have established the diagnosis of lung cancer, the typical imaging tests that are required for this cancer may not yet have been performed. Likewise, in situations in which breast cancer has been diagnosed, biopsies may vary from fine-needle aspirations, which give little information, to excisional biopsies, in which a great deal of information is available. The patient needs to have a clear understanding of the extent of the physician's understanding of the cancer at this point in time. Clarification here will reduce the likelihood of disappointment at a later time, particularly if the cancer is shown to more aggressive than the initial expectation.

Once the exact level of understanding of this cancer is established, the surgeon should turn attention to his or her role in the cancer's management. Will the procedure that is to occur be only exploratory in nature, will it yield information that will be used by other physicians, or is it to be considered the definitive treatment for this disease? This is often an excellent time to introduce the concept of multidisciplinary care, as most forms of cancer are likely to be treated in this manner. The nature of possible adjuvant treatments with chemotherapy, radiation or hormone blockade should be described. If a patient enters a surgical procedure believing it to be definitive treatment and is later referred to multiple other specialists, it may establish a level of distrust toward the surgeon and to other subsequent treating physicians.

Studies have clearly shown that the amount of information that may be processed at an initial consultation varies and that physicians can over-estimate the ability of the patient to retain information (7). As such, it is extremely helpful to indicate a manner in which the patient may communicate questions or concerns in the future. If you feel that the patient will benefit from returning for another visit, or you prefer to speak in person, make that clear at this time. If there is a nurse who is typically responsible for further education, psychosocial support and answering questions, be certain to indicate this and explain how the patient can reach your nurse. Additionally, indicate how available you may be to answer questions outside the setting of the office. It is important that the patient always feels that there is some way in which to communicate with you, whether it is directly with you or through a nurse.

One final comment worth repeating at the end of the initial consultation is that your recommendations at this point are based on the available information. Continually emphasizing to the patient that all of the data are not yet available, helps enormously if there should be an unexpected result.

Diagnosis

When a patient presents with a clinical scenario in which there is a suspicion of cancer without histologic confirmation, the decision to perform a biopsy and the method of doing this will depend on each situation and the needs of the patient. Generally, biopsy options can be either surgical or non-surgical. If a lesion is best treated initially with surgical excision in the event of malignancy, the discussion typically focuses on surgical exploration for the purposes of diagnosis and treatment. Alternatively, if a particular type of cancer will involve multidisciplinary treatment, where resection is not the initial treatment, alternative non-surgical forms of tissue diagnosis are proposed. In either case, the relative accuracy and limitations of the biopsy methods should be reviewed. Two scenarios in particular should be discussed. The first is the possibility that a non-surgical biopsy (e.g. needle biopsy) is either falsely negative or non-diagnostic. Subsequent strategies (i.e. repeat needle biopsy or surgical exploration) should be reviewed. The second scenario is the chance that the immediate pathology evaluation at the time of surgical biopsy is equivocal for cancer. Again, the plan in this event should be laid out prior to the procedure. The more the surgeon demonstrates anticipation of what could occur, the greater insight their patient will gain about their illness. Where subsequent resection entails an extensive, potentially morbid procedure, the decision may be to terminate the initial diagnostic procedure and wait for the final pathology report. In other scenarios, where complete excision is low risk or would be more difficult at a subsequent procedure, excision may be warranted. Such decisions need to be individualized for each person and their surgeon.

If a patient presents with an established tissue diagnosis, the clinician should initiate review of the previous pathology by their institutional pathologists for confirmation of the diagnosis, and the consultation can then proceed to any necessary additional workup. Further workup will vary depending on the clinical scenario and the proposed operation, but falls into two broad categories. The first is the oncology workup—this is best explained to the patient as assessment of the (potential) extent or stage of cancer. The purpose in defining the extent of disease is to allow discussion of appropriate treatments and, ultimately, prognosis (8; 9). For most solid tumours, this entails a variety of imaging and potentially additional non-invasive or invasive tests, depending on the results. The second category of workup is pre-operative—here assessments are made of the potential cardiopulmonary and anaesthetic risks of the procedure. This is highly dependent on the specific procedure, the type of anaesthesia required and the overall performance status and specific comorbid conditions of each patient. For the former, this may entail further specialized tests (e.g. cardiac stress testing) and/or medical consultations. For the latter, the patients should understand what the purpose is of each pre-surgical testing process, which can include blood tests, ECG, chest X-ray and an anaesthesia evaluation.

Pre-operative discussion

Once it is has been agreed that surgery is the next step, discussion of its various aspects is critical to preparation, not only for the patient to be able to give informed consent, but also so that they and their families know what to expect. The key components are: pre-operative preparation, the operative approach, anaesthetic and pain management, potential side-effects, post-operative recovery, length of stay and anticipated discharge.

Pre-operative preparation

There are many important aspects to pre-operative teaching regardless of the procedure. Two key ones include fasting the night before the operation, specifically if general anaesthesia will be administered, and instructions with respect to taking medications. The latter is particularly important with regard to cardiac, diabetic and anticoagulant medications. In addition to verbal instructions, it is very useful to have written materials that patients can use as a reference. Other logistical information, such as knowing what time to report to the hospital, where to park and how to get to the perioperative area are helpful and can decrease any additional anxiety about the procedure. When there are procedure specific instructions, these should also be carefully reviewed with the patient (e.g. bowel preparation for colon resection).

Operative approach

Discussion of the operative approach includes a number of components. Start with the actual technical aspects of the effects of the procedure: the size, number and location of incisions; length of the procedure; use of any specialized equipment; use of prophylactic antibiotics; prevention of deep venous thrombosis. The second is the goal of the operation. It is critical that patients understand the difference between diagnostic, curative and palliative operations in terms of long-term disease outcomes.

Anaesthetic and pain management

Although patients will generally have an opportunity to speak with the anaesthesia team regarding the type of anaesthesia and its associated risks, it is helpful in the pre-surgical discussion for the surgeon to briefly mention the preferred anaesthetic technique and the plan for post-operative pain management. Knowing that post-operative discomfort will be addressed and that they will have opportunities to discuss these issues further with the anaesthesiologist, are very reassuring to patients.

Potential side-effects

It is important for patients who are often focused on the oncology result of a given surgical procedure to understand the potential acute and chronic effects that can result, including the potential for complications. While this may provoke anxiety in some patients, knowing the risks of a given procedure is required for a patient to be able to give informed consent and will ultimately allow them to anticipate what to expect post-operatively. We suggest that this discussion is divided into minor and major categories; review only the most common types of after-effects with the understanding that other less common complications may occur. Avoid minimizing the possibility of complications, as this will undoubtedly lead to patient frustration and anxiety if an unanticipated outcome occurs. Patients are helped by distinguishing between short-term and long-term effects with an idea about the trajectory of recovery ('How long before I am fully recovered?')

Anticipated discharge

Lastly, it is expected that the surgeon discusses the anticipated length of hospital stay and discharge parameters. This is invaluable for two reasons. First, this information allows patients to gauge their expectations about the surgical experience and helps them prepare physically, emotionally and practically for when they leave the hospital. Second, in the setting of rising healthcare expenditures and limitations in resources, this allows for timely discharge planning and the utilization of hospital beds to serve other patients.

Post-operative complications

Patients who have undergone a surgical procedure for cancer will spend varying amounts of time within the hospital. While some procedures, such as a pancreaticoduodenectomy, still require prolonged hospitalization, the majority of procedures make use of relatively short stays and many, including those for breast cancer, are performed on an outpatient basis. Thus, the surgeon may not have had contact with the patient for several days or weeks at the time of the formal post-operative visit. For this reason, this visit is particularly important for the key information exchange that occurs between the surgeon and the patient. It is not unusual for this encounter to be as lengthy as the initial visit.

Surgeons need to clarify in their own minds what they would like to accomplish at the post-operative visit. Typically, this will include an evaluation of the surgical site, a discussion of any complications that may have occurred during or after the procedure, and a discussion of the pathology report. For the most part, it can be helpful, strategically, to address the actual surgical issues prior to discussing the pathology report. Then, the entire focus can be upon the implications and importance of the pathology findings. Patients can pay full attention without undue concern regarding anticipated pain or discomfort from removal of sutures, surgical staples or drains.

When addressing the pathology report, it is generally helpful to have a copy available to share with the patient and the family members present. While it is not necessary to explain each aspect of the report, patients appreciate it when surgeons underline and underscore the important dimensions. This may include highlighting the size of the tumour, the lymph node count and the presence or absence of clear margins. All of this must be cast in a way that the patient can understand its implications for further treatment. For instance, will further surgery be required for involved margins or will the patient need to see a medical oncologist at this point in time? Has your initial understanding of this cancer changed or has the procedure been confirmatory? Additionally, indicating your thoughts on the likelihood of other treatments, based upon these results, is extremely helpful guidance to the patient.

At times, and from a practical standpoint, it is necessary to have an initial discussion of the pathology report by phone with the patient. Particularly for the anxious patient, and in situations where more surgery may be indicated, this can focus the discussion at the time of the subsequent appointment. It is often appreciated when one asks a patient at the time of the procedure whether he or she would like to hear the news about the pathology by phone or rather prefer to wait until the visit. Many will indicate their desire to hear the information sooner rather than later. If you should choose to call the patient, be certain that the phone call is made at a time when you can answer all the questions that the patient has. Simply giving the outcome without explanation will not be helpful whatsoever.

The final component of the post-operative visit should be an outline of the future for the patient. If referrals are necessary, the nature of each referral should be explained in detail, including their timing. If it is expected that the patient will be seeing both a medical and a radiation oncologist, but only one referral is made initially, explain clearly the reasons for this. While it may seem repetitive to outline the course of treatment once again, it is extremely helpful to a patient and will increase satisfaction.

In the management of most cancers, the surgeon remains involved over at least several further visits. However, in some cases, such as a lymph node biopsy to diagnose lymphoma, a follow-up visit may not be necessary. It is important to clarify what the follow-up schedule should be, as well as the rationale for this. Finally, whether there is an expectation that the patient will be seen again or not, declaring your availability to give assistance in the future, whether to answer questions or review concerns, is greatly appreciated.

References

1. Costantini M, Foley K, Rapkin B (1998). Communicating with patients about advanced cancer. *JAMA* **280**, 1403–4.
2. Detmar S, Muller M, Wever L, *et al.* (2001). The patient-physician relationship. Patient–physician communication during outpatient palliative treatment visits: an observational study. *JAMA* **285**, 1351–7.
3. Fallowfield L, Jenkins V, Farewell V, *et al.* (2002). Efficacy of a Cancer Research UK communication skills training model for oncologists: a randomised controlled trial. *Lancet* **359**, 650–6.
4. Fallowfield L, Jenkins V, Farewell V, *et al.* (2003). Enduring impact of communication skills training: results of a 12-month follow-up. *Brit J Cancer* **89**, 1445–9.
5. Razavi D, Merckaert I, Marchal S, *et al.* (2003). How to optimize physicians' communication skills in cancer care: results of a randomized study assessing the usefulness of posttraining consolidation workshops. *J Clin Oncol* **21**, 3141–9.

6. Jenkins V, Fallowfield L (2002). Can communication skills training alter physicians' beliefs and behavior in clinics? *J Clin Oncol* **20**, 765–9.

7. Dunn SM, Butow PN, Tattersall MH, *et al.* (1993). General information tapes inhibit recall of the cancer consultation. *J Clin Oncol* **11**, 2279–85.

8. Piccirillo J, Tierney R, Costas I, *et al.* (2004). Prognostic importance of comorbidity in a hospital-based cancer registry. *JAMA* **291**, 2441–7.

9. Christakis N (1999). *Death Foretold—Prophecy and Prognosis in Medical Care.* The University of Chicago Press, Chicago.

Chapter 41

Communication in non-surgical oncology

Lai Cheng Yew and E Jane Maher

The importance of cancer

A total of 280,000 people are diagnosed with cancer every year in the UK (1). It is estimated that more than one in three people will develop some form of cancer during their lifetime. This risk increases with age, as cancer is primarily a disease of older people. As a result of the ageing population in the UK, by 2025 it is expected that the incidence of cancer will increase by 100,000 per year (1).

The importance of cancer is reflected in the enormous media interest that it attracts. For example, the UK charity, Macmillan Cancer Support surveyed mainstream national newspapers over a 6-month period and found 500 articles mentioning the word 'cancer' (2) (almost three articles per day). There are thousands of websites about cancer that provide easy access to a wealth of unfiltered information, which can be useful but also the basis for the myths that surround the illness. The perception of cancer is hugely influenced not only by the scale of the media attention, but also the language used in situations involving cancer. Patients with cancer are often described as 'victims', 'fighting' a 'battle', and 'surviving' because of a 'positive attitude'. Cancer is perceived as a feared disease because of the mortality associated with it. Similarly, while in the past the diagnosis of metastatic disease implied a rapid demise, many patients with metastatic breast and prostate cancer may have several years of good quality life. Public opinion has not kept up with these changes. The way in which cancer is portrayed by the media creates a frame of reference on which patient–clinician communication is based.

Cancer as a complex illness

There are more than 200 types of cancer—breast, lung, colorectal, and prostate account for over half of all new cases. Different types of cancer have very different illness trajectories, defined not only by the natural history and stage of the cancer, but also patient characteristics and treatment options available. There is considerable variation between different cancer types, such as pancreas versus breast. But, in the majority of cases, cancer care involves numerous clinicians and health-care professionals throughout the patient's cancer journey. In addition, treatments are becoming much more complex, often involving a combination of surgery, chemotherapy, radiotherapy, and biological agents. For all these reasons, communication in cancer is particularly challenging for both the patient and the clinician.

The role of non-surgical oncology

The non-surgical oncologist is involved in almost every patient's cancer journey—either at diagnosis, during treatment, at follow-up, at recurrence, through survivorship, and even at the end of life. The main treatment options offered by this group are chemotherapy, radiotherapy, and biological therapies, all of which can be used in the radical or palliative setting. There are significant acute and late toxicities associated with these treatments, some of which are life-threatening, e.g. neutropenic sepsis.

Many of the treatment regimes in current use have been studied in a much younger population than the typical patients that receive treatment. Also, in cases where there is a choice of treatments, often the non-surgical option is preferred over surgery for older patients, or those with a poorer performance status. These patients are more prone to the acute side-effects of treatment, and because of improved survival rates, some are surviving long enough to experience late side-effects. Therefore, the non-surgical oncologist does not just provide a particular treatment, but has a much more involved role in monitoring toxicities during treatment and in long-term follow-up. Because they can also offer palliative treatments, they will often diagnose and/or treat a recurrence and initiate palliative care. Communication issues will arise at all these stages of a patient's cancer illness, and the non-surgical oncologist must be aware of the complexities of the relationship with the patient.

Frameworks linking communication and outcome

The communication between patient and clinician can be better understood using the framework defined by the US National Institutes of Health (NIH) (3). This links six key functions and seven pathways of communication with measurable health and quality-of-life outcomes. More effective patient–clinician communication can improve health outcomes.

Functions of communication

1. Fostering healing relationships.
2. Exchanging information.
3. Responding to emotions.
4. Managing uncertainty.
5. Making decisions.
6. Enabling self-management.

The six core functions of communication overlap and interact to produce communication that affects health outcomes—primarily survival and quality of life. There is little research on the relationship between communication and health outcomes, but the NIH monograph proposes a number of pathways that help to understand this link. This is based on the idea that the proximal outcomes of communication, essentially immediate outcomes on the functions of communication listed above, and intermediate outcomes, such as adherence to advice and patient empowerment, contribute to the third set of outcomes, those related to health, i.e. survival and quality of life (see Fig. 41.1).

For most patients the outcomes of greatest relevance are the health outcomes—survival and quality of life. The relationship between communication and health outcomes can be mediated by the proximal and intermediate outcomes listed above. For example, a patient who has been given clear information about tamoxifen (effective information exchange—proximal outcome) by a clinician with whom she has developed a rapport (good patient/clinician relationship—proximal outcome) is more likely to take the tamoxifen for the recommended time period (adherence—intermediate outcome), which results in improved survival (health outcome). However, communication can directly affect health outcomes, e.g. a clinician can inform a patient of a normal test result, resulting in reduced anxiety and improved quality of life. Thus, the pathways linking

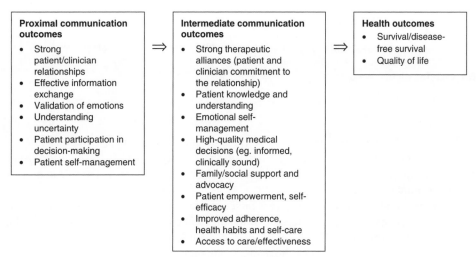

Fig. 41.1 The influence of effective communications on health outcomes.

communication with health outcomes are complex and may or may not involve the proximal and intermediate outcomes as mediators. Figure 41.2 shows how these pathways of communication are thought to be interrelated.

The importance of different communication functions, pathways, and outcomes will vary between cancers, patients, and even during the cancer journey, as the experience of patients and their families is complex and dynamic. For example, at diagnosis, a patient may prioritize information gathering and participation in decision-making (functions 2 and 5), but at the end of life, the patient may need more empathy and a strong relationship with the clinician (functions 3 and 1). The differing communication needs will determine which pathways are more relevant to the appropriate health outcome.

There are a number of factors that moderate the relationship between communication and health outcomes. Moderators interact with an independent variable to predict an outcome, e.g. if a patient trusts his/her doctor, then if the clinician expresses reassurance, the patient will be less anxious than a less trusting patient (Fig. 41.3).

Moderators can be intrinsic or extrinsic to clinicians, patients and their relationship. Intrinsic moderators are individual or relationship characteristics that affect cognitive and affective processes of the patient/clinician, e.g. patient's emotional state, knowledge about the illness, motivation,

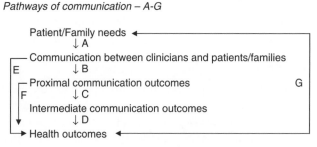

Fig. 41.2 The interrelation of communication and health outcomes.

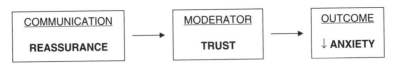

Fig. 41.3 The central role of trust.

health literacy. Extrinsic moderators include cultural beliefs, social support, access to care and disease factors (e.g. stage, type of cancer). These moderators vary in their susceptibility to change, and this is important as those factors which are more easily modified can be targeted in order to improve communication.

The key functions of communication are linked to proximal and intermediate communication outcomes, and distal health outcomes via a number of complex pathways. The relationship between communication and health outcomes is moderated by several factors. Focusing on the modifiable moderators should lead to improved health outcomes.

Communication at the time of diagnosis of cancer

The key communication issues at the time of diagnosis of cancer are breaking bad news, giving information, making decisions about future management, explaining prognosis, and providing emotional support to patient and families. Effective communication is essential at this stage of the cancer journey, as often further diagnostic tests are required to formulate the management plan, and these need to be performed quickly to minimize delay before treatment starts. However, patients are often highly emotional at this time, which makes it difficult for them to retain and assimilate information, and make rational decisions. This problem is further compounded if the initial bad news is poorly communicated, resulting in increased levels of anxiety and a weak patient–clinician relationship. Despite an increase in communication skills training, breaking bad news continues to be something that many clinicians find difficult (4).

Aligning perspectives of a patient–clinician interaction

Communication between patient and clinician can be improved if there is some shared understanding of each other's perspective and the purpose of the interaction is defined. Clinicians often misjudge patients' perspectives, preferences and beliefs about health, particularly when there are racial/ethnicity differences (4). This creates bias and leads to misunderstandings. In some cultures, it is very difficult to accept a diagnosis of cancer. In a recent study by Symonds *et al.*, 48% of South Asian patients agreed with the statement on a questionnaire, 'I don't believe I have cancer' 15 weeks after diagnosis, compared with 31% of white patients. If there is no word for cancer, as in Gujarati or Hindi, understanding of this illness is even more difficult. As well as cultural differences, mismatches in health literacy (understanding health in general and the care process) can be a major barrier to communication (5).

Information sharing

The information given at diagnosis is particularly important as it sets the scene for the patient's cancer journey. Inadequate information can lead to significant anxiety. The majority of patients with cancer want as much information as possible (6). In the UK, access to timely, high-quality information is very dependent on cancer site, e.g. 90% of patients with breast cancer received written information at diagnosis, compared with only 67% of patients with prostate cancer (7). On the other hand, patients can feel that too much information is given at this time, and this is often difficult to interpret making it even harder to make decisions. The clinician has to judge how much detail a patient wants about diagnosis, prognosis, and treatment options. This will vary considerably, even between patients who have cancer of the same site. In addition, some cancers may result in cognitive impairment, e.g. brain tumour, brain metastases. For these patients, communication can be improved by providing information in small chunks, repeating key points, summarizing and checking for understanding, and giving written materials and/or audio-recordings.

Decision-making

Patients must feel that they have had sufficient information to make a decision. For the clinician, it is important that a clinically sound decision is made and that it is consistent with recommendations. However, patients may not want as much information as the clinician gives, and sometimes they prefer a lack of choice (8). Participation in the decision-making process can be an unwarranted burden and patients frequently do not want to take responsibility for the final decision (9). Some patients are more concerned with the personal individual relationships that they form with their clinicians, than the provision of information (10). Whether the patient feels heard and trusts the clinician to act on their behalf may be more important than the degree to which the patient feels they have participated in the decision. Improving the quality of the interaction with the clinician in this way leads to increased satisfaction and reduced anxiety.

Prognosis and uncertainty

Discussing prognosis can be especially challenging, as it raises issues of probabilities and uncertainties. The availability of on-line prognostic tools, e.g. Adjuvant Online, has made it easier to avoid words such as 'small', 'large', 'rare'. However, percentages are often confusing, e.g. quoting 30% of patients with your cancer will be alive in 10 years, leads to uncertainty as the patient does not know which group they will be in. Understanding statistics is difficult for patients, particularly those who have low literacy levels. The example in Box 41.1 illustrates how statistics can be misinterpreted.

The issue of uncertainty is a particular problem for patients with cancer of unknown primary. These patients generally have a poor understanding of their disease and its causes, prognosis, and treatment (12).

Box 41.1 Patient perceptious of probability

In a study investigating consent into a hypothetical trial, 50 patients with cancer were asked to correctly interpret the following statement:

'A particular type of cancer responds to radiation treatment in 10% of cases'

The radiation treatment is about 10% effective in an individual patient: 22%

On average, for 10 out of 100 patients, the tumour will decrease in size after radiation treatment: 46%

There is a 10% chance of survival: 10%

10% of patients are cured: 22%

Sutherland *et al.* (11)

Discussing randomized controlled clinical trials

Discussing randomized controlled trials is one of most problematic areas of cancer communication. Of senior UK clinicians attending communication skills training, 52% acknowledged that providing complex information and seeking consent for clinical trials were their primary communication problems, surpassing breaking bad news (13). Currently only one in three patients approached about clinical trials will consent to randomization. Trials with a 'no treatment arm' are especially difficult to recruit to.

The discussion of clinical trials requires specific skills and understanding of a complex language. Increasingly, the responsibility for giving patients information about trials falls on specialist research nurses. In a clinical trial discussion, the healthcare professional must include an explanation of the standard therapy, reason for the trial, uncertainty about novel drugs/procedures, the concept of randomization, and defining terms such as 'double-blind' or 'placebo-controlled'. If communication is inadequate, patients may fail to understand the experimental nature of the trial and be unclear about treatment options, and, therefore, be unable to give truly informed consent (14).

Randomization is a difficult concept for patients to understand, as the example in Box 41.2 illustrates. Jenkins et al. surveyed 200 patients, 200 oncologists, and 341 people without cancer, and gave them seven descriptions of randomization. The most favoured description of randomization by patients and members of the public was a computer and not the doctor or patient who would decide which treatment was given. The most disliked description (and the one used by more than a quarter of the oncologists) was 'a computer will perform the equivalent to tossing a coin to allocate you to one of two methods of treatment'. This was seen as trivializing the situation and was particularly upsetting in the context of life-threatening disease (15).

Communication during treatment

Once a diagnosis has been made and a management plan decided, it is essential that good communication continues throughout treatment, not least to pick up potentially life-threatening side-effects, such as neutropenic sepsis. Perhaps more importantly, especially for palliative treatments, some idea of quality of life must be ascertained during treatment, as this will be the primary endpoint. Patients must feel comfortable enough to voice their concerns during treatment in order to fully assess their experience. Clinicians are often unable to elicit patients' most important

---

Box 41.2 Patient perceptions of randomisation in trials

In a study investigating consent into a hypothetical trial, 50 patients with cancer were asked to correctly interpret the following statement:

'A process called randomization is used to select your treatment in this clinical trial'

The process will select the best treatment for me: 14%

Each individual patient has exactly the same chance of receiving the drug, or not receiving the drug, as any other participating patient: 66%

One treatment is given one time, another is given another time: 0%

The doctor decides which treatment is the right one for me: 19%

Sutherland *et al.* (12)

concerns, which usually relate to quality of life. Multiple studies have shown that radiotherapy and chemotherapy toxicity scores are a poor measure of quality of life and patient function.

Validated measures of health-related quality of life have been shown to be of use in guiding treatment choices. In a randomized study conducted by Brundage et al., 'surrogate' lung cancer patients were presented with quality-of-life information, in addition to survival and toxicity data, and their preference for chemotherapy was recorded (16). If there was a benefit in quality of life, more patients changed their decision about chemotherapy, and this number increased if the quality-of-life difference was larger. This study shows how health-related quality-of-life data can influence patients' choices.

Quality-of-life data can also be used to show the effect of interventions in communication. Velikova et al. conducted a three-arm randomized trial to look at whether an assessment of quality of life, along with an intervention (feedback from the doctor after review of the quality-of-life results), could improve patient outcome (17). EORTC QLQ 30 questionnaires were used to measure quality of life at baseline and subsequently over a period of six months. There was a significant difference in quality of life between patients who completed questionnaires and those who did not. The difference was even larger for those who had feedback from the doctor. This study clearly shows that a simple intervention, which can easily be performed in clinic, can significantly improve communication and leads to improved health outcomes.

Another intervention shown to improve quality of life is the use of prompts in conversations between healthcare professionals and patients. Aaronson et al. compared the quality of life in two cohorts of patients (18). The first group completed quality-of-life questionnaires at the beginning and end of the study period, but did not receive an intervention. The patients in the second cohort were prompted by the nurses in a series of outpatient visits. These prompts influenced the subjects discussed in the consultations, e.g. symptoms, sexuality. Validated scores of quality of life showed improvement in the group of patients whose conversations were changed by prompts.

Psychosexual functioning

Clinicians are generally good at giving information about diagnosis and treatment (>90% of patients in one study) (19) but less frequently discuss sexual functioning (38%). Patients also may deliberately avoid discussing, or responding to, questionnaire items about sexual wellbeing. The group most at risk of sexual dysfunction are those patients who have had pelvic surgery/radiotherapy and/or hormone manipulation (20). In one study, 82% of women under 50 years old who had surgery and radiotherapy for gynaecological cancer suffered sexual dysfunction (21). Many of these women are depressed or anxious because of chronic sexual problems. When interviewed in one study, women who had undergone major surgery for carcinoma of the cervix or vulva in the previous five years, reported that they would have liked more information on physical, sexual, and emotional after-effects of treatment (22). They also wanted their partners to have been included in the discussions, and a quarter of the partners themselves would have like more information. It is, therefore, very important to identify patients who have psychosexual needs. This subject must be discussed in a suitably private environment, e.g. examination rather than consulting room, and questions should be asked in a sensitive manner. Quality-of-life prompts can help to stimulate relevant discussion, as can introducing non-threatening subjects such as sleep.

Communication and survivorship

Communication skills training tends to concentrate on the issues discussed previously—breaking bad news, giving information about diagnosis, prognosis and treatments, monitoring toxicities from treatment and, to a lesser extent, assessing quality of life. However, as cancer incidence rises and survival rates improve, there are an increasing number of patients living with, and surviving, cancer, who have a specific set of needs that is frequently neglected by clinicians. In the year transition between completion of primary treatment and 'living with cancer', patients often feel abandoned by the hospital system (23). This may have a detrimental effect on recovery rates, as patients and carers often feel unsupported.

In order that patients feel less abandoned once treatment is complete, it is important that they have some understanding of the purpose of follow-up. Currently, most cancers are followed up by a hospital team for around 2–10 years after completion of treatment. However, few recurrences are found by routine surveillance—in breast cancer, most recurrences are self-detected and are usually incurable. Patients also find it difficult to manage the uncertainty aspect of survivorship. Whilst the primary treatment may have 'cured' them, or at least put them into remission, not knowing whether the cancer will return is a continuing cause for anxiety.

The move to living with a chronic illness can be a difficult adjustment to make as patients are more likely to be in poor health and have psychological and functional disability. Many patients have to live with the late side-effects of treatment, which may present some years after initial treatment and can be debilitating. The emotional and psychological burden of cancer can persist long after treatment has finished (24), which may be a contributing factor to patients not being able to work. People younger than 65 years with a cancer diagnosis are six times more likely to not be able to work because of their health, than those without a cancer diagnosis, according to a US study comparing 5000 cancer survivors and 90,000 people without cancer (24). This places an additional financial burden on patients surviving cancer.

Another issue that becomes relevant to survivorship is teaching new health behaviours to not only improve general health but also reduce the risks of specific consequences of cancer treatment. Weight-gain after treatment is a recognized problem, which can result in obesity. The benefits of exercise during and after treatment have been clearly shown (25). Once treatment has finished, interventions to increase physical activity and improve diet can be used to reduce the long-term sequelae of obesity. Another example of reducing late complications of treatment is smoking cessation after chest radiotherapy, in order to preserve remaining lung function. Life-style modification only becomes an issue for patients who survive cancer.

Post-primary treatment support programmes have been shown to improve health outcomes, including quality of life and psychological functioning, and also reduce disability from cancer (26, 27). The emphasis is on helping people to manage their own care. Interventions include giving patients information on recurrence and late side-effects, an assessment of support needs (say at three months post-treatment), and communication with the GP summarizing treatment and any ongoing needs. These measures provide patients with self-management strategies that lead to improved knowledge, better coping behaviour, adherence to treatments, and self-efficacy in symptom management. However, the most effective intervention is participation in self-help and support groups, which provide an environment where patients can share information and experiences.

Communication in end-of-life care

Raising the issue of approaching end of life is difficult for patients and clinicians. Many patients find it hard to ask difficult and sensitive questions about prognosis without prompting (28), and clinicians often wait to be asked (29). A recent randomized controlled trial found that the use of questionnaire prompts resulted in longer consultations, twice as many questions being asked by patients, more end-of-life discussions but also fewer unmet needs (30). If prognosis is estimated, clinicians tend to be over-optimistic (31). A systematic review showed that physicians are generally poor at predicting prognosis in terminally ill patients, with errors (more than double or less than half of actual survival) in 30% of cases (32). Two-thirds of these errors were over-estimates.

One of the reasons why discussing end-of-life issues is so difficult is that many patients are having active cancer treatment in the last few months of life, with as many as 10% receiving active treatment in the last few weeks (32). For these patients, there is no clear cut-off between not having active treatment and the start of end-of-life care (33). End-of-life discussions are often still linked in with the stopping of active treatment, which is too late for effective advance care planning. Oncologists rarely initiate discussions with patients about possibly being in the last year of life (so called 'what if' conversations) during active treatment. This leads to confusion about prognosis and supportive care options for patients. Primary care teams tend not to refer patients for community support until they have received the appropriate signal from the specialist (33). Palliative care and hospice staff may only be peripherally involved in patients' care. Site-specific nurses may be more closely involved with patients, but they often do not see end of life discussions as part of their role (34–36).

Treatment is often initiated in the last few months of life as a way of 'giving hope' to patients. A recent study of the use of second-line palliative chemotherapy in breast cancer found that 'giving hope' was one of the most important aims for oncologists in offering treatment (37, 38). Thus, treatment is acting as a substitute for communication about end-of-life issues. In some countries, in particular the USA, oncologists prefer to use anti-cancer therapy rather than supportive care alone in advanced disease (39). Less than half of European radiotherapists and only 15% of American radiotherapists participated in the terminal care of their patients, according to a survey of the management of NSCLC patients (40). Many oncologists are not involved in the supportive care of their patients and consequently there are fewer end-of-life discussions.

The lack of opportunities to discuss the implications of being in the last year of life can seriously affect quality of life for patients and their carers, and place an unnecessary burden on the NHS. According to the 2004 report, Unclaimed Millions, over half of patients who die from cancer are not receiving the benefits they are entitled to (Disability Living Allowance and Attendance Allowance). This has a significant financial impact on terminally ill patients. Quality of life may also be affected by inappropriate prolongation of active cancer treatment. Delaying the 'what if' discussion may leave patients and carers without the emotional support and information needed to make adequate preparations for death (40–42). Carers often lack understanding of prognosis and also support for themselves, which can result in inappropriate and avoidable hospital admissions of patients with advanced cancer (43).

It is, therefore, of great importance that patients with incurable cancer are given multiple opportunities to discuss possibly being in the last year of life. End-of-life discussions should not be associated only with the withdrawal of treatment or dying, but should be initiated at the start of palliative treatment and regularly reviewed, e.g. every three months. Patients who may be approaching the last year of life can be identified more effectively if the 'surprise' question is asked, i.e. whether the physician would be 'surprised' if the patient died within a year. 'What if' discussions can then take place at the appropriate time and adequate support for end-of-life needs can be provided.

Medical wellbeing and its impact on communication

Effective communication between doctor and patient is dependent on the wellbeing of the doctor. Taylor *et al.* surveyed doctors from various different specialties in the UK in 1994 and

2002, and found that there was an increase in psychological morbidity over time, which was more pronounced in clinical oncologists compared with doctors in other specialties (44). The decline in mental health was due to increased job stress without a comparable increase in job satisfaction. Increased stress and burnout can have a negative impact on communication with patients.

Communication skills training can improve the mental health of physicians (45). In a survey conducted by Ramirez et al., consultants who lacked communication skills training were more likely to suffer from burnout (46). Physicians should also have training that includes coping strategies to help them deal with their own emotions (47). Stress often lasts beyond the consultation itself (46) and therefore it is essential that physicians develop self-awareness and monitor their own wellbeing.

References

1. Cancer Research UK website: **www.cancerresearchuk.org**

2. Cancer in the Media May—October 2000. Reported prepared for Macmillan Cancer Support by BMRB Information Services (2001).

3. Epstein RM, Street RL Jr (2007) *Patient-centered communication in cancer care: promoting healing and reducing suffering.* National Cancer Institute, NIH Publication No. 07-6225. Bethesda, MD.

4. Balsa *et al.* (2003) Prejudice, clinical uncertainty and stereotyping as sources of health disparities. *J Health Economics* **22** (1): 89–116.

5. Davis T *et al.* (2002) Health literacy and cancer communication. *CA Cancer J Clin* **52**: 134–149.

6. Jenkins *et al.* (2001) Information needs of patients with cancer: results from a large study in UK cancer centres. *British Journal of Cancer* **84** (1): 48–51.

7. Tackling cancer: improving the patient journey. National Audit Office, HC 288 session 2004–2005, 25 February 2005.

8. Salmon P and Hall G (2004) Patient empowerment or the emperor's new clothes? *Journal of the Royal Society of Medicine* **97** (2): 53–56.

9. National Breast Cancer Centre and National Cancer Control Initiative. Clinical practice guidelines for the psychosocial care of adults with cancer. Camperdown, Australia: National Breast Cancer Centre; 2003 (cited 20 Nov 2007). Available from url: **http://www.nhmrc.gov.au/publications/symposes/files/cp90.pdf**.

10. Burkitt Wright E, Salmon P, *et al.* (2004) Doctor's communication of trust, care and respect. Qualitative study. *British Medical Journal* **328**: 864–867.

11. Sutherland *et al.* (1990) Are we getting informed consent from patients with cancer? *Journal of the Royal Society of Medicine* **83** (7): 439–443.

12. Boyland L, Davis C (2007) Patients' experience of carcinoma of unknown primary site: dealing with uncertainty. *Palliative Medicine* (in press).

13. Fallowfield *et al.* (2002) Efficacy of a Cancer Research UK communication skills training model for oncologists: a randomized controlled trial. *Lancet* **359** (9307): 650–656.

14. Fallowfield and Jenkins (1999) Effective communication skills are the key to good cancer care. *European Journal Cancer* **35** (11): 1592–1597.

15. Jenkins V, Fallowfield L, Cox A (2005) The preferences of 600 patients for different descriptions of randomization. *British Journal Cancer* **92** (5): 807–810.

16. Brundage MD, Feldman-Stewart D, Leis A, *et al.* (2007) The importance of quality of life information to a lung cancer (NSCLC chemotherapy treatment decision—results of a randomized evaluation. In Proceedings of International Psycho-Oncology Society 9th World Congress of Psycho-Oncology, London, 16–20 September 2007.

17. Velikova *et al.* (2004) Measuring quality of life in routine oncology practice improves communication and patient well-being: a randomized controlled trial. *Journal of Clinical Oncology* **22** (4): 714–724.

18. Aaronson NK, Hilarius DL, Kloeg P, *et al.* (2007) The use of Health-Related Quality of Life (HRQL) assessments in daily clinical oncology nursing practice: a community hospital-based intervention study. In Proceedings of International Psych-Oncology Society 9th World Congress of Psycho-Oncology, London, 16–20 September 2007.

19. Cox A, Jenkins V, Catt F, *et al.* (2006) Information needs and experiences. *European Journal Oncology Nursing* **10** (4):263–72.

20. Basen-Enquist K, Bodurka DC (2007) Medical and psychosocial issues in gynaecological cancer survivors. In *Cancer Survivorship Today & Tomorrow.* (ed. P Ganz). Springer, 114–121.

21. Corney *et al.* (1993) Psychosexual dysfunction in women with gynaecological cancer following radical pelvic surgery. *Br J Obstet Gynaecol* **100** (1): 73–78.

22. Corney *et al.* (1992) The care of patients undergoing surgery for gynaecological cancer: the need for information, emotional support and counselling. *J Adv Nurs* **17** (6): 667–671.

23. Cardy P *et al.* (2006) *Worried sick: the emotional impact of cancer.* Macmillan Cancer Support.

24. Hewitt M *et al.* (2003) Cancer survivors in the United States: age health and disability. *Journal of Gerontology* **58** (1): 82–91.

25. Kirshbaum M (2007) A review of the benefits of whole body exercise during and after treatment for breast cancer. *Journal of Clinical Nursing* **16** (1): 104–121.

26. Coulter A and Ellins E (2006) *Patient-focused interventions.* Picker Institute Europe.

27. Rehse B and Pukrop R (2003) Effects of psychosocial interventions on quality of life in adult cancer patients: meta-analysis of 37 published controlled outcome studies. *Patient Education and Counselling* **50** (2): 179–186.

28. Street R L (1991) Information giving in medical consultations: the influence of patients' communicative styles and personal characteristics. *Soc. Sci and Medicine* **32**: 541–548.

29. Parker S *et al.* (2006) A systematic review of prognostic/end-of-life communication with adults in the advanced stages of a life-limiting illness: patient/caregiver preferences for the content, style and timing of information. *Journal of Pain and Symptom Management* **34** (1): 81–93.

30. Clayton *et al.* (2007) Randomized controlled trial of a prompt list to help advanced cancer patients and their caregivers to ask questions about prognosis and end-of-life care. *Journal of Clinical Oncology* **25** (6): 715–723.

31. Glare *et al.* (2003) A systematic review of physicians survival predictions in terminally ill cancer patients. *British Medical Journal* **327**: 195–8.

32. Earle *et al.* (2004) Trends in aggressiveness of cancer care near end of life. *Journal of Clinical Oncology* **22** (2): 315–321.

33. Lamont *et al.* (2002) Physician factors in the timing of cancer patient referral to hospice palliative care. *Cancer* **94** (10): 2733–2737.

34. Grunfeld *et al.* (2006) Perceptions of palliative chemotherapy: the view of advanced breast cancer patients. *Journal of Clinical Oncology* **24** (7): 1090–1098.

35. Gatellari *et al.* (1999) Misunderstandings in cancer patients. *Annals of Oncology,* **10**, 39–46.

36. Jamal *et al.*, Proceedings EAPC, Budapest 2007.

37. Grunfeld *et al.* (2005) Decision-making for palliative chemotherapy: perceptions of patients with advanced breast cancer. *J Clin Oncology* **24**(7): 1090–1098.

38. Grunfeld *et al.* (2001) Chemotherapy for advanced breast cancer: what influences oncologists decision-making. *British Journal of Cancer* **84** (9): 1172–1178.

39. Maher *et al.* (1992) Treatment strategies in advanced and metastatic cancer: differences in attitude between the USA, Canada and Europe. *Int J Radiat Oncol Biol Phys* **23**: 239–244.

40. Fried *et al.* (2005) Unmet desire for caregiver–patient communication and increased caregiver burden. *J Am Geriatr Soc* **53** (1): 59–65.

41. Goldstein *et al.* (2004) Factors associated with caregiver burden among caregivers of terminally ill patients with cancer. *Journal of Palliative Care* **20**: 38–43.

42. Grunfeld *et al.* (2004) Family caregiver burden: results of a longitudinal study of breast cancer patients and their principal caregivers. *CMAJ* **170** (12): 1795–1801.

43. Higginson *et al.* (1994) Reducing hospital beds for patients with advanced cancer. *The Lancet* **344** (ii): 409.

44. Taylor C *et al.* (2005) Changes in mental health of UK hospital consultants since the mid-1990s. *Lancet* **366** (9487): 742–4.

Chapter 42

Palliative medicine: communication to promote life near the end of life

Ilora G Finlay and Nicola Pease

When does a cancer patient become a palliative care patient?

Ask yourself the survival question: 'would you be surprised if this patient is alive in six months?' (1). If the honest answer is yes, then you need to start to sort out end-of-life care. In many ways, end-of-life care is planning for the worst and hoping for the best.

And what about the patients? It seems that patients know only too well they are getting more ill, not responding to treatment and that their life is rapidly drawing to a close. But it also seems that, unless the doctor has courage and compassion to listen openly and allow the unspoken questions to be voiced, the patient will comply with the conspiracy of silence, harbouring unspoken fears about what might happen and unable to put affairs in order with those closest to him or her.

In this text, the use of a toolkit (2) has been described as a way of coping with difficult consultations. One of the most difficult scenarios is when the whole topic of non-response to treatment—or no treatment options—has to the broached. The U-turn that the oncologist has to do is hard—after all the treatment that a patient has been offered, the message is effectively one that 'it was probably all in vain'. So how can that be offered gently and without devastating both patient and oncologist, without continuing to offer interventions that will do more harm than good and which only serve to make the oncologist feel better because 'something is being done'?

In different healthcare systems, the organization of funding determines how palliative care services link into the oncology services. Two classical models (Figs 42.1 and 42.2) are evident; unfortunately the sudden transition (Fig. 42.1) is imposed by systems that require patients to sign out of oncology treatment in order to access palliative and hospice care. The other option (Fig. 42.2) is seen where a palliative care team works alongside an oncology service and is able to enhance the patient's quality of life during oncology treatments. The latter is common in

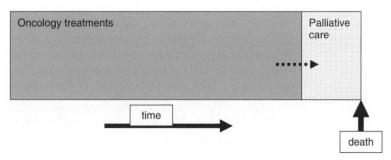

Fig. 42.1 The transition to palliative is abrupt. For example, the patient may have to alter financial insurance cover to obtain the service.

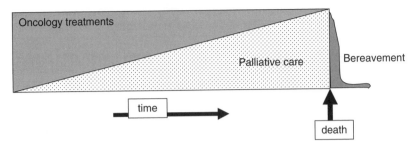

Fig. 42.2 Transition between palliative and active treatments is linked to the patients' fluctuating condition, occurs at any time and represents integrated services.

countries like the UK, Australia and Canada, but not the norm in the USA. However, without information about their own condition, patients cannot make choices on how they want to live in the last phase of their lives.

Transition to palliative care

So how can the situation be raised? The general principle is to get the patient to tell you what they feel is happening, but that may feel easier said than done. Of course it is breaking bad news all over again and will involve the difficulties that entails. The toolkit is given as an explanation in Table 42.1, Box 42.1 and Table 42.2.

Table 42.1 Breaking bad news–the toolkit in action

Tool	Doctor	Patient
Comfort	Do come and sit down Mrs P. Are you comfortable on that chair? Or would you prefer the higher seat?	
		Yes, thank you.
Non-verbal	Looking serious	
Question—open	How have things been?	
		Not so good.
Reflection	Not so good?	
		No, I've been tired all the time and my appetite has gone again.
Reflection	Tired all the time?	
		Yes, I just don't have the energy I had. And I don't think the new tablets suit me; the ache in my back is worse some nights and stops me sleeping.
Question—focused	Does anything else stop you sleeping?	
		Well, worry…

Table 42.1 (continued) Breaking bad news

Tool	Doctor	Patient
Question—focused	About?	
		Everything
Reflection	Everything?	
		Yes, what will happen if this does not work, what about the children, what I should do, what if it's come back...
Reflection	Come back?	
		The cancer.
Question—focused	Do you feel as if it has come back?	
		At times...
Question—focused	And if it has?	
		Do you think it has?
Summarizing (followed by checking back that patient agrees with the summary)	Well, it sounds to me as if you're telling me you feel it has. You're tired, the backache is worse, your appetite has gone and your worries are stopping you sleeping. Is that right?	
		Yes, I do worry a lot. So do you think the cancer is back again?
Partial reflection	I'm sorry to say I share your worries.	
Listening—use of silence		Oh...
Non verbal (confirms the bad news)	Uh huh (nodding slightly)	
		Mmmm...
	So do you think we should discuss what next?	
		Yes.
Summarizing	Let me summarize where I think we are. We both think things might have got worse, and need to check that out. And you feel tired, have back pain and aren't eating well, so we need to find out the cause of those particular symptoms and then do something to improve them.	
		What are you suggesting?
Combination of reflection and summarizing used to spell out a plan	Firstly, perhaps we need to X-ray your back to see just what is going on...	

Box 42.1 The angry patient

Comfort—sit down and try to ensure your eye level is below the level of the person who is angry. Sitting over someone can appear dominating and can worsen the situation.

Listen—the person who is angry will feel validated and more in control if they feel they are being listened to; active listening is the greatest tool to calm a fraught situation. Remember the 80–20 rule = listen for 80% of the time!

Non-verbal communication—the pace can often be slowed by ensuring you are sitting down, speaking slowly, gently and clearly, and using fewer—not more—words. And avoid any aggressive postures—open palms and open posture is less threatening than closed fists and folded arms.

Questions—should be kept as open as possible, exploring what the real concerns are and keeping the discussion focused around the real issues, rather than risk being drawn into side issues.

Reflection—complements active listening. Reflect back key words or phrases to elucidate the misconceptions or fears underlying the anger.

Summarize the points heard—it will reinforce that the person has been listened to and will allow a little breathing space in the flow of words; it also gives you thinking time. And also summarize the plan you jointly evolve with the patient.

Some situations are particularly difficult. For the physician, when there are a lot of 'cross identifiers', such as a patient who is a close colleague or friend, or the same age as one's own children, or a strong reminder of someone close, it can be particularly hard, as the patient's dying forces the physician to confront the frailty of medicine and the inescapability of mortality (3).

The patient or family who is angry threatens one's personal safety boundaries, sometimes actually physically, and often in terms of professional standing, future livelihood, and so on, yet anger is a desperate attempt to gain control; it marks the person who feels out of control. So in this situation the toolkit comes into its own. Working through the different parts is outlined in Box 42.1.

Communicating in the face of delirium

Consent is key to almost all medical decisions. Yet in the face of delirium, it can be very difficult to ascertain exactly what a patient wants done or not done.

The patient may have left an advanced decision outlining a refusal of consent to treatment in a specific situation. In many places these are spoken of as advance directives, but strictly speaking they are not directives because a person cannot direct another to do something to them—you cannot direct someone to kill you, to operate on you if there is no clinical indication, to overload you with fluids or administer some drug that is inappropriate for your condition and so on. So these documents are 'advance refusals' and that term will be used here; in some countries such a document is potentially legally binding and the doctor who treats against the advanced decision of the patient may be vulnerable in law.

But, ascertaining the validity of such an advanced decision can be difficult. Was it made freely and without coercion? Was it an informed decision? And at the time that it was made, did the patient have the mental capacity to make such a decision?

A particular difficulty can arise if the advanced decision does not correspond with the patient's best interest. In this situation the advanced decision is usually seen as being legally binding, but only if it is a valid advanced decision. For an advance decision to be valid, it must specify the treatment that is to be refused, in medical language or lay terms. It should set out the circumstances in which the refusal will apply, including as much detail as possible on the circumstances in which the refusal will apply. And advanced decisions only apply when the person lacks capacity to consent to the specified treatment.

In addition, the patient may have made an advance statement of their wishes in treatment, but an advance statement is not legally binding, although it usually will outline what the patient would like to have done, or where the patient would like to be cared for (such as at home, in a hospice, etc.). Sometimes these are called Preferences in Care documents or Medical Orders for Life Sustaining Treatments (MOLST), depending on the legislative jurisdiction (4, 5). Such documents cannot instruct the clinician to do something to the patient, but can express their clear wishes to be taken into consideration when making a decision in the patient's best interest.

Mental capacity act 2007

In the United Kingdom, the process of taking a decision on behalf of the patient has now been outlined within a legal framework (6). One piece of legislation has been produced in England and Wales, and another in Scotland by the Scottish Parliament. These pieces of legislation, although applying only to the United Kingdom, enshrine best practice in law. They set out some simple steps to be taken in determining capacity for an individual decision and the framework of taking 'best interest' decisions on behalf of the patient. Although the legislation does not apply elsewhere, it provides an important framework applicable anywhere in the world in terms of good clinical practice. The framework has to be underpinned by sound communication with the patient, their family and carers.

Five statutory principles underpin this legislation. First, a person must be assumed to have capacity, unless it is established that they lack the capacity. Second, a person is not to be treated as unable to make a decision, unless all practical steps to help introduce it have been taken without success. Third, a person is not to be treated as if he is unable to make a decision merely because he makes an unwise decision. Fourth, an act done or decision made on behalf of a person who lacks capacity must be done, or made, in his best interests. And, fifth, before the act is done, or the decision made, regard must be had to whether the purpose for which it is needed can be as effectively achieved in a way that is less restrictive of the person's rights and freedom of action.

In assessing capacity, a two-stage test of capacity has been outlined. First, does the patient have a disorder of the mind or brain that is impairing his ability to make a decision? Second, if so, has it made the person unable to make a particular decision? Thus, the test is situation-specific; a person may lack capacity to manage financial affairs or to take a decision over where to move to, but may be able to take a decision over whether he needs more or less analgesia or what he would like to eat. This two-stage test of capacity covers a wide range of situations, such as alcohol or drug misuse, delirium, mental illness, dementia, learning disabilities or the long-term effects of brain damage for whatever reason, such as following surgery and/or radiotherapy.

Capacity may be fluctuating, so the law outlines that everything must be done to try to enhance the person's capacity to take a decision. However, even when capacity is permanently impaired, the clinician must ensure that the patient is communicated with in the language that he can understand, in a calm environment, with comfort addressed and so on, doing everything possible to enhance the capacity that the patient has. Thus, for example, there is an onus on the clinician to ensure that a patient who is deaf has his hearing aid, if needed, that the patient is not sitting in a position where sunlight from the window is obscuring the view of the doctor, that the patient is not distracted, that any information leaflets are written at a reading age and in a language understandable by the patient, with a print font that is legible and that it is relevant to the individual patient. Thus simply giving a patient an information leaflet does not meet their communication needs at all.

In making the decision, there are three stages that should be fulfilled for a decision to be valid. First, does the patient understand the decision they need to make and why they need to make it? Second, can the patient understand information about the decision? Third, can they retain it, use it and weigh it up to make the decision? (7). Of course, this all hinges on the information being presented to the patient in an understandable way and that the decision is being made voluntarily and free from coercion of any sort.

If the patient lacks capacity, there is also a requirement that the decision is put off, if possible, until capacity is regained. If capacity is unlikely to improve, then a 'best interest' decision has to be taken on behalf the patient. The clinician is required to consult with others; for example, those who are family and carers and are likely to know the patient's past and present wishes and feelings, and beliefs and values. This information gathering is important to guide decision-making. Even when the patient lacks capacity, every effort must be made to permit and encourage participation in the decision-making process through communication with the patient.

So, when a best-interest decision is to be taken, it must be taken without prejudice, avoiding the influence of age, appearance, condition or behaviour. All relevant circumstances must be considered and every effort made to encourage and enable the patient to participate in the decision-making, including consideration as to whether the decision could be put off until later. There are special considerations of life-sustaining treatment and, in general, the default option is to work to sustain life.

Sometimes patients will have appointed someone with power of attorney for property and financial affairs, but only to take healthcare decisions on behalf of the patient in the event of a lack of capacity. Such a person, appointed as lasting power of attorney for personal welfare, must have this role formally registered, cannot over-rule an advance decision to refuse treatment and can only consent to refuse life-sustaining treatment on behalf the patient if this has been agreed at the time that the power of attorney was granted.

Discussing death

In general in society death is little discussed. Patients often try to raise the topic of death in different and tactful ways. Questions around assisted suicide and euthanasia are often used to test the clinician's ability to be open and honest and as a way of ascertaining what lies ahead. The way the clinician responds can begin to restore some realistic hope of improved quality of life, which must be accompanied by redoubling efforts at good palliation. But a response that takes the request at face value—and offers to explore the request and process it—gives the subliminal message to the patient that the situation is indeed hopeless and that they would be better off dead.

Here again, the toolkit can be used to explore the reasons behind such a request, as illustrated in the brief dialogue in Table 42.2.

Patients often worry about their potential mode of dying, and benefit from the physician's openness to discuss likely events. Here the physician is wise to keep an emphasis on effective palliative treatments to ameliorate any suffering. Death from liver failure, coma, cardiac events or respiratory failure merit discussion and are further illustrated in this chapter in a subsequent section on communication about palliative treatments.

Table 42.2 Discussing death – the toolkit in action

Tool	Doctor	Patient
Question—open	How have you been?	
		Terrible. I'm fed up with it all.
Reflection	Fed up?	
		Yes, you wouldn't let a dog die like this.
Question—focused	Do you feel as if you are dying?	
		Of course I do and I just want to get it over with quickly.
Reflection	Over quickly?	
		Well, you know, end it all.
Reflection	So can you tell me the specific things that make you feel life is so awful that you want to end it all?	
		Well I can't do what I used to, don't feel like the person I was.
Reflection	Don't feel like the person you were?	
		No, look at me now. I'm a burden. And it frightens me.
Reflection	It frightens?	
		Yes. I'm frightened of being a burden, frightened of what tomorrow holds and frightened of losing my independence and my dignity.
Reflection	So is there anything at all you can think of that would help you feel more independent and with more dignity?	
Silence (listening)	…	
		What if my wife cannot cope?
Reflection	Cope?	
		With my toilet needs.
Question—clarification	Have you spoken about this with her?	
		No, you see we're pretty private about stuff like that.
Summarize	So can I summarize what I think I've heard: you feel so wretched that you want to die, you are frightened of being a burden, frightened that your wife can't cope and worried about some of the intimate aspects of care such as the toilet. Is that about right?	
		Yes.
	And is there anything else?	
		No that's the main things.
Summarize the plan and check back on it (active listening, observing patient comfort)	So, could we try to make sure your privacy is maintained, get support for your wife and look at ways to increase your sense of control over your own care?	
		That would be really helpful…

Spirituality

Clinicians, particularly doctors, can sometimes find it difficult to discuss the issues around spiritual beliefs and concerns. Indeed, some patients feel that it is not the doctor's role to discuss such issues, yet others may not know who to speak to (8). This leaves the clinician walking a tightrope.

Again, the patient can be given openings to discuss spirituality and, if the topic is picked up, the conversation could be pursued (9). Using the principles outlined above, an open question around issues of faith and belief could be phrased along the lines of: 'Are there any faith-based, religious or spiritual concerns you feel we should address?'. In response to this, a patient once asked me if I have a faith. Not wanting to close the conversation either way, nor commit myself (remembering the principle of 'comfort'), I responded that 'at times it was a bit like a sieve'; the response came 'so you're just like me' and the patient went on to explain that, although everyone assumed she had a strong faith, she was full of doubts and internal conflicts. In my response, it was important initially to just simply reflect back words and phrases to demonstrate I was actively listening. I could offer no solutions, no answers and no therapy, yet the patient found this conversation particularly comforting and commented about how helpful it was to simply be listened to and believed, without kindly meant but hollow words with which she could not identify.

In a study of patient's perception of spirituality, patients frequently used analogies to 'being in the same boat', to 'being caught' rather like a fish, and to not wanting to burden those they love with difficult memories (10). As one patient commented, when her son asked her, 'Why are you always laughing and smiling?' she replied, 'Because I do not want you to remember me miserable. I want you to remember me laughing and smiling'. The US National Consensus Project Guidelines for Quality Palliative Care recognise spirituality as a critical component of care (11).

Collusion

In different cultural settings, different families function in unique ways. Wherever they live, they often bring with them their own family traditions. These are not linked to religion, race or local education, so it can be dangerous to make assumptions about the type of person a patient is, or about how their family functions. In some families, the eldest male relative becomes a key decision-maker. This can be quite difficult when the care is being given by others, since this eldest male may live some distance away and often has little insight into the care pressures.

Again, the use of open questions can be helpful to explore what the individual patient wants. Questions such as, 'Are you the type of person who wants me to speak directly to you or are you the type of person who wants me to deal with your family?'. When the patient becomes more ill, confused and loses mental capacity, the focus of decision-making switches.

Many family difficulties arise in the twilight time, when the family desperately want to protect the person they love and so they play an over-optimistic game, fearful that the truth will remove the hope and the patient will lose the will to live (12). Sometimes this is carried to an extreme and the family are compensating for things that have happened in the past.

The patient may have issues in the past that have also been kept hidden. Advancing illness brings with it the fear that some past secrets may be revealed, such as the existence of a second family, previous misdeeds or guilt, or other difficulties.

When dealing with the family who exert a great deal of pressure, it can be helpful to spell out that you are 'not here to make anything more difficult than it is already' and that you recognize that they are wanting to protect the person they love. It is also helpful sometimes to clarify—and thereby help them understand—that the patient knows that he is ill and indeed feels ill; being an intelligent person the patient will realize things are being hidden, and may believe that if nobody will talk about what's happening, the truth must be so terrifying that no one dares voice it (13). Of course, a person who knows that they have been lied to will always find it difficult to trust again, so it is very important that the clinicians do not lie in response to a question.

The family, exerting pressure for clinicians to collude with them against telling the patient the truth, can find it reassuring to know that the clinicians will not suddenly announce the devastating news, but will only respond with gentle honesty to questions from the patient. It is also helpful to spell out that the clinical team are not there to destroy hope, but are there to try to make things easier than they are at present.

The conversation with a patient can then be handled using the toolkit. By simply using open questions, picking up on key words or phrases and reflecting them back to the patient, then listening to the response and reflecting further, the clinician can be secure in only using the words and language of the patient, yet allowing the patient to tell the clinician about the situation.

Denial

Sometimes the patient and the family are tremendously unrealistic, to the point of being in denial over what is happening (14). Denial is a normal defence mechanism in response to major stress, but denial that persists can result in the patient failing to address major areas of concern. Unrealistic, full-scale denial can also present an atmosphere of collusion which, at the end of the day, all comes crashing down as myths and lies are not sustainable in the long term.

Because denial is a defence or coping mechanism, it can be dangerous to simply destroy denial. It is much safer to get the patient to gradually see that their perception of things does not match reality. The concept of 'finding a window on denial' has been used to describe this process. It is as if the clinician is gently feeling (with words) along a solid brick wall (the patient's denial), looking for a chink that can be eventually opened up to reveal a window through the wall. Again, to achieve this, the use of reflection and summarising are key tools. A beneficial question for the patient is: 'Have you thought about what you would want if things did not go quite as well as we all hope?'.

Although denial may not be harmful to the patient, it can be deleterious to others, such as children and the family, who are dependent on the patient and for whom plans for the future must be made.

Making a will

It is surprising how many people go through life without ever having made a will. The clinician can quite simply ask whether there are specific administrative concerns, such as writing a will, that the patient has not addressed. This can be downplayed, because everybody should have written a will as soon as they become adults and have any material possessions at all. This can be quite simply mentioned in terms of 'hoping for the best and planning for the worst', which is something that we all should do.

Inappropriate treatment requests

In the days of the internet, patients and their families can search the web widely, but usually lack the knowledge and experience to be able to interpret what they find. The four ethical principles outlines by Beauchamp and Childress (15) guide decision-making:

1. Autonomy. The autonomy of one person cannot over-ride the autonomy of another, but for a patient to be able to exercise autonomy, the patient must have accurate high-quality information in order to be able to make a decision. Thus, informed consent is intricately linked to the

principle of autonomy. As well as information on treatment side-effects, risks and burdens, the patient also needs to know what will happen without an intervention. For some patients, it is possible to point out that their body will cope better with the disease if the 'worldly or social part' of their body is not exhausted, because the requested treatment is more likely to do harm than good.

2 and 3. Nonmaleficence and beneficence. For every proposed intervention, the potential benefits must be carefully and honestly weighed against the risks and burdens of the treatment. Sometimes, radical medical treatment is indicated even in very advanced disease (e.g. with the testicular tumours), but this is rare.

4. Justice. The principle of justice requires a 'just distribution of resources', remembering that staff are often the key resource in the system, as well as a right of the patient to 'the best treatment within the resources available'.

These different parts of the equation need to be worked through with the family, sometimes using visual prompts and diagrams to help explain why a treatment that looks like a miracle cure may turn out to be more harmful than a placebo.

Preparing for parting

The hardest situation of all is preparing for, and facing, the total finality of death. Children and the family, of all ages, need to be prepared just as much as adults do, if not more. When a grandparent is dying, the children also need to be prepared. Children should be involved in discussions and kept informed as much as possible, although the information given to them must be age-appropriate for their level of mental development.

Younger children have no concept of time and therefore feel that whenever they are told something will happen, it will happen with great immediacy. Therefore, as a general rule of thumb, the younger the child, the more difficult it is for them to anticipate events. But this does not mean the child should not be prepared. The more preparation, the better the child can cope at the time of death and bereavement. Even very small children can understand that their parent is ill and not getting better. In the course of any such conversation, it is really important that the child understands that they have no responsibility for the illness; small children often believe that because they were naughty or caused a parent to be tired, that they somehow have precipitated the disease.

It can be very helpful for children to have a memory box prepared by the person who is dying. The box can contain small items, memorabilia, letters, cards and so on, which help the child in later years to realize that they were deeply loved. Some parents find this a difficult process, preferring to simply designate one or two items to be given to the child after their death and that the child can have as keepsakes.

Communicating about medications and palliation

Myths and misinformation about morphine abound. In the lay press and media, the perception is often repeated that somehow morphine shortens life. This can lead to fear in patients and relatives that starting opioids for symptom control will inevitably be 'the beginning of the end'.

In fact, there is no evidence that morphine, when given appropriately and titrated for symptom control, shortens life (16, 17). However, these deep-seated fears will mean that information about symptom control drugs needs to be given clearly alongside addressing these anxieties.

When starting a patient on analgesia, explain that they will not become tolerant to the analgesia if it is taken before the pain recurs, that they will not become addicted to morphine given for pain relief, but the one side-effect is constipation. A laxative that combines stimulant and stool-softener properties needs to be taken regularly once or twice a day. As the transit time from mouth to anus is about 48 hours, the laxative needs to be taken whether the patient has had a bowel movement or not. Drowsiness can occur with morphine when it is first prescribed; lowering the dose is a simple solution, although some patients report feeling less drowsy when rotated onto a synthetic opioid, such as fentanyl or oxycodone.

Dyspnoea is another deeply distressing symptom (18). The symptom itself causes a ' fight and flight' response of adrenaline. Patients should have it explicitly explained that they will not choke to death, that they will be able to breathe, even though breathing is hard work, and they will not die from lack of air intake. Many patients are enormously relieved when this is spelled out, but very few voice the fear of suffocation—it is almost as though to voice it might make it into a self-fulfilling prophecy and that is too terrifying a thought.

Thus simple explanations over how the body functions and how dying occurs are an important clinical duty. Patients sometimes need to be told that they will simply become quite drowsy, slip into a coma, not lose mental faculties, not lose their dignity, but will then die quietly and gently from the coma, as their breathing becomes shallower and their heart weaker. At the moment of death, nothing sudden or frightening happens.

Relatives need help in thinking who wants to be with a patient when they die, in having enough warning to travel from afar and to be able to come and say their last goodbyes. When there are family travelling from abroad, it may be worth considering with a patient whether it is better to see relatives sooner rather than later, when all can enjoy each other's company. The relatives may also be relieved to be given permission to stay away nearer the time of death and not attend the funeral.

Hope and hopelessness

It is easy when thinking about the end of the patient's life to take the view that there is nothing more that can be done, that interventions may be futile and that the situation is essentially hopeless (19). Such an attitude reflects a false sense of identity in the clinician, since few diseases in medicine are cured; the majority are controlled to some degree by medication, but complications ensue, and eventually patients die of their disease, whatever it is.

So when first meeting a patient and taking their history, clinicians should keep a mental log of the issues that can be improved, the things that can be done to help a patient restore their own sense of personhood and regain a quality to life. Sometimes the issue of hope may be around some very simple physical aspects, such as getting pain under control, having a good night's sleep, getting home or just feeling more in control of medication. At other times, the sense of hope comes from being able to realize unfulfilled dreams and aspirations, modified to take account of the reality of the situation the patient finds himself in. And for some, their hope is for a peaceful natural death in their own bed.

However, if the clinician loses the sense that the patient has personal worth or is not worth working with to improve their current reality, such negative attitudes will be detected by the patient. They will be communicated nonverbally and they will destroy the last vestiges of hope the patient may have. Hope must be realistic, it must be achievable, but it must never be abandoned in communicating with the dying.

References

1. Lunney JR, Lynn J, Foley DJ, Lipson S, Guralnik J (2003). Patterns of functional decline at the end of life. *JAMA* **289**, 2387–92.

2. Noble S, Pease N, Finlay I. The United Kingdom general practitioner and palliative care model in Handbook of communication in oncology and palliative care. Eds. Kissane *et al.* Oxford University Press; 20;ch57: 659–669.

3. Graham J, Ramirez AJ, Cull A, *et al.* (1996). Job stress and satisfaction among palliative physicians. *Palliat Med* **10**, 185–94.

4. Hickman SE, Sabatino CP, Moss AH, *et al.* (2008). The POLST (Physician Orders for Life-Sustaining Treatment) paradigm to improve end-of-life care: potential state legal barriers to implementation. *J Law Med Ethics* **36**, 119–40.

5. Weiner L, Ballard E, Brennan T, *et al.* (2008). How I wish to be remembered: the use of an advance care planning document in adolescent and young adult populations. *J Palliat Med* **11**, 1309–13.

6. Mental Capacity Act 2007, london: HMSO

7. Apelbaum PS, Grisso T (1988). Assessing patients' capacities to consent to treatments. *NEJM* **319**, 1635–8.

8. Pulchalski CM (2008). Spiritual issues as an essential element of quality palliative care: a commentary. *J Clin Ethics* **19**, 160–2.

9. Kissane DW (2000). Psychospiritual and existential issues. The challenge for palliative care. *Aust Fam Physician* **29**, 1022–5.

10. Ballard P, Finlay I, Jones N, Searle C, Roberts S. Spiritual perspectives among terminally ill patients: a welsh smaple. Modern Believing 2000; **41**(2): 30–8.

11. Puchalski CM (2007–2008). Spirituality and the care of patients at the end-of-life: an essential component of care. *Omega (Westport)* **56**, 33–46.

12. Lee A, Wu HY (2002). Diagnosis disclosure in cancer patients—when the family says 'no!' *Singapore Med J* **43**, 533–8.

13. Reich M, Mekaoui L (2003). Conspiracy of silence in oncology: a situation not to be overlooked. *Bull Cancer* **90**, 181–4.

14. Zimmerman C (2004). Denial of impending death. A discourse analysis of the palliative care literature. *Soc Sci Med* **59**, 1769–80.

15. Beauchamp TL, Childress JF (2008). *Principles of Biomedical Ethics*, 6th edn. Oxford University Press, Oxford.

16. Regnard C (2007). Double effect is a myth leading a double life. *BMJ* **334**(7591), 440.

17. George R, Regnard C (2007). Lethal opioids or dangerous prescribers? *Palliat Med* **21**, 77–80.

18. Shackell BS, Jones RC, Harding G, *et al.* (2007). 'Am I going to see the next morning?' A qualitative study of patients' perspectives of sleep in COPD. *Prim Care Respir J* **16**, 378–83.

19. Downman TH (2008). Hope and hopelessness: theory and reality. *JRSM* **101**, 428–30.

Chapter 43

Communication issues in pastoral care and chaplaincy

Peter Speck and Christopher Herbert

The diagnosis of a life-threatening disease can trigger a variety of reactions in the recipient of such news. In addition to a range of emotional and psychological responses, there will come a time for most when questions of a more existential nature arise. Some of these will relate to causality, others to the possible meaning and purpose of the illness, or what the future may hold in terms of the individual's beliefs about what happens when we die. These questions may be difficult to voice and may also be difficult for others to hear and respond to, but they are very much the concern of pastoral and spiritual care, as reflected in the following description:

> Those activities of the Church which are directed towards maintaining or restoring the health and wholeness of individuals and communities in the context of God's redemptive purposes for all creation (1).

If we are to be able to discern and respond appropriately to the questions that arise in the minds of patients, families and staff, it is important that those responsible for the provision of spiritual care can develop a relationship with the person who is ill, to enable the airing of such issues and the exploration of appropriate responses, which will support the person at various stages in the progression of the disease. The UK guidance for supportive care in adult cancer (2) made it clear that all staff in a palliative care setting share a responsibility for spiritual care, even if there are specially designated people appointed to provide for the range of discerned need. This applies whether the setting is within a hospital, a hospice or the community. The implication of this is that the level of communication skills held by all staff should be sufficient to facilitate conversations and explore responses to the illness, to enable assessment of need and referral to appropriate people. The NICE guidance also makes it clear that such assessment should be oft repeated, since the needs frequently change over time.

Assessment tools can be lengthy or insensitive and directive, restricting the ability of the patient to set the agenda. An effective assessment will highlight the issues that are important to the patient and may begin with an open question such as: 'What are the things that are really important to you now?'. Answers may include the person's family, their treatment options, the extent to which they can maintain some control over what happens and so on. The conversation may move to an exploration of what has helped the person cope when life has been difficult in the past. This may reveal the person's own strengths, those of significant people in their life or their beliefs (religious or otherwise). By inviting the patient to explore what is important to them and to review their strategies for coping, the caregiver is indicating an ability and willingness to listen and respond to non-clinical issues. Such a conversation may reveal strong and healthy beliefs that are significant for the patient and for which they wish ongoing support. The conversation may also expose distress and anxieties that may lead to an intervention by a psychologist, social worker or spiritual care provider (3). Sometimes it is more appropriate for a chaplain/spiritual caregiver to work and support the staff member in continuing the conversation, rather than to take over and replace the staff member. The decision as to who should provide for the identified need will depend on the resources available and the patient's choice as to with whom they wish to continue the conversation and whether the patient is cared for at home or in an inpatient setting.

The inpatient setting

Much of chaplaincy in a hospital or hospice is concerned with assessing and meeting the needs of patients, staff and families, whether they are religious or not. Chaplains come from a faith tradition, but are usually able to work with people who are within and outside of their faith group. Because they are used to reflecting on existential issues in a broad way, they should be able to work creatively with many of the questions and concerns raised by people adjusting to a life-threatening illness. This does not mean that they will have easy and ready answers to the issues raised, but by their training and their experience should be able to stay with the tensions, uncertainty and anger voiced by people in such situations.

Pastoral care is concerned with enabling people to grow, to learn, to be sustained and to achieve healing that is more than physical wellness in the context of their beliefs. For those whose belief contains an understanding of a deity or God, then the communication is not only interpersonal but is also with that sense of 'otherness' we frequently term 'the divine or the sacred'. In the context of a religious belief this means that the individual may seek the support of the faith community in terms of prayer, sacrament or other ritual, and counselling for specific areas of concern. Each faith tradition will have its own specific rituals appropriate to times of illness and these may be conducted privately with the sick person or corporately with other believers by the bedside or place set aside for religious worship in the hospital or hospice. This may range from specific acts of prayer, the laying-on of hands for healing, strengthening and blessing, or anointing with oil. There may also be specific rituals appropriate at the time of approaching death, and those used as the body is subsequently prepared for the funeral of the deceased (4, 5). In addition, the individual may wish to explore their belief, their understanding of the deity or what happens after death, and to seek help for areas of doubt or conflict in their faith. It is important not to assume that believers will have no doubts, even after years of faith.

Spiritual caregivers also need appropriate training and supervision to remain sensitive within pastoral relationships, as well as dealing with issues in their own agenda that arise out of the nature of their work. It is, therefore, essential that pastoral caregivers maintain their own spiritual life in order to be able to 'journey' with others—sometimes into very dark places.

Alice was a 33-year-old married woman and mother of two young children. She developed pancreatic cancer with metastatic spread. On admission she was both frightened and very angry. When the chaplain met her, in the course of a general visit to her ward, she was very scathing about what the chaplain represented. After her verbal attack, Alice was surprised that the chaplain re-visited the following day, and she asked how the chaplain could represent a God who 'allowed such terrible things to happen'. This began an exploration between Alice and the chaplain of the nature of God, the problem of suffering and the seeming unfairness of much that happens to us. No easy answers were offered, but neither did the chaplain duck the issues or run away. A mutually respectful relationship developed and Alice realized that the chaplain was able to stand 'the heat' and was not going to offload a religious framework on to her. She began to use these encounters as a safe space, not only to ventilate feeling, but also to explore her fears and review options for her family and their future. As it became clear that her prognosis was very poor, she was also able to use the chaplain to help her, and later her husband, to plan her funeral and discuss how best to prepare her children for her death. This latter need led to a member of the child psychology team joining the chaplain to work with the family as a unit. Alice was still not sure if she really believed in God or could trust God to ensure that in the end it would all work out, but she did feel she could trust the chaplain to conduct her funeral in a way that would not compromise her views and wishes. Alice also created a narrative of her life in which she recorded significant incidents and people who had shaped her and made her what she was. In particular she talked of the love she had for her husband and children, as well as some of her hopes for their future. She also wrote out recipes for dishes that she knew the family enjoyed, so that they could continue to make and enjoy them. In one section, she acknowledged her ambivalence about God, together with the hope that there would be some continuity beyond death, so that she might know her husband and children again. When Alice died, the chaplain conducted the funeral and was joined by the local vicar from the area where Alice and her family lived. This provided an opportunity for the community clergy to relate meaningfully with the family and provide ongoing support over the months following the funeral.

In this example, it is significant that the chaplain was not affronted by the negativity expressed at the first meeting, but felt able to return later and sensitively see whether they could relate, or if the patient really did not wish any further contact. Palliative care is frequently provided by members of a multi-professional team and it is essential that there is good communication between members of that team. The chaplain/spiritual caregiver should be a member of that team, known and trusted by them, so that each can draw on the skills of others in the best interests of the patient and family. In the case of Alice, it was important that the other members of the team did not assume the chaplain was upsetting Alice when they observed some of her angry interchanges. The ventilation and working through of fears, anxieties and anger can be an important feature of pastoral care—as recognized in other forms of therapeutic work. It was also important that the chaplain collaborated with other members of the multi-disciplinary team and the appropriate faith leader in the community.

The community or home setting

Historically, pastoral care developed as part of the role of community clergy who sought to support, educate and provide for the needs of their people in a whole range of life crises. The more specialist work, pastoral care in hospitals, hospices and other institutions, grew out of this background. Whilst there has been some academic research about the pastoral and spiritual care offered by hospital chaplains (as has been illustrated in the previous section), less academic research has been carried out about what constitutes good pastoral care in the more diffuse settings of patients in the community, in nursing homes or in their own domestic settings.

It would be incorrect to deduce from this that pastoral care is not actually being offered outside hospitals. In practice, indeed, Christian churches and other faith groups in the United Kingdom have been providing pastoral care for centuries. In the seventeenth-century *Book of common prayer*, for example, a specific order of service was created entitled 'The visitation of the sick'. This service is prefaced with the rubric:

> When any person is sick, notice shall be given thereof to the Minister of the Parish; who, coming into the sick person's house, shall say...

Two hundred years later, manuals for Church of England parish priests written in the early nineteenth century, as well as encouraging a sacramental ministry to the sick, exhorted clergy to carry out pastoral work with appropriate decorum:

> The assistance given by the minister to his sick parishioners, should not be confined to prayer and conversation; much aid may be afforded them through books. There are many small tracts he [sic] may give away, and some larger works he may lend, when occasion calls for them (6).

This book does not reveal what the reactions of any possible beneficiary of such earnest endeavours might have been.

Over a century later, in the 1960s, a series of influential books on the provision of pastoral care were produced. Amongst them were *The pastoral care of the dying* (7), written by a highly regarded hospital chaplain, Norman Autton, and *Sick call* (8), written by Kenneth Child, a former hospital chaplain and parish priest. The latter book was designed to provide:

> ...a simple handbook for the newly ordained priest or deacon on sick visiting (9).

In the 1980s, a new series of books providing advice on pastoral care were produced. Amongst them was *Letting go: caring for the dying and bereaved* (10); whilst this volume was designed as a practical text, it was addressed, significantly, not only to clergy but also to lay people, and marked a significant shift in the perception of who actually offered pastoral care.

In 1992 Christopher Moody wrote *Eccentric ministry: pastoral care and leadership in the parish* (11) in which he questioned previous pastoral role models for the clergy, the professionalism of the nineteenth century and the counselling and community-worker models of the twentieth century. Whilst acknowledging that such models in the last decades of the twentieth century continued to exist, he nevertheless championed a view of the Church, which saw its raison d'être as interacting with local communities, but in ways that were more culturally sensitive:

> ...the contemporary situation of cultural diversity requires us to travel light.... There is a great danger otherwise that we [the book is addressed to the Church] will become increasingly estranged in a cultural ghetto, sustained only by our own sense of exile, rather than reviving a sense of being on pilgrimage towards something new (12).

Three years after Christopher Moody's book was published, David Stoter, then the Manager of the Chaplaincy Department and Bereavement Centre, Queen's Medical Centre, Nottingham, gave voice to a concept in pastoral care that had become increasingly popular: spirituality. He wrote (13):

> Spiritual care was, until recent years considered to be mainly the responsibility of the hospital chaplain or a minister of religion, priest or religious leader and requests for help were usually referred to the appropriate person for attention, and the matter was then thankfully left in their hands.... Things are now changing radically, however, and there is currently a surge of interest in caring for the whole person and looking after their physical, emotional, social and spiritual needs.

It is interesting to note the delightful tension between the job description of the author as 'manager' (a word that can conjure up a mechanistic, task-orientated occupation) and the content of the book, *Spiritual aspects of health care*, which emphasizes the necessity for a truly holistic, patient-centred approach to pastoral care.

> Healing...[is] concerned with whatever is happening within the person who is in the process of being cured, or who is beginning the journey of coming to terms with deteriorating health or with the prospect of death. Healing is about journeying towards wholeness of mind, body and spirit as an entirety (14).

Spiritual care, a central theme of Stoter's book, is defined as:

> ...that integrating power or force in total patient care which signals the overwhelming need to recognise the person who is suffering and, by extension, to recognise the suffering in family, among friends and indeed for the professionals involved as well (15).

In such a scenario, the key component is the creation of good partnerships between everyone involved in the accompaniment of the patient on his or her 'journey'.

This very brief survey of the literature surrounding Christian pastoral care, from the sixteenth to the twentieth centuries, reveals that the language brought to our understanding of care is constantly changing, influenced deeply by culture and context. The major metaphors of the sixteenth century, for instance, were about illness as God's 'visitation', in which sickness was seen as being for the trying of patience, for an example to others, for the testing of faith or as a sign that things needed to be corrected. In the twentieth century, the metaphors changed; the notion of sickness as a journey, a pathway or a pilgrimage became paramount. In the twenty-first century, one of the most recent Christian liturgical expressions of how sickness is understood includes the word 'wholeness'. The title of these services is 'A celebration of wholeness and healing' (16) but whilst it focuses on the needs of the individual, it also points out that prayer for healing.. *needs to take seriously the way in which individual sickness and vulnerability are often the result of injustice and social oppression* (17). In brief, then, the language used to describe sickness and pastoral reactions to it, and the struggle to discern whether or not any sickness might have some kind of moral purpose or outcome, has undoubtedly changed across the centuries in the United Kingdom. However, the central questions for the patient, as has been argued at the beginning of this chapter, have remained essentially the same: 'Is there any purpose?', 'What is my destiny?', 'What am I for?', 'Is hope of any kind of a chimera a reality?'.

In a hospital setting these questions can be very sharp, not least because the normal mundane matters of getting on with life are suddenly stripped away. In these circumstances the sensitivity of chaplains and all the medical staff need to be of a high order. Whilst the questions themselves may be stark, the actual setting in which they can be addressed, the hospital ward, for example, may not be immediately conducive to the patient opening up his or her soul to someone who will listen. But it is the quality of listening that is absolutely vital; giving serious, uncluttered attention to the patient is so important.

Unfortunately, that kind of attention seems to be in short supply. If I (CH) may be anecdotal for a moment, a few days ago I was visiting a friend in hospital. The nurse came to the bedside to take blood pressure and temperature readings. The equipment used was state-of-the-art but the nurse gave the patient not a single moment of attention. Not a single word was exchanged. The eyes of my friend pleaded for attention but the nurse, not having looked at the patient, did not register the unspoken questions. It was pitiful—but apparently not untypical in that particular hospital.

Communication skills begin not at 'skills' level but much deeper, with the basic attitude of one human being to another. The message, unspoken but of intense power, that the nurse gave to my friend was that she, the patient, did not matter. It was very hurtful. If the attitude is wrong, then clearly real communication is going to be difficult. Had the nurse actually given the patient undivided attention, even if only briefly, the levels of stress would have been alleviated.

The setting where this event happened was in an orthopaedic ward; how much more sensitivity is required when the patient is receiving palliative care. Then total and compassionate attention will be amongst the most important gifts to be offered.

The best forms of pastoral care, therefore, require the caregiver to have a basic, paradigmatic attitude that regards the other person as having absolute worth and thus being someone to whom absolute attention should be given. If that is the foundation, the rest can follow: how to listen deeply, that is, how to listen not only to what is said but also to what is unsaid; how to discern when it is right to keep silence, and not be harassed into talking endlessly to the patient; how to discern when it is right to speak, and then what might or might not be said. This can sometimes be easier in the context of the person's own home, without some of the distractions or interruptions that can occur in the busy inpatient unit.

If pastoral care and communication skills are thought of as being like a quarry face in which various geological layers are exposed, the bottom layer should be the largest one, that is, the basic attitude towards the other person; above that lies the layer of listening with attention; then should come the ability to judge when silence is best; and only near the top should words themselves feature. Where such layered communication skills are exercised, and where the fundamental attitude to the patient is one in which that patient's human value is treated with absolute respect, as happens in many hospices, then true pastoral care and deep human learning can, and does, take place—and the effect on patients, staff and patients' families can be transformative.

Conclusion

Pastoral care, wherever it is offered, requires the caregiver to focus on, and relate to, the whole person who is before them. It is to be distinguished from counselling, since the encounter takes place within the context of a belief system held by the pastoral carer, and which may or may not be shared by the recipient of care. The essence of the communication is the creation of a safe space within which the person can explore such issues as: personal worth and value, the possible purpose of what is being experienced, the opportunity to access strength and the power to rise above (transcend) the here and now experience, thereby sustaining hope in a future. Being a recipient of palliative care is but one life event for which pastoral care can be a resource, complimentary to other aspects of care, and requiring careful attention to the sensitive use of communication skills.

References

1. Campbell A (2002) Pastoral care. In: Carr W (ed.) *The new dictionary of pastoral studies.* SPCK, London.
2. NICE: National Institute for Clinical Excellence (2004) *Improving supportive and palliative care for adults with cancer.* **www.nice.org.uk.**
3. Speck P. (2004) Spiritual issues in palliative care. In: Doyle D, Hanks GWC, MacDonald N (eds). *Oxford textbook of palliative care,* 2nd edn. Oxford University Press, Oxford.
4. Speck P. (2003) Spiritual/religious issues in care of the dying. In: Ellershaw J, Wilkinson S (eds). *Care of the dying: a pathway to excellence.* Oxford University Press, Oxford.
5. Cobb M. (2005) *The hospital chaplain's handbook: a guide for good practice.* Canterbury Press, Norwich.
6. Elder Brother (1882) *A manual for the parish priest, being a few hints on the pastoral care, to the younger clergy of the Church of England; from an elder brother,* 2nd edn. FC & J Rivington, London.
7. Autton N. (1966) *The pastoral care of the dying.* SPCK, London.
8. Child K. (1965) *Sick call: a book on the pastoral care of the physically ill.* SPCK, London.
9. Child K. (1965) *Sick call: a book on the pastoral care of the physically ill.* SPCK, London, p.2.
10. Ainsworth-Smith I, Speck P. (1982) *Letting go: caring for the dying and the bereaved.* SPCK, London.
11. Moody C (1992) *Eccentric ministry: pastoral care and leadership in the 'parish.* Darton, Longman & Todd, London.
12. Moody C (1992) *Eccentric ministry: pastoral care and leadership in the 'parish.* Darton, Longman & Todd, London, pp.130–1.
13. Stoter D (1995) *Spiritual aspects of health care.* Mosby, London, p.iv.
14. Stoter D (1995) *Spiritual aspects of health care.* Mosby, London, p.156.
15. Stoter D (1995) *Spiritual aspects of health care.* Mosby, London, p.156.
16. Common Worship (2000) *Pastoral Services.* Church House Publishing, London, p.13.
17. Common Worship (2000) *Pastoral Services.* Church House Publishing, London, p.11.

Chapter 44

Communication in oncology pharmacy: the challenge of treatment adherence

Venetia Bourrier and Brent Schacter

Introduction

As with other professions, pharmacists have experienced a change from traditional drug-oriented services, including distribution and preparation, toward patient-oriented services (1). Many professional organizations and societies believe that pharmacists have a pivotal role in the provision of information in oncology, hospice and palliative care; pharmacists should be integral members of interdisciplinary teams (2). High-quality cancer care requires both traditional and expanded pharmacist activities, including a variety of clinical, educational, administrative and support responsibilities. In this chapter, we describe the pharmacists' roles and responsibilities in the provision of care to patients with cancer, with a particular emphasis on communication and the promotion of patients' treatment adherence.

Professional knowledge and skills

Pharmacists practicing in oncology and palliative care require a broad, integrated knowledge and a strong commitment to optimally meet patients' needs. The scope of this knowledge covers pharmaceutical, medical, research, management, basic and social sciences, humanities and even population health areas of expertise (3).

The pharmacist's skills include communication, collaboration, problem identification and resolution, critical thinking, self-assessment and ethical decision-making. Oncology pharmacists need to think analytically, clearly and critically, while solving medication problems during daily practice. They need to systematically find, appraise and apply information to make informed, evidence-based decisions. Use of retrieval techniques to access necessary information is vital. In communicating information about medications, pharmacists need to structure the material in systematic categories, avoid jargon and carefully go through the rationale, dose, mode and timing of administration and potential side-effects for each medication. To do this effectively, each pharmacist is responsible for their continuing competence in this specialty practice area (3).

Pharmaceutical care

In recent years, a paradigm shift towards a patient-focused, rather than a disease-focused, approach has occurred. Fortunately, the profession has moved from the traditional distribution services towards patient-oriented and clinical pharmacy services. In oncology, pharmacists established central services for the compounding of cytotoxic drugs and began to offer clinical services for therapeutic drug monitoring. Pharmaceutical care concepts were introduced to optimize individual drug therapy (1).

Recognition of the numerous risks to patients associated with complex and multiple medication therapies led to a conceptual framework for an advanced pharmacy practice philosophy. In 1990, Hepler and Strand introduced the concept of 'pharmaceutical care' to advance the development of the profession (1). Pharmaceutical care is defined as the 'direct, responsible provision of drug therapy for the purpose of achieving definite outcomes that improve a patient's quality of life' (2). A patients' quality of life, during and after chemotherapy, has emerged as an important outcome alongside tumour responsiveness. Consequently, patients need to be offered an appropriately indicated, effective, safe and convenient drug therapy. To limit therapy-associated toxicity, supportive care became an integral part of anti-cancer systemic therapy. In the palliative setting, medication therapy is the cornerstone of most symptom control management.

In 1998, the Fédération International Pharmaceutique (FIP) extended the Hepler and Strand definition, describing pharmaceutical care as a 'collaborative process that aims to prevent or identify and solve medicinal product and health related problems. This is a continuous quality improvement process for the use of medicinal products' (1).

One goal is to provide seamless continuity of care to individual patients. Pharmaceutical care is a needs-based approach in which the pharmacist is responsible to the cancer patient. Key principles include achieving each patient's autonomous consent, prioritizing their needs and establishing a covenant for care (3).

The care process

Pharmaceutical care can be structured according to the SOAP method, in which *S*ubjective information and *O*bjective parameters for the patient are *A*nalysed to create an individual care *P*lan. In collaboration with the prescribing physician and the patient, the goals of the individual's drug therapy are defined and added to the plan. To ensure continuous review of the care plan, regular appointments with the pharmacist are established throughout treatment. This plan needs to be re-evaluated and adjusted according to the patients' response and needs (1).

Treatment of a cancer patient is complex and the selection of therapy—chemotherapy, hormone and other therapies—belongs to the prescribing physician in consultation and agreement with the patient. The medication record, if complete, provides an overview of the drug history of the patient and is required to discern the patient's situation. The oncology pharmacist should interview cancer patients for the purpose of obtaining medication histories (3). A comprehensive medication history should contain information relating to:

+ adverse drug reactions, including allergies;
+ past and currently prescribed medication therapy, including the names of the medications, doses, frequency of administration, indications and duration of therapies;
+ non-prescription medication use;
+ use of complementary or alternative therapies;
+ compliance with prescribed medication regimens;
+ name of physician(s) and community pharmacies (3).

For the cancer patient, the oncology pharmacist should identify, prevent and resolve drug-related problems (DRPs) including, but not limited to:

+ taking or receiving a non-cancer treatment medication without valid indication;
+ need for pharmacotherapy that has not yet been prescribed, especially for supportive care of predictable treatment-related toxicities;
+ taking or receiving a medication for an inappropriate indication;

* taking an inappropriate dose of an indicated medication;
* experiencing an adverse drug reaction, including drug-induced disease and/or drug sensitivity;
* therapeutic complications;
* experiencing a drug–drug, drug–food, drug–lab test interaction, or allergy to a drug or class of drugs;
* not taking or receiving a drug prescribed and/or non-compliance due to lack of understanding;
* failure to fill a prescription due to lack of money;
* drug dependency;
* other habits or practices that may lead to drug-related problems (3).

A number of these problems can be detected just from analysing the patient health record. This information provides a realistic picture and assessment of the patient.

Pharmaceutical care in oncology is a continuous process. The oncology pharmacist should assess the patient for development of drug-related problems throughout the entire treatment protocol and beyond, if feasible. The oncology pharmacist should evaluate:

* the cancer patients' response to treatment and achievement of the therapeutic outcomes (especially with drug therapies directed to symptom management);
* adverse effects from drugs, including allergies and toxicities (especially serious, life-threatening or unexpected toxicities from cancer chemotherapy);
* changes in the clinical condition of the cancer patient (including altered kinetics of drug absorption, distribution, metabolism or disposition) that necessitates an alteration in drug therapy or dosage;
* changes in patient status leading to a delay or discontinuation of therapy;
* patient hospitalization (3).

Target populations for pharmaceutical care

As a consequence of limited resources, it is impossible for oncology pharmacists to provide pharmaceutical care to all oncology and palliative care patients. Those patients with complex drug regimens, chronic diseases and who need to be frequently hospitalized, benefit most from pharmaceutical care. These characteristics apply to many oncology patients (1). Some criteria for identifying cancer patients who would most benefit from pharmaceutical care include (3):

* patients whose clinical state or condition may affect medication absorption or disposition, alter dosage requirements or predispose them to adverse drug reactions or medication toxicity;
* patients with organ dysfunction (hepatic or renal) that may affect chemotherapy drug metabolism or elimination;
* patients with other co-morbidities that may limit drug dosing (e.g. cardiac dysfunction with anthracyclines) or that may affect outcome from systemic therapy (e.g. diabetes, COPD, etc.) where age, weight or physiologic parameters are important factors in determining appropriate medication therapy;
* patients on multiple drug therapies in addition to the drugs used for cancer treatment;
* patients who are taking non-cancer medications that have a narrow therapeutic index (e.g. digoxin, aminoglycosides) or drugs that have a high likelihood for drug interactions with cancer treatment drugs;

+ patients taking investigational, special access or compassionate release drugs; and,
+ patients taking medications in doses greater or less than recommended in the treatment regimens or by the manufacturer.

Communication to achieve seamless pharmaceutical care

In the ambulatory setting, the continuous monitoring of medication use is helpful, given the number of medical practitioners that cancer patients tend to see (1). Seamless pharmaceutical care helps when patients are transferred from one clinical service to another. When a cancer patient is discharged from the hospital or ambulatory care facility to the community, the oncology pharmacist should provide a written summary of the patients' medication history and specific outcome, as well as communicating with primary care practitioners, as needed. Electronic linkages facilitate this communication via an electronic health record. The desirable outcome provided by seamless care is enhanced consistency of care, fewer medication-related problems and improved quality of life (3).

The multidisciplinary team—a triangle of care

Good working relationships with physicians, allied healthcare providers, nurses and community healthcare providers, are fundamental. Sharing information appropriately ensures patient safety and optimal treatment outcomes. A fundamental feature is that pharmacists accept responsibility for the patient's pharmacotherapeutic outcome alongside physicians. As depicted in Fig. 44.1, the triangle of care ensures that the patient and their medication needs are at the apex and the main focus of these efforts (1).

In oncology, the goal of treatment is either cure or slowing disease progression, while palliating symptoms and reducing the incidence of adverse effects, organ toxicity and drug resistance (1). When feasible, the assignment of dedicated pharmacists to specific disease-site groups, facilitates this focus. The specific practice of pharmacists on healthcare teams can be defined within a scope-of-practice document or a similar tool or protocol developed by the healthcare organization. This

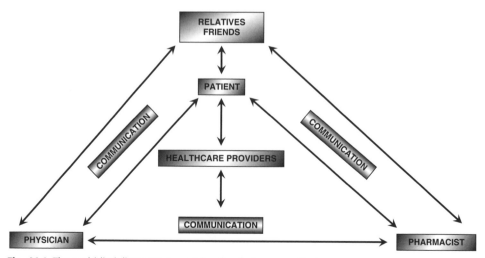

Fig. 44.1 The multidisciplinary team—a triangle of pharmaceutical care.

document can include referral and communication guidelines, including the documentation of patient encounters and the methods and processes for sharing patient information with appropriate members of the multidisciplinary team (2). The visible presence of pharmacists during inpatient care rounds and close by ambulatory clinics, in interdisciplinary team conferences and in informal discussions, is vital (3).

Medication safety and quality

Tragic accidents involving cytotoxic drugs have generated widespread publicity and public concern. The absence of a pharmacist's overview has reportedly contributed to three children's deaths from vincristine overdoses and to two deaths and one serious injury from vinorelbine overdose (4). The set up of central services for compounding cytotoxic drugs and the standardization of chemotherapy order forms were some of the first pharmacy contributions to decrease prescribing and dosing errors and to increase safety in handling cytotoxic drugs (1). In one study of pharmacists' interventions in the treatment of haematology–oncology patients between October 1995 and May 1996, 503 interventions included 85 (17%) to correct prescribing errors. Physicians accepted 97% of the pharmacists' recommendations (4).

Over time, cancer chemotherapy has evolved from being delivered primarily in inpatient settings to outpatient clinics because of greater convenience and lower cost. Each organization should establish a minimum acceptable level of pharmacist responsibility for outpatients. This should include prospectively reviewing orders, screening laboratory test results, providing drug information, counselling patients and reviewing drug storage. Investigational drug protocols should only be initiated at sites where comprehensive pharmaceutical services are available (4).

The generally narrow therapeutic range of anti-cancer drugs means a particular risk for the patient with respect to drug safety. Institutions should establish dosage limits for anti-neoplastic agents, set up dose-verification procedures that stress multiple independent checks and work to standardize the prescribing vocabulary (5). Hiring specific 'safety pharmacists' ensures that safety checks and quality system processes are incorporated into all pharmacy procedures. The ultimate focus of any medication safety pharmacist is the safety of each individual patient (6).

Poor communication among physicians, pharmacists, nurses and other healthcare providers can lead to medication errors. Alert and knowledgeable patients who know that they can contact a pharmacist for advice can be the last line of defence against medication errors. Failure to heed patient concerns has led to serious errors, which could have been prevented (4). All healthcare providers should cooperate in identifying potential problems and solutions. Multidisciplinary discussions should take place after a medication error and routinely as part of quality improvement efforts. If caregivers work together as a team, most errors can be contained. A system of reporting all errors ensures that practitioners learn from their mistakes; each error should be reviewed by a multidisciplinary team with the ultimate goal of system-wide improvements (4).

Treatment guidelines and evidence-based care

Clinical practice guidelines (CPGs) provide evidence-based recommendations regarding the treatment of different diseases and symptoms. Proper selection and application of the guidelines require an understanding of their purpose, rationale, development methods, critical evaluation, potential implementation strategies and their limitations.

The implementation of CPGs can contribute to improving patients' quality of life and can reduce unnecessary drug costs (1). CPGs, especially those of high quality, are a key component in a practice model that integrates evidence with clinical expertise and the patient's values (7). Therapeutic or CPGs involving medications should be elaborated through a multidisciplinary team approach with physicians, pharmacists and other healthcare professionals. However, no matter how CPGs are developed, they are meant to be a guide to healthcare decisions and not dictate them.

Many potential barriers exist that preclude oncology practitioners from implementing such recommendations into their practice. These barriers include:

+ lack of familiarity or awareness that a CPG exists;

+ disagreement with the guideline recommendations;

+ fear of cookbook medicine and loss of autonomy;

+ time constraints or lack of personnel to implement the CPGs effectively;

+ lack of input into CPGs during their development or adaptation for use.

To overcome the first barrier—a lack of familiarity and awareness—the pharmacist must make every effort to be familiar with available CPGs and where to locate them. Various sources exist, including peer-reviewed journals, which are searchable through MEDLINE, EMBASE, Google or Yahoo.

In the event that oncologists are unaware of particular CPGs, strategies such as academic detailing (a process by which the pharmacist visits a physician to provide a 10 to 15 minute educational intervention on a specific topic) or in-service education should be instituted. Algorithms outlining specific treatment protocols should be made easily accessible so that physicians can consult them while providing care.

When a physician disagrees with a guideline recommendation, the pharmacist could locate, evaluate and share the evidence that supports the improvement in patient outcomes or lowering of the cost. For instance, Dranitsaris *et al.* showed prospectively that implementation of evidence-based anti-emetic guidelines, with the support of pharmacists, promoted more clinically appropriate use of 5-HT3 antagonists, which improved patient care, outcomes and reduced costs (1). While there is great uniformity in CPGs developed to date, there is more diversity in the specifics of the clinical pathways that can be used to realize a guideline. Clinical pathways, such as specific chemotherapy regimens, drug doses and schedules, schedules for imaging studies and follow-up parameters, provide a more comprehensive approach to patient management.

Direct patient care consultations and counselling

Oncology pharmacists should be available in both inpatient and outpatient settings for all patient care consultations requested by cancer patients, their families, physicians, nurses and other healthcare providers. These consultations typically involve tasks of patient education, ascertaining medication histories, medication reconciliation or a complete pharmaceutical care evaluation. The communication of educational information throughout anti-cancer therapy includes side-effect counselling and management and proper handling techniques.

Cancer chemotherapy drugs have a high probability of toxicity, making it essential that patients adequately understand their correct use. As a standard, all patients should be seen at least once by the oncology pharmacist (3). He or she should counsel patients and family members to address anxieties about drug therapy, provide information required for safe and appropriate drug therapy, offer ideas for the prevention and/or management of potential side effects and promote compliance (3). In doing this, the pharmacist should be sensitive to the emotional aspects of the burden of cancer, providing empathic support as the conversation unfolds. Discretion is important in discussing adverse events—ask the patient how much information they desire and tailor the content to each individual's needs. The goal is to adequately educate patients to render treatment safe, without creating fear.

Verbal instructions should always be supplemented with written information, such as medication information sheets. Other counselling devices, such as compliance aids and audiovisual material, should be utilized where available. Written information should cover the following aspects of each medication:

- the name of the medications and its purpose (specific patient treatment regimen);
- physical appearance and storage requirements;
- route of administration, dose and duration of therapy;
- potential side-effects and precautions;
- action to be taken in the event of a dosage omission;
- possible adverse and/or toxic drug reactions and methods for prevention;
- special consideration:

    potential drug–drug interactions;

    drug–food interactions;

    drug–disease interactions;

    drug–herbal interactions;
- prescription refill information;
- when to call the physician or go to an emergency department (e.g. when a potentially serious adverse drug reaction occurs or a side-effect persists greater than 24 hours);
- any other information regarding access or coverage of the medication.

In the event that the patient is receiving cancer chemotherapy in the home using ambulatory infusion pumps, they should be informed of procedures for handling cytotoxics and waste products, and made aware of the expected length of the infusion. In addition, home spill kits should be provided to these patients (3).

The oncology pharmacist should evaluate the effectiveness of counselling on the patients' medication knowledge through checking questions and/or follow-up. Telephone follow-up programmes are beneficial. In addition, the pharmacist should reinforce relevant medication knowledge through repeat counselling on later visits. All medication consultations should be documented by the pharmacist in each patient's health record (3).

Medication order review (triage)

Prior to dispensing any medication, the pharmacist should verify the medication order against the treatment protocol, the patient's medication profile and the patient's health record. In the absence of a specific treatment protocol, pharmacists wisely check the prescription against two independent literature sources (3).

The oncology pharmacist should check the following:

- the patient's name, diagnosis, identification number (e.g. health insurance number, or hospital unique number) and location;
- age, gender, allergy or medication intolerance, or history of adverse drug reaction;
- weight, height and body surface area for all chemotherapy patients;
- signature of authorized prescriber, whether written or electronic;
- critical laboratory values or clinical criteria, which must be monitored (according to pre-defined criteria) in order to proceed safely with chemotherapy treatment;

- the name of the medication, formulary status and chemotherapy protocol;
- dosage, number of doses or cycle number, dosage interval;
- dosage form, frequency and route of administration and complete directions for use;
- planned stop date, given the duration of treatment;
- cumulative doses of selected drugs;
- date order was written, name of physician and license number;
- date and time of the planned treatment;
- therapeutic duplication;
- drug–disease incompatibility, drug compatibility;
- significant drug–drug, drug–food or drug–herbal interactions;
- planned use of supportive therapies (e.g. anti-emetics, hydration, etc.);
- check that all appropriate prescriptions for medications for use at home have been written (e.g. oral oncology drugs, corticosteroids, anti-nauseants, haematopoietic-stimulating factors, etc.);
- laboratory results to determine adequate organ function, drug serum concentration (where appropriate) and need for dose modifications;
- for parenteral admixtures: correct intravenous fluid, final volume and concentration, stability and potential incompatibilities and rate of administration; and
- name of chemotherapy regimen or, if research, protocol and patient study numbers (3).

Medication triage checklists, such as illustrated by Fig. 44.2 can assist the pharmacist with this triaging function. Time may be needed to resolve any questions regarding the chemotherapy order with the prescriber and document the resolution in the patient's health record. Telephone or verbal orders for chemotherapy should not be allowed or accepted (3). Effective and comprehensive medication order review can detect potential medication errors and ensures increased patient safety.

Medication-use evaluation (MUE)

Medication-use evaluation (MUE) encompasses the goals and objectives of drug-use evaluation (DUE) with an emphasis on improving patient outcomes and quality of life (QOL). Oncology pharmacy programmes should coordinate, in conjunction with the medical oncology service, the Oncology Drug Advisory Committee (or equivalent) and/or the Pharmacy and Therapeutics committee, a system for the ongoing evaluation of drug use (3). In the past decade, DUEs have been focused on expensive and new chemotherapy agents. MUE involves the following:

- development of oncology drug use criteria to promote optimal therapy;
- evaluation of approved oncology drugs against predetermined criteria;
- identification of problem areas (e.g. overuse of expensive anti-emetics);
- education to correct patterns of inappropriate use and evaluation of the impact of these educational programmes;
- adherence to established external standards (professional practice regulations, hospital or programme accreditation, legal requirements).

Results of DUEs should be communicated to the MUE team or programme and problems identified should be resolved. The frequency of evaluation depends on the need and economic impact (3).

Chemotherapy orders checklist

Name of Patient: ID#:

Treatment protocol:

Verified protocol against the disease/diagnosis	
Verified protocol against the intent of treatment (i.e. Adjuvant/metastatic/palliative)	
Verified that non-formulary approval or special approval granted if applicable	
Verified that blood counts adequate to proceed with treatment	
Calculated BSA based on most recent weight	
Checked doses against BSA or weight (if weight-based)	
Checked if doses appropriate for protocol	
Initialled all calculations and dose checks	
Checked doses against pharmacokinetic parameters (assessed patient's renal and hepatic function)	
Checked for appropriate pre-medications and supportive care therapy	
Checked route of administration	
Checked allergies/past hypersensitivities/possible drug interactions	
Hypersensitivity reaction treatment form included	
Verified if any special infusion vehicles, administration sets or special precautions required	
Verified that order is correctly entered into computer system	

N/A= not applicable

Comments: _____

_____

_____

Pharmacist signature: _____ Date: _____

Fig. 44.2 Medication triage checklist.

Research initiatives

Initiation of, and participation in, clinical and/or health services research is appropriate for oncology pharmacist's practice. Such research improves the knowledge base and expertise of oncology pharmacy practice (3). To facilitate research initiatives, knowledge of epidemiology, statistical analysis, research protocol development and critical appraisal of the literature is helpful. Presentation and/or publication of results are an integral component of the research process (3). In addition, the oncology pharmacist should be involved in clinical trials and should have a working knowledge of all aspects including trial design, approval and implementation methodology at their practice site (3).

There are specific recommendations for oncology pharmacists involved with clinical trials at their practice sites, which are:

- Follow the standard pharmacy department policies and procedures for management of clinical trials. Oncology trials may differ from other clinical trials in their expected toxicities and number of early-phase studies. Involving the pharmacist in a thorough review of each protocol is helpful, but technical issues may be incorporated into general pharmacy operations or managed by a technician.

- Where possible, ensure written informed consent has been obtained from the patient prior to initiation of the study treatment.

- When the pharmacy is in possession of code-breaking information, (randomization lists), the procedure for revealing the treatment code should be clearly outlined in department trial procedures.

- Oncology pharmacists should provide drug information, in the form of a data sheet, on all investigational agents used at their practice site.

- The oncology pharmacist or designate should ensure that clinical trial drugs are received, stored and dispensed by the institutional pharmacy whenever possible. They should maintain an accurate record of drug dispensed, returned to the sponsor, or destroyed.

- The pharmacist should monitor the dose, adverse effects, compliance and concomitant medications using the pharmaceutical patient care model.

- Oncology pharmacists should take part in tumour board meetings.

- All information pertaining to a particular trial should be organized in a format, which allows for easy set-up and retrieval of information (manual, binder or computerized).

- Pharmacists involved in clinical trials should also actively participate in pharmacy societies that are associated with relevant clinical trials consortium (3).

Clinical trials are a significant component of oncology pharmacy practice at most tertiary cancer treatment centres. To engage community-based sites in research, the pharmacist should develop methods to ensure continuity of care between the sites (3). In certain centres, a formalized process through resource impact committees exists to review the impact of clinical trials on service provision, education and training.

Other specialty pharmacy practices

Clinical pharmacy practice in paediatric oncology

Paediatric oncology pharmacists should offer pharmaceutical care that takes into consideration the unique clinical characteristics of the paediatric patient and their diagnosis that may impact on drug side-effects and acute and long-term toxicities (3). The majority of paediatric cancer patients (approximately 75%) will be cured. Consequently, issues arising from long-term survival, such as health-related quality of life and late effects like the development of second malignancies, are important. In addition, most children with cancer are treated within the context of multi-centred clinical trials.

Families are extensively involved in the treatment of their dependant children and thus should be included in all treatment-related discussions. The families and healthcare providers are important partners in achieving desirable pharmaceutical care outcomes for paediatric cancer patients (3). As with adults, seamless care is very important since patients move back and forth from clinics and community settings to hospital over the course of the treatment programme. Communication between pharmacists regarding the paediatric patients care plan is crucial.

Pharmaceutical care in these children is aimed at maximizing both short- and long-term outcomes. The pharmacist contributes by determining appropriate dosages, delivery techniques, formulations and routes of administration for drugs used in treatment regimens. Since dosing accuracy is very important in the treatment of children, the pharmacist should triage all drug orders with reference to dosing guidelines and track the cumulative doses of cytotoxics (3).

The paediatric pharmacist should be aware of how parameters like age and organ function influence both acute and long-term toxicities. Dose setting also affects complications like nausea, infection, constipation, and so on. Care plans are adjusted to reflect these organ functions (3).

Clinical pharmacy practice in community oncology

Cancer patients may be geographically resident in rural communities, where community oncology programmes provide treatment closer to home. Such outreach programmes may operate via the concept of 'shared care.' A cancer centre oncologist may retain overall responsibility, while care is delivered by the multidisciplinary team (family physicians, surgeons, nurses, pharmacists and support staff) in the rural or community setting. Here the role of, and communication from, the community liaison pharmacist (who is usually at the tertiary centre) to the team in the community is crucial. He or she can be directly involved in the triage of orders, which, if electronically entered at the tertiary centre, ensures the highest level of patient safety and seamless care.

Conclusion

With the knowledge that has accumulated within their discipline, pharmacists have expanded their clinical role to offer enhanced pharmaceutical care to cancer patients. The implementation of this pharmaceutical care improves the communication between healthcare providers to enrich the function of the multidisciplinary team. Beneficial outcomes include increased treatment adherence and optimal care for patients, with ultimately satisfaction enjoyed by the whole healthcare system.

References

1. Liekweg A, Westfeld M, Jaehde U (2004). From oncology pharmacy to pharmaceutical care: new contributions to multidisciplinary cancer care. *Support Care Cancer* **12**, 73–9.
2. Lipman AG (2002). ASHP statement on the pharmacists' role in hospice and palliative care. *Am J Health-Syst Pharm* **59**, 1770–3.
3. **https://www.capho.org** (2004). *Canadian Association for Pharmacy in Oncology Standards of Practice for Oncology in Canada*. Version 1 1–55.
4. Cohen MR (2007). Preventing medication errors in cancer chemotherapy. In: Cohen MR, *Medication Errors*, 2nd edn. American Pharmacists Association, Washington DC.
5. Cohen MR, Anderson RW, Attilio RM, *et al.* (1996). Preventing medication errors in cancer chemotherapy. *Am J Health-Syst Pharm* **53**, 737–46.
6. Turple J (2008). Practice spotlight: medication safety pharmacist. *Can J Hosp Pharm* **61**, 273–4.
7. Gaebelein CJ, Gleason BL (2007). Evaluating and implementing practice guidelines. In: *Contemporary Drug Information: An Evidence Based Approach*. Lippincott, Williams & Wilkins, New York.

Chapter 45

Psychosocial programme development

Barry D Bultz, Paul B Jacobsen, and Matthew Loscalzo

There are always challenges to the initiation of new programmes in healthcare, especially given the propensity for politics to dominate decision-making in the healthcare system. Consequently, programmes that may intuitively be in the best interest of our patients, even those supported by good science, often have to wait. Clearly then, we must learn to effectively communicate who we are, what we do, and how we can improve healthcare outcomes in a biopsychosocial world.

In psychosocial oncology these communication issues are ubiquitous. From primary treatment centres to academic/tertiary care facilities to rural settings, psychosocial oncology faces many of the same issues of visibility and acceptance. In developing countries, psychosocial oncology is faced with an even greater challenge because of the need to compete with primary treatments such as chemotherapy and radiation therapy which are limited and underfunded.

The goal of this chapter will be to discuss the impact of the psychosocial aspects of cancer and why psychosocial programme development should be considered as a key piece of the armamentarium in the fight against cancer. Also, this chapter will highlight communication strategies that might prove helpful for the development of psychosocial oncology programmes.

Background

In the brief history of specialized cancer care, recognition of the patient experience (1–3) has recently gained the attention of healthcare system administrators, providers, patients, and the advocacy community.

The growth and development of psychosocial oncology was triggered by the landmark text *On death and dying* in 1969 by Elizabeth Kubler-Ross (4). Prior to Kubler-Ross's book, talking about death and dying had been a subject that not only received little attention but had been conspicuously avoided in an attempt to spare the patient depression, anxiety, and loss of hope. Silencing feelings of distress was the conventional therapeutic approach employed to enhance the patient's outlook, quality of life, and coping skills in face of the life-threatening encounter with cancer.

Kubler-Ross's book was the catalyst to change clinical cancer practice in North America and most European countries. It rapidly caught the attention of healthcare providers, the academic community, and popular press, filling a gap in our knowledge about end-of-life experiences. In so doing, Kubler-Ross popularized, if not created, a new discipline in healthcare—palliative care and psychosocial oncology. In the 40 years since her pioneering work, there has been increased attention in research to the many facets of pain and symptom management in the care of all patients, and particularly cancer patients. So transformational was the work of Kubler-Ross that it resulted in a change to medical education to include the challenges for those facing a terminal illness. Thus, it seems inconceivable today that a cancer centre might not include a palliative care service incorporated into a cancer programme.

Since the popularization of *On death and dying*, academic psychology, psychiatry, social work, and nursing, began researching the emotional impacts of cancer on the patient, beginning with diagnosis, and moving through treatment, recurrence of disease, and survivorship. Through rigorous research, the emerging field of psychosocial oncology investigated new intervention strategies to improve quality of life and the patient experience across the illness trajectory. Today, many countries acknowledge the importance of open communication around cancer, and the impact and limitations of biomedical treatments. Unfortunately, despite the current evidence of need, most, if not all, psychosocial oncology programmes are poorly staffed and funded (5). In one of the few psychosocial staffing surveys completed across a nation, a survey of Canadian psychosocial oncology programmes in 2000, found that the overall dedicated funding for psychosocial care was less than 3% of cancer centre operating dollars (5) and that, by contrast, at least 5% of operating dollars was dedicated to cleaning of the facility (6, 7).

Today, the discipline of psychosocial oncology and its benefits in patient care remains poorly understood by medical colleagues. Unfortunately, optimal psychosocial patient–staff ratios have not been established, nor have standards or guidelines received broad-scale endorsement by cancer care facilities or third-party funders. This is surprising given that the abundance of good research addressing the benefits of psychosocial treatments, patient testimonials, and the desire for more services. In contrast, where hospital administrators and insurers have avoided/sidestepped the responsibility of appropriated funding for the psychosocial aspect of patient care, advocacy group and cancer foundation campaigns have been able to raise many millions of dollars to ensure that patients receive the benefit of psychosocial support and interventions. While this is a positive voice for the emotional care of the cancer patient, this speaks to the need for effective and innovative communication strategies to ensure the integration of psychosocial care into the hospital/cancer care system.

The importance of standards

The identity of psychosocial oncology is not yet fully established. There is a need to establish how psychosocial oncology functions as a discipline, is accepted by the medical community, and, perhaps most importantly, is funded. In comparison to medical or radiation oncology, medical physics or nursing, there are no uniform ways that psychosocial oncology exists, be it departments, services, or programmes. How best to provide services and to communicate the science of best practice in psychosocial oncology is an ongoing challenge. In response to these challenges the Canadian Association of Psychosocial Oncology (CAPO) (8) attempted to standardize psychosocial oncology programmes in cancer facilities. CAPO developed standards 'to assist cancer facilities, program leaders and practitioners in the delivery of psychosocial care' (8). The writing of these standards 'came about from recognition that psychosocial oncology standards are required to ensure that the basic principles and quality of care in the domain of psychosocial oncology are consistently applied and available to people living with cancer' (8). These standards serve as a well thought-out guide for psychosocial care and programme development, and have subsequently been endorsed by several key Canadian cancer stakeholders.

The patient journey: the prevalence of distress

A number of large studies exist that identify distress as a significant challenge to cancer patients (9–12). Despite the compelling research indicating a high incidence of distress in cancer patients, communicating these findings seems to have little consequence in facilitating adequate patient–staff ratios when establishing psychosocial oncology programmes or in healthcare payment plans.

Nonetheless, sharing the magnitude of the problem with administrators and colleagues is critical in creating a better understanding of the place of psychosocial oncology in each institution. In fact, the prevalence of patient distress has begun to garner the attention of policy makers and may, with the branding of distress as the 6th vital sign in cancer (6, 7, 13–15), create a common messaging platform to communicate the scope of the challenges facing patients.

Role of distress screening

There is general agreement that the percentage of cancer patients who initiate a request for psychosocial care represent a small fraction of those who are distressed (10). Consequently, psychosocial programmes face the challenge of identifying the larger population of patients who are distressed but have not sought help. To address this challenge, a number of governmental and professional organizations have recommended that cancer patients be routinely screened for the presence of heightened psychological distress (15–17). Several arguments can be made for implementation of routine screening for distress. First, evidence suggests that heightened distress is associated with a number of negative outcomes, such as poorer adherence to treatment recommendations (18), worse satisfaction with care (19), and poorer quality of life (20). Second, heightened distress is highly treatable. Numerous randomized controlled trials show that psychological distress, including anxiety and depression, can be alleviated by pharmacological and non-pharmacological interventions (21). Third, heightened distress is common. Prevalence estimates derived from large-scale studies typically exceed 30% (11, 12). A fourth, and perhaps most important, reason to screen routinely is evidence that heightened distress often goes unrecognized by oncology professionals (11).

Although routine administration of a screening measure would address the problem of under-recognition of distress, clinicians seem reluctant to use these tools (22). The format and length of many existing tools may be a barrier; the time required for administering, scoring, and interpreting these measures favours use of more informal but less reliable methods. To address this, several ultra-short screening tools have been developed, such as the single-item Distress Thermometer (16). A recent systematic review concluded that these ultra-short tools have psychometric properties that favour their use for screening purposes (22).

It is tempting to believe that greater recognition of distress through implementation of routine screening will lead directly to less psychological suffering. Unfortunately, the evidence does not support this view. For example, a recently completed randomized trial found no difference in health-related quality of life, relative to usual care, in comparison to those patients randomized to screening (23). These and others studies (24, 25) have taught us that information about heightened distress provided to treating clinicians must be accompanied by specific actions on their part for screening to make a difference.

This evidence, that screening alone does not improve quality-of-life outcomes, points to the need for psychosocial oncology programmes. Patients identified as distressed need to be referred to professionals who have the requisite skills to identify the source(s) of patient distress and apply the appropriate interventions in a timely manner. This view is consistent with conclusions of a recent US Institute of Medicine report (26) on meeting the psychosocial health needs of cancer patients. The report identified three components as being fundamental to the delivery of effective care:

(1) the identification of psychosocial needs through activities such as routine screening;

(2) the development and implementation of a plan that links patients with needed psychosocial services, and coordinates psychosocial and biomedical care; and

(3) follow-up and re-evaluation.

Clearly, this model of care will need to be operationalized in different ways given the resources available and the volume of patients seen in any particular setting. Nevertheless, it serves as a useful model for planning a new psychosocial oncology programme or evaluating the adequacy of existing programmes, and may lead to a better understanding of staffing ratios required to address patient needs.

Keys to successful programme development

The primary factor contributing to the successful development/expansion of a psychosocial oncology programme is institutional support. Ideally, the leadership of an institution will recognize the need for such a programme and seek to recruit individuals to develop it. More typically, a group of individuals will be seeking to convince the leadership of an institution that such a programme is needed. Regardless of how the development process is initiated, it is incumbent on those involved to identify the goals of the proposed programme and to enumerate the resources necessary to achieve those goals. One useful approach is to identify and examine existing psychosocial programmes that are operating successfully elsewhere.

The most important resource for programme development is personnel. Consideration of the programme's goals should guide selection of the disciplines to be represented in the programme (e.g. psychiatry, psychology, social work, and/or pastoral care) and the number of professionals from each discipline needed to launch the programme. For example, programmes that seek to offer a comprehensive array of psychosocial services and to assist all patients identified as distressed will require a greater number of professionals from a greater number of disciplines than programmes that are more narrowly focused. Additional resources that need to be considered include support personnel (e.g. appointment schedulers) and space (both for seeing patients and for staff offices). Programmes that are started with insufficient resources to meet their initial goals are not likely to succeed, since they will quickly produce dissatisfaction on the part of patients, programme staff, and referring clinicians. One useful strategy, particularly in establishing a programme where one does not already exist, is to have a modest set of goals and to then expand those goals based on the experience gained in the first few years of operation. Initial success, even if limited, is more likely to generate support and enthusiasm for the programme than lofty expectations that go unmet.

Given the limited resources generally available for development of psychosocial programmes, it is essential to maximize their use. A key objective must be to have all psychosocial professionals working together in a collaborative fashion. Toward this end, the roles and responsibilities of each professional as defined, in part, by their areas of expertise and professional training, need to be clearly outlined. Often, this begins with an initial evaluation of programme needs in order to determine what mental health disciplines need to be involved in patient care. In addition to limiting duplication of effort across disciplines, this approach maximizes the utilization of each professional's skill set.

Communicating advances in psychosocial research

Psychosocial oncology, like all other areas of healthcare, must be evidence-based in order to gain institutional and funding support. Fortunately, there have been many studies demonstrating interventions that are effective in helping patients and their families cope with the diagnosis and treatment of cancer. With continued research in psychosocial care there is an ever-increasing body of knowledge outlining the benefits to patients and the cost-offsets for healthcare providers. Part of the role of psychosocial oncology must be to share these findings with colleagues in medicine and with the public.

Fortunately, there is a vast audience with an appetite for things relating to cancer. Within the academic institution, formal channels exist in the form of rounds, grand rounds, internship and residency training, and advisory and board meetings. Being 'at the table' with administrators and other decision-makers presents a unique opportunity that must be seized. Speaking to colleagues and other health providers at local, national, and international meetings can be seen as essential in the development of psychosocial oncology. Educating patient groups and the media is another effective tool to promote the value and impact of psychosocial oncology.

Making the business case for psychosocial care

Psychosocial programme development appears to be easier to accomplish within the not-for-profit sector, where the goal is generally to create value by enhancing the social good (27). In this sector, funding for psychosocial programmes almost always comes from institutional resources, philanthropy, or billing for services. Given that in private healthcare systems, mental health professionals are reimbursed for services at significantly reduced rates when compared to medical or surgical services, strong institutional support and philanthropy are usually essential if a programme is to develop. In nationalized systems the cost-efficacy case needs to be made to build up a service.

In the for-profit sector, making the ethical/compassionate case should be one of the main drivers, rather than a typical business model where profit is the primary metric. Effective arguments should include: hospital/cancer centre accreditation; patient safety; risk management; cost savings to the institution; quality patient care; patient satisfaction; regulatory compliance; and perceived competitiveness in the market place. These points represent the most compelling motivations for institutions to support the development of psychosocial programmes. We call these the psychosocial domains of value.

While fundraising and philanthropy enhance many cancer services, these funds often are not directed to psychosocial programmes. Given that well over 90% of the budget for psychosocial programmes is allocated to personnel, fund raising should be linked to specific programmes that will enhance one of the above domains of value. Consequently, it is important for psychosocial programme leaders to have a firm grasp of what truly motivates support by the administrators of hospitals who have many competing interests and departments.

In the American system, most, if not all, hospital-based psychosocial oncology programmes are often poorly insured and are, therefore, seen as a dollar drain on the institution. However, evidence suggests that timely and appropriate psychosocial care can, in fact, reduce costs. Therefore, in developing a psychosocial programme, a strong business plan is necessary to demonstrate credibility in the domains of service, research, and education. Great psychosocial programmes grow because they provide relevant, targeted, and highly visible services that are helpful to the cancer experience of the patient and add prestige to specific key constituents. Physicians in leadership roles, administrators, nurses, and patients and families can all be important advocates when lobbying for funding for psychosocial programmes. Although in clinical care the patient and family are the priority, in programme development they provide a relatively weak voice in bids for funding.

In the National Health Service in the UK, the problems are not that different. Insufficient, appropriately-trained personel exist, leading to few applicants, even when posts are established. Posts need to be justified in the competitive funding environment of service commissioning.

How to engage key stakeholders?

Regardless of the particular constituency, it is necessary to understand what motivates stakeholders as they relate to psychosocial care. In simple terms, why should other stakeholders care about you and your existence? What do they have to gain, or lose, with the implementation of a psychosocial oncology programme? How can these programmes enhance patient care, improve compliance, and perhaps even enhance survivorship? It is always important to remember that a new or evolving psychosocial oncology programme is extremely vulnerable to resistance or opposition. Therefore, it is essential at the outset to build bridges with other programme leaders and to highlight the value added by the psychosocial programme. It takes a great deal of time and effort to create a new programme but very little effort to undermine one.

Unfortunately, patients do not develop strategic plans or create hospital budgets. This is done by cancer centre boards, cancer centre directors, upper-level hospital administrators, and leaders of medical and nursing departments. Therefore, it is necessary to know when new strategic plans are being developed and to be relentless about the importance of psychosocial oncology. For example, promoting the benefits to the hospital of having universal psychosocial screening of all new patients or creating a mandatory support services orientation class for all new patients will highlight what the programme will do in a measureable way. It is also essential that psychosocial leaders be part of the ongoing advocacy and education of all decision-makers at the institution. Psychosocial leaders can use clinical skills in the leadership arena to further the programme through knowledge, data, and persuasiveness.

Communication strategies with nursing

Psychosocial teams who do not engage nursing from the beginning do so at their own peril and simultaneously lose powerful allies. Most referrals for psychosocial support are generated in some way by the nurse at the bedside. Nurses also care very deeply about helping people avoid unnecessary suffering. The psychosocial team can easily build meaningful relationships with nursing by evaluating what they value. Nurses at the bedside care about making patients feel safe and comfortable. They are also committed to ensuring that their patients and family members get the best medical and psychosocial services possible. It can be helpful to teach the nurses how to identify and refer for distress, depression, anxiety, demoralization, and other common problems.

What do physicians want from the psychosocial programmes communication strategies?

Except when there is a financial crisis within the institution, physicians are the most influential stakeholders in psychosocial programme development. Physicians in leadership positions are very sensitive to the hospital's stature in the community, market competitiveness, and quality care. Patient satisfaction is also a highly valued domain. They want to be sure that patients receive the best services possible, in the most efficient and cost-effective way possible; therefore, it is important that the psychosocial programme focus on these areas. Physicians who are clinically focused are much more concerned with the quality of direct services to patients and families. A smooth-flowing and organized clinic, where patients and families are supported, and distress is prospectively managed by the psychosocial team, is highly valued. Psychosocial services have become highly specialized and are tailored to the changing treatment regiments. It is, therefore, best to have an assigned psychosocial oncology professional who has expertise in the specific cancers treated in a particular clinic. This ensures that psychosocial interventions are evidence-based, and state-of-the-art. This model also supports the highest levels of team functioning. Because cancer clinics tend to be high stress and emotionally charged environments, it is a great benefit to the patients, physicians, and nurses to have a team member who is knowledgeable about that setting and is built into the system of caring. Physicians may not have the time or the skills necessary to manage complex psychosocial problems. They may see these issues as a distraction and as a misuse of their time. This reluctance on the part of physicians provides a unique opportunity for the psychosocial team. While the physicians seldom hold the unrealistic expectation that the psychosocial team will 'fix' the distressed patient or family member, they do expect that the psychosocial professional will improve the patient experience within the healthcare setting, benefiting all stakeholders.

A necessary role of the psychosocial team is in educating physicians about the psychosocial perspective in an ongoing disease process. By far, most of the education will be as result of case-based role-modelling by the mental health professional. For example, the mental health professional can demonstrate the ability to enable the patient and their family members to focus their distress to meaningful communication, which under the best circumstances can be replicated by the physician. Mental health professionals can demonstrate to physicians, through role-modelling with actual situations in the clinic, the process of engaging emotionally upset patients by:

(1) taking the time to listen and to allow for emotional ventilation;

(2) repeating back what you think you heard, so the patient or family member can fill in key areas;

(3) giving emotional support and praise for putting concerns into words;

(4) focusing on defining with maximum clarity the problem situation;

(5) developing a meaningful plan of action with the patients, family, and healthcare team; and

(6) clearly defining a follow-up plan and evaluation of effectiveness.

What do hospital administrators want from the psychosocial team: communication strategies?

Hospital administrators are essential partners in creating any successful psychosocial programme. They tend to see themselves as caring individuals who bring order and fiscal discipline to institutions. So the psychosocial team must be able to communicate with administrators about the psychosocial benefits to patients and the institution. Benefits about public image, being a compassionate facility, and cost-savings are some of the key discussion points that seem to attract administrators' attention. Any programme without clear objectives, benefits, and identified liabilities will raise the suspicion of administrators. Since psychosocial care may be seen as a 'soft' science by some, it is necessary to ensure that goals and objectives are clearly stated, and that benefits to the institution are repeatedly communicated.

Hospital administrators need to understand how the psychosocial programme supports the vision and mission of the institution. The psychosocial oncology programme must be seen as the 'connective tissue' of the healthcare system and must be perceived as essential for the institution to reach its goals. Effectively identifying and addressing barriers to medical care is a key role. Through systematic screening, and the management of patient anxiety, depression, and emotional distress, the psychosocial team can reduce unnecessary hospitalizations and re-admissions, expensive diagnostic tests and procedures, litigation, patient dissatisfaction, disruptions (agitation, angry or crying outbursts), and hospital systems and staff burn-out. This is an environment where the psychosocial team can clearly demonstrate to administrators and others the value of psychosocial management of complex problems. The benefits to the patient, family, healthcare staff, and to the system overall are many and are objectively measurable.

Summary and conclusions

Cancer will affect almost 40% of our population over the course of their lifetime and 35–45% of these will suffer from clinically significant distress (10, 12). These figures, combined with ever-increasing survival rates and life-expectancies, make quality of life a salient issue for cancer survivors. Thus, the need for psychosocial care to help patients adjust and cope with the chronic sequelae associated with cancer and its treatments has never been greater.

Despite significant advances in clinical care, research, and education, programme development in psychosocial oncology still has a 'hard row to hoe'. Given the 'soft science' argument waged against psychosocial oncology, it becomes increasingly imperative to communicate clearly about the benefits of psychosocial care from an evidence-based perspective, focusing on the value added in the care of the patients, and the benefits to the healthcare team and the institution. However, with the increased attention to the patient experience, coping, and quality of life over the past three decades, psychosocial oncology has begun to play an increasingly central role in comprehensive cancer care. Clinicians, researches, and educators must continue to work diligently to demonstrate the benefit of psychosocial oncology in reducing patient burden, enhancing quality of life, and reducing healthcare costs. Like Sisyphus from Greek mythology continually struggling to push a bolder uphill, psychosocial oncology continues to face challenges in gaining a place as a core service in cancer care.

References

1. Stanton AL. Psychosocial concerns and interventions for cancer survivors. *J. Clin. Oncol.* 2006 Nov 10; **24**(32): 5132–5137.
2. Zimmermann T, Heinrichs N, Baucom DH. 'Does one size fit all?' moderators in psychosocial interventions for breast cancer patients: a meta-analysis. *Ann. Behav. Med.* 2007 Nov–Dec; **34**(3): 225–239.
3. Rehse B, Pukrop R. Effects of psychosocial interventions on quality of life in adult cancer patients: meta analysis of 37 published controlled outcome studies. *Patient Educ. Couns.* 2003 Jun; **50**(2): 179–186.
4. Kubler-Ross E. *On death and dying.* New York: Macmillian; 1969.
5. Bultz BD. *Changing the face of cancer care for patients, community and the health care system. Report to the Romanon commission on the future of healthcare in Canada.* 2002.
6. Bultz BD, Carlson LE. Emotional distress: the sixth vital sign–future directions in cancer care. *Psychooncology* 2006; **15**(2): 93–95.
7. Bultz BD, Carlson LE. Emotional distress: the sixth vital sign in cancer care. *J. Clin. Oncol.* 2005; **23**(26): 6440–6441.
8. Canadian Association for Psychosocial Oncology. *National Psychosocial Oncology Standards for Canada.* 1999. Available at: http://www.caps.calfinalstandards.cfm
9. Jacobsen PB, Donovan KA, Trask PC, *et al.* Screening for psychologic distress in ambulatory cancer patients. *Cancer* 2005; **103**(7): 1494–1502.
10. Carlson LE, Angen M, Cullum J, *et al.* High levels of untreated distress and fatigue in cancer patients. *Br. J. Cancer* 2004; **90**(12): 2297–2304.
11. Fallowfield L, Ratcliffe D, Jenkins V, *et al.* Psychiatric morbidity and its recognition by doctors in patients with cancer. *Br. J. Cancer* 2001 Apr 20; **84**(8): 1011–1015.
12. Zabora J, BrintzenhofeSzoc K, Curbow B, *et al.* The prevalence of psychological distress by cancer site. *Psychooncology* 2001; **10**(1): 19–28.
13. Holland JC, Bultz BD, National comprehensive Cancer Network (NCCN). The NCCN guideline for distress management: a case for making distress the sixth vital sign. *J. Natl. Compr. Canc Netw.* 2007 Jan; **5**(1): 3–7.

14. Bultz BD, Holland JC. Emotional distress in patients with cancer: the sixth vital sign. *Community Oncology* 2006; *et al.* (5): 311–314.

15. Rebalance Focus Action Group. A position paper: screening key indicators in cancer patients-Pain as a 5th vital sign and emotional distress as a 6th vital sign. Canadian Strategy for Cancer Control Bulletin. *Can Strategy Cancer Control Bull* 2005; **7**(Supplement): 4.

16. National Comprehensive Cancer Network. NCCN practice guidelines for the management of psychosocial distress. *Oncology* (Williston Park) 1999; **13**: 113–147.

17. National Institute for Clinical Excellence (NICE). *Guidance on cancer services: improving supportive and palliative care for adults with cancer.* London: NICE 2004.

18. Kennard BD, Stewart SM, Olvera R, *et al.* Nonadherence in adolescent oncology patients: preliminary data on psychological risk factors and relationships to outcome. *J. Clin. Psychol. Med. Settings* 2004; **11**: 31–39.

19. Von Essen L, Larsson G, Oberg K, Sjoden PO. 'Satisfaction with care': associations with health-related quality of life and psychosocial function among Swedish patients with endocrine gastrointestinal tumours. *Eur. J. Cancer. Care. (Engl)* 2002 Jun; **11**(2): 91–99.

20. Skarstein J, Aass N, Fossa SD, *et al.* Anxiety and depression in cancer patients: relation between the Hospital Anxiety and Depression Scale and the European Organization for Research and Treatment of Cancer Core Quality of Life Questionnaire. *J. Psychosom. Res.* 2000 Jul; **49**(1): 27–34.

21. Jacobsen PB, Donovan KA, Swaine ZN, *et al.* Management of anxiety and depression in cancer patients: toward an evidence-based approach. In: Chang AE, Ganz PA, Hayes DF, *et al.* (eds). *Oncology: an Evidence-Based Approach.* New York: Springer; 2006, pp.1552–1579.

22. Mitchell AJ. Pooled results from 38 analyses of the accuracy of distress thermometer and other ultra-short methods of detecting cancer-related mood disorders. *J. Clin. Oncol.* 2007 Oct 10; **25**(29): 4670–4681.

23. Rosenbloom SK, Victorson DE, Hahn EA, *et al.* Assessment is not enough: a randomized controlled trial of the effects of HRQL assessment on quality of life and satisfaction in oncology clinical practice. *Psychooncology* 2007 Dec; **16**(12): 1069–1079.

24. Boyes A, Newell S, Girgis A, *et al.* Does routine assessment and real-time feedback improve cancer patients' psychosocial well-being? *Eur. J. Cancer. Care. (Engl)* 2006 May; **15**(2): 163–171.

25. McLachlan SA, Allenby A, Matthews J, *et al.* Randomized trial of coordinated psychosocial interventions based on patient self-assessments versus standard care to improve the psychosocial functioning of patients with cancer. *J. Clin. Oncol.* 2001 Nov 1; **19**(21): 4117–4125.

26. Institute of Medicine (IOM). *Cancer care for the whole patient: meeting psychosocial health needs.* Washington, DC: National Academics Press; 2008.

27. Collins J. *Good to great and the social sectors: a monograph to accompany good to great.* New York: Harper collins; 2006.

Chapter 46

Communication challenges with the elderly

Ron Adelman and Michelle Green

Introduction

With the present explosive growth of the elderly population and its extensive use of health services (1), surprisingly little is known about how physicians communicate with older patients. Relatively few studies have focused specifically on physician–older patient communication. This chapter first highlights some distinct aspects of the physician–older patient encounter that influence communication. The authors then describe a range of communication issues that may have particular meaning for health professionals caring for older patients who are diagnosed with cancer or life-threatening disease, undergoing treatment for this, or requiring palliative approaches that provide symptom relief.

There is a controversy about when 'old age' begins; that is, nothing magical occurs at the chronologic age of 65 that marks an individual as older. The age of 65 was not derived from a biologic process; it was defined by social demographic data. Even so, the age of 65 is generally perceived as the beginning of old age. However, it is clear to gerontologists that the process of aging starts decades earlier in life, before reaching the age of 65, and an individual's chronologic age often is not an accurate predictor of function.

If one conceptualizes the ageing population to include individuals from 65 years of age to death, old age may encompass a span of as many as 35 years or more. Thus, some gerontologists view the elderly patient population as being composed of several age cohorts: the young-old (individuals 65 to 74 years old), the middle-old (individuals 75 to 84 years old), and the old-old (individuals 85 years and over). Each of these age groups has its own unique historical perspective and may have different social support and psychological needs, as well as different types of medical problems. For instance, the old-old are more likely to have cognitive impairments, poorer physical health, fewer financial and social resources, and are less likely to be consumer-oriented than the young-old cohort (2). In addition, the majority of older patients have below-basic literacy levels and significant problems with health literacy (3). The combined effect of greater consumerism and a higher level of health literacy among young-old than the old-old are likely to result in different interactions with physicians. Given the heterogeneity among elderly individuals, it is difficult and, indeed, hazardous to make generalizations about older patients (4). By utilizing the geriatric assessment instruments (e.g. measuring cognitive, psychological, functional status), an older patient can be evaluated for his or her unique level of function. These concepts have begun to be integrated in oncologic geriatric care to better determine appropriate medical interventions for older individuals with cancer (5).

Also, with improved health status and recent more positive social perceptions of ageing, many in the field of ageing consider individuals in their sixties and early seventies to be in late middle age. Compared to younger adult patients, however, communication with the older patient is likely to be complicated by ageist attitudes, sensory deficits, cognitive impairment, functional limitations, and the frequent presence of an accompanying relative or caregiver in the medical visit.

Attitudes toward age and ageing

Ageism, defined as the system of destructive false beliefs about older people, is one of the last 'isms' to be acceptable in Western society. It is pervasive in the medical care system (6). Ageism in the medical encounter may result in the disregard of medical problems of older people and inappropriate misattributing their problems to 'normal' ageing (7). Physicians may be less likely to recommend preventive regimens or treat medical problems or psychiatric problems aggressively when the patient is older (8, 9). Some physicians spend less time with older patients or may be inattentive to older patients. Physicians may consider elderly patients more 'difficult' to deal with than their younger counterparts (2).

The origins of ageist beliefs are multifactorial. Our fears of our own ageing and death, a subject still taboo in many societies, play a large role in the development of ageist attitudes. In Western societies, preoccupied with productivity and youth, fears of obsolescence and physical and mental losses foster an ageist perspective. Distinct from other -isms, such as sexism and racism, ageism has a dangerously personal focus; we all become old—that is, if we are fortunate enough to survive. If an individual has become old and has incorporated significant dislike for ageing or older people, this older person then becomes the object of his or her discrimination. This self-directed prejudice has ominous implications for successful ageing; that is, older people themselves may be ignorant about normal ageing or have preconceived ageist attitudes that affect medical care. For example, when an older individual believes that depression or impaired memory is part of normal ageing, he or she will not readily seek medical attention and possible treatment will not be pursued.

Ageist bias is relevant especially in the context of medical care, as these attitudes may cause health providers and patients to discount or deny needs for care. It is likely that healthcare professionals are more susceptible than the lay person to the development of ageist attitudes (6). By definition of their work, physician trainees are primarily exposed to the most vulnerable elderly populations: the ill, the frail, the confused, the demented, and the hospitalized. Robust older people are generally not in the patient sample they are exposed to. Ageism, therefore, may be an occupational hazard of the health professional and can undermine medical care. For example, one study documented how older women with breast cancer are treated less aggressively than their younger counterparts (9). Still, little is known about how subtle negativism about older patients by health providers' influences their medical care.

Geriatric medicine

Older patients often have multiple medical problems that mask one another or make the treatment process for any one disease more difficult. Common diseases often present atypically in older people, yet many physicians have not been taught specific diagnostic skills for evaluating the geriatric patient. For example, classic signs of coronary artery disease, such as chest pain or shortness of breath on exertion, may be more difficult to track in an older person with severe osteoarthritis who cannot walk well.

Older patients usually have accumulated longer medical histories than younger patients. Considerable expertise is required to distinguish important and pertinent clinical problems in an initial evaluation. Many geriatricians acknowledge that it may take two or three visits to assess the geriatric patient adequately. The tasks of geriatric medicine are quite challenging; not only is it important to obtain a comprehensive medical history, but it is essential to secure a social and psychological history as well. This task can be daunting given the time constraints of contemporary medicine. To be able to access the personhood of the older patient amidst all this data collection requires exemplary interpersonal skills on the part of the physician. Additionally, accessing the patient's perspective on goals of care and their wishes, including advance decisions, is an important task of the geriatric medical encounter.

Treatment of the older patient is made more complex by the coexistence of multiple medical problems, the increased risk of adverse drug effects in older people, and the risks inherent in polypharmacy. Also, one of the major differences between the care of older patients is the decrease in reserve in the older patient should something go wrong. Homeostatic reserve has a much wider breadth in younger patients compared to their older counterparts (10). As some frail elderly patients may be homebound and have difficulty returning for routine follow-up office visits, evaluation of ongoing treatment and the early recognition of new problems become much more compelling.

Finally, setting goals for treatment and care may also be more challenging with the elderly patient. Many of the problems encountered in geriatric medicine cannot be solved. For example, many cancers will become chronic care issues. However, the inevitable decline of the elderly patient spells a need for balanced and realistic goals for the physician, patient, and the patient's family or other designated healthcare proxy. As mentioned earlier, knowing the patient's wishes and having a dialogue that enables discussion and revision of approaches to care with time are pivotal to the rendering of holistic care.

The aggressive curing instinct that develops in medical training is not always appropriate in geriatric practice. The physician instead must be able to recognize the time at which more treatment is perhaps unjustified, and must help patients and families come to terms with this difficult reality. However, symptom relief is always critical at any stage of an older patient's illness. Palliative care encompasses symptom-relief for any stage of illness; that is, strategies to relieve multidimensional symptoms from chronic illness, from life-prolonging therapy such as radiation and chemotherapy, as well as for symptoms at the end of life. Acceptance of death and skills in helping a patient die comfortably, and attend to the affected significant others, are prerequisites for the physician caring for older patients. These abilities require special insight, self-awareness, and training and will be discussed in greater detail later in this chapter.

Sensory deficits

Hearing is obviously an important component of communication. Presbycusis, or decreased hearing of higher frequency sounds, is one of the most common and significant sensory changes that affect older people. The incidence of sensorineural hearing loss increases each decade so that by the seventh and eight decades 70–80% of older adults are affected (8). This prevalence makes hearing loss a significant factor to address in older patient–physician communication. In the office setting, amplification with a reasonably priced microphone and headset can enhance communication. Establishing good visual contact, reducing background noise (as listening is more difficult with competing sounds), rephrasing rather than repeating misunderstood phrases, and pausing at the end of a topic may also facilitate communication. To optimize verbal communication, it is helpful for the physician to stand two to three feet away from the patient and to speak at normal to *slightly* louder levels (8). Hearing loss is an important predictor of function for older people, with far greater implications than the immediate inability to communicate in the medical encounter. Recognition and discussion of this fact in the medical visit are important elements of comprehensive geriatric care. For those older patients who use hearing aids, it is important to remind patients to always wear them to medical visits. Perhaps, most importantly, the physician should ask the patient the best strategies for communicating within the clinical setting.

Vision loss also has a large impact on patient–physician interaction, because visual clues are vital in communication. After age 65, there is a decrease in visual acuity, contrast sensitivity, glare intolerance, and visual fields. Older patients who experience visual loss are twice as likely to have difficulty with basic activities of daily living (ADL) and instrumental ADLs, as compared with those who have normal vision (8). Because a large percentage of elderly people are visually compromised, effective communication strategies for these individuals need to be addressed in the medical visit. Sitting close to the older patient with visual loss is one such strategy. The medical office can help compensate for visual loss through environmental supports, such as improved illumination and the use of contrasting colours in décor and signage. Also, paying attention to the size of print in patient information handouts or any other communication, such as appointment cards and letters, can make a significant difference for the visually impaired older patient.

Cognitive impairment

A common myth about old age is that ageing is synonymous with cognitive decline. The incidence of dementia among older people in their sixties is low (e.g. the rate of moderate to severe dementia is about 2% among persons 65–69 years of age); however, the incidence of cognitive dysfunction progressively increases with age (11).

There is a broad range of cognitive loss among individuals with dementia and unless the physician is trained to uncover this problem, it can be missed in those patients with mild or even moderate loss. Obtaining an accurate assessment of the patient's cognitive status is essential to assure optimal communication and medical treatment. At times, geriatricians perform a brief mental status examination as part of an initial assessment. As most patients are sensitive about such testing, it is imperative to prepare the patient before performing the examination. Stating that these tests are performed for all patients or, 'it's only a screen, don't worry about getting the answers correct' can be reassuring. Incorporating the mental status examination into the physical examination so that these questions appear as a routine part of the neurological examination may make the test less threatening for the older patient. Such a screen is included in comprehensive assessment of the geriatric oncology patient.

If a patient has some cognitive impairment, the physician's approach to the older patient must be modified. Unfortunately, some health providers falsely assume that a diagnosis of mild cognitive impairment (MCI) or dementia means that the patient's capacity is impaired in all dimensions of human intellect, emotion, and behaviour. This might be termed 'dementiaism'; that is, inappropriately stereotyping patients with any cognitive impairment as being incompetent and incapable of participating in their care (2). All dementias are not the same: major differences exist between mild and severe dementias, and the type and range of losses among individuals varies widely. Each patient with MCI or dementia requires careful evaluation and an individually tailored approach and treatment plan. Patients who have early dementia often are concerned or upset about their cognitive problems and are more sensitive to the physician's responsiveness and attitude. Attending to the patient's perspective is often important. When a cognitively impaired patient is upset with mental status testing during the first visit, it is wise to abandon the test and focus on developing a relationship with the patient. The physician can always return to testing in future visits when a greater degree of trust has been established. Communication skills with cognitively impaired individuals require knowledge of how the disease progresses for individual patients and the changing needs of individuals over time. As communication with the patient becomes more difficult, the physician must establish a solid relationship with the patient's family or significant other to provide the most appropriate and sensitive care for the patient.

Functional deficits

Many older patients have functional limitations and problems with basic and instrumental activities of daily living (ADLs). These limitations may make the logistics of a medical consultation difficult (e.g. getting to the room, moving from chair to examination table etc). Indeed, in a healthcare system where domiciliary visits are not undertaken, these frail older patients may be seen so infrequently that visits to the doctor are emotionally and physically taxing, and the patient may have generated an extensive agenda addressed during the visit.

Allowance for functional deficits may extend the duration of the medical encounter (i.e. helping the patient move onto an examination couch or assisting with undressing and dressing). Few consulting rooms are equipped with appropriate equipment to help patients manoeuvring in a small examining room and there is little research that examines whether and how physicians make allowances for functional deficits. Yet it is clear that those patients with functional deficits, who visit the doctor unaccompanied, do require special provision from the service.

By contrast, when a domiciliary visit is undertaken, a great deal of information can be gleaned from seeing the patient's home, how they live, and how they function in their own setting.

Third persons in the medical encounter

One major characteristic that distinguishes the geriatric medical consultation from other encounters is that often the older patient is accompanied by a third person (e.g. spouse, adult child, or professional caregiver); various studies have found that 20–57% of elderly patients are accompanied by a third person to a medical visit (12). Indeed, in a study of initial contacts with geriatric medicine, 50% came independently, 30% with a third person, and 15% with two or more individuals accompanying the patient (unpublished).

The third person (or additional persons) may either facilitate or inhibit the development and maintenance of a trusting physician–patient relationship. The third person probably plays multiple roles during the visit depending, for example, on the duration of the encounter, the particular content of the interaction, the health status of the patient, and the needs of the accompanying individual.

Three major roles for the third person have been conceptualized: the advocate, the passive participant, and the antagonist roles (13). When the third person is supportive of the patient, that person is considered an advocate. This person actively encourages and empowers the patient. The passive participant is a third person who is present but minimally involved in the encounter, with scant knowledge about the patient and is generally disengaged from the interactional dynamics of the visit. The antagonist is a third person who works against the patient on either overt or covert levels. This individual may be openly hostile and rude to the patient, and the patient's agenda is either discounted or ignored. The antagonist tries to take advantage of the patient or the physician or both. These potential roles have not yet been empirically validated. To examine the dynamics of dyadic versus triadic visits, Greene et al. (14) compared a matched sample of two-person and three-person encounters. It was noted that, although the content of physician talk was not different in dyads or triads, patients in triads were frequently referred to as 'she' or 'he' by physicians, patients raised fewer topics overall in triads than in dyads, patients were less responsive to topics they raised themselves and were less assertive in triads than in dyads, and less shared laughter and joint decision-making took place in triadic than in dyadic encounters. This study demonstrates that the presence of a third person in the medical encounter with an older person and his or her physician is likely to influence the interactional dynamics of the encounter. Indeed, no matter how minor the involvement of the third person during the visit, his or her presence may change the basic content and process of the encounter. Many geriatricians believe it essential to spend some time in every encounter alone with the patient, often easily achieved during the physical examination part of the visit. This enables private time for a patient to reveal important issues that may not be raised in multi-person encounters.

Strategies for improving the physician–older patient relationship

How can an effective and empathic relationship develop between an older patient and his or her physician? What specific components of communication help to create such a relationship? In this section, the authors describe some approaches that physicians and patients may employ to improve communication. These strategies are derived from the authors' analysis of the empirical literature to date and clinical experience in geriatric care (RA). Few data exist correlating interactional processes with health outcomes for older patients; therefore, these recommendations represent the authors' perspectives on how physicians and older patients can develop a positive relationship at the present level of understanding.

Understanding the patient's perspective

A non-ageist approach is critical for the development of the physician–older patient relationship (2), and must recognize the remarkable heterogeneity of the elderly population (4). Each patient (whether older or younger) must be seen as an individual with specific needs and different concerns and beliefs. A physician is non-ageist when he or she pays attention to issues such as health promotion for the older patient (indicating optimism about the older patient's future), and to anticipatory care (i.e. allowing planning for an active future) covering prevention of falls, avoiding medication non-adherence, and decreasing caregiver stress.

Getting to know the older patient as a person is the best antidote to ageist behaviour. When a physician perceives the older patient as a person with a defined history of accomplishments as well as future goals, ageist stereotypes are likely to be abandoned. An excellent method to incorporate this framework into practice is to conduct a life review. Often this oral history gives a fascinating glimpse into the patient's world and the patient's identity, encompassing the history of the past century, as well as providing a means of determining what is important to the patient. Accessing this narrative history to the patient's story may be time-consuming initially, but it is worth the time extended because it gives a formidable jump-start to the development of trust, which is unfortunately missing so often in the medical encounter. The simple act of listening can be poignant for the patient, as well as the physician. Indeed, through the very act of listening to an older patient's life history, the physician comes to understand the patient's present life, value system, achievements and failures, and this knowledge assists in the diagnosis and treatment of current problems. Allowing for, and supporting, the patient's presentation of self, i.e. the patient's disclosure of his or her identity, undoubtedly improves the relationship (14). To reiterate, the more one knows a patient, the less the patient is relegated to a stereotype.

A physician who makes a house call and sees the severely functionally impaired or hospice patient in his or her own environment has an added opportunity to cement their relationship. The effort of making a home visit, which is relatively unusual in contemporary practice, is likely to have special meaning for a homebound older person. The home visit gives the physician a unique opportunity to examine family dynamics, functional status, living conditions, and gain a glimpse at the patient's identity. In addition, the physician may see photographs, paintings, and memorabilia that invite the physician to learn more about the patient's life. Being a visitor or a guest in another's home changes the power dynamics of the medical visit and allows the patient to exert more control in the encounter. This levelling of the interactional playing field may make it easier for the patient to express his or her perspectives about medical care and treatment, and perhaps enable more joint decision-making.

Studies show that physicians often do not give patients a chance to introduce their concerns (15), and patients' questions are given low priority in medical encounters (16, 17). In one study, Greene *et al.* (18) found that physicians were more responsive to the topics they raised themselves, as compared to the topics that older patients raised. Furthermore, when older patients are able to initiate discussion of their issues, they are not addressed as thoroughly as when physicians raise the issue. Moreover, there is a lack of concordance between the older patient agenda for the visit and the physician agenda for the visit (19), even though a focus on patient-raised issues or the 'patient-centred' approach is essential to establishing rapport.

Patients need encouragement to participate fully in the consultation, although not all older patients feel comfortable in this role. Before seeing the doctor, patients should be asked to list and prioritize their problems and their questions, to consider whether they wish to have a trusted family member or friend accompany them and, during the consultation, to ask for clarification of any aspects that are unclear. After the visit, telephone follow-up can facilitate understanding and will expose difficulties with, or intolerance of, medication or other concerns.

Integrating the psychosocial into medical decision-making

The psychosocial domain is a core element of geriatric medical decision-making, because older patients tend to have multiple medical and psychosocial problems. Some of these problems may be embarrassing and uncomfortable for the patient to raise, so the physician must create an environment in which patients feel safe to raise difficult subjects such as loneliness, depression, anxiety, abuse and neglect, caregiver burden, fears about death, concerns about family members, advance directives, memory loss, incontinence, sexual dysfunction, or addiction, e.g. alcohol, drugs, gambling; these highly personal topics will only be raised when the patient feels the physician can be trusted with such disclosures. It is important to emphasize that the physician need not have the expertise to treat these problems—it is, however, essential that the physician make the appropriate referral to a professional with the appropriate skills.

How does the physician create the safe atmosphere to a consultation? First, physicians must assure patients that all information is confidential; when patients understand that their privacy will be preserved, they are likely to be more disclosing. In addition, physicians must strive to be non-judgmental, which is no easy task when patients' attitudes differ significantly from those of the physician.

Physicians should provide continued support and encouragement to patients as they reveal their embarrassing or emotionally taxing concerns, allowing the patient to talk without interruption, verbally acknowledging distress, and being attentive to such non-verbal cues as tear-filled eyes, voice alterations, or trembling hands. The physician's duty is to try to assist the patient by providing informational, instrumental, or emotional support. This support may be as basic as letting the patient know that the physician is available to listen again at the next visit. The experienced physician realizes that intimate questions may be revisited over time. By raising unresolved issues over time, the physician reveals his or her engagement with the patient's ongoing story, which may be clinically and interpersonally useful. Sensitive timing in raising personal issues is part of the art of medicine; for example, asking an older patient about do-not-resuscitate orders during a first medical visit may not be appropriate for many patients.

Obviously, the physician alone cannot provide all the support needed to meet psychosocial needs, so appropriate referral to a social worker or other health professional becomes an important skill in geriatric medicine.

Attention to sensory and functional limitations

All medical premises must accommodate wheelchairs and those who accompany the patient, and have suitably adapted toilets for disabled patients. The physical environment of a practice sends powerful messages to older people, particularly those with functional deficits, and many doctors' offices are not designed with older patients' needs in mind. Older patients' needs must be considered in the planning, construction, furnishing, and equipping of all medical environments. On a domiciliary visit, the doctor can observe whether the apartment or house accommodates the older patient's functional limitations and can spot how adapting the environment to a patient's functional status could allow a patient to continue to live independently.

Communication between older patients and their providers about cancer

Cancer has a disproportionately high incidence and toll on the elderly population. Sixty per cent of all cancers and 70% of all cancer deaths occur in people aged 65 and over (21). Middle-old and old-old patients grew up in the era in which cancer was almost always a death sentence and, for some, the word 'cancer' denotes pain and certain death. Because of this history, older patients often have an inordinate fear of cancer, which can result in denial, lower attendance for cancer screening and, possibly, non-adherence to cancer treatment regimens. Thus, it is important for the clinician to determine older patients' beliefs about cancer. The clinician may specifically ask the patient: What do you know about the disease?, What are your concerns/fears/beliefs about treatment?, What are your short-term and long-term goals for care?. The notion that each type of cancer is different and that many cancers are treated like a chronic disease may be a revelation for older patients and needs to be discussed.

Ageism and cancer

In addition, there is an extensive literature that documents the occurrence of ageism in the treatment and care of older patients with cancer, manifested in a variety of ways. Older patients are frequently excluded from clinical trials, despite the recommendation of the FDA in 1989 to include older patients (22). This exclusion means that clinicians do not have sufficient data to determine whether to treat or how to treat older patients with cancer. Many in the medical profession assume that life-prolonging treatment is more a priority for younger than older patients (23). They assume that older cancer patients cannot tolerate aggressive surgery or chemotherapy (22). However, research demonstrates no significant differences in outcomes for older and younger patients who participate in clinical trials (22).

Ageism in the medical profession often guides diagnostic and treatment decisions. For example, Litvak and Arora (24) found that older women with breast cancer are 'understaged, underdiagnosed, and undertreated' in comparison to younger women; Faiella (25) concurs that women with breast cancer are treated less aggressively; and Bouchardy et al. (26) found that older patients with breast cancer less frequently receive breast-conserving surgery, axillary node dissection, and adjuvant radiation therapy, chemotherapy and hormone therapy. Thus overall, older women with breast cancer are not given optimal treatment. With respect to other cancers, Fuchshuber (27) reported that older patients are less likely to receive surgery for lung, liver, pancreas, oesophagus, and gastric and rectal cancer. Peake *et al.* (28) found that older patients with lung cancer are undertreated. Chemotherapy is less likely to be offered to older patients with stage III colon cancer or to older women with ovarian cancer (29).

What is it about ageing and cancer that results in prejudicial management and treatment? Bouchardy *et al.* (26) suggest that patients' co-morbidities, lesser life-expectancy, and poorer functional status may affect physicians' decisions.

Penson and colleagues (23) consider the assumptions that clinicians make about older patients, like the belief that older patients value symptom-relief over life-prolonging treatment, will not tolerate chemotherapy well (25), despite literature to the contrary (28), carry risks associated with surgery, or lack long-term benefits from treatment (27).

Diagnosis

The communication literature on diagnosis of cancer focuses most frequently on the delivery of bad news to patients. This literature describes communication between physicians and patients of all ages. We do not know if older patients have different needs at this crucial time, although there is some indication that older individuals cope psychologically with the diagnosis of cancer as well, if not better, than their younger counterparts (2, 5). While some suggest that older patients are less interested in knowing their diagnosis than younger patients (14), others note that patients still desire information, but do not want to be as actively involved in decision-making about treatment (5). In one community sample, 88% of older individuals wanted to be told whether they have cancer (15). Because of these differences in attitude and knowledge, physicians need to evaluate their older patients' understanding and expectations about the disease.

Regardless of age, individual patient preferences for information and support need to be ascertained. As previously mentioned, since many cancers have become chronic diseases, communication skills are needed to support a long-term relationship between the older cancer patient and the physician. Caring for a patient with cancer occurs in stages; it is a dynamic process and patient needs will change over time. A longitudinal perspective on communication about cancer is likely to be the most effective and realistic; recognizing that communication must continue from the delivery of bad news through what may be difficult treatments to either survivorship or death. Of note, Hagerty *et al.* (30) recognize that communicating prognosis involves more than the delivery of 'bad news'. Consideration must be given to how much information to provide and whether to present statistically-derived survival data and anticipated life-expectancy.

Treatment

Although treatment for cancer should be based on physiologic rather than chronologic age (17), older patients receive substantially less aggressive or appropriate cancer treatment than younger patients (2, 18). Breast cancer patients older than 70 years are less likely to receive appropriate surgery for their condition than patients 50–69 years (19). Elderly patients with non-Hodgkins lymphoma, and those with breast cancer, are much less likely to receive sufficient chemotherapy doses to promote the best chances for survival (20). Nordin *et al.* (3) discuss the age-based inequality of care in gynaecologic oncology, which results in poorer prognosis for older women. Furthermore, there is evidence that older cancer patients in nursing homes receive less adequate pain-management than younger cancer patients (21).

There is no difference in younger and older patients' desire for surgery that will offer a possibility of cure from cancer (3). Getting the most effective treatment is equally important to older and younger women with breast cancer (2). Older women, like their younger counterparts, wish to be involved in decision-making about treatment (2).

Although treatment for many cancers may be different in an older population because of the course of the disease, co-morbidity, and the toxicity of regimens, treatment decisions must be individually tailored and take into account the older patient's life-style, preferences, and concerns about quality of life (31). While there is some indication that older patients prefer a less active role in medical decision-making (22) and consider their visits less participatory than younger patients (23), physicians must ascertain older patients' desire for involvement in treatment decisions (14).

Patients may not be known well by the surgeon or oncologist who is recommending life-altering treatment. Communication about patients' values, preferences, and life circumstances needs to be integrated into decisions about appropriate treatment and care. Given the extended period of treatment, ample time exists to develop a supportive relationship. In some practices, the bulk of care during treatment may be delegated to non-medical staff, such as nurses and physician assistants. A full-scale research agenda regarding communication between these health professionals and older patients is needed.

Older cancer patients may be concerned about becoming a burden to their family; their caregivers may be elderly themselves and thus require significant informational and instrumental support. If the caregiver has functional impairments or limited vision or hearing, the role may be more challenging and impact on both the patient's and caregiver's own health. The physician needs to be open to discussions about the burden of care and approaches for alleviating these stressors. Communication about referrals to social work and other social service agencies may be key at this time. For more frail older patients, it may be important to make certain that follow-up plans are clearly understood and organized in advance, e.g. arranging for post-chemotherapy phlebotomy in the home (21).

Survivorship

As previously mentioned, the notion of surviving cancer may not be one that is seriously considered by those older patients who may conceptualize the diagnosis as meaning the end of life. Therefore, to think about being a cancer survivor and living a full and meaningful life after diagnosis and treatment may require negation of a firmly held belief of many years. The physician must be prepared to communicate the realities of a good prognosis (as well as a poor one) to the older cancer patient.

The dearth of research investigating health professional–older patient communication about cancer is partially explained because such study requires grounding in multiple disciplines (including communication, sociology, psychology, and medicine). Many of the research questions require a multidisciplinary approach. The following reflects some of the research questions that require investigation:

(a) How do different age cohorts of older individuals perceive cancer? For example, do young-old cancer patients have a more optimistic and consumerist approach than their old-old counterparts? What are older patients' perceptions and fears about treatment and prognosis? How do these perceptions influence the identification of symptoms, coping with the disease and adherence to treatment regimens?

(b) How does health literacy of older individuals affect communication with health professionals and older patients' ability to follow recommended treatment regimens?

(c) Are there ageist biases in cancer screening, detection and treatment? How do these biases affect screening recommendations, diagnosis, care and physician–older patient communication?

(d) What are older patients' preferences regarding the amount and type of information they receive about a diagnosis of cancer and subsequent treatment? How can physicians identify older patients' preferences for participation in decision-making about cancer treatment?

(e) What are the emotional, instrumental, and informational supports needed by older individuals? How can physicians best respond to these needs?

(f) How does physician specialty (i.e. primary care, oncology, and surgery) influence the quality of communication with older cancer patients?

(g) How does the setting of care (e.g. outpatient practice, inpatient, nursing home) and physician reimbursement (salaried, capitation, fee-for-service) influence communication between physicians and older patients?

Research that encompasses the multiple levels of meaning in cancer care demand qualitative and quantitative approaches to capture the essential communication processes. Ultimately, these research findings must be translated into medical education and training, which will improve care of the older cancer patient.

Communication issues in palliative care

Well-developed communication skills are critical to provide effective palliative care. Duggleby and Raudonis (32) describe some of the special communication needs in palliative care, including recognition that older and younger patients describe pain differently. Quality of life also has a different meaning. While these authors acknowledge that communication with older patients in palliative care requires different skills, few studies specifically examine older patient–healthcare professional interactions surrounding palliative care. There is a clear need to develop evidence-based recommendations for older patients (33).

Communication skills include the ability to direct a patient/family meeting to discuss advance planning and goals of care. About 70% of family physicians who provide palliative care report no training in communication (34) and doctors in training have been found to be inadequately prepared to deal with end-of-life care decision-making (35).

When called to make an inpatient palliative care consultation, the palliative care clinician is often meeting the patient and family for the first time. From the personal experience of one author (RA), one tactic that seems to engage patients is, on first meeting, to ask open-ended questions that focus on the patient's identity. This approach often is well-received and opens up a non-medicalized, 'lifeworld' perspective that gives the patient permission to present personal aspects of his or her self. Communication-based research needs to uncover effective strategies for this initial and important engagement with patients and families. Anecdotally, often families, particularly when the older patient is unable to speak for him or herself, have an urgent need to paint the picture of the older patient's identity to make certain that their loved one is perceived as a person to respect and attend to.

Another strategy, which is unexpected and under-utilized, is the use of humour to engage the patient. Dean and Major (36) conclude that humour may play an important role in humanizing medical care, including end-of-life care.

Even with the increased interest and medical education initiatives that focus on dying and death, discussions about death in the medical encounter are infrequent and uncomfortable for physicians and unsatisfactory for patients. Death continues to be a taboo subject in medical practice, resulting in very few patients being enrolled in hospice programmes or being enrolled too late to obtain the full benefit of the programme. In fact, as many older patients are likely to be unaware of programmes such as hospice, physicians need to inform patients and their families about this service in a timely way. Also, some older patients may have frightening memories of loved ones who had great pain and suffered considerably when dying. They need to be reassured by their physicians that they will not be abandoned and informed about the availability and efficacy of current palliative care interventions.

Common barriers to effective communication with terminally ill patients about dying include a pervasive social and personal denial of death, patients' fears about the dying process and death, and physicians' and other heath professionals' discomfort and anxiety about such discussions. In addition, families may have limited experiences with death and may possess unrealistic expectations about the healthcare system's ability to restore a patient's health, even when the patient has a terminal illness. Overcoming these barriers is very dependent on clinicians' communication skills, which, in turn, improve the quality of life for the terminally ill patient. Central to this approach is to better understand the meaning of the illness for the patient, whatever his or her age might be.

Much of the focus has been on communicating about advance directives. Through focus groups of patients with chronic and terminal illness, family members and health professionals, Wenrich (37) identified other skills for communication with terminal patients, including talking with patients in an honest and straightforward way, being sensitive to when patients are ready to talk about death, picking up non-verbal cues and creating an appropriate physical environment. In addition, Tulsky (38) suggests strategies to communicate with hope, including eliciting patients' realistic short-term goals.

When a patient is terminally ill, the team is catapulted into one of the most emotionally significant and inescapable rites of passage in an individual's life. How can the palliative care team access the patient's perspective and that of the family at this crucial time? Attention to the patient's personhood and his/her presentation of self, as described by Greene et al. (14), can enable the patient's identity to emerge. Dy *et al.* (39) concur that 'personalization' is a key element of patients' satisfaction at the end of life.

It becomes important to reframe the care goals so that patients, families, and healthcare professionals recognize what can be achieved in the patient's remaining days. Care goals at this stage can include pain-management and symptom-relief; sharing last words with significant others; giving a loved one permission to die, bringing meaning and closure to one's life; and reassurance that the individuals being left behind will be fine. Understanding the cultural and religious context for care at the end of life is critical for the patient and family comfort, and must be specifically elicited. When older patients do not have family, the significance of the team's involvement is even greater. If an older patient is socially isolated, often recruiting a volunteer to spend time with the patient can be helpful.

Palliative care team communication

When a patient is hospitalized, optimizing care involves its personalization in the depersonalized hospital environment. With overburdened physicians, too few nurses, and ever-increasing bureaucratic demands, individualized, supportive care is difficult to provide. In the contemporary hospital, it is often the palliative care team that enables this level of attentive care to occur.

When a palliative care team has been called in to see a patient, not only must the team communicate well with the older patient and family members, but it must also be skilled in communicating with other members of the patient's care team (e.g. oncologist, primary nurse, social worker, primary care physician, medical resident). Palliative care teams may be formal, as in an academic setting in which often nurses, physicians, and social workers compose the team, or more informal, with appropriate teams forming as needed, for example, consultation with a chaplain or a psychiatrist. During major family meetings, where goals of care are being discussed, the palliative care team wisely includes the patient's primary care physician whenever possible. After all, part of the purpose of an inpatient palliative care team is to train physicians to better deal with the manifold issues involved in communication, such as discussions about terminal illness, symptom relief and goals of care. It is ironic, perhaps, but eminently understandable, that 'specialists', i.e. the palliative care team, sometimes have to be called in to perform duties that all physicians should be aware of and trained in.

Proper preparation for patient/family meetings is an important task of the palliative care team. Preparation requires adept discussion about goals of care with the primary care physician and other appropriate disciplines. The objectives of a family meeting need to be defined in advance (see Chapter 16) and the interdisciplinary team members need to be in agreement about the goals. At the start of the conference, a team member should present the goals of meeting and the role of the palliative care team. It is often most appropriate for the palliative care team member who is working most closely with the patient/family to lead the discussion. It is fruitful to ask the patient (if present) and each family member to define his/her understanding of the patient's illness near the start of the meeting. This overall strategy facilitates the patient/family to voice their concerns, thoughts and feelings and allows staff to gauge the patient/family members' perspectives. Otherwise, the professionals may dominate talk and the critical perceptions of the patient and family remain unspoken (at least until later in the meeting).

Conclusion

Attending to communication issues is critical for effective geriatric medical care in all stages of the continuum through health and disease. Given the often negative perceptions of the elderly and the great heterogeneity of this population, it is imperative that health professionals assess each older patient as an individual. The impact of a cancer diagnosis and treatment, as well as a terminal illness, have a powerful effect on the lives of older people. Health professionals who care for the elderly with sensitivity to their personhood, their medical status, and psychosocial needs will have a profound influence on the quality of older patients' lives.

References

1. Adelman RD, Greene MG, Ory MG (2000). Communication between older patients and their physicians. *Clinics in Geriatric Medicine* **16**, 1–24.
2. Adelman RD, Greene MG, Charon R (1991). Issues in physician-elderly patient interaction. *Ageing and Society* **11**, 127–48.
3. Gazmararian J, Williams M, Peel J, *et al.* (2003). Health literacy and knowledge of chronic disease. *Patient Education and Counseling* **51**, 267–75.
4. Haug M, Ory M (1987). Issues in older patient-provider interactions. *Research on Ageing* **19**, 3–44.
5. Extermann M, Hurria A (2007). Comprehensive geriatric assessment for older patients with cancer. *Journal of Clinical Oncology* **25**, 1824–31.
6. Greene MG, Adelman RD, Charon R, *et al.* (1986). Ageism in the medical encounter: An exploratory study of the doctor-elderly patient relationship. *Lang and Comm* **6**, 113–24.
7. Greene MG, Hoffman S, Charon R, *et al.* (1987). Psychosocial concerns in the medical encounter: A comparison of the interactions of doctors with their old and young patients. *Gerontologist* **27**, 164–8.
8. Cobbs EL, Duthie EH, Murphy JB (eds) (1999). *Geriatrics Review Syllabus*, 4th edn. *A Core Curriculum in Geriatric Medicine*. Kendall/Hunt, Iowa.
9. Greenfield S, Blanco DM, Elashoff RM, *et al.* (1987). Patterns of care related to age of breast cancer patients. *JAMA* **257**, 2766–70.
10. Hazzard W (1994). Introduction: the practice of geriatric medicine. In: Hazzard WR, Bierman EL, Bass JP, *et al.*, eds. *Principles of Geriatric Medicine and Gerontology*, 3rd edn. McGraw Hill, New York.

11. Costa Jr PT, Williams TF, Sommerfield M, *et al.* (1996). *Recognition and initial Assessment of Alzheimer's Disease and Related Dementias.* Clinical Practice Guideline No.19. Rockville, MD, US Department of Health and Human Services, Public Health Service, Agency for Healthcare Policy and Research, AHCPR Publication No. 97–0702.

12. Prohaska TR, Glasser M (1996). Patients' views of family involvement in medical care decisions and encounters. *Research on Aging* **18**, 52–69.

13. Adelman RD, Greene MG, Charon R (1987). The physician–elderly patient–companion triad in the medical encounter: The development of a conceptual framework and research agenda. *Gerontologist* **27**, 729–34.

14. Greene MG, Adelman RD, Rizzo C, *et al.* (1994). The patient's presentation of self in an initial medical encounter. In: Hummert M, *et al.*, eds. *Interpersonal Communication in Older Adulthood.* Sage, California.

15. Marvel MK, Epstein RM, Flowers K, *et al.* (1999). Soliciting the patient's agenda: have we improved? *JAMA* **281**, 283–7.

16. Frankel R (1990). Talking in interviews: a dispreference for patient-initiated questions in physician-patient encounters. In: Psthas G, ed. *Studies in Ethnomethodology and Conversation Analysis.* Washington DC: The Interactional Institute for Ethnomethodology and Conversation Analysis and University Press of America.

17. West C (1984). *Routine Complications: Troubles Talk Between Doctors and Patients.* Indiana University Press, Bloomington.

18. Greene MG, Adelman RD (1996). *Responsiveness of Physicians and Older Patients to Self-Initiated And Other-Initiated Topics in First Medical Visits.* Presented at the 5th Kentucky Conference on Health Communication. Lexington, Kentucky.

19. Greene MG, Adelman RD, Charon R, *et al.* (1989). Concordance between physicians and their older and younger patients in the primary care medical encounter. *Gerontologist* **29**, 808–13.

20. Stewart MA, Brown JB, Weston WW, et al. (1995). *Patient-Centered Medicine: Transforming the Clinical Method.* Sage, California.

21. Yancik R. (1997). Cancer burden in the aged. *Cancer* **80**, 1273–83.

22. Townsley C, Selby R, Siu L (2005). Systematic review of barriers to the recruitment of older patients with cancer onto clinical trials. *Journal of Clinical Oncology* **13**, 3112–24.

23. Penson R, Daniels K, Lynch T (2004). Too old to care? *The Oncologist* **9**, 343–52.

24. Litvak D, Arora R (2006). Treatment of elderly breast cancer patients in a community hospital setting. *Arch Surg* **141**, 985–90.

25. Faiella E, Gulden P (2007). Battling ageism in cancer negligence cases. *Trial*

26. Bouchardy C, Rapiti E, Fioretta G, *et al.* (2003). Undertreatment strongly decreases prognosis of breast cancer in elderly women. *Journal of Clinical Oncology* **21**, 3580–7.

27. Fuchshuber P (2004). Age and cancer surgery: judicious selection or discrimination? *Annals of Surgical Oncology* **11**, 951–2.

28. Peake M, Thompson S, Lowe D, Pearson M (2003). Ageism in the management of lung cancer. *Age and Ageing* **32**, 171–7.

29. Elkin E, Lee S, Casper E, *et al.* (2007). Desire for information and involvement in treatment decisions: Elderly cancer patients' preferences and their physicians' perceptions. *Journal of Clinical Oncology* **25**, 5275–80.

30. Hagerty R, Butow P, Ellis P, *et al.* (2005). Communicating prognosis in cancer care: a systematic review of the literature. *Annals of Oncology* **16**, 1005–53.

31. Hurria A, Cleary TA, Adelman RD (2006). Cancer in the frail elderly. In: Muss HB, Hunter CP, Johnson KA, eds. *Treatment and Management of Cancer in the Elderly.* Informa Healthcare/Taylor & Francis, New York.

32. Duggleby W, Raudonis B (2006). Dispelling myths about palliative care and older adults. *Seminars in Oncology Nursing* **22**, 58–64.

33. Parker S, Clayton J, Hancock K, *et al.* (2007). A systematic review of prognostic/end-of-life communication with adults in the advanced stages of a life- limiting illness: patient/caregiver preferences for the content, style, and timing of information. *Journal of Pain and Symptom Management* **34**, 81–93.

34. Alvarez MP. (2006). Systematic review of educational interventions in palliative care for primary care physicians. *Palliat Med* **20**, 673–83.

35. Gorman TE, Ahern SP, Wiseman J, *et al* (2005) Residents' end-of-life decision making with adult hospitalized patients: a review of the literature. *Acad Med* **80**, 622–33.

36. Dean R, Major J (2008). From critical care to comfort care: the sustaining value of humour. *Journal of Clinical Nursing* **17**, 1088–95.

37. Wenrich MD, Curtis R, Shannon SE, *et al.* (2001). Communicating with dying patients within the spectrum of medical care from terminal diagnosis to death. *Arch Intern Med.* **161**, 868–74.

38. Tulsky J (2005). Beyond advance directives: importance of communication skills at the end of life. *JAMA* **294**, 359–65.

39. Dy S, Shugarman L, Lorenz K, *et al.* (2008). A systematic review of satisfaction with care at the end of life. *Journal of the American Geriatrics Society* **56**, 124–9.

Chapter 47

Issues for cognitively impaired elderly patients

Andrew Roth and Christian Nelson

Introduction

As established in the previous chapter, there are very real and practical difficulties of communication with older cancer patients (1). Cancer increases in prevalence steadily as people get older and it occurs in many different body sites. Communication difficulties become compounded with elderly patients who have to deal with multiple deficits, including sensory losses and physical frailty (2). These issues become extremely challenging and frustrating when those older patients have cognitive deficits and begin losing, or have lost, aspects of their autonomy and independence. We see these challenges at various times of the cancer experience as particularly:

◆ the need to make treatment decisions soon after diagnosis, including the complex choice of whether to treat or not treat the cancer, depending on the overall health and multiple medical co-morbidities of the patient and likely life-expectancy;

◆ informed consent issues for medical procedures;

◆ dealing with healthcare proxies, especially when there is no other family or supportive family member around;

◆ dealing with issues of independent living;

◆ when dementia is present at diagnosis or arises in the midst of chronic treatment for cancer; and

◆ dealing with confusion or delirium in the general ward setting.

These matters touch most medical caregivers: oncologists, nurses, ancillary services staff such as physical and occupational therapists, dietitians, psychiatrists, psychologists, and social workers. Staff face these situations in all oncology settings: ambulatory clinics, inpatient wards, and specialty treatment and procedure areas, such as radiation oncology and MRI scans. The challenge for oncology staff is to know how to communicate appropriately with patients in various circumstances. Physicians can work together with the older patient to improve the quality of communication during the medical encounter. Benefits of improved communication also include enhancement of trust, improvement in the accuracy of information and understanding, while decreasing the frequency of mistakes (3).

Unfortunately, there has been little research done in the area of communicating with elderly cancer patients who have cognitive deficits. This chapter may, therefore, raise more questions for future research than it can answer. In the first part, we review the small communication literature from the fields of geriatric psychiatry and cognitive disorders. Second, we focus on case studies and attempt to provide practical solutions for common problems that arise with communicating with the elderly who are cognitively impaired.

Background on the cognitively impaired with cancer

The encounter between the clinician and the cognitively impaired elderly patient with cancer and their family brings a number of communication challenges that are specific to this population. Not all health professionals are sensitive to specific issues in geriatric oncology care; there are challenges for clinicians conducting interviews with patients while family members are present in terms of patient autonomy; the importance of communicating as a multidisciplinary team increases significantly to make sure that explorations of disease prognosis and treatment recommendations are consistent and appropriate; and, lastly, issues of informed consent with the cognitively-impaired are complicated and can lead to misunderstanding and inappropriate treatment (4).

Dialogues between physicians and their elderly patients are often marked by ineffective communication, as a result of characteristics of the physician and/or patient, and circumstances that can make these encounters particularly challenging. Despite a recent focus on communication in medical and cancer care, even patients without cognitive deficits report significant levels of unmet needs, particularly in the following realms of communication: information provision, psychosocial support, and response to emotional cues. These issues are particularly relevant to older patients. While studies with older patients with cognitive problems are sparse, those in other clinical populations give us some idea as to issues we need to be aware of within the geriatric oncology community (5). Attending to the unmet needs of cancer patients, information provision, and promotion of patient compliance, have been found also to be correlated with provider behaviour patterns (6).

There have been randomized, controlled communication trials (7, 8) in younger patients, but none in older cancer patients. Razavi et al. (8) reported significant changes in doctor use of emotional words. The content of the training programme and the benefits of the reported changes are not clear. Jenkins et al. (7) showed that communication skills training is a successful means of altering some doctor consultation behaviours and attitudes. Finally, Jenkins and colleagues (9) conducted a pre-post study of training in discussing randomized, controlled trials of cancer therapy. In video-taped interactions with actors before and after the training, improvements were noted in several desirable outcomes.

In addition, ethical questions about treatment options arise. For instance, is it appropriate to suggest surgical treatment for a newly diagnosed lung cancer in a patient with dementia? Should one embark on a rigorous chemotherapy regimen in a patient who has a good Karnofsky Performance score but with slight cognitive problems that may be the harbinger of Alzheimer's disease, and may be exacerbated if a medication like Dexamethasone is required? Anxiety often makes these decisions more difficult, yet patients' anxiety levels have been found to be significantly reduced when the clinician was flexible and responsive to the individual patient's needs for information and emotional support (10).

Ageing is impacted by physical, psychological, and social factors. Physiologic changes accompanying ageing include functional and sensory deficits (see Chapter 42). The elderly tend to view the medical encounter from more traditional, biomedical perspectives, and take a more submissive role when interacting with physicians. From a social perspective, they are more likely than their younger counterparts to live alone, have less money, and be less educated; and the older the patient, the more likely that he/she will be accompanied by a companion at the medical visit. Decisions about who is an appropriate supplementary historian, while protecting patient confidentiality, are issues to be considered. Conflicting information that may flow from partial cognitive deficits can also complicate treatment planning. Attending to these challenges of older cancer patients is crucial for providing optimal care.

Recent research has demonstrated that first impressions do count a lot (11). Successful communication in initial consultations may positively influence a patient's psychological health over a long period of time. Alternatively, poor initial communication can have adverse effects longitudinally as well. Key challenges to effective physician–older patient communication include: physical, cognitive, and language changes; time; off-target verbosity; the managed care environment; and companions present during medical encounters. The bulk of the responsibility for effective communication between physician and older patient lies with the physician.

Physician behaviour in medical interactions has far-reaching implications in terms of both patient satisfaction and compliance with treatment recommendations. However, because of the physiological, psychological, and social challenges the elderly bring, it may be more difficult for physicians to negotiate quality communication with the elderly.

Over the past twenty years, medical schools have gradually introduced communication skills training in recognition of the vital role it plays in optimal patient care (see Chapter 7); however, less time has been devoted to the problems of elderly patients. The most effective method for learning communication skills is observation of ideal and effective communication strategies, followed by rehearsing the skills in role-play, receiving immediate feedback on performance to permit modification, and then repeating the practice. In this way, the trainee has the opportunity to hone his or her own communication patterns without negative experiences. This positive experiential process has been recognized as the central component in successful acquisition of communication skills.

Exemplary clinical predicaments

When cognitive deficits are so clear and severe that it has been deemed by a physician, and understood by family, that the patient does not have decisional capacity, direction to a healthcare proxy is fairly straightforward. Unfortunately, it is the ambiguous and perhaps unstable nature of the cognitive problems that lead to complicated decisions, such as in the case scenario in Box 47.1.

Important in these situations is ensuring that appropriate informed consent is obtained before moving ahead with treatment. Too often in hospital situations this is not considered until a patient refuses care. Especially when patients or family members have sensory deficits, it is important to take the time to explain the information in language that the patient can understand, and

---

Box 47.1 Case scenario illustrating the loss of capacity and consent

Mr Burke is an 80-year-old married man, who has prostate cancer, for which he had a prostatectomy six years ago. His Prostate Specific Antigen (PSA) has been increasing and he now has a metastatic lesion in his spine that explains some of the back pain he has complained about for the last few months. He is on Atenolol for hypertension and was recently started on Aricept, by his primary care physician, for forgetfulness. Mr Burke comes to the consultation with his 77-year-old wife who has a mild form of Alzheimer's disease. Their grown children live in other states and are not with them today. They were referred by Mr B's urologist for discussion about possible hormonal therapy and radiation therapy. In the session, you discover Mr B and his wife have difficulty hearing, and seem not to fully understand the treatment options as you try to describe the pros and cons of each option. They are very uncertain about which option to choose.

then check with the patient, or have the patient paraphrase your discussion to ensure the patient understands the information. Patients should be able to clarify the need for the treatment, the side-effects or complications from the treatment, as well as the risks of refusing the treatment. When considering capacity, the more life-threatening nature of the disease and treatment proposed, the higher the standard of cognition for the patient to understand the need for the treatment, potential side-effects and complications, and risks of refusal.

The specific suggestions and skills that may help a clinician accomplish these important tasks range from simple suggestions to more complicated plans such as organizing joint consults with multiple disciplines. Some of the basic suggestions include providing written information that is easy to understand and written at a grade level appropriate for the audience, using simple phrases, and taking frequent breaks in the conversation to clarify (e.g. have the patient paraphrase) the plan. If possible, it might benefit the patient to meet with the larger treatment team to help clarify decisions for treatment. This may be beneficial if the patient has worked with one specific doctor with whom they have developed a trusting relationship. These issues become all the more challenging if the patient does not speak English and translators are needed. Reaching out to additional family members when capacity is questioned is important.

Working with multiple clinical staff and maintaining appropriate communication between these staff may be specifically important in working with cognitively impaired elderly patients. For example, on an inpatient service, there is a need for accurate information to be handed on from one shift to another and from one specialty to another, as staff cannot rely on the patient to give accurate information. The problems of evaluating changes and monitoring responses to various treatments is heightened if each of the healthcare professionals does not have the same understanding of what is going on with a patient. Some professionals may not realize that patient input may be misleading. Direct verbal communication, as well as accurate and clear charting, is imperative. Charting documentation of 'dementia' when there are other reasons for cognitive changes can lead to a less aggressive treatment approach, either for primary cancer treatment, co-morbid medical problems, or even ancillary care, such as physical or occupational therapy. Home aide services are often reliant on patients to give direction to aides. Depending on the degree of cognitive deficits, direction may be able to be given adequately to optimize a patient's autonomy and independence. In addition, nursing aides can be taught to improve their communication skills with cognitively impaired patients (12).

Relatives' views and interpretations of medical issues and how much they are allowed to participate in helping patients make decisions are clearly of concern (e.g. Box 47.2). Often, cognitive changes are not static, though they may be stable for some time, depending on the cause and trajectory of the illness and other factors; it is important for a clinician to distinguish reversible from irreversible changes in cognition, as these can impact treatment decisions and prognoses significantly. Relatives or caregivers bring their subjective bias to the situation, which may or may not be relevant to the patient's primary needs. The relatives or caregivers may only see the patient at selected times or may be overwhelmed and frustrated with caregiver burden. As a result, it is important to be able to elicit accurate information from the patient's perspective, as well the relative or caregiver.

To do this, the following suggestions or skills may be helpful. Consider seeing the patient alone first, in order to understand their perception of the situation and if there is anything they want to disclose to you without the caregiver or relative in the room. There are times that this need is not perceived until you have met with the family member and reviewed the situation. It may also be important to maintain structure and limits during the consult, attempting to remain neutral, while listening and considering all perspectives and concerns. There are times when a family member may be domineering and pushing a specific course of treatment or management; it is

Box 47.2 Case scenario illustrating a dominant caregiver

Ms Rusk is a quiet, proud 83-year-old, widowed woman with non-Hodgkin's lymphoma, who was treated with chemotherapy about three years ago that has now recurred. She lives alone, but comes in with her 42-year-old divorced daughter, who was successfully treated for breast cancer five years ago. The patient has been having more difficulty ambulating, with two recent falls, and the daughter feels the patient requires an assisted living situation, which the patient refuses. The daughter does not let her mother fully answer questions and dismisses her mother's answers with 'You always say that; but you are always wrong'. The daughter believes her experience with breast cancer has made her an expert on the needs of cancer patients. Though the patient cannot concentrate on the newspaper like she used to (she used to read the *New York Times* from cover to cover), she recalls what she does read. She has multiple somatic complaints that do not have clear medical aetiologies, and she feels depressed.

important to continue to use your clinical judgment and perhaps request consultations from other services, such as patient representatives or social workers, to help understand and better manage the situation. There may also be gains by teaching caregivers of those with cognitive deficits how to communicate better with their loved ones (13).

Assessment of depressive symptoms is important in elderly cancer patients who present with new onset concentration problems. Sometimes these deficits are a result of the depression in what used to be called pseudo-dementia, and what is now known as syndrome of dementia in depression. Even though this scenario may eventually result in a definitive dementia diagnosis, treating the depression now could alleviate the mood and cognitive difficulties and allow for improved communication. The most notable signs of pseudo-dementia may include lack of motivation in answering questions or giving information, depressed affect that accompanies the cognitive decline, is more common with late-onset depression, and less likely to have language impairment and to confabulate than those with true dementia—these diagnostic entities may be better evaluated with validated instruments and treatment algorithms (14).

Another prominent issue that often arises when dealing with cognitively impaired elderly patients is loss of independence (Box 47.3). A glaring example of this is the decision to take away driving privileges when a patient becomes too frail, impaired by disease or medication or cognitive changes, and where the medical team's responsibility lies in this decision process.

Box 47.3 Case scenario illustrating loss of independence

Mr Mayo is a 73-year-old man with metastatic lung cancer who lives in a small rural town. He comes in with his wife, who is very concerned that her husband gets lost more frequently while driving his car. He is taking a low dose of OxyContin for bone pain. She is concerned that his reflexes are slower. Though she has talked with their children and primary care physician, they are all cognizant of Mr Mayo's desire to maintain his independence through driving, especially since there is no public transportation in their town. Mrs Mayo has not driven in thirty years, but volunteers to restart if her husband will give up the keys. They argue in the physician's office.

Suggestions for this type of clinical encounter might include a range of possibilities from assessment to discussion of loss of autonomy and its consequences. Usually, a multidisciplinary approach, with inclusion of family, is helpful in resolving these situations. At times, a work-up for cognitive problems, including Mini-Mental Status Exam (MMSE), neuro-psychological evaluation, and occupational therapy evaluation, may help clarify the deficits to help determine what constraints are necessary. In the specific example of driving, an evaluation by the Department of Motor Vehicles may provide supplementary information to make this decision. As patients lose their independence, it is important to discuss new ways of maintaining activities; for example, investigating alternatives to the patient having to drive himself.

Many of these suggestions come from our clinical experience of working with these issues and patients in a large cancer centre (See Table 47.1). Although several interventions have targeted improvement of elderly patients' communication skills to help them in medical visits, interventions aimed at improving physician interactions with older patients have yet to be widely explored. In fact, there is a remarkable dearth of geriatric communication training programmes in the oncology setting, despite the fact that cancer occurs primarily in the elderly. Attention given to enhancing clinician–patient communication skills with elderly cancer patients and their families could optimize the healthcare delivered to older patients, and improve the sensitivity and effectiveness of cancer clinicians in communicating with elderly patients.

Cognitive impairment in the cancer patient

Clinicians would do well to understand a number of issues with the elderly:

(a) identifying and handling anxiety and depression in the frail elderly and understanding their impact on clinical care;

(b) awareness of confidentiality and privacy of information;

Table 47.1 Cognitive Issues in the Elderly

Issues	Strategies and skills
◆ Informed treatment decisions.	◆ Giving written information that is easy to understand and grade level appropriate for the audience.
	◆ Using simple phrases.
	◆ Taking breaks in conversation to clarify understanding.
	◆ Having patients paraphrase their understanding.
	◆ Joint meetings with treatment team.
◆ Working with family members.	◆ Consider meeting with the patient alone.
	◆ Maintain limits and structure during consult.
	◆ Act as advocate for the patient with aggressive family members.
	◆ Consult from patient representative and social work.
	◆ Suggesting ways family members or caregivers can communicate more effectively with the patient.
◆ Loss of independence.	◆ Multidisciplinary approach to assess cognitive, emotional, and physical deficits.
	◆ Consider DMV evaluation for question of driving capacity.
	◆ Discuss alternatives for activities, additional supports and resources.

(c) normalizing and managing the diminishing and actual loss of independence;

(d) problems with co-morbid illnesses and physical disabilities (mobility, hearing, vision) and the interaction these concerns have with diminished cognitive abilities;

(e) treatment adherence related to understanding treatment goals; and

(f) degree of cognitive deficits and how they impact decision making.

Addressing these subjects would heighten sensitivity to relevant issues in the elderly, thereby challenging attitudes that often stereotype the elderly and compromise optimal care and compassion. Clinicians could be made more aware of the range of attitudes about the elderly that influence the information shared with their patients, in turn influencing treatment choices. Devising methods for communicating appropriately with cognitively compromised patients would ease the concerns of clinicians, patients and families.

Pain

Additionally, staff could be informed about the components of frailty and co-morbidities that interfere with effective communication with elderly patients coping with cancer. For instance, assessment of pain in cognitively impaired patients can be very difficult. A pain-assessment checklist has been found to be helpful in identifying painful situations in seniors with severe dementia (15).

Interviewing training

In-service training with oncology staff, highlighting the common issues of independence and confidentiality when the elderly patient with cancer presents with relatives and care providers, may be useful. For instance, it is important to learn how to conduct interviews while maintaining neutrality, when family members do not give patients sufficient leeway in asking questions. This could help the staff obtain sufficient data, assist patients to make their own decisions when suitable, and may make possible more appropriate communication.

Often clinicians are not adept at exploring roles and relationships in interviews or know how to show how these dynamics may impact illness and care provision. Observing various interactions among the oncologist, patient, and patient family members may give helpful insight into how to improve outcomes of care for both the patient and the family. Addressing the needs of third parties in a clinical consultation, responding to their questions, nurturing their role as care providers, and optimizing constructive communication, are key components to better outcomes with patients who have compromised concentration.

Team approaches

As important as creating an optimal team-based approach to communicating with an older patient about complicated treatment options may be in general, it is imperative in working with cognitively compromised patients. For example, rather than meeting with a patient and family members on three separate visits, a surgeon, radiation oncologist, and medical oncologist may be present together to introduce cancer treatment options to a patient and spouse, or adult child. Teams could learn how to clarify the role of each team member, know who will address which needs of the patient and family, and be certain that the role of nursing and psychosocial team members is clarified so that these domains are not neglected by the team. Though not always well-defined, there are differing roles and responsibilities of a multidisciplinary team attempting shared care of a patient needing multimodal treatments. It is important not just to think about communication from the standpoint of interactions between staff and patient, but also amongst the team. The goals of team communication, the contributions of designating a case coordinator and using nursing and allied health practitioners, to achieve seamless care are worthy pursuits.

The role of psycho-oncology

Often liaison with psycho-oncologists, familiar with the nuances of cancer care as well as treatment of psychiatric and cognitive disorders, can help educate the interdisciplinary team, as well as optimize cognitive and psychological functioning to allow for better outcomes. Psychiatrists can also assist in evaluations for capacity to make treatment decisions with cognitively impaired patients, including understanding and judgmental capacity in reasoning about a choice. They can also assist with identifying the role of surrogate decision-makers in this setting. Ethically and medico-legally, clinicians are involved in achieving and documenting informed consent with the cognitively impaired.

Recognizing when powers of attorney, healthcare proxies, or court appointed guardians are necessary, and which hospital resources are available to assist in these measures will relieve the tension surrounding very stressful situations. In addition, focus on appropriate communication techniques through life stories can increase overall well-being and quality of life in persons with dementia (16), and help them satisfy their spiritual needs (17). It is helpful to provide communication strategies to staff dealing with cognitively impaired patients with dementia in the hospice setting (18).

There is also benefit in teaching communication strategies to caregiver spouses to enhance communication and the quality of interactions with simple techniques (for instance, using simple sentences), rather than those that do not seem to help (slow speech) (19), or using questions necessitating a yes/no response rather than open-ended questions (20). In addition, innovative means of communication, such as video-phones with cognitively impaired patients may allow for improved focus and attention when families are not near by (21).

Conclusion

Cancer is a disease of ageing—the field of oncology must focus on better care of the elderly, and the elderly with cognitive deficits in particular, as the population of each country grows older. Educating oncology nurses, physicians, and families, will not only benefit those working and training at major cancer centres, but will also be useful for others working in the field. The need for randomized studies of communication interventions in older cancer patients is imperative.

References

1. Greene MG, Adelman RD (2003). Physician–older patient communication about cancer. *Patient Educ Couns* **50**, 55–60.
2. Adelman RD, Greene MG, Ory MG (2000). Communication between elderly patients and their physicians. *Clin Geriat Med* **16**, 1–24.
3. Bruschi P (1998). Prescription for effective communications with older patients. *J Med Soc New Jersey* **95**, 43–5.
4. Extermann M, Hurria A (2007). Comprehensive geriatric assessment for older patients with cancer. *J Clin Onc* **25**, 1824–31.
5. Lerman C, Daly M, Walsh WP, *et al.* (1993). Communication between patients with breast cancer and healthcare providers. Determinants and implications. *Cancer* **72**, 2612–20.
6. McCormick WC, Inui TS, Roter DL (1996). Interventions in physician–elderly patient interactions. *Res Ageing* **18**, 103–36.

7. Jenkins V, Fallowfield L (2002). Can communication skills training alter physicians' beliefs and behaviour in clinics? *J Clin Oncol* **20**, 765–9.

8. Razavi D, Delvaux N, Marchal S, *et.al.* (2002). Does training increase the use of more emotionally laden words by nurses when talking with cancer patients? A randomised study. *Br J Cancer* **87**, 1–7.

9. Jenkins V, Fallowfield L, Solis-Trapala I, *et al.* (2005). Discussing randomised clinical trials of cancer therapy: evaluation of a cancer research UK training programme. *BMJ* **330**, 400.

10. Schofield PE, Butow PN, Thompson JF, *et al.* (2003). Psychological responses of patients receiving a diagnosis of cancer. *Ann Oncol* **14**, 48–56.

11. Nussbaum JF (1998). Physician–older patient communication during the transition from independence to dependence. *J Oklahoma State Med Assoc* **91**, 504–8.

12. Bourgeois MS, Djikstra K, Burgio LD, *et al.* (2003). Communication skills training for nursing aides of residents with dementia: the impact of measuring performance. *Clin Gerontol* **27**, 119–38.

13. Small JA, Gutman G (2002). Recommended and reported use of communication strategies in Alzheimer caregiving. *Alzheimer Dis Assoc Disord* **16**, 270–8.

14. Alexopoulos GS, Borson S, Cuthbert BN, *et al.* (2002). Assessment of late life depression. *Biol Psychiat* **52**, 164–74.

15. Fuchs-Lacelle S, Hadjistavropoulos T (2004). Development and preliminary validation of the pain assessment checklist for seniors with limited ability to communicate (PACSLAC). *Pain Manage Nurs* **5**, 37–49.

16. Acton GJ, Yauk S, Hopkins BA, *et al.* (2007). Increasing social communication in persons with dementia. *Res Theory Nurs Pract* **21**, 32–44.

17. Ryan EB, Martin LS, Beaman A (2005). Communication strategies to promote spiritual well-being among people with dementia. *J Pastoral Care Counsel* **59**, 43–55.

18. Thompson PM (2002). Communicating with dementia patients on hospice. *Am J Hosp Pal Care* **19**, 263–6.

19. Small JA, Gutman G, Makela S, *et al.* (2003). Effectiveness of communication strategies used by caregivers of persons with Alzheimer's disease during activities of daily living. *J Speech Lang Hear Res* **46**, 353–67.

20. Small JA, Perry J (2005). Do you remember? How caregivers question their spouses who have Alzheimer's disease and the impact on communication. *J Speech Lang Hear* **48(1)**, 125–36.

21. Savenstedt S, Zingmark K, Sandman PO (2003). Video-phone communication with cognitively impaired elderly patients. *J Telemed Telecare* **9** Suppl, S52–4.

Chapter 48

Communicating with children when a parent is dying

Cynthia W Moore, Michele Pengelly, and
Paula K Rauch

When a parent with dependent children is diagnosed with a life-threatening illness, it is common
for a significant part of their distress to be associated with worries about their children. The
family-centred care approach has stimulated a new focus on addressing patients' wishes to support their children's coping. This is a deveopment in its early stages, and the initiatives vary widely
across settings. While there are not yet data to support a particular approach, it is important to
highlight lessons learned from existing initiatives. This chapter draws on the clinical experience
from two different programmes: one an innovative programme spearheaded by nurses at a
regional oncology centre in South Wales, and the other a parent-guidance programme offered by
child psychologists and child psychiatrists at a major academic cancer centre in Boston.

In the Welsh programme, child-friendly space has been created in the hospital setting, which
includes toys chosen by a play therapist to be fun and therapeutic. The setting offers parents
an opportunity to spend quality time with their children, while facilitating play as a means of
helping children express anxieties. The creation of the children's room has allowed important
family events, such as birthdays and Christmas, to be more comfortably celebrated together in
the cancer centre. And, the staff's appreciation of the importance of the patient's family is clearly
communicated (1).

In addition to the children's room, a family tree is utilized as an assessment tool for taking a
parenting history. A family tree helps clinicians focus on the patient as a person, who is connected
to a family. Its use avoids the reductionism of a narrow focus on the disease process, or a long list
of predetermined questions that might inhibit the free expression of the patient's self-generated
family concerns. By noting names, ages and gender of children in the family tree, the clinician
delivers the message that the team has real interest in the patient's family.

At the Massachusetts General Hospital Cancer Center PACT (Parenting at a Challenging Time)
programme, child psychiatrists and psychologists provide free guidance to parents with cancer
about communication and children's coping. Between two- and three-hundred new families a
year receive first-time consultations and many benefit from repeated meetings at critical points
during the course of the illness (2). Information about the programme is provided to each new
cancer patient in the form of a brochure with guiding principles for supporting children's coping
along with information on how to access the programme. This allows the patient to self-refer, or
for any member of the treatment team to engage the PACT clinicians. Individual clinical consultations are supplemented with a book (3) written by the PACT team, and a website (4), which
includes additional educational information.

While quite different in focus, both of these programmes share an appreciation for the
complexity of parenting with cancer, and provide direct support for parents around some of

their concerns. Both also promote open communication—between healthcare professionals and parents, and parents and their children. This chapter draws upon the authors' collective experiences in these two different settings, to inform healthcare professionals about family communication about illness, so they are better prepared to address parents' concerns.

Review of literature

Communication and children's adjustment

A body of research examining the effects of parental cancer on children's functioning has begun to take shape. Studies indicate that a number of children coping with parental illness experience depressed and anxious mood, poor concentration, intrusive thoughts, school difficulty, sleep problems and somatic complaints (5–10). Efforts are underway to identify family processes and individual factors that predict poorer outcomes for children.

Some research suggests that communication about the illness has the potential to affect children's adjustment. For example, a study of the long-term adjustment of 116 grown daughters of cancer patients found that many identified inadequate communication about the cancer as an impediment to their eventual adjustment (11) Adolescents with a parent diagnosed with cancer two to six years earlier tended to be more anxious or distressed when they felt unable to discuss the illness with their parents or received little information from parents (12, 13). And 6–12-year-olds, pre-adolescent and adolescent children, who were uninformed about the parent's cancer, were more anxious than children from the same families who had been told the parent's diagnosis (14).

Research assessing the relationship between family communication style and distress, with multi-item questionnaires, yields murkier results. Watson *et al.* (10) did not find a restricted communication style to be associated with children's emotional or behavioural problems in families with maternal breast cancer. A study of 80 families that assessed children's adjustment a year after completion of the parent's treatment, did not find that mother's report of poorer communication, or the child's report of their ability to ask questions, their knowledge or satisfaction with the information provided, were associated with children's adjustment (8) However, the strength of any relationship between children's adjustment and family communication may have been attenuated by the length of time since the completion of the parent's treatment. There was a trend towards a relationship between children feeling able to ask questions, and better adjustment; 70% of children who felt able to ask questions had good adjustment, versus only 47% of children who felt unable to ask questions.

A study of 212 children, aged 11–18 years, with a parent with cancer, also examined the relationship between communication and distress. Communication was poorer for some adolescents who had a parent with recurrent disease or a parent receiving more intensive treatment. Time since diagnosis did not affect communication patterns, but communication during the acute phase of the illness was not assessed. Adolescents who had negative feelings about communication with either parent, or who tended not to share feelings with parents, reported more intrusive thoughts and feelings about the illness, greater efforts to avoid thinking about the illness and greater overall distress (15).

These studies measured general family communication style, rather than the openness of communication about the parent's illness. Studies have yet to determine how closely these two types of communication are related. A focus only on restricted communication may obscure a finding that both too little and too much information about cancer is detrimental to children; there is a layer of distorting results if families with 'just right' levels of openness are conflated with those who have difficulty judging when children have enough information.

Content of family communication about illness

Barnes *et al.* (16, 17) interviewed 32 women with breast cancer, and found variability in the extent to which children were told about the illness. Only 50% of children learned their mother had cancer soon after she received the diagnosis, and 19% still didn't know even after she had surgery or radiation therapy (17). Older children received more information at the time of diagnosis and were also more likely to learn the mother had cancer. Interestingly, mothers with less education tended to mention cancer specifically, and to share more information with children at initial diagnosis, than better-educated mothers. More open mothers felt the child had a right to know, wanted to keep the child's trust and hoped that talking would alleviate the child's anxiety. Those who disclosed less, wanted to avoid facing difficult questions, including questions about death, wished to protect the child and to preserve special family occasions, and believed that the child would not understand the illness (16). Another interview study with mothers with newly diagnosed breast cancer found that few mothers addressed feelings when telling their children about cancer (18). Over-disclosure about the cancer and over-reliance on children's questions to guide the discussion were two extremes that needed work.

Interviews with children suggest that they value being able to talk with parents about cancer. In a sample of children whose mothers had breast cancer, about 33% of the 6–12-year-olds, and 25% of the 13–20-year-olds mentioned that talking about the cancer helped. In contrast, only 6% of the younger and 11% of the older children reported that *not* talking or thinking about the illness helped (19). Kristjanson *et al.*'s (20) interviews with 31 adolescents with mothers with breast cancer suggested that, for them, knowing whether their mothers would survive was most important. A number also felt it helpful to know how serious the illness was, the side-effects of treatment, how to help their mothers and what the range of normal adolescent responses looked like. However, each adolescent's need for information varied, depending on family and personal characteristics. This suggests that an individualized parent or family guidance approach may be better suited to meeting the unique needs of each child in a family, than a group 'one size fits all' model.

These studies together emphasize the value that parents and children place on open communication about illness, as well as the need for professional support to parents about how best to talk to children about cancer. This need is increasingly recognized, as evidenced by a recent review that found that helping children to understanding the parent's somatic illness and medical treatments was a consistent priority for interventions (21).

Children's reactions to parental illness and death: a developmental model

Conversations with children about parental illness must be developmentally appropriate, or they risk being confusing or misattuned to children's real worries. Other articles have detailed children's understanding of, and reactions to, illness based on stage of development (2, 22, 23). Highlights are summarized in Table 48.1.

The importance is evident, across age groups, of maintaining regular routines and expectations, to promote children's sense of security. Additionally, children will benefit from having family time that feels 'normal' and is not always focused on the parent's illness. Parents may need help in recognizing the many ways that reminders of illness impinge on their child's life, and learning how to retain a sense of normality.

Children at any age may have temporary fluctuations in their behaviour or mood following a change in a parent's medical status. However, these are usually not expected to last more than

Table 48.1 Children's conceptualization of parental illness and death

Child's understanding and reactions	Guidance for parents
Infants and toddlers (0–2 years)	
◆ Aware of parent's absence, but not the reasons ◆ Sensitive to disruptions in their routine and caregivers' distress	◆ Provide consistent caregivers, routines and settings
Preschoolers (3-5 years)	
◆ Aware of the absence of a loved person ◆ Explanations for illness and death are often inaccurately self-centered or self-blaming ('I got mad at Daddy, and made Daddy sick'). ◆ Egocentric questions are common ('When can you play with me again?') ◆ Limited concept of time creates need to tie events in the future to concrete markers (a birthday, Halloween) ◆ Concrete thinkers, so euphemisms like 'Mommy is in Heaven now,' are misunderstood ◆ Death understood as prolonged separation; may believe the deceased is alive elsewhere ◆ Do not appreciate that death is irreversible, and may offer 'solutions' to death, such as trying a new medicine or replacing old batteries	◆ Explore child's understanding of the illness and/or death; dispel guilt by correcting misconceptions and reassuring the child that nothing they did caused the illness or death ◆ If a parent is withdrawn, explain that the parent is sad or worried, and why, and that the child did not cause the adult's distress ◆ Provide concrete descriptions of death (his body does not work anymore: he can't see, hear, or feel anything; his heart stopped pumping and he stopped breathing) ◆ Be patient in repeating that the deceased will not come back ◆ Maintain consistent caregivers, preschool attendance, play dates, meal times and bedtime rituals during illness and after a death
School-aged children (6–12 years)	
◆ Simple cause and effect logic promotes curiosity about causes of illness and death, but may have significant gaps in understanding, e.g. may believe that cancer is contagious, or cancer is always caused by smoking ◆ May believe that stress causes or maintains illness, and be extremely concerned about 'stressing out' the parent with less-than-perfect behavior, poor school performance, or even talking about worries ◆ Worry about the health of other important adults ◆ Understand that death is final and irreversible, but do not fully appreciate that it is universal ◆ Better understand the physical aspects of death, but may struggle to comprehend the spiritual aspects ◆ May experience guilt about things they did or did not do with or for the deceased	◆ Provide a simple explanation of the diagnosis and treatment of an illness, and clear, accurate information about causes of death ('Mom's cancer had spread to so many places in her body, and there just weren't any medicines that helped anymore') ◆ Dispel misconceptions regarding causes of illness or death, as well as contagion ◆ Maintain predictable routines and expectations ◆ Maintain school as an island of normality ◆ Somatic complaints are common; ask for updates from school about frequency of visits to the nurse ◆ Help put guilt and other concerns in perspective by thinking together about the entire relationship rather than only the recent past

Table 48.1 (continued) Children's conceptualization of parental illness and death

Child's understanding and reactions	Guidance for parents
Adolescents (13–18 years)	
◆ New capacity for abstract reasoning promotes adult-like worries (e.g. about family finances, the well-being of siblings) as well as questions about justice, and the meaning of life and suffering	◆ Provide information about the illness and treatment, and clear, accurate information about causes of death
◆ Egocentrism and emotional immaturity may still cause them to focus on the personal effects of illness or loss in ways that can feel selfish to adults	◆ Remember that adolescents may seek information from other sources, such as the internet, and encourage them to check the accuracy of this information with parents
◆ Understand that death is final, irreversible and universal	◆ Respect adolescent's wish for privacy and control over dissemination of information about an illness or loss, as much as seems reasonable
◆ May feel anxious about their own mortality, e.g. susceptibility to a heritable illness	◆ Encourage conversations and relationships with appropriate non-parental adults
◆ Sensitive about how a loss sets them apart from peers	◆ Do not expect adolescents to assume adult responsibilities
◆ Conflictual relationships with either parent may produce resentment, guilt, or regrets, that complicate adaptation to the illness and grief	◆ Watch for evidence of risk taking behavior or substance abuse in response to the illness or death

a few weeks or to cause significant ongoing impairment. Should a child exhibit difficulty in more than one setting (home, school/daycare, with peers), or for more than several weeks, a conversation with the paediatrician, and perhaps an evaluation with a mental health professional, would be warranted.

Guidelines for talking about a parent's terminal illness and death

Although the approach to talking to children about illness and death must take into consideration the child's developmental level, certain general goals guide most of these conversations. Conversations should balance warmth and openness, with care not to overwhelm a child with more than she needs to know. In timing the conversation, the goal is to prevent the child both from being caught unawares by significant events, and from being made too anxious for too long about events far in the future. Often, a child's questions in response to a 'news bulletin' provide a guide for further discussion.

Family conversations about a parent's chronic illness have different goals at different times, but address a number of common themes. Most families will find they need to share information about the diagnosis, treatment progress and changes in prognosis; to discuss how treatment will affect a child's day-to-day life; to problem-solve around some area of family life that isn't working well; and simply to provide reassurance and an opportunity for children to express their feelings. Some families will also need to discuss a parent's impending death, or address children's worries about a parent's death, even when the parent is medically stable.

When these conversations are handled sensitively, they teach children a number of important lessons. Open communication signals to children that they are a valued part of the family, worthy of being included in age-appropriate decision-making. This feeling of 'family as team', on which each member has an important role to play, may reduce a child's sense of isolation. Parents are encouraged to have conversations that actively inquire about, and validate, children's feelings and reactions to illness, whether positive or negative. Children need to feel confident that their worries will not be taken lightly, and that adults will do their best to help them manage their worries. Finally, allowing children to hold on to hope, even when a death is imminent, may be more helpful than working too hard to help the child see 'the truth.'

Talking about initial diagnosis

Parents frequently express concern about having the first conversation with children in which they confirm a cancer diagnosis. They worry that their children will feel overwhelmed with fear or sadness, and that they will be unable to cope with their children's feelings. This fear can inhibit communication, so it is important to help parents set the stage for these conversations. Children tend to feel most comfortable hearing distressing news when they are in a comfortable place, usually home, where they can react without fear of embarrassment. There is no single 'just right' time to talk, but parents may plan the conversation for a time when there will be time for talking as a group, as well as individually with each child. Ideally, the child will be free after the conversation to make some choice about what to do next—whether calling a friend, engaging in a solo activity or engaging with the parent.

Often parents struggle with whether to simply tell children that they are 'sick' or whether to specify the name of the illness. They fear burdening their children, especially when the child has experienced a cancer-related death. Parents are reassured to learn that, frequently, their own worries are different than their children's. The word 'cancer' may not carry the same frightening connotation for children as for adults.

Children are likely to overhear conversations between parents and doctors, friends and other family. Without direct communication, it is difficult to know what the child has heard but isn't talking about. An atmosphere of openness allows parents to feel more confident that their children will ask questions, rather than keep concerns private.

Parents may find it easiest to begin by recapping any unusual events from the past weeks, explaining the events and checking with children about their understanding and reactions:

> You might remember that I've had a few doctors' appointments in the past couple of weeks, and that sometimes you've gone to a friend's house after school since I haven't been home. The doctors have been trying to understand why I have [whatever symptom may have initiated the process]. They just told me that I have something called [breast, colon, etc.] cancer. I am feeling sad, and wish I didn't have [—], but there are treatments that my doctors expect will [cure, contain] the cancer. I'm going to do everything I can to get better. You will probably have questions and feelings about this and I want us to talk about them together as they come up.

For a younger child, a parent might simply say:

> I am sick with something called cancer. I'm going to be visiting the doctor a lot and taking medicine to get better. Some days, Mrs Smith will bring you to preschool instead of me.

Talking about a change in treatment

To an adolescent or a school age child, the parent can say something such as:

> My doctors told me recently that the medicine I've been taking/treatment I've been getting isn't working to shrink the cancer. It turns out the cancer has spread, or metastasized. I'm upset about that because I had hoped this treatment would really help. But, my doctor has suggested a new kind of medicine that I'm hopeful will work better.

Parents can go on to let the child know when and where the new treatments will occur, and how this will affect the child's routine.

Some children will ask, 'But what if this medicine doesn't work, either?'. Parents may want to be hopeful, while acknowledging the uncertainty:

> Well, that's a possibility, but right now I'm optimistic that this new medicine [or treatment] will help a lot. If it turns out that this doesn't help, I'll work with my doctors to figure out another kind of treatment that might work better. And, I'll let you know how this goes.

They may also want to underscore their confidence in their medical team, so that the child is less likely to feel worried that better care would be found elsewhere.

Talking about the end of active treatment

Learning that active treatment options have been exhausted is extremely painful, and parents may struggle with whether to share this information with their children. With younger children, or very anxious children, as long as the parent is not facing death within a few months, it may be better to wait. But for adolescents and children who ask many questions, a conversation may be helpful. Parents might say:

> You know I have tried quite a few different kinds of treatments for cancer—radiation, several chemotherapy medicines, surgery, more chemotherapy—and none of them worked as well as we hoped. The cancer has continued to spread [or grow]. My doctors just told me that we have run out of treatments that might even slow down the cancer. I will still go see them, but the medicine they will be giving me is just to make sure I am comfortable and not in too much pain.

Or with a younger child:

> You probably remember that I have tried several different kinds of medicine to get better from cancer. None of them has been able to keep the cancer from getting worse. I just found out from my doctors that there aren't any more medicines to even try that could make my cancer better. So now the medicine I take will just be to make sure I don't have too many aches and pains.

Soon after this point, adults may also need to discuss the possibility of a referral to a hospice, home care with hospice or inpatient treatment. It may be helpful to talk with older children about how these different options would look and to elicit their feelings and concerns about the options. For example, some children have great difficulty seeing a parent in a hospital bed at home. A temperamentally inflexible child may be unsettled by the frequent comings and goings of nurses. On the other hand, some anxious children prefer that everyone stay under one roof together and are reassured by frequent check-ins with the ill parent.

Talking about imminent death

Adults often wonder about how to facilitate children's saying good-bye to a dying parent, and at what age such a conversation becomes appropriate. In part, it depends upon what is meant by 'saying good-bye' and the dying parent's ability to be responsive to the child. For a toddler or preschool child, saying good-bye might mean giving the parent a kiss and saying 'night-night' as he has every evening, without awareness that this may be the last time he receives a kiss in return. For a 6–12-year-old child, it might mean telling the parent the best and worst parts of her day, and hearing in return the parent's love and pride in her. For an adolescent, saying good-bye might entail simply saying, 'I love you' to a parent with whom the adolescent had argued frequently.

If children are made aware that a parent is not likely to survive much longer, these kinds of final conversations with the parent become more likely. Parents, in return, can say how much they love the child and also that they forgive the child for any conflict or difficulties in the relationship and recognize that the child loves them in return. Ideally, these conversations will happen gradually, rather than in one afternoon. While there is no definitive time at which to tell a child that a parent will die, parents will want to do so early enough so that talking is not prevented by sudden declines in cognitive function or mental status. However, telling children too far in advance can serve to heighten anxiety, establish an expectation for good behaviour over an impossibly long period of time and be confusing for a child who sees the parent continuing to function reasonably well. Sharing feelings aloud can be encouraged by simply saying that it is important to do so in case things do not go as everyone hopes. It is often unclear how much longer a parent will have the capacity for these conversations, so adults can suggest to children that time with the ill parent is precious and it is important for them to say what needs to be said soon.

Not all children will want to see a parent who is close to death. If caring adults take the time to try to understand and alleviate any concerns the child may have, the child may be amenable to visiting after all. Children express concerns about being in the hospital and feeling frightened of the strange people and equipment there; fear that they will have trouble remembering a parent as healthy if they see the parent looking extremely ill; and fear that they will be embarrassed if they cry in front of other people outside the immediate family. Often, providing very clear descriptions of what the child may see, hear and experience, reminding children that they may leave the parent's room at any time with a designated adult, limiting other visitors while children are there and normalizing a variety of emotional responses, will allow the child to feel well enough prepared.

Talking about death with children

Death is commonly referred to euphemistically. We speak of someone 'passing on' or 'passing away', 'being called to be with God', 'going to Heaven' or 'going to live in the sky', or 'being taken by the angels'. Even when adults disagree about the spiritual meaning of death, we share a common understanding that death is the end of biological life. Children lack this shared understanding and thus rely on clear explanations from adults about what has occurred. Once again, development plays an important role in the child's ability to comprehend and process the news of a parent's death (see Table 48.1 for a summary). Hearing death described solely in spiritual terms may be confusing for children, as it was for a 5-year-old who resolved to become an astronaut so he could visit his father who now 'lives in the sky'.

In addition to a clear description of the death, children may need reassurance that adults are available to care for them and to love them, that much about life will remain constant and that they will not always feel so sad. Their questions may range from the concrete ('What will happen to Mom's clothes and credit cards?') to the philosophical ('Do you think Dad somehow knew it when I got that goal in hockey?').

Talking about the funeral

Adults can prepare children for a funeral by describing what they are likely to see and hear during the rituals, and the kinds of emotions that may be expressed by mourners. For example, the child may see a large wooden box, called a casket or coffin, in the middle of the church. The casket (coffin) holds the dead body. People may be crying during the service because they are sad and miss the person who died.

Family members may disagree about whether younger children should attend a parent's funeral. It may be helpful to provide them with the option of leaving the service early, by identifying in advance an adult to stay with each child. Families may also wish to take the opportunity presented by having many friends and relatives together to request that stories about the deceased be put in writing. These create a legacy of memories of the parent that children may appreciate even more as they get older.

Challenges to communication

The child who 'holds it all in'

Some kinds of children, and children's reactions to illness, frequently elicit greater concern from parents. The child who is not talking much about feelings about the parent's illness is one such child. Parents worry that he or she may be experiencing significant inner turmoil and bearing the burden alone, but feel stymied about what to do. It can first help to ascertain whether the child's reticence about the parent's illness is consistent with his style more generally. When prompted, many parents recognize the unwillingness to talk as the child's long-standing style in response to stressful situations. Understanding this response as stemming in large part from the child's temperament, and not the intensity of the child's suffering or the parent's inadequacy in properly explaining things, can reduce parents' anxiety. Next, the clinician can assess the child's functioning in a variety of arenas—school, friendships, hobbies, sleep, relationships with family members—to better gauge the impact of the parent's illness on the child's day-to-day life. If the child's functioning has remained stable in these areas, parents can be reassured that these are good signs. If not, or if the child's silence is unusual for him, greater concern is warranted.

The child with special needs

Communicating with children with pre-existing mental health issues or developmental delays may pose a particular concern for parents. Transitions and ambiguous situations often pose a challenge for these children. When we consider with parents how to share information with these children, we find that parents are often well aware of communication strategies that have been successful in the past. Parents benefit from reminders about their own expertise in dealing with their child, and assistance in generalizing strategies for communication to a new area. They may think about previous challenges and successes; these may guide decision-making about the current situation, including making use of the people who know the child best.

The child with a difficult temperament

Children who are emotionally intense, less flexible and slow to warm up to new settings and people, may have a more difficult time with adjustments to routines. Parents should utilize strategies that were effective in supporting the child's adaptation to normative changes, such as a new school year. Sometimes parents describe children as 'not wanting to hear anything about the illness'. The parents are willing communicators but the child is far from a willing partner, so parents may feel they shouldn't say anything to the child. While it makes sense to avoid sharing too much detail, almost all children benefit from knowing the basics about the illness, treatment plans and progress made, even when they would prefer to block it out. A 'just the facts, ma'am' style may be best suited for these children. Parents can provide brief, low-emotion news bulletins, focusing on the aspects of the situation that will most impact the child.

Teens heading to college/adolescents with high-stakes tests

Parents worry about sharing bad news with adolescents who are facing normative but stressful challenges, such as high-stakes exams, college applications or choosing a college. They fear that talking about the illness, the child will be knocked off his or her developmental track and perhaps not recover. Many parents express how loathe they are to have their illness interrupt the child's trajectory and, therefore, greatly minimize the gravity of the situation or hide it altogether. The clinician might explore with parents the nature of the challenge the child is facing. Is it a one-time event occurring soon, like a college entrance examination? Is it a one-time decision with long-term consequences, like choosing a college? Or a much longer term challenge, like 'getting through his junior year?'. Often it makes sense to support a parent's wish to hold back certain information until after a big test or a major event, unless doing so would deny the child an opportunity to interact meaningfully with a parent who could die or lose cognitive function imminently. However, withholding information that could affect an adolescent's choices about the future, while well-intentioned, can backfire and lead to the adolescent feeling babied, excluded or duped, once the full story is apparent. Deciding whether to go across the country to one's first choice college or stay close to home to be near an ill parent can be an excruciating decision—but an adolescent can gain maturity from having wrestled with the various aspects of the question.

When parents express concern about the impact of illness on a child for a long period of time ahead ('his whole junior year'), the clinician may remind the parents how difficult it will be to keep things secret, and talk about the potential loss of trust between parents and child. Some parents may also explicitly give the adolescent permission to not concern him or herself with the parent's illness, and some adolescents will be able to focus on their own goals. Those who are not, may benefit from increased support and close monitoring of their functioning over time, such as asking other adults who know the adolescent well to regularly check in with him or her, and having a low threshold for exploring counselling options.

The child with a poor relationship with the sick parent

Disagreements between adolescents and parents about rights and responsibilities are typical, and tend not to disappear even after a parent is diagnosed with a life-threatening illness. Parents may express the wish that their adolescents 'step up to the plate' and assume a number of new responsibilities that parents can no longer manage, while adolescents frequently wish for less, not more, responsibility, as they adjust to the many changes wrought by the parent's illness. The challenges inherent in the parents' specific expectations, and the degree to which the adolescents have already mastered the skills needed to meet these expectations, help predict the degree of frustration and disappointment experienced by both generations. Clinicians can help parents remember that adolescents normally need a great deal of peer interaction and support, and that, under stress, this may be intensified. Just because an adolescent is spending more time with his friends than at home does not mean he does not care about the ill parent, though it may feel so to the adults. In addition, parents can be helped to include the adolescents in decision-making about new expectations, and to consider carefully how they can match what they need with what the adolescent can reasonably manage.

Sometimes parents describe conflict with adolescents as very intense, prolonged or concentrated. For example, one mother described how her husband and 16-year-old son 'really go at' yelling, name calling and stopping just short of becoming physically aggressive. Other families do cross that line and admit to having fights that get physical or, at the other extreme, fights that result in estrangement. Under these circumstances, clear communication becomes more challenging, yet perhaps even more critical. In an ideal world, the family would begin in family therapy treatment to focus on both the content of the disagreements and the way they are played out. In the far-from-ideal circumstances that usually surround serious illness, however, many families are unable to commit the time and resources to pursuing this option. The best the clinician may be able to do is to reframe the divide for the parents, and to help the parents reframe it for the adolescent. Parents may fail to recognize an adolescent's love hiding under anger but, with guidance, may be able to look beyond the acting out and see their child as frightened, mad at the unfairness of the world and struggling to contain his sense of vulnerability. The father who fought frequently with his 16-year-old was able to tell his son before he died that were their time together longer, he was confident that they would have worked out their differences. He also said that he loved his son and believed that his son loved him.

The child with a poor relationship with the well parent

When children have a poor relationship with the well parent, they may experience guilt for feeling that the 'wrong parent' got sick. They may worry about the loss of the parent who best understands them, and find fault in the well parent's care for the ill parent. The situation may be further complicated by the ill parent's lack of full faith in the well parent's ability to raise the children in the way they would wish. In this case, we often encourage the parents to build a support team for the children, ideally made up of people who can provide some of the same qualities as the ill parent, who know the children well and who will be tolerated by the surviving parent. We may also talk with parents about their differing roles in the family and highlight how, over time, these roles can become polarized and somewhat rigid. One father of two sons was able to accept coaching from his wife about how to talk to his older son about ongoing academic difficulties, and to see his son through her eyes, not as lazy, but as struggling.

Hoping for the best versus planning for the worst

Sometimes communication difficulties stem not from anything about the child, but from disagreement between the parents. For example, views about how best to manage living with a serious illness may become polarized. One parent may focus on hoping for the best, while the other may find comfort in planning for the worst. The planner may feel frustrated at not having the partner's input on the many 'what-ifs' and the positive thinker may feel that the focus on 'the negative' will not help their health. The clinician can help by pointing out how each person has taken on one part of the emotional work, and by dividing the labour this way, the couple cannot benefit from their joint expertise. Sometimes balancing the discussion, by suggesting they each think about what they would want the other to know if anything happened suddenly, creates enough of a shift in focus to allow the ill parent to consider the less optimistic possibilities. Another tactic is to ask the couple to switch roles, so the well parent expresses his or her wishes for the spouse and children if he or she were to die first. Afterward, the ill parent can do the same. The clinician can also encourage the well parent to seek others to discuss worries with, and to prioritize their concerns and questions. For example, knowing details about the family's finances may be critical, but discussing funeral arrangements could be postponed. In this way, the ill parent is spared some of the less pressing worries.

Parents may also differ in their willingness to share details about the illness and prognosis with children. Sometimes the parent wishing for less openness has a history of parental illness or loss him or herself. The intense feelings imbued in those memories fuel the insistence on sparing the children from worrying before they have to. Sometimes helping this parent think through what went well and less well during their own childhood experience with a parent's illness will suggest that ignorance about the situation, rather than knowing too much, caused anxiety. It may also help to think about the parent's developmental level at the time of their parent's illness, compared to their child's, and contrast the types of concerns children at each stage are likely to feel. For example, a mother who had lost her own father as an adolescent recalled her sadness at realizing that he wouldn't be able to attend her high school graduation, or college graduation, or wedding. Her children, who were younger, were more concerned with the fact that their father was no longer able to make his special chicken enchiladas or take the boys skiing.

Sometimes, the ill parent doesn't refuse permission to have the illness talked about, but only says positive things him or herself about prognosis. In this case, the well parent may be able to share with the children the idea that the parents differ in how they are dealing with uncertainty, that neither way is right or wrong, but that there are certain parts of the medical story that the children need to at least hear about:

> Mom is putting all her energy into getting better and is not even going to think about the possibility that she won't…but the doctors did let us know that the cancer has spread. She will be taking a new kind of medicine that we hope will slow it down.

The impact of divorce

Divorced or estranged parents frequently present with complicated issues. How much medical information to share, how much financial information to share, how to talk about plans for the children and how to make necessary adjustments to child care arrangements, are common sources of confusion and conflict. Almost always, trust between the parents is fragile at best, thus coordinating conversations about these painful areas requires exquisite sensitivity and frequent reminders of how hard the work is, and how much the clinician admires the couple for attempting to do it.

We suggest to estranged parents that there is information that both parents need to have, in order to sensitively assess how the children are coping, and answer their questions with a reasonable amount of accurate detail. Also, children may have difficulty keeping secret the information they are struggling to process, and instructing them 'don't tell your father about any of this' creates a burden. At the same time, we make clear that we respect each parent's wish for privacy about personal issues, and try to clarify and address whatever fears each one has about having these health-oriented conversations.

Children with divorced parents may worry about access to a deceased parent's extended family. Their grieving can be made more difficult without the active support of adults, who loved the parent, in helping them remember the deceased parent's positive qualities and memorializing him or her. In addition, they may have practical concerns such as where they will live, what school they will go to and how often they will see their friends. As hard as it is to think about potential changes in a child's life, having both parents participate in this planning is usually beneficial to the child. Parents may have an easier time accomplishing this advance planning when reminded that parents without serious illnesses also have to plan for the unexpected. They may talk to children about their concerns by saying, 'Even though I am at the beginning of my treatment and we expect it to work, I wonder if from time to time you have worries about what would happen if I died'.

Challenges for grandparents

Grandparents can be a wonderful, stable source of support for families dealing with parental cancer, but this is not an easy job. If staying temporarily with the family, they need to learn and to adapt to the family's routines, walk the line between being actively supportive and intrusive, and at the same time manage their feelings of anxiety and sadness at their own child's illness. Several sources of concern are frequently described, when grandparents care for grandchildren in these circumstances. First, they are likely to be much less familiar with the children's temperaments and personalities than the parents, and may be less familiar with the normal range of typical behaviour for a given age. Thus they may suggest that their grandchildren are not reacting normally, and raise the parents' anxiety. Grandparents may benefit from information about children's normal reactions to parental cancer, and particularly the idea that a child may 'get' the idea that the parent is really sick, but continue to enjoy playing and activities.

Perhaps because of lingering generational differences, grandparents may be less enthusiastic about open communication with children about parental illness. They may be a significant influence on conversations with a child when a parent is nearing the end of life. Thus, it may be helpful to talk with parents about who else in the family system is influencing their communication with children, and to engage grandparents or other extended family members in a conversation about what they believe children should know and why. During a parent's illness, or after the death of a parent, it is not uncommon for grandparents to try to soften the impact for children by reducing expectations of the child, or 'treating' the child with later bedtimes or extra dessert, for example. While in small doses, this might help everyone feel a little better, these kinds of changes to routines can have a downside in the long run. Children will benefit more from stable routines, which can create a sense of security, as well as from consistent age-appropriate expectations.

Challenges to professionals

Talking with our patients about their children can be emotionally draining. However, enormous gains in rapport and trust can accrue from asking about, and addressing, parenting concerns, precisely because these are such affect-laden issues. Clinicians can start by making the effort to ask parents about their children, to learn a bit about child development and to identify or create some resources for these families.

Case example 1

Mr Lopez was a 43-year-old diagnosed with a recurrence of colon cancer after a 3-year remission, about to begin chemotherapy. He and his wife had two children, Mario (4 years old), and Juliana (8). They had recently told them that, 'Dad isn't feeling well, but is going to the doctor to get medicine so he can get better'. They had avoided using the word 'cancer,' because they did not want to frighten their children. As he began to face the prospect of losing his hair soon, Mr Lopez felt uncertain about how to discuss this.

The parents were asked about recent changes in any of the children's behaviour or mood, and reported a few mild difficulties. Mario was losing his temper over 'nothing'. Juliana had visited the school nurse a few times recently with stomach-aches, and was also more whiny than usual.

It was suggested that, while the Lopez's desire to protect their children was understandable, telling the children more might help them feel more secure. They were probably overhearing conversations among adults, but not benefiting from the opportunity to get questions answered. Both were probably picking up on adults' worry and sadness. They decided to tell the children:

> Dad went to see his doctor, as you know, and recently learned he has colon cancer. Juliana, you might remember that he had this when you were younger, when Mario was a baby. He is working now with a team of doctors who are experts in caring for people who have colon cancer. He will be getting special medicine, called chemotherapy, to shrink the cancer. This medicine might make Dad tired and uncomfortable, but it works really well at fighting cancer. The medicine will also make Dad's hair fall out, but it will grow back in when he stops taking it. Some things at home may be a little different for a while—Juliana will be getting a ride to gymnastics with her friend Katie, and Mrs Smith will care for Mario on Dad's chemo days so Mom can go with him. But lots will stay the same. We're a good team, and we'll figure out together how to manage this.

Then, they would address the children's questions and feelings, first together, and then later individually at times they knew each child would be most likely to talk. Mrs Lopez was worried that she might cry during the conversation. She was reassured to hear that her being tearful would not harm her children if she could explain that this news is sad and a little scary for her, but that she is confident that Dad is getting the best care he can. Suggestions were also made about concerns typical for preschool and school-age children, so the parents could think in advance about how to address these.

Case example 2

Mrs Taylor was a 51-year-old diagnosed with advanced ovarian cancer. She and her husband had been open about her treatment and disease progression with their 13-year-old son, Jonathan, all along. When her oncology team felt that she would likely die shortly, Mr Taylor asked for help in deciding what to tell Jonathan. After talking to the team, he told Jonathan that:

> Mum is very ill and not getting better. Her cancer is in many places in her body. Even though the doctors have done everything they can, she will not be able to live much longer. She will stay in the hospital so the doctors can continue to give her medicine so she is not in pain. We don't know exactly what will happen in the next few days, but probably Mum will sleep more and more as her body stops working. If you would like to say anything special to her, today would be a good time to do it. But, we can continue to visit even when she is mostly sleeping. Would you like to come in to the hospital with me?

Jonathan was sad and worried, but decided that he would like to go to the hospital to be close to both of his parents. He was able to talk with his mother and tell her how much he loved her. However, as the day went on he became more and more distressed. A specialist oncology nurse asked if there were aspects of his mother's care he did not understand, and he focused on the biological side of death. Mrs Taylor had been started on a subcutaneous syringe driver to administer analgesics and anti-emetic drugs. The device administered a set dose of medication over a 24-hour period. Jonathan had misunderstood the information he had been given and believed that his mother would die as soon as the syringe from the driver was empty. He had been sitting with her, frightened to leave her side. The nurse was able to clarify the purpose of the medication and reassure Jonathan that the team was doing everything they could to keep his mother comfortable as possible, for as long as possible.

References

1. Pengelly M (2006). Family matters in acute oncology. *Cancer Nurs* **5**(**3**), 20–23.
2. Moore CW, Rauch PK (2006). Addressing parenting concerns of bone marrow transplant patients: opening (and closing) Pandora's box. *Bone Marrow Transplant* **38**, 775–782.
3. Rauch P, Muriel A (2006). *Raising an Emotionally Healthy Child When a Parent is Sick*. McGraw-Hill, New York.
4. http://www.mghpact.org
5. Welch AS, Wadsworth ME, Compas BE (1996). Adjustment of children and adolescents to parental cancer: Parents' and childrens' perspectives. *Cancer* **77**(**7**), 1409–1418.
6. Siegel K, Karus D, Raveis VH (1996). Adjustment of children facing the death of a parent due to cancer. *J Am Acad Child Adolesc Psychiatry* **35**(**4**), 442–450.
7. Birenbaum LK, Yancey DZ, Phillips DS, *et al.* (1999). School-age children's and adolescents' adjustment when a parent has cancer. *Oncol Nurs Forum* **26**(**10**), 1639–1645.
8. Nelson E, While D (2002). Children's adjustment during the first year of a parent's cancer diagnosis. *J Psychosoc Onc* **20**(**1**), 15–36.
9. Visser A, Huizinga GA, Hoekstra HJ, *et al.* (2005). Emotional and behavioural functioning of children of a parent diagnosed with cancer: a cross-informant perspective. *Psychooncology* **14**, 746–758.
10. Watson M, St. James-Roberts I, Ashley S, *et al.* (2006). Factors associated with emotional and behavioural problems among school age children of breast cancer patients. *Br J Cancer* **94**, 43–50.
11. Leedham B, Meyerowitz BE (1999). Responses to parental cancer: a clinical perspective. *J Clin Psychol Med Settings* **6**(**4**), 441–461.

12. Nelson E, Sloper P, Charlton A, *et al.* (1994). Children who have a parent with cancer: a pilot study. *J Cancer Educ* **9**(1), 30–36.

13. Grant KE, Compas BE (1995). Stress and symptoms of anxiety/depression among adolescents: Searching for mechanisms of risk. *J Consult Clin Psychol* **63**, 1015–1021.

14. Rosenheim E, Reicher R (1985). Informing children about a parent's terminal illness. *J Child Psychol Psychiatry* **26**(6), 995–998.

15. Huizinga GA, Visser A, van der Graaf WT, *et al.* (2005). The quality of communication between parents and adolescent children in the case of parental cancer. *Ann Oncol* **16**, 1956–1961.

16. Barnes J, Kroll L, Burke O, *et al.* (2000). Qualitative interview study of communication between parents and children about maternal breast cancer. *BMJ* **321**, 479–481.

17. Barnes J, Kroll L, Lee J, *et al.* (2002). Factors predicting communication about the diagnosis of maternal breast cancer to children. *J Psychosom Res* **52**, 209–214.

18. Shands ME, Lewis FM, Zahlis EH (2000). Mother and child interactions about the mother's breast cancer: An interview study. *Oncol Nurs Forum* **27**(1), 77–85.

19. Issel LM, Ersek M, Lewis FM (1990). How children cope with mother's breast cancer. *Oncol Nurs Forum* **17**(3, Supplement), 5–12.

20. Kristjanson LJ, Chalmers KI, Woodgate R (2004). Information and support needs of adolescent children of women with breast cancer. *Oncol Nurs Forum* **31**(1), 111–119.

21. Diareme S, Tsiantis J, Romer G, *et al.* (2007). Mental health support for children of parents with somatic illness: A review of the theory and intervention concepts. *Families Systems & Health* **25**(1), 98–118.

22. Rauch PK, Muriel AC (2004). The importance of parenting concerns among patients with cancer. *Crit Rev in Oncol/Hemat* **49**, 37–42.

23. Pettle SA, Britten CM (1995). Talking with children about death and dying. *Child Care Health Dev* **21**(6), 395–404.

Chapter 49

Creative arts in oncology

Marilyn Hundleby, Kate Collie, and Linda E Carlson

Creativity can be such a great comfort. It is uniquely ours, can never be taken away and can be used anywhere. In times of illness, this source of comfort can become a lifeline (1, p.7).

Creative therapies integrate physical, emotional, and spiritual care and enable people with cancer to respond creatively to the challenges they face. Opportunities to engage in creative expression enable people with cancer to mourn, grieve, celebrate life, be empowered to endure their situation, and find meaning in what they are experiencing. They may tap into abilities and talents they never knew they had, and find that their own healing powers are mobilized in this way (2–5).

Creativity can light the pathway to well-being by generating new insights, activating inner strength, and rekindling joy. Particularly in the case of group interventions, isolation can be reduced (6). Feelings of mastery, purpose, and control are generated at a time of devastating loss of control. There is also evidence of physiological benefits (7, 8).

Through the process of creating, people with cancer can learn to transform their feelings, sometimes long hidden, into constructive energy. As stated by one patient in the Cross Cancer Institute *Arts in Medicine* programme:

> When we are engaged in the process of creating, challenging emotions such as anger, fear and sorrow are put into a more realistic and balanced perspective. These feelings become transformed into a healing energy that allows us to move forward with life (1, p.7).

The arts facilitate communication between patients and healthcare personnel by bringing understanding and insight on the part of patients that can then be communicated to the care team, and by making it possible for patients to express things that would be impossible to put into words. The arts give concrete form to feelings that might not be recognized without opportunities for non-verbal creative expression. Words may be inadequate to express the depth and breadth of emotion that comes from hearing the words, 'You have cancer'. However, it may be possible to express the complexity of these emotions with images, sounds, or movements. The arts also have an important role to play when emotions that are easy to recognize are difficult to discuss, or when an emotional topic is hard to face. Difficulties discussing illness and death can be circumvented with the arts when words are not used (9–11).

In recent years, the number of art programmes for people with cancer has increased dramatically in North America. Some of the best known programmes are the *Art for Recovery* programme at the University of California in San Francisco Comprehensive Cancer Center, the *Creative Journey* programme at the Memorial Sloan-Kettering Cancer Center (12), the art programme at the Shands Cancer Hospital at the University of Florida (13, 14), and the *Arts in Medicine* programme at the Cross Cancer Institute in Edmonton, Canada (1).

As interest in the use of creative arts in oncology has increased, so have efforts to assess the benefits. This new area of research is producing promising results. For example, in a simple pre-post questionnaire study that looked at the effects of one session of bed-side art therapy for controlling common cancer symptoms in 50 patients with a variety of types of cancer, the participants reported significantly decreased levels of eight of nine symptoms, including pain, anxiety, and tiredness—in spite of the exertion required for the art therapy session (7). In a study of a bed-side art therapy intervention for family members of cancer patients that used a pre-post single-group design, over a 6-month period the 40 caregivers reported decreased levels of stress and anxiety, and more positive emotions after completing the activities (15). A follow-up study noted similar reductions in anxiety and stress in a larger sample of family caregivers (16). A non-randomized study of 60 patients undergoing chemotherapy for cancer showed that those who had four or more sessions of art therapy, had less depression and fatigue at post-test than those who had fewer than three sessions (17).

A small randomized study of the effects of individual weekly art therapy during radiotherapy sessions for women with non-metastatic breast cancer showed that women who participated in the programme evidenced greater increases in coping resources compared to those in a treatment-as-usual control group (18). Another study of breast cancer patients randomly assigned 30 women to either four sessions of individual art therapy or a wait-list group that received the sessions after the post-assessment (19). Pre- and post-questionnaires showed improvements in anxiety, depression, anger, and confusion compared to the control group. In exit interviews, women reported increased self-awareness and connectedness with their feelings, and increased insight around issues they thought needed attention (time for self-care, reflection, and quiet), and also said they felt less helpless and happier than before.

In a large and rigorously designed study of a *Mindfulness-Based Art Therapy programme*, the participants (93 women with cancer) showed significant decreases in distress and improvements in health-related quality of life over the 8-week programme, compared to a randomly assigned treatment-as-usual group (20).

Other creative modalities have also been investigated. For example, in a randomized study about expressive writing, cancer patients who wrote about their cancer experience reported significantly less sleep disturbance, better sleep quality and sleep duration, and less daytime dysfunction than those who wrote about a neutral experience (21). In a mixed-methods study of an *Authentic Movement* dance programme, the 33 participants (women who had completed treatment for breast cancer) who were randomly assigned to an immediate 6-week group programme showed differential improvement in vigour, fatigue, and somatization compared to a wait-list control group. The women were interviewed and given the opportunity to provide written feedback (22). Most reported positive experiences with the programme, especially with regard to social support, self-awareness, positive feelings about their bodies, and awareness and appreciation of their own strength, sensitivity, and knowledge.

In a qualitative study, 17 women with breast cancer were interviewed about their use of art therapy or art making to address their psychosocial needs (23). A narrative analysis yielded four storylines showing that creative expression was experienced by the women as a safe haven where emotions could be expressed and resolved and insights about cancer could emerge, resulting in increased vitality. Other qualitative studies about the use of the arts in cancer care also illustrate links between expressing emotion, reinforcing identity, gaining new insights, and overall vitality and courage (e.g. 3, 24).

These studies and others like them have identified promising directions for future investigations into the potential benefits of arts-based interventions for people with cancer. More research is needed, especially large, randomized trials of specific approaches that show promise and studies focusing on a range of types of cancer (not just breast cancer). The relationships between creative expression, increased self-awareness, and improved communication with care providers should be explored fully.

The Cross Cancer Institute *Arts in Medicine* programme

The *Arts in Medicine* programme at the Cross Cancer Institute in Edmonton, Alberta, Canada is a well-established creative arts programme in a regional cancer centre (1). The programme brings together psychologists, art therapists, and professional artists to facilitate creative arts classes for cancer patients, their families, and professional staff. The art forms that are used include, but are not limited to: photography, painting, clay sculpture, soapstone carving, fibre arts, journal writing, poetry, collage, dance, drama, and music. The programme is a psychologically-based and planned supportive self-therapy. Participants are provided with creative materials, instruction in the art form being used, thought-provoking meditations, a safe and encouraging environment, and opportunities for recording personal experiences and insights. A professional therapist attends each class to assist participants in drawing out insights and solutions from their creative experiences and those of others in the group, which can then be used to help them cope with the challenges they each face.

Participants are encouraged to enrol in a creative modality that suits them. Those who wish a quiet or contemplative experience may choose to paint icons, create a mandala, or develop highly personal images using coloured pencils. Individuals involved in photography classes work by themselves and then share their photographs and reflections in the weekly sessions. Clay sculpture offers participants a very personal encounter as they dig into the clay and mould something with their bare hands.

Creating art, reflecting upon it, and writing about the experience within a group, permits patients to more fully communicate the depth of emotion they feel. As with any professionally-facilitated psychosocial group, it is important that a safe and supportive environment be maintained by the professional therapist, in which rapport, unconditional positive regard, trust, confidentiality, and safety are assured. Previous experience with the particular art form is not necessary for the participants, as the central focus is on the process of creating rather than the quality of what is created. Initially, many participants will say 'I'm not creative,' or 'I'm not artistic,' and will feel hesitant until they discover that they have creativity that can be nurtured, even if they have no previous artistic skill. Many remarkable art pieces are created, often to the amazement of the person involved. It is the individual's experience (some refer to this as their journey) of creating their art that is most important.

Integrating the arts into psychosocial care is a powerful way to visibly demonstrate personal strengths and accomplishments. Tangible affirmation of this is shown when patients make such comments as 'I created this. I did this!'. This feeling of mastery is conveyed as patients become more assertive and self confident in communicating needs to medical staff, and to family and friends.

Arts in medicine process

Group size, composition, and time

Most groups consist of eight to ten participants who meet together for two hours every week for six weeks. Groups are typically comprised of patients and family members. The majority of participants tend to be female cancer patients. A registered psychologist or social worker co-facilitates each class, with a local artist specializing in the art form being used. Doctoral and practicum students from related faculties often participate in the classes, assisting the group leader and gaining a greater understanding of the emotional aspects of cancer. Time is allotted as follows: a 5- to 10-minute period of meditation begins each class, followed by a hands-on experience. The last 20 minutes are devoted to written reflection, concluded by group discussion of the overall process.

One- or two-day retreat programmes have proven beneficial for individuals who are unable to commit to the regular six-week programme due to work obligations or travel distance to the cancer centre. Classes in soapstone carving and photography have been successful in attracting male participation, and have become popular elements of the curriculum.

Materials

We have found it imperative to provide high-quality art materials. Having beautiful materials, be they brushes, paints, beads, yarns, or art papers, subtly communicates to patients that their time and work is important and valued. Many people have commented on how this gives them an added sense of self-worth. High-quality materials also contribute to the success of what is ultimately created, which can lead to beneficial feelings of mastery.

Meditation

Similar to *Mindfulness-Based Art Therapy*, each creative arts session begins with a meditation. This is important for setting the tone and quieting the mind. It brings about focus and preparation for the process of creating. Initially, attention is given to breathing. Then, over the next few weeks, participants become more attuned to what is commonly known as 'being present' or being 'in the now'. As Kabat-Zinn (25, p.64) states, 'It allows us to cultivate, refine and deepen our capacity to pay attention and to dwell in present-moment awareness'. Within the creative process, patients experience the calm that comes from being in the moment. After experiencing this form of mindfulness, many patients have reported a sense of serenity and calm. They are encouraged to use the same technique at home as a means of breaking away from worry, anxiety, and fear.

Writing

At the conclusion of each class, participants are invited to write about their experience. At first, most participants would prefer to avoid writing; however, over time there is a recognition and appreciation of the importance and therapeutic benefit of self-reflection. Taking 15 minutes in silence to write contemplatively, allows participants to go deeper into their psychological and spiritual experience. Written expression often solidifies personal insights and illustrates how creative work can be a great teacher. Expressive writing may take the form of prose or a stream of consciousness writing. This provides yet another avenue for participants to come to grips with problems and challenges, to see new possibilities, and to adopt a more helpful perspective.

Group discussion

Writing is followed by a group discussion led by a professional therapist, in which participants share their experiences, writing, thoughts, vulnerabilities, and resiliency to the issues they are facing. In the context of group discussion, feelings and coping strategies are shared, as participants learn to navigate the challenges and milestones of treatment and beyond. Rapport develops and participants teach and learn from one another through their stories, analogies, and varied life experiences.

Case report 1

The following example unveils the unexpected, anticipatory grief of a mother who comes face-to-face with her concerns about leaving her young daughter without a mother. The creation of a small soapstone bear (Fig. 49.1.) portrays this mother working through her complex existential issues and multifaceted emotional concerns. Anticipatory and complicated grief reactions, losses of many types, changes to body image, feelings of diminished control, as well as sadness, fear and anxiety are all addressed through her creative expression.

At age 43, diagnosed with inoperable, stage 4, non-small-cell lung cancer, the patient describes her journey during this one-day soapstone carving retreat:

> One desperately needs an outlet—someone, some programme, or some group to talk deeply about what it is you're going through. It took a day to create this bear. We had all the material and support we needed in terms of being gently moved in a direction that might open up more channels of communication about the process of coping with this disease. It was a matter of taking your piece of stone, carving it into not just a bear, but *your* bear. Carving the bear that is inside of you, that represents something very special to you. In essence, the process is about finding out what kind of journey your bear is on.
>
> My chunk of soapstone was very small and it reminded me of a child, so naturally I thought about my five-year-old daughter. The bear turned out to be a little bear, balancing a ball on the top of her nose. The ball represents the world, and the ball for my daughter, is her needing to juggle her new world, which will be a world without me.
>
> It is a very difficult thing, going inside your self. It is one of the first steps in moving from that place of, 'I'm dying, I'm dying' to 'I'm living for today'. I'm carving a bear, and this is what I'm doing today. It is quite a process because it does force you to look under the surface of things. This process took me to a place of immense sadness, it took me to a place of incredible happiness, and it took me to just about the entire spectrum of emotions. This was a defining moment. It's hard, but that's not why you don't do it. Sometimes we think, 'Oh, I can't think about that right now', but at some point you have to think about it, and boy do things become so much easier when you think about it. I'm amazed at how little time is spent on nurturing the person who has the disease. Arts in medicine can be so beneficial in allowing oneself to connect—because I was all over the place.

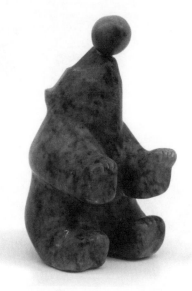

Fig. 49.1 Using the creative arts and humanities.

Case report 2

Following a radical mastectomy, a patient found it extremely difficult to adjust to the changes to her youthful body. Even after re-constructive surgery, she struggled with the addition of her new breast, which she described as 'red and angry'. Arlene began by talking with a psychologist and then writing about the loss of her breast in a letter to her body. Finally, she decided to enrol in a clay sculpting class, which was being offered for 2 hours each week. Here she talks about her experience with clay (see Fig. 49.2):

> My husband never had a problem with my body, regardless of the surgeries. I was the one who had the problem. When I looked in the mirror, I didn't look like the cover girl in the *Sports Illustrated* magazine—even if I had two perfect breasts. I blamed all the ugliness on my breast surgery. I felt so unfeminine. I didn't want my husband to touch my breast. In fact, he hadn't touched my breast in three years! He wasn't allowed. It just didn't make me feel nurtured or sexually awakened in any way. It just didn't.
>
> As I worked with the clay, sculpting a torso, something surprising happened. Initially, I had decided not to put breasts on her, but then I decided I wanted to sculpt breasts. Riding to work one morning on the Rail Transit, I was thinking about my sculpture. The phrase 'just let me bloom' popped into my head. The words came from nowhere, but they became the title of my piece. They also gave me the idea of having a rose come forth from the top of the torso, just like I was blooming in all my glory.

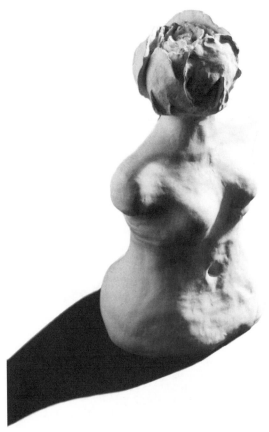

Fig. 49.2 Using the creative arts and humanities—'Just let me bloom'.

I let this piece absorb so much of me, all the emotions that I had stored up for several years. That is why it is so powerful. I still tend to get emotional when I look at her. It was like 'giving it up'—taking the sad, upsetting feelings and working them out into something beautiful. I can now say, 'Wow, this is beautiful and this piece represents me. If this is beautiful, then I'm beautiful!'.

It was after the fifth week of the six-week sculpting programme, when my husband and I were lying in bed and I told him, 'You can touch my breast now'. I had come to the place of acceptance and feeling whole again. Previously, I never thought of the reconstructed breast as *my* breast. It was just a form, an 'add-on'. But as I worked with the clay, shaping it, stroking it—it became me. The whole form, whether or not she looked like me, became me.

Conclusion

The clinical and research evidence of the multi-dimensional benefits of arts-based modalities suggests that care teams in oncology settings could benefit from the implementation of creative arts programmes—to facilitate patients' ability to communicate with their care teams and to process difficult emotions that could interfere with effective communication regarding their cancer treatments.

The provision of opportunities for creative expression can change patients' views of the cancer treatment centre from a place to be feared, to a supportive and enriching environment that patients are less likely to avoid. Collaboration between professional artists in the community and oncology-based therapists is the preferred approach for creative interventions, to maximize participants' exploration and communication throughout their difficult cancer journey. Required investment in space, supplies, and trained personnel for arts programmes in oncology are minimal, compared to the cost of other types of programmes, but have the potential to greatly improve the treatment experience for patients.

Acknowledgements

Dr Linda E Carlson holds the Enbridge Research Chair in Psychosocial Oncology at the University of Calgary, co-funded by the Canadian Cancer Society Alberta/NWT Division and the Alberta Cancer Foundation.

Dr Marilyn J Hundleby and Dr Kate Collie acknowledge the Alberta Cancer Foundation and the Alberta Cancer Board for continued funding of the *Arts in Medicine* programme at the Cross Cancer Institute. We thank Dr Ceinwen Cumming for her assistance with this chapter.

References

1. Hundleby MJ, Abbott S. *Cancer and the Art of Healing.* Edmonton, AB: Alberta Cancer Foundation; 2006.
2. Bailey SS. The arts in spiritual care. *Semin Oncol Nurs* 1997; **13**(4): 242–247.
3. Predeger E. Womanspirit: a journey into healing through art in breast cancer. *Advan Nurs Sci* 1996; **18**(3): 48–58.
4. Malchiodi CA. Using art therapy with medical support groups. In: Malchiodi CA, ed. *Art therapy handbook.* New York, NY: Guilford Press; 2003, pp.351–361.
5. Dreifuss-Kattan E. *Cancer stories: creativity and self-repair.* Hillsdale NJ: Analytic Press; 1990.
6. Gabriel B, Bromberg E, Vandenbovenkamp J, *et al.* Art therapy with adult bone marrow transplant patients in isolation: a pilot study. *Psychooncology* 2001; **10**(2): 114–123.
7. Nainis N, Paice JA, Ratner J, *et al.* Relieving symptoms in cancer: innovative use of art therapy. *J Pain Symptom Manage* 2006; **31**(2): 162–169.

8. Trauger-Querry B, Haghighi KR. Balancing the focus: art and music therapy for pain control and symptom management in hospice care. *Hospice Journal* 1999; **14**(1): 25–38.

9. Luzzatto P. Musing with death in group art therapy with cancer patients. In: Waller D, Sibbett C, eds. *Art therapy and cancer care*. Maidenhead UK: Open University Press; 2005, pp.163–171.

10. Miller B. Art therapy with the elderly and the terminally ill. In: Dalley T, ed. *Art as therapy: an introduction to the use of art as a therapeutic technique*. London, UK: Routledge; 1996, pp.127–139.

11. Wood MJM. Art therapy in palliative care. In: Pratt M, Wood JM, eds. *Art therapy in palliative care: the creative response*. London UK: Routledge; 1998, pp.26–37.

12. Luzzatto P, Gabriel B. The creative journey: a model for short-term group art therapy with posttreatment cancer patients. *Art Therapy: Journal of the American Art Association* 2000; **17**(4): 265–269.

13. Lane MT, Graham-Pole J. Development of an art programme on a bone marrow transplant unit. *Cancer Nurs* 1994; **17**(3): 185–192.

14. Lane MT, Graham-Pole J. The power of creativity in healing: a practice model demonstrating the links between the creative arts and the art of nursing. *NLN Publ* 1994; (14–2611): 203–222.

15. Walsh SM, Martin SC, Schmidt LA. Testing the efficacy of a creative-arts intervention with family caregivers of patients with cancer. *J Nurs Scholarsh* 2004; **36**(3): 214–219.

16. Walsh SM, Radcliffe RS, Castillo LC, *et al*. A pilot study to test the effects of art-making classes for family caregivers of patients with cancer. *Oncol Nurs Forum* 2007 Jan; **34**(1): 38.

17. Bar-Sela G, Atid L, Danos S, *et al*. Art therapy improved depression and influenced fatigue levels in cancer patients on chemotherapy. *Psychooncology* 2007 Nov; **16**(11): 980–984.

18. Oster I, Svensk AC, Magnusson E, *et al*. Art therapy improves coping resources: a randomized, controlled study among women with breast cancer. *Palliat Support Care* 2006; **4**(1): 57–64.

19. Puig A, Lee SM, Goodwin L, *et al*. The efficacy of creative arts therapies to enhance emotional expression, spirituality, and psychological well-being of newly diagnosed Stage I and Stage II breast cancer patients: a preliminary study. *The Arts in Psychotherapy* 2006; **33**: 218–228.

20. Monti DA, Peterson C, Kunkel EJ, *et al*. A randomized, controlled trial of mindfulness-based art therapy (MBAT) for women with cancer. *Psychooncology* 2005 May; **15**(5): 363–373.

21. de Moor C, Sterner J, Hall M, *et al*. A pilot study of the effects of expressive writing on psychological and behavioral adjustment in patients enrolled in a Phase II trial of vaccine therapy for metastatic renal cell carcinoma. *Health Psychol* 2002; **21**(6): 615–619.

22. Dibbell-Hope S. The use of dance/movement therapy in psychological adaptation to breast cancer. *The Arts in Psychotherapy* 2000; **27**(1): 51–68.

23. Collie K, Bottorff JL, Long BC. A narrative view of art therapy and art making by women with breast cancer. *J Health Psychol* 2006; **11**(5): 761–775.

24. Reynolds F, Lim KH. Turning to art as a postive way of living with cancer: a qualitative study of personal motives and contextual influences. *The Journal of Positive Psychology* 2007; **2**(1): 66–75.

25. Kabat-Zinn J. *Coming to ourselves: healing ourselves and the world through mindfulness*. New York, NY: Hyperion; 2005.

Section E

Education and training

Section Editor: Barry D Bultz

A focus on education in communication is the key to changing culture and practice from a strictly biomedical model to 'whole personal care'. Without formalized training, we are left to use old habits that are often based on antiquated assumptions and beliefs. Through formalized training, new objectives and opportunities emerge to empower patients and caregivers to improve healthcare experiences. This section provides an overview of the principles of communication skills training, and outlines the training requirements of all the key players in communication training and the teaching thereof. Guidelines for learner-centred communication, and training for health professionals and patients, are described in detail. We also provide suggestions for training facilitators and simulated patients who play an essential role in shaping healthcare professionals' behaviour to be more effective and compassionate as they practice their craft.

Chapter 50

Learner-centred communication training

Suzanne M Kurtz and Lara J Cooke

Introduction

In the last 20 years, medical education and the broad profession that it serves have taken on communication education and training as an important component of the curriculum. In many countries, substantive communication training has become a requirement for accreditation of undergraduate schools and residency programmes across all specialties. Continuing Education (CE) offerings on communication are widespread. Undergraduate, residency, and CE programmes have developed a variety of approaches for enhancing communication in healthcare. These advances notwithstanding, formal communication training is still a relatively recent development in medical education.

The overarching purpose of this chapter is to explore ways of implementing learner-centred, experiential communication teaching in palliative care and oncology. Drawing parallels between effective physician–patient communication and effective communication teaching, we discuss building on the learner-centred approach as a means for moving toward the emerging paradigm of relationship centred education and care. The chapter offers evidence-based best practices regarding what to teach in clinical communication curricula and how to teach it. In the process, we consider how communication teaching can enhance accuracy and efficiency, as well as the 'culture of compassion' that is so significant to the practice of medicine in palliative care and oncology.

Because how we think about communication has a major impact on how we communicate in medical and educational contexts, this chapter begins by examining assumptions and (mis)perceptions that students, residents, physicians, and medical educators frequently hold about communication. Next, we look at the goals, approaches, paradigms, and first principles that inform decisions about what is worth teaching in communication education and training. Finally, we offer specific strategies and techniques for teaching communication effectively in medicine. We combine these elements into an organizational structure around which to develop more comprehensive, systematic, and coherent communication programmes from undergraduate, through residency, and on to continuing education. This structure is a crucial foundation for experiential learner-centred education.

How we think about communication influences what we do

The process of initiating a communication programme at any level in medical education inevitably prompts certain questions from learners and faculty alike. Three of the most persistent of these questions reflect underlying assumptions that have a major impact on how we teach communication and the degree to which learners will engage in such training.

A: Isn't communication in medicine just an optional add-on in an overcrowded curriculum, a social skill in which learners are already adept? One learner's succinct comment on this is representative: 'Hey, I'm good to go socially—I don't need communication training'. However, an extensive body of research supports an alternative point of view (1, 2). Literature indicates that there are major problems with communication in medicine and that more effective communication improves medical consultations substantively by increasing accuracy and efficiency; enhancing supportiveness, trust, collaboration, and partnership between physician and patient; and reducing conflicts, complaints, and malpractice litigation. Research also shows that more effective communication improves outcomes of care, including understanding and recall, follow-through and adherence to treatment plans, symptom relief, physiological and psychological outcomes, patient satisfaction, and physician satisfaction. More effective communication enhances coordination of care and reduces costs. Communication in medicine is not the same as social skill—it is a crucial component of clinical skill that should be taught as rigorously and intentionally as medical technical knowledge, physical examination, and medical problem solving.

B: Can communication skills really be taught? The literature provides an unequivocally positive response to this question. Several comprehensive reviews outline models of communication training that have resulted in specific, measurable improvements in physicians', residents', and medical students' communication performance (2–4). Communication is not an innate talent; it is a learned skill or, more accurately, a series of learned skills.

C: Is it really necessary to teach communication—won't physicians and other caregivers get it through experience anyway? Unfortunately, when it comes to communication in medicine, experience may be a poor substitute for formal education. While experience is often an excellent reinforcer of habit, it tends not to discern between good and bad habits. Consider, for example, a series of studies showing that without ongoing reinforcement, communication skills may deteriorate from the time students enter medical school to when they begin practice (5–7). On measures of empathy, medical students who have been trained, perform better; however, empathy skills have been shown to decline over time and are measurably lower at the end of medical training than at the beginning (8). Furthermore, it appears that communication skills may be relatively entrenched by the time residents complete their training—that is, more experience probably does not improve communication skills (6, 9). Deficiencies in communication skills have been delineated across the continuum of medical education, including at the level of residency and practicing clinicians. Physicians interrupt their patients' opening statements within the first 30 seconds, on average, despite the fact that 'spontaneous speaking times' for complex medical patients average less than 2 minutes (10–13). Physicians use closed-ended questions in an effort to structure and expedite interviews, but unfortunately this results in as little as 50% of the relevant patient concerns being elicited during some interviews (14, 15). The result is a failure to discuss key patient concerns, perspectives, and agendas during the medical interview. This in turn has a negative impact on both patient and clinician satisfaction with medical interviews (16). Studies measuring the use of patient-centred communication behaviours in primary care senior residents showed that these behaviours (e.g. checking for patient understanding, responding to patients' emotional cues) occur in only 58% of recorded interviews (17). Experience alone is not sufficient; explicit communication training is necessary.

Acknowledging these questions and responding to the underlying assumptions they reflect, puts communication skills teachers in a position to initiate programmes with strong credibility that have an essential element needed to motivate adult learners and even reluctant participants. That element is relevance.

Deciding what is worth teaching

A number of factors affect how we conceptualize communication teaching and make decisions about what is worth teaching in communication education.

Goals of communication teaching

At the most basic level, what we decide to teach depends on the outcomes we are trying to achieve through communication education. We draw our goals directly from research evidence and have applied them to communication programmes at all levels of medical education and in a variety of contexts. At more senior levels, we expect deeper mastery of skills and more mature development of attitudes and capacities (compassion, integrity, mindfulness, etc.). Contexts and problems become more complex as learners advance, but the goals of training remain constant. Regardless of whether the learners are medical students, residents, or practicing physicians or surgeons with years of experience, the outcomes we are aiming for invariably include (2):

* promoting relationships of collaboration and partnership;
* increasing:

    accuracy

    efficiency

    supportiveness
* enhancing patient and physician satisfaction and
* improving health outcomes.

The ultimate goal of ensuring that we improve every physicians' communication skills in practice to a professional level of competence dictates that communication curricula focus not only on what learners understand cognitively (knowledge) but also on their communication skills and behaviours (competence), what they choose to do in practice (performance), and what happens to patients as a result (outcomes) (18).

While the above goals fit all learners, different educational levels do lend themselves to different emphases. Medical students spend less time on explanation and planning than on history-taking, presumably due to the paucity of their medical expertise and their lack of confidence regarding information giving (19). In contrast, residents' responsibilities give them the opportunity to reinforce effective information-gathering skills and to add an emphasis on explanation and planning skills. Despite this shift, residents often receive little training in the communication skills related to explanation and planning (19). If this gap is not addressed during residency or medical school, difficulties with explanation and planning are likely to persist into medical practice and in many cases go unchecked (6, 17). Underscoring this gap, one study demonstrated that 70% of malpractice cases include four problems related to explanation and planning: deserting the patient, failure to understand the patient's perspective, devaluing the patient's views, and delivering information poorly (20). We suggest that residency training is the time and place to add a focus, not only on explanation and planning but also on communication between colleagues or with other members of the healthcare team.

In oncology and palliative care — where long-term care, high stakes, and a bewildering array of serious issues are the norm — there can be no doubt that it is important to develop communication skills. The relationship between the physician, healthcare team, patient, and patient's significant others will determine, to a large extent, the degree to which patients comprehend and adhere to complex medical treatment regimes. The effectiveness of oncologists' and palliative care specialists' communication will also impact the extent of emotional suffering, anxiety, and uncertainty experienced by patients with cancer or those at the end of life.

Given what we know about the importance of communication in healthcare generally, and in oncology and palliative care in particular, we need to make communication professionals out of everyone who goes into clinical practice. We can achieve this goal, but only if we extend communication education from the early years of medical school, through clerkship, into residency and beyond.

Skills vs. attitudes and capacities vs. issues

The debate is ongoing about how best to bridge the gap between doctors' communication behaviours during consultations and the behaviours that research has shown to make a positive difference in the outcomes of care for each of the players. Three primary views on how to structure communication training and education have emerged from the debate:

(1) The skills perspective structures learning around three types of communication skills: what doctors say (content skills), how they say it (process skills), and what they are thinking and feeling (perceptual skills). These skill sets are interdependent; a weakness in any of them results in a weakness in all. Skills-based programmes give primary attention to the development of process skills, since they are the least emphasized in most medical curricula, and secondary attention to content and perceptual skills, since they are the focus of other parts of the medical curriculum.

(2) The attitude perspective focuses teaching on preparation of the inner ground; that is, on enhancing attitudes, capacities, intentions, assumptions, and psychological factors that influence how doctors communicate. Here the rationale is that these underlying factors block effective communication and attending to these factors will improve communication.

(3) The issues perspective suggests that we structure learning around specific communication issues, such as delivering bad news, death and dying, obtaining informed consent, communicating treatment risks and benefits, and reducing error, as well as issues related to gender or culture and to communication with children, geriatric patients, neurologically compromised patient, etc.

Without preparation and development of the 'inner ground' of intentions and capacities, the masterful use of skills becomes manipulation. On the other hand, the best of intentions and the most well-developed capacities are essentially useless if we do not have well-developed skills to demonstrate or apply them in practice. The dilemma in using issues as the primary focus is inefficiency. This perspective can promote the mistaken notion that each issue requires a different set of skills, when in fact the same communication process skills are useful in responding to each of these issues. The context changes from issue to issue, the content of the communication changes, the skills may need to be applied with greater intentionality, intensity or mastery, but the skills themselves remain the same.

The historical perspective: the shot put vs. the frisbee approach

Another take on what to teach comes from a brief look at the long history of communication training in academe. From this vantage point, what we end up teaching in communication programmes (and how we teach it) boils down to two basic perspectives that Alton Barbour (21) has metaphorically dubbed the 'shot put approach' and the 'frisbee approach'. The first was in vogue literally from the time of the ancient Greeks to the middle of the twentieth century. It defined communication as the well-conceived, well-delivered message. Effective communication consisted of content, delivery, and persuasion. As when throwing a shot put, all the speaker had to do was put together a message, deliver it, and his job was done.

In the 1940s the focus began to shift toward interpersonal communication and the frisbee approach. As Barbour suggests, two new concepts are central to this approach; both are significant to medicine and especially relevant to palliative care and oncology. The first concept is confirmation, which RD Laing (22) defined as recognizing, acknowledging, and endorsing the other person. The second concept is mutually understood common ground. This common ground, of which both parties in the interaction are aware, is a necessary foundation for trust, which is in turn the basis for authentic relationships. Decades ago, SJ Baker (23) called this idea 'reciprocal identification' and pointed out that people reach mutual understanding of common ground primarily by talking with each other about it. His model offers an excellent remedy for moments of discomfort, defensiveness, or conflict: simply (re)establish some sort of mutually understood common ground. Establishing mutually understood common ground does not mean that people agree but that they understand each other. In medicine, this can be as straightforward as a mutual understanding of the reasons for the patient's visit or of the next steps physician and patient will take. In the frisbee approach the message is still important, but the emphasis shifts to interaction, feedback, and relationship.

Shifting paradigms in medical (and educational) practice

Shifts in the predominant paradigms for conceptualizing healthcare (including physician–patient interaction) and those that help us conceptualize education (including teacher–student interaction) have followed a similar pattern. In education, a shift has occurred from teacher-centred education, wherein teachers held control and told essentially passive students what to think and do, to learner-centred education. The latter places emphasis on the learner's perspectives and learners take a much more active, participatory role: learners assist in setting their own objectives and experiential activities, which demand high levels of learner participation. Both teachers' and learners' agendas and contributions are important.

Similarly in healthcare, we have moved from doctor-centred care, wherein the physician held most of the control hierarchically and told essentially passive patients what to do, to patient-centred care (24). The latter has required that doctors understand their patients, as well as their patients' disease. Patient-centred care placed new emphasis on eliciting and responding to the patient's perspective regarding the patient's thoughts, beliefs, feelings, and expectations, as well as the effects of illness on their lives. Building on patient-centred care, a third paradigm shift is in progress. Called relationship-centred care (25), it sees relationship as central to all healthcare and healing, including the clinician's relationship with patients, self, colleagues, and communities.

Principles of effective communication and teaching

The 'first principles' of communication provide another way to frame the content of communication curricula. Not surprisingly, the 'first principles' of effective communication are identical to the first principles that characterize effective teaching.

Effective communication and teaching:

+ Ensure interaction, not just transmission of a message.
+ Reduce unnecessary uncertainty, e.g. about roles and responsibilities, a patient's prognosis, the patient's expectations for the visit, etc.
+ Require planning and thinking in terms of outcomes. Effectiveness can only be determined in the context of the outcomes you and the other(s) are working toward.
+ Demonstrate dynamism by engaging authentically with the other and also remaining flexible, developing a deep enough repertoire of skills to allow different approaches with different people or contexts.
+ Follow a helical rather than a linear model. Once and done is never enough. Effective communication, like effective teaching and learning, requires reiteration, coming back around the helix at a little higher level, taking feedback to your communication (or efforts at teaching or learning) into account at each turn. The helix serves as an excellent model for curriculum development.

Special considerations regarding communication issues in oncology

A recent survey of 394 oncology patients (26) sought to determine the information needs and experiences of cancer patients in the United Kingdom. The vast majority of patients wished for complete disclosure of information in the cancer setting. In addition, while most patients indicated that they received adequate information about their diagnosis, initial tests, and prognosis, fewer patients reported having discussions about clinical trials and psychosocial issues. In a field where delivering bad news is an essential skill, and in some cases, where clinical trials may represent the only hope for medical treatment, it is essential that addressing these shortfalls be a part of any new communication curriculum.

Another recent study investigated oncologists' communication patterns in relation to patient characteristics. Siminoff *et al.* (27) showed that physicians' communication style was more likely to be oriented towards establishing rapport and relationship building when interacting with patients who were younger, white, affluent, and had more education. Similarly, patients who were younger, had higher educational levels, and were more affluent, were more likely to engage in relationship-building conversation with their oncologists and were more likely to ask questions. While it is doubtful that these findings are unique to the area of cancer care, this study underscores the need to build in activities that attune residents and practicing clinicians to the possibility of differences in the quality of communication between oncologists and patients with varying demographics.

Choosing effective strategies for teaching communication in medicine

The comprehensive reviews of communication education referred to earlier in this chapter (2–4) identify experiential, learner-centred education as a best-practices approach to teaching and learning communication in medicine. This approach is the most efficacious way to teach communication, if what you are looking for is engaged learners who effectively enhance or change their behaviour, deepen their understanding, are able to apply both skills and understandings in real interactions with patients or others, and sustain their learning over time (2—see especially pp.63–72).

Learner-centred, experiential education

Experiential, learner-centred education follows the premise that learning is at its best when the following criteria are met:

- the learner sees the relevance of the content;
- the content is presented in a goal or task-oriented light;
- there is opportunity for considerable autonomy and self-direction on the part of the learner; and
- the individual learner's prior knowledge and level of experience are recognized and acknowledged as legitimate (28).

As is the case in patient- and relationship-centred care, learners are active and interactive participants in their own learning process and in that of their peers. Couple this with problem or inquiry-based learning, in which learners have the opportunity to apply theoretical understanding to real-life situations and problems, and you have participatory, learner-centred, experiential education. The agendas of both learner and facilitator are important. The facilitator has considerable responsibility in structuring the learning sessions and guiding learners to stretch their comfort zones, experiment, and move beyond what they already know how to do. Learners have the responsibility to prepare for, and participate in, experiences and discussions. Feedback in this kind of learning is interactive: a conversation between all the participants rather than a lecture.

What it takes to enhance communication skills and change behaviour

Research indicates that knowledge about communication skills and capacities, and about their relative importance in caring for patients is very useful, but generally not sufficient to change behaviour effectively. Several other elements emerge from the research that are essential if we want to enhance communication skills, change behaviour in practice, and sustain that learning over time (2):

♦ systematic delineation and definition of skills;

♦ observation of learners communicating with simulated and actual patients;

♦ video (or at least audio) recording of the interaction for later review;

♦ well-intentioned and detailed descriptive feedback;

♦ repeated practice and rehearsal of skills in a safe setting;

♦ active small group or one-to-one formats for learning.

Given this list of essentials, and the responsibilities and time pressures in clinical practice, it becomes clear that some dedicated time for communication training away from clinic or ward is essential. Fallowfield *et al.* (29) provide one example of a dedicated programme that incorporates many of the essential elements. The authors conducted a controlled, randomized trial of an intensive, 3-day, experiential communication workshop for 160 oncologists in the United Kingdom. Participants in the programme were directly observed, video-taped, and received feedback on their consultative skills. Participants showed between 30 and 50% improvement in specific, measurable communication skills, such as use of open-ended questions, summarizing, and use of empathetic statements. Not only did the authors demonstrate that their programme was efficacious, in a 1-year follow-up study, they were able to demonstrate that the effects were also enduring (30).

Identifying the communication skills to teach and learn

A quick reread of the bulleted list above reveals that all of the essential elements depend for implementation on our ability to delineate and define the skills. Numerous models have been developed to identify the skills that are the focus of many communication programmes. For example, the Maastricht's Maas Global (The Netherlands), the Segue Model (USA), Patient-Centered Care (Canada), the Model of the Macy Initiative in Health Communication (USA), and the Calgary–Cambridge Guides (Canada and England). Most effective programmes are based upon models such as these.

Skills models and the feedback instruments through which they are presented constitute a particularly important part of the organizational structure. They summarize the communication skills curriculum and allow us to deconstruct communication. Used as guides to structure observation and feedback, the instruments help us identify individual learner's specific strengths and weaknesses and enable more systematic, concrete learning. As Faldon *et al.* (31) indicate, comprehensive models overcome two problems: over-confident learners are introduced formally to unique aspects of medical interviewing; and learners who lack confidence are offered a lifeline.

So, what specific communication skills are worth teaching? As an example, we will examine more closely our own highly evidence-based Calgary–Cambridge Guides (C–C Guides) (1, 2, 32). As is true of most instruments, the C–C Guides have gone through numerous iterations (in this case over the last 30 years) that drew on the work of medical colleagues in Australia, Canada, England, the Netherlands, the United States, and elsewhere. Riccardi and Kurtz (33) published an earlier version. Many students, faculty, and patients have added their feedback and suggestions. The C–C Guides have enjoyed widespread international recognition and have, to our surprise, been translated into numerous languages. The guides and the Calgary–Cambridge approach to teaching communication apply equally well to a variety of disciplines and levels. Communication programmes in nursing and allied health professions, teacher education, and veterinary medicine are employing the guides with minor modification. In fact, we use the exact same guides with learners at every level of medical education because there are no 'basic' or 'advanced' skills. There are only varying degrees of mastery and sophistication in applying the skills, and varying expectations for how far learners at different levels will take a given case.

The C–C Guides form the backbone of the curriculum. The 71 items on the process guides provide a useable summary of the research literature on what makes a difference in doctor–patient communication. To make this comprehensive list more manageable and memorable, the skills are organized around the framework in Fig. 50.1, plus subheadings in each section that represent the aims clinicians need to accomplish within each task. This framework corresponds directly to the tasks that are undertaken in any consultation: initiating the session, gathering information (including communication skills associated with physical examination), providing structure, building relationship, explanation and planning, and closing the session. With the exception of

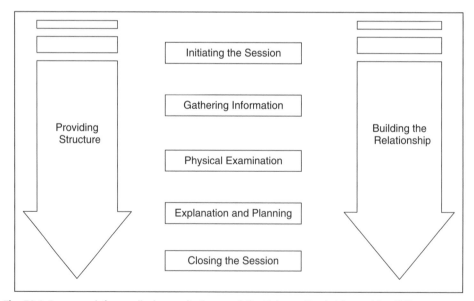

Fig. 50.1 Framework for medical consultations and the Calgary–Cambridge guides (32).

Kurtz S, Silverman J, Benson J, & Draper J (2003). Marrying Content and Process in Clinical Method Teaching: Enhancing the Calgary-Cambridge Guides. *Academic Medicine*. Vol 78, No 8/August, 802-809.

relationship building and providing structure, which occur throughout the consultation, all the tasks occur more or less sequentially in any given interaction. In essence, the guides comprise a four-page summary of the content of the communication programme.

Although only a few pages in length, the Guides have several advantages. They delineate and define the skills that make up effective doctor–patient communication, offering guidance with considerable flexibility for personal style and varied contexts. They provide an accessible summary of the evidence regarding doctor–patient communication and present a common language for labelling and referring to specific behaviours. The Guides make transparent the skills-content of the course; since the same instrument is used for both feedback during learning sessions and summative assessment, the Guides also help to make evaluation transparent. They provide a basis for consistent teaching and feedback, and form a common foundation for communication programmes at all levels of medical education.

Putting the other essential elements into play

As other chapters in this book demonstrate, consultations that provide the experiential basis for communication training can include interactions with various 'patients'. Simulated patients are trained to portray specific situations (ideally based on real cases) that course organizers select or that learners bring to the table, based on situations they have encountered. Learners role-play situations they have experienced. Volunteer patients replay their real medical problems. Actual patients participate through their ongoing care. Learners can work with live consultations or use video-tapes of consultations. Video-taping is an invaluable part of the programme that offers learners a check and balance for their own perception and self-assessment, a feedback and teaching tool for the group, and a way to focus on specific points of strength or weakness.

Pairs or small groups of learners guided by an expert facilitator or coach, work especially well because they offer the opportunity for individual practice, as well as the benefits of gaining feedback from the perspective of others. With trained, simulated patients (or in some cases with volunteers and during video review) where the facilitator or a fellow learner takes on the role of the patient in the interview, learners can 'rewind' parts of the interview to give the original interviewer a chance to try an alternate communication approach or to see how a colleague would handle the situation. Small groups that meet regularly are best able to develop a place of trust that enables the experimentation and mistake-making that are hallmarks of experiential learning. One-to-one formats are also useful, but these have the disadvantage of potential power struggles and fewer points of view.

Agenda-Lead Outcome-Based Analysis (ALOBA): a protocol for feedback and facilitation

Teaching and learning communication skills are substantively different from other clinical skills. Communication is more complex than simpler procedural skills; so many more variables influence it. Although it is not a personality trait, communication is closely bound to self-concept. To put it another way, no one is invested in how they palpate a liver before they learn how to do it, but we are often heavily invested in our communication skills and the connection we perceive those skills to have with our personal style. Unlike procedural skills, which have an achievement ceiling, you can always improve on communication skills. Even if you are exemplary one day, the next a variety of distractions—or the variety of people you get to communicate with—can make you feel awkward and inept.

The idea of communication training is to enhance what learners already do well, expand each learner's repertoire of skills, work with applying comfortable skills in more complex circumstances, and break habits that serve neither clinician nor patient well. While focusing on communication process skills, and the content and perceptual skills that interact with them, learners and facilitators also need to keep the ongoing development of right capacities and attitudes in mind. Perfecting skills without developing the inner ground of capacities, such as respect, integrity, and compassion, amounts to manipulation. Capacities are relatively useless without refinement of the skills that are needed to demonstrate those capacities.

Agenda-Lead Outcome-Based Analysis (ALOBA) is a protocol developed for giving feedback and facilitating experiential, learner-centred, problem-based sessions (2); it maximizes participation and learning of the entire group, reduces defensiveness, and enhances learning. ALOBA begins by greeting the group and, in the initial meeting, getting to know each other briefly and agreeing on rules of conduct (confidentiality, participation, attendance, experimentation, etc.). Next the facilitator prepares the group to observe an interaction that will be the basis for individual feedback, as well as a gift of 'raw' material for the entire group's learning. Before the interaction begins, the facilitator asks for the agenda of the learner who is about to interact with a patient, engage in a simulation, or share a video. For example, the facilitator might ask: 'What do you want us to watch for?', 'What do you want feedback on?'. The group then observes the interaction and makes concrete and specific notes on the interaction using the C–C Guides. The learner or the coach may call 'time-outs' during the interaction to get ideas if problems arise or try something over, but time-outs are generally kept to a minimum. Once the observation is complete, the facilitator, in true learner-centred fashion, again requests information about the learner's perspectives and insights before allowing others to weigh in with their ideas on the interaction: 'How do you think that went?', 'What are your feelings about the interaction?', 'Anything else you'd like us to look at now regarding the interaction?'.

Spotting skills and discussing feedback is the next step. After the group and the patient (if present) respond to the learner's agenda, others may point out things the learner may not have thought to ask about. By offering well-intentioned, descriptive feedback that is as concrete and specific as possible, the group is essentially holding up a mirror to reflect what they saw or heard. The facilitator and all group members are responsible for ensuring that the feedback is balanced between reinforcing what worked and discussing problem areas and next steps to make the interaction even better. The group offers alternative approaches and participates in 'rewinds' to try them out.

The outcome-based part of ALOBA comes into play when trying to determine what communication skills and approaches would be most effective. Instead of trying to evaluate what is good or bad or attempting to reach consensus about the 'best' approach, ALOBA urges consideration of the outcomes the learner was trying to accomplish at a given moment as well as the outcomes the patient was trying to work on. The facilitator or a group member might ask: 'What were you trying to accomplish just then?', 'And what was the patient needing or working on?', 'Was what you were doing getting at both sets of outcomes?', 'What else would be an effective way to work toward those outcomes?'. With communication skills, effectiveness can only be determined in the context of the outcomes sought by the various players in an interaction.

Figure 50.2 offers a graphic representation that facilitators have found useful as a quick reference guide for how to run a session using the ALOBA approach (2). The protocol is not cast in stone; it is intended as a flexible guide, a framework that facilitators can adapt to their learning groups' changing needs and purpose. Note how closely the ALOBA protocol resembles the tasks on the C–C Guides (Fig. 50.1). Not surprisingly, the skills required to effectively facilitate a session using ALOBA are the same as those listed in the C–C Guides, but are here applied to the learner group.

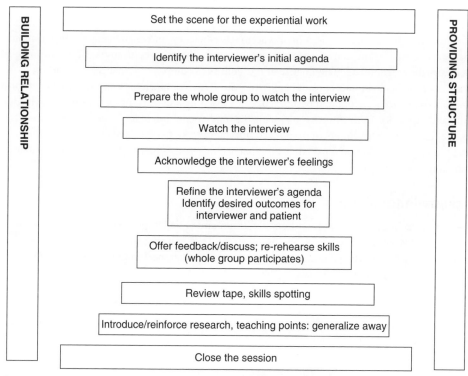

Fig. 50.2 How agenda-led outcome-based analysis works in practice (p.133, 2).

*From: Kurtz SM, Silverman JD, Draper J (2005) *Teaching and Learning Communication Skills in Medicine, 2nd Ed.* Radcliffe Publishing: Oxford (UK) & San Francisco. 133.

Modelling and the informal curriculum

In communication training and education, as in the teaching of other clinical skills, there is most definitely a place for the traditional apprenticeship strategy of modelling on the part of more experienced practitioners. Modelling can have a profound effect on attitudes, as well as communication skills. It can influence behaviour in extremely valuable ways and sometimes, inadvertently, in adverse ways. Obviously clinicians model communication skills and attitudes whenever they interact with a patient. They may be less aware of what they are inadvertently modelling as they interact with colleagues or other staff and of what learners pick up from how experienced clinicians treat the learners themselves. The point here is that those of us whom learners observe or who interact with learners, either as teachers or as role models, need to become more aware of what we are contributing to this informal, hidden curriculum (34).

Optimal learning occurs when the formal curriculum, consisting of experiential learning opportunities, structured around a strong organizational framework, and a model that delineates communication skills, combines forces with informal curricular interventions during daily practice that are associated with modelling to advantage. Such interventions include cueing, observation, guided reflection, explicit commentary, and questions regarding what we are modelling—the very same interventions that we bring to bear when teaching other clinical skills.

Summary

Quality communication training enhances accuracy, efficiency, and relationships—three elements that are essential to the delivery of quality healthcare. Effective communication training also facilitates the creation and maintenance of the 'culture of compassion' that is so important to the practice of medicine in oncology and palliative care. To accomplish these ends, we have set forth evidence-based foundations and best practices for teaching and learning clinical communication skills and capacities. In addition to enhancing the implementation of individual programmes, this chapter calls for the development of more comprehensive, systematic, and coherent communication training in oncology and palliative care that extends from undergraduate, through residency, and on to continuing education.

Acknowledgements

We wish to acknowledge Drs Jonathan Silverman and Julie Draper, who are co-authors with Dr Kurtz of two companion books that discuss in greater detail many of the concepts, approaches, and research findings offered here. Listed as the first two references in this chapter, the books are a primary source for these materials.

References

1. Silverman J, Kurtz S, Draper J (2005) *Skills for Communicating with Patients*, 2nd Edition. Oxford and San Francisco: Radcliffe Publishing.

2. Kurtz S, Silverman J, Draper J (2005) *Teaching and Learning Communication Skills in Medicine*, 2nd Edition. Oxford and San Francisco: Radcliffe Publishing.

3. Fallowfield L, Jenkins V. Current concepts of communication skills training in oncology. *Recent Results Cancer Res* 2006; **168**: 105–112.

4. Aspergren K (1999) Teaching and learning communication skills in medicine: a review with quality grading of articles. *Med Teacher* **21** (6): 563–70.

5. Maguire P, Fairbairn S, Fletcher C (1986a) Consultation skills of young doctors: 1—benefits of feedback training in interviewing as students persists. *BMJ* **292**: 1573–76.

6. Maguire P, Fairbairn S, Fletcher C (1986b) Consultation skills of young doctor: II—most young doctors are bad at giving information. *BMJ* **292**: 1576–8.

7. Helfer RE (1970) An objective comparison of the pediatric interviewing skills of freshman and senior medical students. *Pediatrics* **45**: 623–7.

8. Poole AD, Sanson Fisher RW (1979) Understanding the patient: a neglected aspect of medical education. *Soc Sci Med* **13A**: 37–43

9. Ridsdale L, Morgan M, Morris R (1992) Doctors' interviewing technique and its response to different booking time. *Family Pract* **9**: 57–60.

10. Dysch L, Swiderski D (2005) The effect of physician solicitation approaches on ability to identify patient concerns. *J Gen Intern Med* **10**: 267–270.

11. Langewitz W, Denz M, Keller A, *et al.* (2002) Spontaneous talking time at start of consultation in outpatient clinic: cohort study. *BMJ* **325** (7366): 682–3.

12. Marvel MK, Epstein RM, Flowers K, *et al.* (1999) Soliciting the patient's agenda: have we improved? *JAMA* **281** (3): 283–7.

13. Beckman HB, Frankel RM (1984) The effect of physician behaviour on the collection of data. *Ann Intern Med* **101**: 692–6.

14. Roter DL, Hall JA (1987) Physicians' interview styles and medical information obtained from patients. *J Gen Int Med* **2** (5): 325–349.

15. Stewart MA, McWhinney IR, Buck CW (1979) The doctor patient relationship and its effect upon outcome. *J R Coll Gen Pract* **29**: 77–82.

16. Roter DL, Stewart M, Punam M, *et al.* (1997) Communication patterns in primary care physicians. *JAMA* **277** (4): 350–6.

17. Campion P, Foulkes J, Neighbour R, *et al.* (2002) Patient centredness in the MRCGP video examination: analysis of large cohort. *BMJ* **325** (7366): 691–2.

18. Miller GE (1990) Commentary on clinical skills assessment: a specific review. National Board of Medical Examiners' 75th Anniversary. *Philadelphia*: 48–51.

19. Kauffman DM, Laidlaw TA, Macleod H (2000) Communication skills in medical school: Exposure, confidence, and performance. *Acad Med* **75** (Suppl 10): S90–S92.

20. Beckman HB, Markakis KM, Suchman AL, *et al.* (1994) The doctor-patient relationship and malpractice. *Arch Int Med* **154**: 1365–70.

21. Barbour A. Making contact or making sense: functional and dysfunctional ways of relating. Paper presented for Humanities Institute Lecture 1999–2000 Series, University of Denver, 2000.

22. Laing R (1961) *The Self and Others*. Pantheon Books, New York.

23. Baker SJ (1955) The theory of silences. *J. Gen Psychology* **53**: 145.

24. Stewart MA, Brown JB, Weston WW, *et al.* (2003) *Patient-Centred Medicine: Transforming the Clinical Method*, 2nd Edition. Radcliffe Medical Press, Oxford.

25. Beach MC, Inui T and the Relationship-Centereed Care Research Network (2006) Relationship-centred care: a constructive reframing, *J Gen Intern Med* **21**: S3–8.

26. Cox A, Jenkins V, Catt S, *et al.* (2006) Information needs and experiences: an audit of UK cancer patients. *Eur J Onc Nurs* **10**: 263–272.

27. Siminoff LA, Graham GC, Gordon NH. (2006) Cancer communication patterns and the influence of patient characteristics: Disparities in information-giving and affective behaviours. *Patient Education and Counseling* **62**: 355–360.

28. Knowles MS (1984) *The Adult Learner—A Neglected Species*. Gulf, Houston, Tex.

29. Fallowfield L, Jenkins V, Farewell V, *et al.* (2002) Efficacy of a Cancer Research UK communication skills training model for oncologists: a randomized controlled trial. *Lancet* **359**(9307): 650–656.

30. Fallowfield L, Jenkins V, Farewell V, *et al.* (2003) Enduring impact of communication skills training: results of a 12-month follow-up. *Br. J Cancer* **89**: 1445–1449.

31. Faldon J, Pessach I, Toker A (2004) Teaching medical students what they think they already know. *Ed for Health* **17** (1): 35–41.

32. Kurtz S, Silverman J, Benson J, *et al.* (2003) Marrying Content and Process in Clinical Method Teaching: Enhancing the Calgary–Cambridge Guides. *Acad Med* **78** (8): 802–9.

33. Riccardi VM, Kurtz SM (1983) *Communication and Counseling in Healthcare*. Charles C. Thomas: Springfield, IL.

34. Suchman AL and Williamson PR (2003) personal communication.

Chapter 51

Facilitating skills practice in communication role-play sessions: essential elements and training facilitators

Carma L Bylund, Richard Brown, Barbara Lubrano di Ciccone, and Lyuba Konopasek

Rationale for role-play

Experiential role-play work is the most essential component of a communication skills training program (1). In facilitator-led role-play sessions, learners act out simulations of consultations, frequently using an actor taking the role of the patient. In such sessions, learners are able to attempt the use of new skills within the safe environment of a confidential and constructive practice session. Without such practice and feedback on communication skills, a learner's sustained behaviour change in clinical settings is improbable (1, 2).

The success of communication skills training programmes is dependent on adept facilitation, wherein skilled facilitators engage learners and conduct role-play sessions in a learner-centred fashion. In order to ensure a high standard of instruction, facilitators must be trained to lead these sessions.

In this chapter, we begin by describing common variations on role-play sessions. Then, we delineate the important elements of facilitating skills practice in a role-play session. Third, we outline processes that are helpful in conducting train-the-trainer programmes and in sustaining a core of competent facilitators. Finally, we end by identifying areas for future research and development in facilitation.

Role-play variations

The principles discussed in this chapter are applicable to different types of communication training situations. Two important variations of role-play are the size of the group and who plays the role of the patient (trainee or actor). Whatever form the role-play session takes, the skills practiced remain very similar and few changes in teaching strategy are required.

Small group vs. fishbowl role-play sessions

The term 'small-group role-play' will be used to describe 2–3 learners working with a facilitator and a simulated patient. The term 'large-group role-play' or 'fishbowl' describes training with a role-play demonstrated in front of an entire training group, often in a larger room. Both small group and fishbowl role-plays are examples of experiential learning.

Small-group sessions are usually preferable for skills acquisition as they allow each learner dedicated time in the role of physician. However, small-group sessions require more facilitators and actors, and may not be feasible for programmes with fewer resources. In some cases the logistics of the training module may also make small-group sessions unrealistic. For example, a communication skills module on conducting a family meeting (3) would involve a group of simulated patients to play the roles of a family; it is unlikely most communication skills training programmes have the resources and space to support several small-group sessions of this nature.

Rather than practicing skills, fishbowls are particularly useful for demonstrating and analysing skills. The focus on analysis may be preferable for training experienced learners rather than novices, as experienced practitioners bring a wealth of practical knowledge to the group, as they have all previously struggled with these communication issues. Fishbowls give more people the opportunity to observe a specific encounter and then participate in the feedback session. This allows the group, rather than just the instructor, to influence the learning and the attitudes of participants. Fishbowls can also be used to introduce the role-play process immediately before the group is broken down into small-group role-plays. A debriefing of the observed activity follows each type of role-play, although more time is generally spent on debrief in fishbowls.

It is useful to consider practical considerations, such as resources, the skill level of learners, and the specific learning objectives when designing a communication skills training session and choosing which type of role-play session to use.

Actors versus learners as simulated patients

In any role-play session it is necessary to have a 'patient' for the learner to interact with. In some training sessions, actors are hired to play the patient's role; in others, fellow trainees play that role. It is critical to the success of any role-play session that the scenario and environment are as authentic as possible, so that the learners are able to suspend disbelief and fully engage in the role-play. Therefore, actors are generally preferable (4) as they can be trained ahead of time to play a role in a particular way. However, using actors involves significant resources (e.g. money and time). Furthermore, playing and debriefing the role of patient can be valuable in training physicians in patient-centred communication techniques. For clarity in this chapter, we use the term simulated patient (SP) to denote the person playing the role of the patient, whether that be an actor or another learner.

Essential elements of facilitating role-play sessions

A competent facilitator provides the foundation for successful communication training. The facilitator's goal is to achieve a consistent and reliable experience for learners across role-play groups. The personal style that each facilitator will bring into the process should not alter the basic guidelines for facilitation. The aim is to create a learner-centred experience and this is achieved by prioritizing the learner's agendas and needs. The processes of communication skills training and the corresponding facilitation skills that we have adopted are based on principles of adult learning theory. Adult learners need to understand the reason why they should learn something even before starting to learn it, and they need to be actively engaged, not only in the theoretical, but in the participatory and practical settings as well. Optimal learning conditions that satisfy many of these principles include: self-initiation, self-direction, realistic learning solutions, internal motivators, problem-centred organization, a variety of resources, and the opportunity to receive and offer feedback (5).

Guidelines and role-play rules can be effective in helping to set expectations and standards for the group. Some useful training rules include the following (6):

* Confidentiality. Reinforce the rule that 'what happens in the group stays in the group' and discourage discussions outside the role-play.

* Inclusiveness. The facilitator ensures that each participant has an opportunity to participate in the role-play and in the feedback session.

* Stopping. Only the facilitator or the learner in the hot seat can stop the role-play at any time. Emphasize that when the facilitator stops the role-play, this is not indicative of poor performance.

* Feedback. Starting with the learner, the facilitator solicits positive (reinforcing) feedback first and constructive alternatives later.

* Flexibility. Learners should feel free to make adjustments to written role-play scenarios in order to meet their needs, but should make sure that adjustments are consistent with the rest of the role-play.

* The practice principle. Practice, particularly re-running a particular segment, is not remedial or punitive. Instead, role-play is an opportunity to try new skills and to compare different methods of communication.

Sequence of strategies for facilitating small group role-play

In this chapter, we outline a series of strategies for facilitation of small-group role-play. These strategies are based on the Memorial Sloan–Kettering Cancer Center (MSKCC) facilitation guidelines (6), which were developed based on best practices in literature and other training materials (1, 7, 8). Here we outline a series of tasks that facilitators in their programme should demonstrate in group sessions (6). The basic teaching tasks that facilitators use during group sessions fall into the following categories:

(1) start the session;

(2) structure the group's learning;

(3) run the role-play;

(4) facilitate the feedback process; and

(5) close the session.

We outline each of these tasks and the individual steps associated with them in Box 51.1. Although these tasks were developed for a programme that uses small-group role-play sessions and professional actors, the principles can be applied to other types of role-play sessions as well.

Start the session

The facilitator spending time at the beginning, introducing role-play and helping the participants to feel comfortable, is an important task that contributes to a smooth role-play session. This can be done through making introductions, reviewing the rules and processes of role-play and giving feedback (8), normalizing anxiety, and requesting a volunteer to begin the role-play. This step is essential in creating a safe and supportive learning climate with learners, who have not previously participated in role-play work in communication skills training.

Structure the group's learning

The facilitator should take several preparatory steps to structure learning. Learners should be given time to read copies of the role-play scenario and discuss any questions that they might have.

Box 51.1 Comskil facilitation tasks

1. Start the session.
   - Make introductions as appropriate.
   - Establish or reinforce rules of role-play.
   - Confidentiality.
   - Inclusiveness.
   - Stopping rules (time out).
   - Feedback (learner first, positive first, constructive alternatives).
   - Flexibility.
   - Normalize the anxiety created by being observed.
   - Determine first learner to participate in role-play.
2. Structure the group's learning.
   - Distribute the copies of role-play scenarios.
   - Allow time to read scenarios.
   - Discuss patient's potential needs.
   - Adjust role-play scenario to meet a learner's goals, if necessary.
   - Discuss goals for this interaction both generally and specific to individual learners.
   - Agree on starting place.
   - If necessary, inform actor ('off-stage') of beginning scenario or other instructions.
3. Run the role-play.
   - Instruct learner to invite patient(s) in.
   - Note commencement time.
   - Watch closely and take notes.
   - Notice both non-verbal and verbal behaviour.
   - Look for key moments when the interaction shifts.
   - Stop the role-play after 3–4 minutes.
   - Manage time allocation for each learner fairly.
4. Facilitate the feedback process.
   For the feedback component, the actor may or may not be present. The facilitator's task here is to create a supportive environment in which descriptive and balanced feedback is offered.

Elicit feedback from the learner:
   - What was going well?
   - What problems were faced?
   - What help would the learner like from the group?

Elicit feedback from other group members.
   - Encourage participation from the entire group.
   - Elicit feedback from simulated patient (if appropriate or helpful).

> ### Box 51.1 (continued) Comskil facilitation tasks
>
> Utilize video playback to provide further opportunities for reflection.
>
> Reinforce communication skills.
>
> Provide opportunities for the group to resolve problems.
>
> Use feedback to suggest strategies for moving forward.
>
> Try out suggestions.
>
> Rapidly acknowledge conflict or inappropriate criticism or feedback.
>
> Return to Steps 2–4, as needed.
>
> 5. Close the session.
>
> De-role the actor (as appropriate).
>
> Establish major issues, learning, and questions.

If necessary, the facilitator can make adjustments to the role-play scenario as written. The group should discuss the potential needs of the patient that they are about to meet.

Another role of the facilitator is to give the SP appropriate direction. Speaking privately with the SP before a role-play segment helps to ensure that they fully understand the scenario. Facilitators can also use this time to give the SP specific instructions (e.g. the intensity of emotion desired or a particular cue to be given).

Eliciting individual learning goals is a significant part of structuring the group's learning. During the goal-setting, the facilitator will ensure that the learner has reviewed the role-play scenario and identified specific skills that the he/she would like to practice. Successful goal-setting should not be overwhelming or uncomfortable, instead it should help learners to identify their own 'learning edge', which has been defined by Fryer-Edwards and colleagues as 'the place where the learner can work that will be challenging but not overwhelming' (8, p.640).

Run the role-play

Once the learner and the SP are clear on the starting point, the facilitator should start the role-play. During the role-play session, the facilitator should carefully observe and take notes. The facilitator should also note the amount of time that has passed and look for the appropriate stopping place. Factors influencing the decision to stop a role-play include: if the learner's objective has been met and whether enough data has been gathered for meaningful feedback. Generally, this is about 3–4 minutes. Exceptions to this may include, if the learner's goal has been accomplished in less time (i.e. eliciting the patient's agenda) or, alternatively, if the goal is more complex (i.e. explaining a complicated, randomized clinical trial). As facilitators gain experience, they are able to more effectively make judgments about the appropriate length of each role-play segment and how it best meets the learner's goals.

When the role-play segment is ended, the facilitator should instruct the SP whether to stay in the room for the feedback discussion (this is usually only relevant if the SP is an actor). If the learner chooses to replay the segment again and the SP is present for the feedback discussion, it may impact the way the SP plays the character. The SP leaving the room promotes a more standardized approach. However, at other times, having the SP stay in the room to participate in the feedback is useful because well-trained SPs can give valuable feedback. As the facilitators gain experience, their judgment about using SP feedback improves.

Facilitate the feedback process

Facilitating feedback is the most complex and time-consuming process. The facilitator's task here is to create a supportive, stimulating, learner-centred environment, in which all group members' opinions are valued. The facilitator should first ask the learner to give feedback on his or her own performance in order to promote self-assessment. Starting with the positive feedback is recommended (e.g. 'What do you think you did well in that consultation?') (7). Other members of the group should generally be invited to give feedback before the facilitator gives feedback. The facilitator should work to maintain a balance of positive and constructive feedback during this time. Focusing on positive behaviours may seem counter-intuitive to group members, but the reinforcement of such behaviours is critical for the learner who is playing the role of clinician, as well as the learners who are observing. The facilitator should ask the learner to identify what problems or challenges he or she faced in the interaction; the facilitator can then elicit the help of the group in coming up with ways to address the problem or challenge. Throughout the feedback process, the facilitator should reinforce the communication skills that were taught in the earlier didactic session through reinforcing and naming what was observed (7).

Occasionally, communication skills training programmes have the resources to offer video-playback as part of the learning process. Video-recording the role-play and reviewing specific sections in the feedback session are valuable in allowing learners to observe and reflect upon their own performance. Suggested strategies include selecting specific portions of the video-recording to show, pausing the video to ask questions (e.g. 'What did you think when the patient said that?'), and observing nonverbal communication.

At times during feedback sessions, a learner who was observing may make an inappropriate critical comment or a conflict may arise. This has the potential to become a 'critical incident' and must be responded to quickly (9). An excerpt from the MSKCC Facilitator Training Booklet (6) follows:

> Occasionally, a learner will become acutely distressed as a result of role-play and feedback. We term this a 'Critical Incident' because of its potential to demoralize and impede learning—a harmful outcome. Facilitators carry the key responsibility to both recognize and respond to such an event. The aim is to ameliorate the distress and re-establish a constructive learning environment as quickly as possible.

> Empathic support for the learner is the key strategy to be applied by the facilitator should the learner appear distressed. For instance, the facilitator might state, 'I sense you were upset by what occurred. How did you feel?' or 'I sense you are discomforted by those comments—they seemed too critical.' When learners experience the support of a facilitator in this manner, they are likely to rally and work constructively with feedback that was clumsy or insensitive. A skilled facilitator will turn awkward moments prophylactically into creative opportunities, keep the learning environment safe and prevent major critical incidents from occurring.

> (9, p.7)

After sufficient feedback has been given through group discussion, the facilitator's task is to provide a segue to the next role-play segment in a learner-centred manner. In some cases, the learner may want to replay the segment, trying out some of the suggestions that were given. A facilitator might say, 'You've heard a couple of suggestions for doing that differently. Would you like to try it over using some of these ideas?'. The process of replaying a segment of a consultation more successfully can be a significant learning moment. Alternatively, the learner may choose to move forward with the consultation, picking up where he/she left off. The facilitator should ensure that the SP and learner understand the next role-play and then cycle through the tasks of run the role-play and facilitate the feedback process again.

Paying close attention to the amount of time available in the role-play session, and ensuring that each learner (in small-group sessions) has a chance to take the role of the physician, is a difficult yet important task. When it is time for a new learner to take the role of the doctor, the facilitator should go back to the task of structuring the group's learning and then cycle through the tasks again.

Facilitators should be flexible and adaptable to the group's needs. Flexibility usually relates to identifying learning edges and responding to them. For instance, in one role-play session on discussing prognosis in our programme, members of a small group decided that they wanted to see how a patient would respond with varying prognoses. As each learner took a turn as the physician, he/she offered a different prognosis—ranging from a 10% chance of cure to a 90% chance of cure. A few other examples of such flexibility follow:

- Instead of having a third learner do the same role-play scenario that two learners before have done, the group can work together to come up with a way of adjusting the role-play.

- A learner may be encouraged to offer up a real-life scenario that he or she has found particularly problematic.

- The facilitator may have the SP play the emotion differently for each learner (e.g. highly emotional versus muted).

- If one learner is struggling with a portion of the consultation and another learner who has been observing has an idea about how to handle it, the facilitator can switch learners for a few moments for the observing learner to demonstrate.

- The learner may want to try a particular technique that has not been suggested in the module.

Close the session

The final task at the end of a role-play session is to provide closure to the session. The facilitator can do this by summarizing some of the important points in the group's learning, asking group members to state what they found to be the most useful new skill they learned, and taking time to discuss any questions the group might have (8). Additionally, this is a good time to 'de-role' the SP (if a professional actor), by taking them out of role, introducing them, and thanking them for their time. Especially in cases where the SP has been asked to stay in role during feedback, this is an opportunity to normalize relationships, particularly if there has been a tense encounter between the SP and a learner as part of the role-play (e.g. anger module). Relating out of the context of the role-play is important to avoid persistent negative feelings.

Training and sustaining competent facilitators

As facilitators play such a key role in the success of communication training programmes, effectively training facilitators is vital. We also propose that more attention be given to continued assessment and development of facilitators.

Training facilitators

A well-used method of training facilitators for communication skills training programmes is a train-the-trainer workshop. The train-the-trainer model is grounded in the education literature and is often referred to as 'the cascade model'. One group trains another group, who then trains another group, thus the education is 'cascading' downward (10).

Effective facilitator training programmes follow a basic principle of first ensuring that the facilitator trainee is trained in the *content* of the workshop that they will be facilitating and then in the *process* of facilitation. Train-the-trainer workshops can range in time intensity, depending on what facilitators are being asked to do. For example, the New York Presbyterian Hospital had residency training directors come together for a full day of training to learn how to lead two different 1-hour communication seminars with their residents or fellows. During that day of facilitator training, residency directors were taught, and at the same time participated in, the modules they would teach. Following that, they were taught how to give effective feedback. Other training programmes, such as the programme at MSKCC, invites facilitator trainees to first participate in the full training programme (18 hours) as learners and then to participate in a separate workshop on training facilitators (6). Participating first as a learner allows facilitator trainees to become familiar with the content of modules that they will later facilitate. This experience also provides future facilitators with an opportunity to observe how effective facilitators conduct the small-group exercises, establish goal-settings, and elicit and provide feedback. Participating as learners in training also adds to credibility as a facilitator because they can relate first-hand to the anxiety or apprehension that a learner might feel.

As the content of what a facilitator may teach will vary from programme to programme, the remainder of this section is focused on the facilitator training workshop itself: the process of training facilitators in the essential elements of good facilitation.

We recommend that, where possible, a 2–3 hour workshop be set aside to focus solely on the facilitation process. In order to train effective facilitators, sufficient time must be given to explain and demonstrate important facilitation tasks, as well as allowing facilitator trainees some time to practice and give feedback (6). As such, this final workshop should mimic other communication training workshops—providing a didactic session, as well as small-group practice time, including opportunities to observe and analyse video-recorded sessions.

In the MSKCC programme, our facilitator training module begins with an overview of important educational principles. We then move into a detailed discussion of the Comskil facilitator tasks (Box 51.1). To illustrate each of these tasks, we show videos of a simulated small-group role-play session. Following the didactic portion of the training, we move into small groups—each group having a facilitator trainer and 2–3 facilitator trainees. Each facilitator trainee then gets a chance to practice facilitating a small group, with his or her fellow trainees playing the roles of learners. The facilitator trainer performs a higher-order facilitation process, occasionally stopping the small-group session and leading a feedback session on the facilitator trainee's performance as a facilitator. In our experience, this practice time is essential for facilitators to feel prepared for their first facilitation experience. This workshop has improved facilitators' feelings of self-efficacy in their ability to facilitate role-play (6). With a large group of facilitator trainees, the fishbowl technique may be useful in teaching the skills of observation and giving feedback around communication skills.

Facilitator feedback and assessment

The end of the training module for facilitators should not mark the end of their training. Instead, we view the process of training as lasting through the trainee's first few experiences as a facilitator. Novice facilitators need support and feedback as they work toward achieving competence as facilitators. Several strategies that we have found useful in supporting facilitators include:

- ◆ Pair up novice facilitators with more experienced facilitators in a co-facilitator model. The novice facilitator can then take a turn at facilitating one or two learners, without being responsible for the entire session. Novice facilitators appreciate having a more experienced facilitator to back them up.

- ◆ Conduct briefing and de-briefing sessions with facilitators before and after the workshops. Briefing sessions allow time to review facilitator guidelines and role-plays for the current module. Debriefing sessions are a time to discuss any problems that may have been faced by the facilitators and brainstorm possible solutions.
- ◆ At each session provide copies of facilitator tasks and possible question prompts (e.g. Box 51.2).
- ◆ Provide support with video equipment, if applicable.

Assessing novice facilitators' performance and giving them feedback is also a means of support. For instance, in the MSKCC programme, we audio-record novice facilitators three times during their first nine times facilitating. We code these audio-recordings, using a coding system we developed based upon the tasks described above (11). Feedback letters that describe strengths and offer areas of improvement are then provided to the facilitators before their next training session.

Future areas of research and development for facilitation skills

As communication skills training programmes become more integrated into all levels of medical education, there should be ample opportunities for further research and development into facilitating skills practice in role-play sessions. Three particular areas we see for growth include: examining different methods of training and supporting facilitators, identifying the impact of using a co-facilitator model, and establishing measures for treatment fidelity in communication skills training intervention studies.

First, exploring different methods of training and development for facilitators will be fruitful. For instance, it is unclear if facilitators' improvement over time is due to practice alone or if

---

Box 51.2 Question prompts for communication skills facilitators

You aimed to do X in that interaction. How successful were you in achieving that aim?

Which communication skills or process tasks were useful to you in achieving that aim?

What exactly did you do that achieved that aim?

What was the most difficult part of that interaction?

Is there a part you would like to explore further?

What was your goal when you said that? What were you trying to achieve?

How did the patient respond when you said that? (Verbally and non-verbally)

What were you thinking/feeling at that point?

Would you like some feedback from the patient?

Were there any communication skills or process tasks you could have used?

We have had x suggestions for ways of tackling that issue—which would you like to try?

You set out to do X, but you feel it didn't quite work out. What made it hard?

Are there any ways to get around those difficulties?

How did you know that worked? What did you notice?

Adapted, with permission, from the Medical Psychology Research Unit, University of Sydney.

periodic feedback can assist in improving facilitation skills. If feedback is helpful, questions about the frequency, method, and content of the feedback should be explored.

Second, much of the work written about facilitation assumes a single facilitator model. However, in some programmes, the supply of facilitators is sufficient to use a co-facilitator model. For instance, a programme may choose to use a co-facilitator model that pairs a medical or surgical facilitator with a psychiatrist or psychologist facilitator. Questions regarding the added benefit of using co-facilitators and how to best train facilitators to work in such a model could be explored.

Finally, in terms of researching communication skills training as an intervention, future work should prioritize the issue of treatment fidelity—ensuring that all subjects in an intervention are getting reliable and valid treatments (12). Since multiple facilitators are often involved in a training programme, systems for ensuring competence and adherence to the facilitation model are key.

Conclusion

Role-play work is vital to effective communication skills training. Facilitators for such role-play work need to be trained in providing a learner-centred approach to this activity. Effective facilitation includes beginning and structuring the session, running role-play, facilitating feedback, and closing the session. Through continued support, feedback, and assessment, facilitators can improve their skills and provide standardized and competent training.

References

1. Kurtz S, Silverman J, Draper J. *Teaching and Learning Communication Skills in Medicine*. Abingdon: Radcliffe Medical Press Ltd; 1998.
2. Lane C, Rollnick S. The use of simulated patients and role-play in communication skills training: A review of the literature to August 2005. *Patient Education and Counseling* 2007; **67**: 13–20.
3. Gueguen JA, Bylund CL, Brown RF, *et al*. Conducting family meetings in palliative care: Themes, techniques and preliminary evaluation of a communication skills module. *Palliative and Supportive Care* 2009; **7**(2): 171–179.
4. Knowles MS. *The Adult Learner: A Neglected Species*. Houston, Texas: Gulf; 1978.
5. Green M, Ellis P. Impact of an evidence-based medicine curriculum based on adult learning theory. *Journal of General Internal Medicine* 1997; **12**: 742–750.
6. Bylund CL, Brown RF, Lubrano di Ciccone B, *et al*. Training faculty to facilitate communication skills training: Development and evaluation of a workshop. *Patient Education and Counseling* 2008; **70**: 430–436.
7. Baile WF, Kudelka AP, Beale EA, *et al*. Communication skills training in oncology. Description and preliminary outcomes of workshops in breaking bad news and managing patient reactions to illness. *Cancer* 1999; **86**: 887–897.
8. Fryer-Edwards KA, Arnold RM, Baile WF, *et al*. Reflective teaching practices: an approach to teaching communication skills in a small-group setting. *Academic Medicine* 2006; **81**(7): 638–644.
9. Finlay I. Rules of role-play—guidance for tutors. In: *Diploma in Palliative Medicine*; 2000; Cardiff University; 2000.
10. Bax S. The social and cultural dimensions of trainer training. *Journal of Education for Teaching* 2002; **28**(2): 165–178.
11. Bylund C, Brown R, Diamond C, *et al*. Development of a method of treatment fidelity for communication skills training interventions. *Psycho-Oncology* 2008; **17**: S198.
12. Borrelli B, Sepinwall D, Ernst D, *et al*. A new tool to assess treatment fidelity and evaluation for treatment fidelity across 10 years of health behaviour research. *Journal of Consulting and Clinical Psychology* 2005; **73**(5): 852–860.

Chapter 52

The role of the actor in medical education

Paul Heinrich

Introduction

The world of medical education has been transformed over the past 40 years through the use of members of the public in role-playing to teach and assess clinical and communication skills. Howard S Barrows began to use 'programmed patients' in the early 1960s, and in a sustained creative burst, pioneered most of the subsequent applications of the method (1). Programmed patients were employed to teach, demonstrate, assess in laboratory and clinical practice settings, and to provide constructive feedback to medical students. The technique was extended by a number of research clinicians, such as Paula Stillman and Robert Kretzschmar, who involved members of the public as patient instructors of basic clinical skills and as gynaecological teaching associates (GTAs) in pelvic examinations (2, 3). The technique spread extensively through the USA and into a number of other countries including Canada, the UK, Australia, the Netherlands, Switzerland, Israel, the Ukraine, Russia, Spain, Brazil, and China (1).

These surrogate patients have undergone a number of name changes that reflect the variety of functions that they fulfil, including programmed patients, professional patients, simulated patients, pseudo patients, standardized patients, patient partners, and patient instructors. They are most commonly referred to as SPs, an abbreviation that covers the more general term of simulated patient and the standardized patient for examination purposes.

A large number of papers have documented communication training programmes utilizing SPs and have reported on student satisfaction with the method (4–12). Others have described the approaches taken to recruitment, training, and the effect on the SPs of repeat performance, especially when undertaken over a prolonged period and in simulation of intense scenarios (13–20). The reliability and validity of simulation as an assessment tool has also been verified in a succession of studies since the 1990s (21–23).

Numerous researchers have questioned the need to restrict the role of the SP to professional actors. SPs are now routinely recruited from a wide pool, which includes retirees, past patients, nurses, and drama students (24). Variety in the recruitment pool has been shown to be justified beyond financial considerations, as the performance demands are not always advanced, and many of the simulation tasks are well within the grasp of most people.

In this chapter, however, I will refer to those who play the roles of SPs as actors. The role of an SP requires at least a basic level of acting—the ability to enter into a hypothetical reality for a period of time, the ability to reproduce behaviour according to a predetermined script, and the readiness to access one's personal repertoire of behaviour to act as one would if one were to find oneself in a particular situation. Higher levels of acting, as demonstrated by professional actors, involve moving as oneself into situations beyond personal experience and empathically recreating experiences as someone other than oneself. Many of the discussions over whether SP performance is actually acting or not (5, 15–18) can probably be traced to an unsophisticated view of performance and lack of differentiation between levels of acting.

Despite the universality of the term SP, from the beginning they have been trained to carry out a variety of tasks, each of which presupposes a distinctive mode of performance. Many of the variations in attitude to recruitment, training, and development of scenarios, can be seen as responses to the differing requirements of these performance modes. For example, an actor who is working within an assessment context performs quite differently than someone who is called upon to demonstrate a skill or to respond in an emotionally authentic manner.

We shall first explore the notion of different modes of performance, which determine the subsequent decisions on recruitment, training, feedback, and debriefing.

Virtually all models of simulation with SPs consist of three distinct roles:

1. Actor. Usually the role of the patient, performed by an SP. The role is reality and clinically based in that the characterization and actions are derived from an actual or a classic patient. Barrows was insistent that a specific case study be faithfully reproduced in full detail (24). Based on a recognizable clinical reality, the performer possesses the discipline and understanding to control and direct their actions in line with predetermined guidelines, and the ability to reproduce this SP behaviour over successive occasions. Not all students or members of the public are comfortable or capable of performing in this way, though many can carry out simpler repertoires, such as memorizing a short list of symptoms and questions for clinical examinations. Those who can perform these tasks have at least moderate levels of acting ability, and simply act as they themselves would if they found themselves in the situation. Professional actors are usually employed for longer and more demanding roles.

2. Role-player. A role-player, usually a learner or examinee, who acts as they would in real life. The role-player is almost always aware that the patient is an actor and that they are performing within a hypothetical situation. Clinical training, knowledge acquisition, and past experience are sufficient to enable the role-player to carry out the designated task. This role, which requires the imagination to act as one does in real life, is not an acting role as such; however, it does require a basic level of comfort with the desired performance. The role only becomes acting when the students are asked to make an imaginative leap and pretend to be a doctor with experience and knowledge beyond their present capacities.

3. Educator. A watching educator or group of educators who design the simulation, set the rules and criteria of behaviour, observe the actions of the role-player, and provide feedback of one kind or another. This feedback may be in the form of a formative or summative assessment at the conclusion of the performance; facilitation of the learning process either during or afterwards; post-performance guidance in video-review of the consultation; or supervision of the event.

The mode of performance determines the nature of each of the three roles and the interaction among them. The selected mode also sets in motion a series of decisions that affect, amongst other things, the design of the scenario; the choice of casting of the actor; the training of the actor; the role and preparation of the role-player; the role and preparation of the educator; the nature of feedback and debriefing subsequent to performance; and the sustainability of performance over time. As these factors are largely determined by the mode and its underlying purpose, it is important first to clarify the nature of each mode of performance before discussing some of the implications for design and training.

Assessment

Since the inception of their use, SPs have been used in medical education to assess clinical and communication skills, either as separate activities or in tandem. The practice has become widespread in North America through the impetus of Barrows, Stillman, and others (1, 2, 5), and the inspiration of early education centres such as the Morchand Centre at Mt Sinai. The Association of American Medical Colleges (AAMC) and the American Medical Association (AMA) have recommended the use of SPs, and national examinations of clinical competency have been established by the Medical Council of Canada (MCC) and the National Board of Medical Examiners (NBME) in the USA. The Macy Foundation provided financial support in setting up eight consortia for propagation of the technique and for mutual support (28), and the Association of Standardized Patient Educators (ASPE), internet networking, and annual SP trainer conferences have fostered strong ties among medical schools with SP programmes.

Actors performing as SPs in an assessment capacity work within frameworks requiring standardization of roles and reliable reproducibility so that all students are given the same communication challenge. The actors must be able to:

+ work within scenarios that significantly prescribe their behaviour;
+ repeatedly reproduce the same role;
+ recover quickly with minimal rest periods between encounters;
+ maintain focus; and
+ rate the students according to predetermined criteria on some form of checklist or rating scale.

The interaction may be brief and focused on the performance of a clinical skill, or it may extend up to an hour as a simulation of a full consultation with a patient. Extended simulation demands a conscious grasp of the many performance factors at play in reproducing a realistic recreation of real-life, which is the study domain of the professional actor.

The educator takes the role of objective assessor and views the encounter either in real time as a passive observer in the room, through a viewing mirror from another room, or on video-tape at a later time. The students attempt to match their behaviour to skill sets that are taught as the appropriate responses to the encounter.

Audit

Audit is a special case of assessment. Instead of bringing a doctor in to assess clinical or communication skills in an educational centre, educators send the actors into the doctor's own clinical practice in the guise of one of the doctor's patients (26–31). Doctors usually volunteer for a future visit by an SP as a follow-up to communication skills training workshops. Barrow tested this practice of actor as undercover agent (31) and found it to be effective (24).

Ideally, in an audit situation, the medical professional has given consent for the exercise well beforehand, so that memory and expectation fade into a low index of suspicion. Audit mode is a form of invisible theatre (32) in which the doctor is unaware of the artifice, and depends for its success on careful planning and thorough preparation. The device requires that the clinician be unable to differentiate between the actor and other patients in the practice. Actors need to be well-cast to match closely the social types and stereotypical behaviour of the patient population in question, and they need to appear with realistic props, which include perfectly realized documentation.

Professional actors are ideal for this kind of performance, as they are already trained to be aware of the large number of performance factors at play in recreating realistic performance and to be able to manipulate their behaviour to match the expectations of the clinician. However, with longer training and good casting, non-professionals should be able to manage the illusion as standard interactions between doctors and patients fall within fairly prescribed boundaries. The actors do not need to enter into the persona of someone other than themselves, they simply need to act as they would were they in that situation and had those symptoms.

The educator's main focus is that of auditor or inspector. Unlike other modes, the educator cannot be present at the interaction or view it at a later period, but is represented in the encounter by the actor as undercover agent. Feedback is based on carefully prescribed criteria that determine the actor's script for action and the nature of the items in the actor's report on the interaction.

Experiential learning

Whereas assessments measure skills already acquired, experiential learning creates an environment in which students extend their expertise. The learning event may take the form of an encounter with an individual student, a small group, or a 'fishbowl' interaction with 20 or more participants. The performance takes place within a contained environment, designed for safety of exploration; the opportunity for learning from one's own interaction with the actor; time to temporarily step out from the interaction to receive feedback; and the opportunity to test out heretofore untried decisions and actions. Experiential learning facilitates gaining confidence and skill to expand one's personal repertoire or to personalise a line of action sanctioned as professional best practice.

The educator's role is now that of facilitator of the students' learning. The scope of the workshop depends largely upon the facilitator's own understanding of the learning process, experience in the role of a facilitator, and comfort with ambiguity and uncertain outcome, in that no two learners will come up with exactly the same solution to the situation. These factors will tend to place the facilitator somewhere along an interventionist spectrum from active coach, through watchful umpire, to dispassionate time keeper. Maximizing the experience for the learners is the key focus for the facilitator and the choices made by the role-player are the cues for educational intervention.

The emphasis of performance is marked less by standardization and reproducibility as by the ability to improvise within clearly defined boundaries with a major focus on authentic personal response to the students' words and actions.

Demonstration

Actors are often called up to perform within a demonstration mode, either live and in real time before an audience of medical students or professionals, or in a video-taped interaction as part of a training module as a trigger for discussion. Demonstration usually takes one of four forms:

(1) The actor produces simple, exemplary behaviour as an ideal model for imitation and study.

(2) The performance is cautionary, portraying behaviour that produces disastrous consequences.

(3) The simulated consultation can be a finely nuanced 'slice of life.' The doctor's performance is not meant to be an exemplary model, but shows something of the complexity of clinical practice with scope for possible improvements in various places. These dramatizations provide rich blends of interactions that reward close observation and reflection.

(4) Or the performance could be in any one of a number of comic modes that laughably render inappropriate behaviour self-evidently inadequate and unsupportable.

The existence of these four distinct forms of portrayal suggests matching form to specific educational aim.

Professional actors and traditional approaches to scripting and rehearsal are most appropriate for this kind of performance. The scriptwriter may be a clinician with a dramatic sensibility, or a non-medical scriptwriter with close access to a clinician experienced in the particular interaction.

The script can also be workshopped with the actors from a rough scenario outline. Experience at the Pam McLean Centre of the University of Sydney has demonstrated that medical professionals are able to play the role of the doctor on camera if well-cast and if workshopped into the role. Workshopping reduces the tendency to the wooden or stereotypical behaviour often displayed by doctors thrust with a script before lights and cameras.

Instruction

As early as the 1970s, Stillman recruited members of the public as subjects upon whom students could practise routine, specific, physical examination skills. Around this time, Kretzschmar also introduced the use of gynaecological teaching associates (GTAs) for pelvic examinations (2, 3). These patients were trained to identify clinical best practice, as exemplified by experienced physicians, and used those criteria to assess student practice. Both Stillman and Kretzschmar quickly expanded the role to include the communication skills used in conjunction with the examinations. These early experiments established the basic template for the expansion of the technique to other centres. Patients playing this role of student instructor are trained in specific clinical examination and communication skills (33–38).

Within a short period of time, researchers established three main streams of patient instructors:

(1) healthy members of the public who were able to act as subjects for routine examination skills, where physical findings were not necessary;

(2) patients with stable chronic findings, such as aortic stenosis, asthma, or arthritis (1); and

(3) SPs who are able to simulate physical findings.

Barrows reported that SPs could realistically simulate such findings as lid lag, lid ptosis, wheezing, shortness of breath, carotid bruit, loss of hearing and vision, Babinski sign, and asymmetrical deep tendon reflexes (24).

Professional actors have not traditionally been necessary for this mode of performance, even when simulation of symptoms was added to the formula. The motivation to be involved in the teaching of young doctors is a strong prerequisite for this kind of SP. The roles of actor and educator fuse in this mode, with the educator imparting some of their knowledge to the actor who is able to stand in as proxy. The educator functions as recruiter, trainer, and supervisor.

The rest of the chapter examines the implications of the mode of performance for recruitment, preparation and training, performance, feedback and debriefing, and the effects on the actors.

Recruitment

Barrows identifies only two essential requirements for an SP—intelligence and motivation (24). Intelligent and motivated applicants most likely possess a third necessary factor, a basic level of comfort with performance.

Professional actors are valuable recruits in several capacities. They are trained to identify the many dynamics of performance at play in common human interactions. In assessment situations that are complex, multifaceted, and of lengthy duration, they can apply these insights to the medical consultation and reproduce the interaction with a high degree of similarity over many performances. In audit situations, they do not need to be schooled in the basics of performance and can quickly learn the nature of the interaction and the criteria by which they are to assess the behaviour of the clinician. The major drawback of the use of actors in audit is financial. In experiential learning workshops they are skilled in authentic interaction with a partner; in accessing and reproducing true emotional states at will; in recognizing and describing the impact of their partner's behaviour; and in producing convincing recreations of a range of patient types and responses. In demonstrations they can play both patient and clinician roles. On the other hand, instructional roles and simpler assessment situations can be more that adequately performed by acting students, amateur actros, or members of the public who are comfortable with public interaction.

Recruits from the world of medicine present a mixed bag. In general, medical clinicians and educators are not a first choice as SP for most modes. In assessment or learning, the educator or clinician may be known to the student and may hinder the student's ability to accept the simulated reality. Even where the educator is unknown, often an extensive medical knowledge will affect their ability to empathize and respond as would a patient. Most medical students already have acquired the same problem of medicalization. In the case of demonstrations of communication skills, many doctors and nurses can be rehearsed into playing the clinical role. The role is already known to them through extended practice in real life, and the rehearsal task involves making their usual behaviour known to them so that they can reproduce it comfortably. Our experience shows that many clinicians can reproduce an appropriate version of exemplary behaviour, and the more skilled can manage slice of life. Clinicians tend to drop into comic mode if they portray cautionary behaviour, perhaps as a form of self-protection from the criticism of peers. A small percentage of doctors with natural abilities as performers, often from surgical, intensive care, or anaesthetic specialties, are able to play across the spectrum.

Nursing is also a source of recruitment for assessment. Their nursing experience provides them with an extensive library of patient and clinical encounters to draw upon for experiential learning workshops and demonstration videos, either as patients or in clinical roles.

Non-medical members of the public are a source for SPs in simpler assessment situations that require no more than comfort with performance, alert minds, the ability to learn a simple script of words and actions and to repeat them accurately over many encounters, and a lack of personal agenda from past negative experiences with the medical world. As instructors, the possible need for physical findings or the readiness to expose oneself for pelvic or genital examination limits the pool. Actors or artist models are a potential source for the latter. Non-professionals perform as auditors, provided that they are chosen for their fit to the population profile of the relevant clinicians' practice, are naturally comfortable with performance, and are given more extensive training than would be required by professional actors.

Training for performance

Typecasting is a safe and wise option in most cases, given that the interaction is brief and initial impressions are powerful. Gender, age, ethnic background, physique, or personality type may be an essential requirement to produce the illusion of clinical reality. Elements of the patient's personal and social history, which are not clinically essential, can be left to the actor, as long as the actor's choices do not lead the interaction in a direction counter to the purpose of the exercise.

Rehearsals can mostly be relatively short, as the actor, whether lay person or professional actor, does not rehearse to become a character in any rounded sense but appears as a patient playing her view of the patient's role in a brief and focused encounter. Inexperienced SPs may require longer rehearsal because of the need to be orientated to the mode of performance and to learn their role.

In all cases, the nature of the performance and the desired outcomes determine the training of the actor. Instruction requires the time to learn how to give an experiential tutorial, assessment, the specific elements of the examination or history, and experiential learning, the range of options possible in an open interaction where the actor follows the lead of the student. Audit requires extensive preparation, especially where non-professionals are recruited as SPs because invisible theatre demands a cool head acquired through command of many variables of performance.

In most cases, SPs follow scripts that are produced from the point of view of the patient and written in plain language. Scripting requires conscious effort by educators to abandon their own medical view of the events. In the case of demonstration, the script will be either provided as a written text or workshopped by the director and actors into final form. All other modes are improvisational, scenario-based performance, the number of whose fixed elements are determined by the purpose of the exercise. In these modes, the script takes the form of units of action to be played more or less in a prescribed sequence, with a small number of verbatim elements. In most modes, the performance is built on an illness narrative that proceeds from presenting symptoms through significant events up to the role-play consultation, including any prior interactions with other doctors. The actor rehearses the overall shape and direction of the interaction, essential sequences of history-giving and questioning, and specific questions or verbatim wording where required.

In instruction, the scripting depends upon the degree to which the actor teaches the skill or responds to the students' actions. The script for the former lays down a series of actions for the actor, while for the latter the actor rehearses responses to a menu of possible stimuli from the student. Training for assessment differs from that for experiential learning in that the actor's behaviour needs to be far more prescribed, with specific actions and words being rehearsed. The interaction is more formal and less reactive to the individual style of the student. These prescriptions are particularly at play in the clinical examination setting, and put performance within reach of a large pool of potential SPs. In assessment of a full consultation, the frame can loosen but still not reach the flexibility of performance of most experiential learning workshops, due to the demand for standardized responses. In experiential learning there is greater latitude in training as facilitators vary greatly in their approach and objectives, and standardization is relinquished in favour of student-centred learning.

Training also needs to incorporate some level of medicalization of the actor. In reality, patients gradually become medicalized through experience with the medical system. The patient may have knowledge of medications, tests, scans, anaesthesia, operations, and may have researched on the internet or read booklets on medical procedures. The actor needs this information and experience in order to play the part with any conviction and credence. Where the patient is still naïve, it may be important for the actor not to be so. Many scenarios require the actor to recognize how well a student performs in relation to approved standards, in which case the actor needs knowledge of how those standards translate into practice. If students regularly experience difficulties in certain parts of the interaction, it helps the actor to know this in advance. The more professional the actor, the more likely he can internalize this knowledge and direct his performance while still having his character respond in ignorance of these facts.

Feedback

Training also needs to include rehearsal of feedback, which provides another source of complexity and adds further levels of concentration to the performance. The actors must split their focus to carry out three simultaneous tasks: remain spontaneously open to the interaction with their partner; direct their performance in accordance with the overall script; and remain alert to the specific behaviours to be reported in feedback. This third task alters according to the mode of performance. For example, in assessment and audit, the feedback required will include a checklist, rating scale, or report in which the student or doctor's behaviour is judged according to objective, predetermined criteria. These criteria are developed over time in research and need to be communicated clearly to the actors and practised in rehearsal. Checklists require a sudden and major shift in focus for the actor from what can be intensely subjective performance to detached critique; clarity and practice are required.

In instruction, feedback is of two kinds—objective matching of the student's actions to a model of clinical best practice, and subjective response to how the student handles, relates to, and communicates with the SP. In experiential learning, feedback takes place in three ways:

(1) The actor's responses within the interaction to the student through words and body language provide immediate feedback to the role-player and observers of the impact of the student's actions. This form of feedback is potentially the most direct, yet is most often left out of discussions on feedback.

(2) The actor is able to give feedback in character during timeout breaks in the interaction to guide the student in assessing their performance and directing it forward.

(3) After the interaction, the SP can give general feedback according to broad guidelines set out by the facilitator.

In a setting of learning, feedback takes the form of considered and constructive response to the choices of the role-player rather than the objective assessment of successful performance of external criteria in the examination setting. Feedback can include any number of factors, such as the impact of the student's manner and language, whether they block or facilitate communication, the ability to elicit personal concerns, and the extent to which they share ownership of the consultation.

On method acting

The debate over the relative merits and safety of method versus technique approaches to SP performance (13, 15–18) is a little overstated, as most modern actors borrow skills from a wide range of sources. Method is mostly an internal approach to performance, while technique refers to working from outside behaviour to inner motivation. For instance, an actor wishes to pick up and drink a glass of water. Using method, the actor reminds himself that he is thirsty. He remembers how dry his mouth is when thirsty, and recreates that sense of dryness. He feels thirsty and reaches over to pick up the glass to quench his thirst. The audience reads his motivation into the action and believes it. Using technique, the actor knows that he does not have to do all that internal recreation for such a simple matter. He allows his gaze to pass over the glass while he continues talking with the doctor. Then, a moment later, he reaches out for the glass and drinks it. His noticing of the glass provides sufficient motivation for his action and the doctor believes that he is thirsty. Method has real value as a rehearsal technique; however, it is not always intended for use in performance itself. For instance, an exercise such as emotional memory (39) is a valuable rehearsal technique by which the actor goes back to personal trauma to obtain empathic access to emotions experienced by patients on receiving bad news. Once the actor has accessed the emotion in rehearsal, technique is often sufficient to trigger the emotional reality in performance. Constant return to one's own library of distress can become very emotionally draining. Lack of experience or training in acting may be responsible for reports of subsequent distress after intense or emotional performances (13, 16–20).

The fact remains that the more intense and demanding roles as an SP can take their toll. In general, professional actors tend to possess the techniques and resources to safely enter and debrief from their roles. Cool down after acting is an intrinsic part of the performance process, and less experienced performers would benefit from opportunities offered by educators for times of debriefing afterwards. The impact of emotionally intense roles or of scenarios that demand that the actor vicariously experience emotional pain or existential turmoil over their own mortality is still unknown and the capacity of actors to manage these roles over an extended period of time varies. Capacity over the long term is probably a function of a number of variables and not just acting style alone. A wise course is to provide the actor as wide a range of roles as possible.

Conclusion

Various studies have exhibited confusion as to whether medical simulation should even be considered acting. Acting has erroneously been interpreted purely as the aesthetic drama of the stage. In fact, drama constitutes a continuum from simple role-play to professional acting, and medical simulation falls within the scale of this continuum. The patient role is always an acting role, which is one-third of the educational triad of actor, role-player, and educator. The tasks of each of these three players, and the relationships among them, change according to the demands of the specific performance. Some of these roles are playable by untrained members of the public, while other, more demanding roles, require actors who are trained to recreate complex behaviour.

This chapter distinguishes among five different modes of performance that have developed in medical education. Actors perform in:

(1) assessment;

(2) audit;

(3) experiential learning;

(4) demonstration; or

(5) instruction mode.

The uniform designation of standardized patient obscures the distinctly different nature of each mode of performance. Recognition of these distinctions clarifies the nature of the decisions that need to be made in relation to recruitment, training, performance, and the specific kind of feedback required within each mode. It is hoped that this proposed taxonomy of performance may contribute clarification for future uses of medical simulation.

References

1. Wallace P (1997). Following the threads of an innovation: the history of standardized patients in medical education. *Caduceus* **13**, 5–28.
2. Stillman P, Sabers D, Redfield D (1976). The use of paraprofessionals to teach interviewing skills. *Pediatrics* **57**, 769–74.
3. Kretzschmar R (1978). Evolution of the gynecology teaching associate: an educational specialist. *Am J Obstet Gynecol* **131**, 367–73.
4. Meier R, Perkowski L, Wynne C (1982). A method for training simulated patients. *J Med Educ* **57**, 535–40.
5. Barrows H (1993). An overview of the uses of standardized patients for teaching and evaluating clinical skills. *Acad Med* **68**, 446–51.
6. McManus I, Vincent C, Thom S, *et al.* (1993). Teaching communication skills to clinical students. *BMJ* **306**, 1322–7.
7. Baerheim A, Malterud K (1995) Simulated patients for the practical examination of medical students: intentions, procedures and experiences. *Med Educ* **29**, 410–413.
8. Greenberg L, Ochsenschlager D, O'Donnell R, *et al.* (1999). Communicating bad news: a pediatric department's evaluation of a simulated intervention. *Pediatrics* **103**, 1210–17.
9. Razavi, D, Delvaux N, Marchal S, *et al.* (2000). Testing health care professionals' communication skills: the usefulness of highly emotional standardized role-playing sessions with simulators. *Psychooncology* **9**, 293–302.

10. Smith P, Fuller G, Kinnersley P, *et al.* (2002). Using simulated consultations to develop communication skills for neurological trainees. *Eur J Neurol* **9**, 83–7.

11. Rosenbaum M, Ferguson K (2006). Using patient-generated cases to teach students skills in responding to patients' emotions. *Med Teach* **28**, 180–2.

12. Bosek M, Li S, Hicks F (2007). Working with standardized patients: a primer. International *J Nurs Educ* **4**, 1–12.

13. Naftulin D, Andrew D (1975). The effects of Patient Simulations on Actors. *J Med Educ* **50**, 87–89.

14. Meier R, Perkowski L, Wynne C (1982). A method for training simulated patients. *J Med Educ* **57**, 535–540.

15. Davies M (1989). The way ahead: teaching with simulated patients. *Med Teach* **11**, 315–320.

16. Woodward C, Gliva-McConvey G (1995). The effect of simulating on standardized patients. *Acad Med* **70**, 418–420.

17. Woodward C (1998). Standardized patients: a fixed-role therapy experience in normal individuals. *J Construct Psych* **11**, 133–148.

18. McNaughton N, Tiberius R, Hodges B (1999). Effects of portraying psychologically and emotionally complex standardized patient roles. *Teach Learn Med* **11**, 135–141.

19. Bokken L, van Dalen J, Rethans J (2004). Performance-related stress symptoms in simulated patients. *Med Educ* **38**, 1089–1094.

20. Bokken L, van Dalen J, Rethans J (2006). The impact of simulation on people who act as simulated patients: a focus group study. *Med Educ* **40**, 781–6.

21. Van der Vleuten C, Swanson D (1990). Assessment of clinical skills with standardized patients: state of the art. *Teach Learn Med* **2**, 58–76.

22. Vu N, Barrows H (1994). Use of standardized patients in clinical assessment: recent developments and measurement findings. *Educ Research* **23**, 23–30.

23. Swartz M, Colliver J (1996). Using standardized patients for assessing clinical performance: an overview. *Mt Sinai J Med* **63**, 241–9.

24. Barrows H (1987). *Simulated (Standardized) Patients and Other Human Simulations*. Health Sciences Consortium, Chapel Hill, NC.

25. Morrison L, Barrows H (1994). Developing consortia for clinical practice examinations: the Macy Project. *Teach Learn Med* **6**, 23–7.

26. Burri A, McCaughan, Barrows H (1976).The feasibility of using the simulated patient as a means to evaluate clinical competence of practicing physicians in a community, in *Proceedings of the Fifteenth Annual Conference on Research in Medical Education*, 295–9. Association of American Medical Colleges, Washington DC.

27. Woodward C, McConvey G, Neufeld V, *et al.* (1985). Measurement of physician performance by standardized patients. *Med Care* **23**, 1019–27.

28. Rethans J, Drop R, Sturmans F, *et al.* (1991). A method for introducing standardized (simulated) patients into general practice consultations. *Br J Gen Pract* **41**, 94–6.

29. Baerheim A, Malterud K (1995). Simulated patients for the practical examination of medical students: intentions, procedures and experiences. *Med Educ* **29**, 410–13.

30. Beullens J, Rethans J, Goedhuys J, *et al.* (1997). The use of standardized patients in research in general practice. *Fam Pract* **14**, 58–62.

31. Glassman P, Luck J, O'Gara E, *et al.* (2000). Using standardized patients to measure quality: evidence from the literature and a prospective study. *Jt Comm J Qual Improv* **26**, 644–53.

32. Boal A (1985). *Theatre of the Oppressed*, 126–147.Theatre Communications Group, New York.

33. Csikszentmihalyi M, LeFevre J (1989). Optimal experience in work and leisure. *J Pers Soc Psychol* **56**, 815–22.

34. Moneta G, Csikszentmihalyi M (1996). The effect of perceived challenges and skills on the quality of subjective experience. *J Pers* **64**, 275–310.

35. Anderson K, Meyer T (1978). The use of instructor-patients to teach physical examination techniques. *J Med Educ* **53**, 831–6.

36. Smilansky J, Foley R, Runkle N, *et al.* (1978). Instructor plays patient: an alternative to the case presentation method. *J Fam Pract* **6**, 1037–40.

37. Barley G, Fisher J, Dwinnell B, *et al.* (2006). Teaching foundational physical examination skills: study results comparing lay teaching associates and physician instructors. *Acad Med* **81**, 95–7.

38. Raj N, Badcock L, Brown G, *et al.* (2006). Undergraduate musculoskeletal examination teaching by trained patient educators–a comparison with doctor-led teaching. *Rheumatology (Oxford)* **45**, 1404–8.

39. Stanislavski C (1984). *An Actor Prepares*, 155–81. Theatre Arts Books, New York.

Chapter 53

Training patients to reach their communication goals: a concordance perspective

Carma L Bylund, Thomas A D'Agostino, and Betty Chewning

As the volume of literature in this book suggests, improving clinicians' communication is currently the subject of much scholarship throughout the world. Improving clinicians' communication is necessary, but not sufficient to achieve the best possible communication in a clinical encounter. This chapter is focused on an area that has received much less emphasis—training patients to be good communicators. The physician–patient interaction is a dynamic, socially-constructed, and reciprocal process (1, 2) that relies on at least two participants. Effective communication in a physician–patient relationship, therefore, requires both parties to be actively involved and competent communicators. Moreover, patients' communication may influence physicians' responses (3). Thus, to fully understand and improve physician–patient communication requires a focus on both sides of the interaction.

Such a focus is particularly important given that patients face many challenges in their clinical consultations, including physicians' ethnic or cultural biases (2), interruptions (4), lack of empathic communication (5), minimal tolerance for patients' desires to talk about internet information (2), and a lack of physician–patient concordance (1, 6). Despite the research and teaching efforts that have gone into physician training, patient communication training must also be addressed in order to achieve optimal physician–patient communication. Considerable research has indicated that there is room for improvement in patients' communication skills, including asking questions (7), explicitly stating concerns (8), and verifying information (9). The ineffective use of these skills may contribute to patients' misunderstanding of information given to them (9) and/or lack of adherence to a treatment plan (10).

This chapter begins with a review of studies of patient communication training, both in and out of the oncology setting. We then move to an explanation of the concept of concordance in the physician–patient relationship and how concordance provides a fruitful conceptual grounding for patient communication training. We close with a call for further interventions and research in this area.

Review of patient communication training studies

Published studies on patient communication training in the cancer setting are sparse. Consequently, we have chosen to review literature on patient communication training more broadly. Patient communication training studies differ in both method and content of training.

Method of training

We have expanded upon the definition of Parker and colleagues (1) in describing the methods of patient communication training. The three methods of training present in the literature are material only, material plus coaching, and group interventions.

Materials only

Materials-only communication interventions include those in which patients are given written materials to use on their own. Such methods usually include the use of question prompt-lists, which have been shown to increase the number of questions patients ask their oncologist, particularly around the topics of tests, treatment, and prognosis (7, 11). Cegala and colleagues expanded the focus of materials-only interventions beyond just question asking by developing a patient communication training booklet that has been used in intervention studies (9, 12, 13). The booklet is formatted like a workbook, with examples and spaces for notes. The content of the workbook focuses on the PACE curriculum, which will be discussed below.

Materials plus coaching

The second type of intervention category is materials plus coaching. This method involves the use of a one-on-one intervention in which a researcher interacts directly with a patient to discuss specific strategies or skills that the patient can use during consultations. Such methods may utilize some elements described in materials-only interventions (e.g. question prompt-sheets), but differ in that they also include a component of rehearsal or coaching (1). For instance, Brown and colleagues compared patients who were randomized to receive either a question prompt-list or a question prompt-list plus an individualized coaching session (11). Similarly, Cegala and colleagues have tested an intervention comparing patients receiving the communication training booklet described above with patients who receive the booklet and also have individual coaching prior to consultation (9, 12, 13). The coaching process involved asking patients if they experienced any problems using the training booklet, going over the booklet page by page, helping patients organize how they would approach the consultation, and briefly examining the booklet for evidence of usage (i.e. written notes, underlining) (13).

Group-based interventions

The third patient communication intervention method found in the literature is group-based interventions. Following, we summarize three articles that have described the development and evaluation of such community-based interventions.

First, Tran and colleagues (15) described a community education forum provided to patients and potential patients (not limited to cancer) with the aim of improving active patient communication. Entitled *How to Talk to Your Physician*, the 2-hour programme was presented by two co-educators, a physician, and a non-physician, in the effort to establish the collaborative nature of the physician/patient interaction. A typical forum involved attendees receiving a 20-page orientation guidebook and engaging in an interactive discussion facilitated by the co-educators, including trigger-videos, provocative questions about patient–physician interactions, and suggestions for improving communication (15). Second, Fisch and colleagues conducted a 1-day workshop called *My Life, My Choice*, held to educate cancer patients and family members about improving communication with their cancer care providers (16). The 8-hour workshop made use of a combination of lectures, as well as both large- and small-group discussions facilitated by healthcare professionals. Finally, Towle and colleagues (17) designed and implemented interactive workshops offered to seniors at a community centre (non cancer-specific) with the goal of promoting active participation of patients in consultations. The workshops were 2 hours in duration and involved participants receiving a booklet of communication skills, which were then modelled by simulated physicians and patients.

Content of training

Many patient communication interventions focus almost exclusively on patient question-asking. Although these communication skills are critically important to effective physician–patient communication, other training interventions have included additional skills in order to develop more comprehensive communication training interventions.

The programme developed by Cegala and colleagues (18) proposes that effective patient communication involves four components. Often referred to as PACE, these components are: Presenting detailed Information, Asking questions, Checking understanding, and Expressing concerns. Presenting detailed Information involves being prepared before the consultation to give a focused and extensive breadth of information about symptoms, history, reasons for visit, needs, expectations, an so on. Asking questions pertains to having a preset list of questions prepared that will deepen or clarify understanding of any information, treatments, tests, or diagnoses that may be presented in the consultation. Checking understanding is a form of information verification, which can involve skills such as asking the physician to repeat or clarify information that is unclear, repeating aloud the information that is provided to improve retention, or summarizing the information back to the physician in order to check understanding. Finally, Expressing concerns aims to bring to light any conflicts or concerns (e.g. religious, cultural) that may hinder treatment or the physician/patient interaction. Through open expression of these concerns, a mutual effort of resolution or accommodation can be reached. Towle and colleagues also used Cegala's PACE in their group-based workshops for seniors (17).

A different patient communication training curriculum was designed and utilized by Fisch and colleagues (16). The direct-to-consumer, community-based workshop for cancer patients and their families was divided into three sessions. Session 1 was entitled *Getting Through the Diagnosis/Prognosis Phase* and involved presentation and discussion of skills relevant to reviewing healthcare insurance, choosing the right physician, and slowing down to verify diagnosis, seek second opinions, and clarify information. Session 2, *Exploring Treatment Options*, consisted of informing patients of issues or barriers to understanding and then skills training to overcome these barriers. Often, problems such as being flooded with information, losing sense of control within a consultation and unfamiliar jargon can hinder understanding. This session helped inform patients of such issues that they may not be aware of, as well as teaching skills like asking questions and bringing support that can help to overcome such barriers. This session also aimed to expand patients' knowledge regarding the important aspects and points related to exploring treatment options. Finally, session 3, *Asking the Difficult Questions*, focused on dealing with terminal illness and death. Patients were provided with information and skills regarding emotional responses that they may encounter, coping with such emotions, informing loved ones, preparing for death, and self-assessment of faith, life, and final goals.

Still another patient communication training curriculum has been developed and used in community educational forums (15) by Tran and colleagues. These forums, entitled *How to Talk to Your Physician*, make use of presentations, a guidebook with question checklists, discussions, and tips for improving patient/physician communication. Most relevant to effective patient communication training are the tips for improving patient/physician communication. These are similar to Cegala's concept of PACE, but use an 'ABC' mnemonic to improve recall. The tips include: Asking questions to receive information; Being prepared for each visit; and expressing one's Concerns.

Outcomes of patient communication training

With only a few comprehensive patient communication training programmes published to date, our report on outcomes is limited. The outcomes reported in these studies can be divided into three types: patient self-efficacy, observations of patient skill usage, and patient adherence.

One simple outcome that can be assessed is how the communication training programme affected patients' self-efficacy. Results of the community education forum described by Tran *et al.* (15) indicated that, independent of facilitator and forum site, participants' confidence levels in their ability to communicate effectively with their physician increased. The finding that an increase in confidence was consistent across diverse community settings, suggests that the efficacy of the forum could be replicated across different communities. Furthermore, this effect was independent of the facilitator. However, post-intervention evaluations were given immediately following the forum, so it is unclear if the change in patient confidence levels was sustained over time.

An important and pragmatic outcome of patient communication intervention studies is the extent to which the intervention changed the patient's behaviour. Cegala and colleagues found that, compared to patients receiving materials-only or standard care, patients who received materials plus coaching were significantly engaged in more effective and efficient information-seeking, provided physicians with more detailed information about their medical condition, and used more summarizing utterances to verify information they received from physicians (9). Similar results were repeated in a study involving older patients (13). Patients receiving materials plus coaching engaged in significantly more information-seeking and provision, and obtained significantly more information from physicians.

If indeed a communication training programme can improve communication skills, then it follows that this should have some effect on more distal outcomes—such as treatment adherence. Cegala and colleagues found that, compared to patients receiving materials-only or a control group, patients who received materials plus coaching were significantly more compliant overall (12).

Other research has shown the importance of considering patient characteristics, such as race and culture, when formulating patient communication training programmes. In one such study, subjects received either a 14-page communication workbook 2–3 days pre-visit, a 2-page patient communication handout in the waiting room, or received standard care. There were significant differences in the effect of intervention on Caucasian patients and African-American patients. The workbook had a significant effect on Caucasian patients, compared to minimal or no effect on African-American patients. In particular, workbook-trained Caucasians asked more questions, obtained more information, had greater delayed recall, and greater adherence than their Caucasian counterparts in either of the other two groups. No such differences were found for African-American workbook-trained patients (14).

In sum, the limited literature on comprehensive patient communication training interventions indicates promising findings of the effect of these interventions on patient outcomes. Additional studies are necessary to continue to build an evidence base for effective patient communication training programmes.

One particular limitation of the current research in this area is a lack of a unifying theoretical or conceptual model. Descriptions of the studies reviewed here do not articulate a theoretical or conceptual framework to support their curriculum. Grounding communication training programmes in such a framework is useful in providing coherence to the curriculum, a rationale for the skills being taught and the assessment of those skills (19). To move patient communication training work forward, we advocate adopting concordance as a conceptual framework.

Concordance as a conceptual framework for patient communication interventions

Our approach to patient communication training is founded upon the same perspective that good provider communication is founded upon—concordance, or a shared agreement between the clinician and patient. Training for both clinicians and patients should be directed at attaining the goal of concordance. Current communication training programmes that are focused on patient-centredness and shared decision-making (20) attend to the clinician's role in achieving concordance. We believe that patient communication training programmes that are grounded in the notion of concordance will be the most effective in producing a good physician–patient relationship.

The concept of concordance with respect to regimen decision-making was introduced in 1997 by the Royal British Pharmaceutical Society. Joining calls for greater patient centred care and shared decision-making, concordance was introduced as a cooperative communication style to decrease the continuing 30–50% medication non-adherence rates. Concordance is defined as 'an agreement reached after negotiation between a patient and a health care professional that respects the beliefs and wishes of the patient in determining whether, when, and how medicines are to be taken' (21). Rather than a one-way transmission, the concordance framework depends on a two-way process, usually cooperative, where shared meaning is negotiated between the two participants (22). In this model, more attention is paid to mutual responsibility of both actors for the effect and effectiveness of the transaction. An underlying assumption is that the context and history of the conversation participants (physician and patient), as well as the other person's behaviour will influence each person's behaviour (22). The final product of the healthcare encounter is an agreed upon regimen to address the patient's health quality-of-life priorities. We propose that concordance can be present in, and should be the goal of, any physician–patient consultation, even when there is no need for a specific decision to be made or a regimen to be decided upon. Indeed, if we think of physician–patient communication as something that happens over a course of many individual consultations, it becomes clear that concordance transcends a discrete visit.

As Pollock (23) discusses, 'People seek to contain the disruption of illness, to reduce its significance and engage in lives that are fulfilling and, as far as possible, normal' (p.146). However, to do this implies a partnership with clinicians during the healthcare encounter that respects the patient's priorities and quality-of-life preferences. It is helpful to view the encounter as a communication pathway in which a clinician may offer options and ask for patient preferences; patients may or may not initiate or give preferences in response to provider requests; both parties offer rationales; and agreement is, or is not, reached on the final regimen (24). The concordance perspective recognizes that a patient may quite appropriately choose to delegate the decision role to the clinician; however, in one recent observational study, this occurred in only 7% of visits (25).

At its best, regimen agreement is sought during the encounter by a clinician who communicates much needed expertise and information and by a patient who communicates priorities, concerns, symptoms, and preferences. From this perspective, the patient's responsibility for observation, self-reflection, and communication is central to the communication framework. Patient, as well as provider, training is needed for the potential partnership process to result in concordance. While providers need training to offer options and ask for patient preferences, patients in turn may even need help recognizing that the clinician gave an option or the opportunity to state a preference. In a recent observational study, patients under-reported the number of times a physician was observed presenting them with an option or asking their preference (25).

Returning to the communication curriculum that Cegala and colleagues have developed (18), we see how each of these four skills is important to reaching concordance. First, patients need to be able to present information in a clear way in order for physicians to offer the right choices. Second, patients may need more information before offering a preference and, therefore, need to be able to ask questions. Third, patients may have concerns or criteria relevant to the decision that inform a preference or inform what the physician recommends. Learning how to effectively express concerns may be important. Fourth, in order to ensure that decisions are being made based on a shared understanding of information, patients should check their understanding of the information. These correspond with the four PACE skills (18). An emphasis that we believe should be added to this curriculum is training patients to articulate a clear preference when one is held.

The concordance concept of an encounter in which a decision is to be made involves negotiation in the transaction, where each party exchanges rationale and expertise to reach a mutually agreeable recommendation for care. The clinician who makes the decision without the input of the patient, does so in the dark. Expectations can be established to have the patient monitor regimens and report either qualitatively or systematically at the next visit. For example, the use of a side-effect monitoring tool assisted shared decision-making in a study of patients with cancer (26, 27). Monitoring is not simply about adverse effects or symptom relief, but how well the intervention serves the patient's quality-of-life priorities. It can inform not only the ongoing regimen decisions, but the administration of care, such as scheduling chemotherapy to minimize disruption in order to maintain a quality life (28). While clinician behaviours are critical to encouraging this involvement, patient training itself can help patients to expect to play these roles with reasonable self-efficacy.

Future areas of research

As noted by the National Cancer Institute in its recent monograph on communication in cancer care, the patient–physician interaction is a dynamic process with importance placed on the skills and approach of both parties. Improvement of communication, through skills training and intervention, may transform patients from passive recipients to active participants in care (29). With the idea of concordance in mind, we propose that future research should examine the following six broad research questions about cancer patient communication training.

RQ1: What is the acceptability and effectiveness of a concordance-based curriculum?

Developing and piloting a cancer patient communication training curriculum based on concordance can inform us of the usefulness of this as an approach to training. Such a curriculum would not replace, but would add to, the rigorously-tested components of the PACE framework. By establishing with trainees that the goal of their communication should be concordance with their clinician, the PACE skills can be put into a larger context providing a greater rationale for the skills.

RQ2: What are the most effective methods for training patients in communication skills?

Future research should compare the methods of training described above. For instance, studies could examine if the more economical group-based intervention is as effective as materials plus coaching. Within group-based interventions, there is a need to understand the best type of teaching. We know in physician training that experiential, role-play work is important to learning (30), but there is little written about role-play work in patient interventions. It is important to determine if role-play is an acceptable and effective component of patient communication interventions. Alternative types of instruction, such as trigger-videos, may be more acceptable and easier to facilitate, but it is unclear if it would be as effective as role play. Interactive media formats (e.g. DVDs, web-based programmes) should be explored as an alternative method and tested for their effectiveness.

RQ3: What patient outcomes can be improved by patient communication training?

Determining relevant outcomes and establishing measures of outcomes of patient communication training is essential. Conceptually, we find it helpful to think of these outcomes on a continuum, from proximal to distal. First, the most proximal outcome, and easiest to measure, is participant self-efficacy. Through self-reports given pre-training, immediately post-training, and later post-training (e.g. 6 months), self-efficacy can easily be assessed. Additionally, it is worth exploring whether current measures of cancer patient self-efficacy (31, 32) are valid outcome measures for patient communication training. If patients feel they have the ability to enact effective communication skills, the next logical outcome to be measured is whether they perform those skills in a clinical setting. Audio-recording and subsequent coding of patient–physician interactions allows for assessment of this outcome (13, 33). Patients' use of good communication skills should then lead to physician–patient concordance, an outcome which can be measured as well (34). Further, research has shown that when physicians and cancer patients are concordant about the emotion and information content of a consultation, patient satisfaction increases (35). Similar to this, more distal outcome of patient satisfaction would be patient adherence (12) and reduced anxiety (36).

RQ4: Which patient populations can benefit the most from patient communication training?

Given the characteristics and difficulties faced by certain populations, patient communication may best serve certain groups of individuals in terms of improving medical care and health outcomes. Research findings suggest that, compared to younger patients, older patients experience more difficulty actively interacting in medical consultations. Communication interventions have been shown to significantly increase older patients' information-seeking and provision, as well as receiving information from physicians (13). Given the prevalence of health disparities, an important aim of future research will be to examine the effectiveness of patient communication training as one way to decrease barriers caused by a lack of individual skills. In other words, patient communication training does not address care being denied or not available, but it can address care not being actualized because of inadequate patient communication skills. Research has shown that certain minorities and ethnic groups may be less responsive to communication intervention (33). However, lack of responsiveness may be better explained by method and/or content of intervention. For example, as discussed by Post *et al.* (33), African-American culture tends to be more oriented towards kinship and relations, making them less responsive to materials-only interventions. Minority populations may, therefore, benefit from tailored communication interventions that meet their specific needs, while maintaining consideration of, and sensitivity to, cultural and ethnic issues.

RQ5: Are there areas or topics of physician–patient communication that are particularly challenging, which may require focused patient communication training?

Two areas in particular that may benefit from focused communication training for patients are discussions about internet information and discussions about complementary and alternative medicine (CAM). Studies have shown several reasons why these discussions can be challenging for both physicians and patients. Some oncologists report that internet information has a harmful effect on the physician–patient relationship, particularly when patients directly challenge physicians or when patients have too much information (37). After reading cancer-related internet information, some patients become aware of conflicting medical information, and become overwhelmed, nervous, anxious, and confused (37–40). Discussions about internet information are unique in that they often include face-threatening messages and patients sometimes simply choose not to have the discussion because of these issues (41). Teaching patients how to approach these discussions in a collaborative way that acknowledges the physician's authority (42) may be a fruitful area for patient communication training and research.

Physician–patient discussions about CAM can also be fraught with challenges. Oncologists and their patients often hold very discrepant views on CAM, which creates barriers to effective communication (43). The National Center for Complementary and Alternative Medicine has recently begun a campaign to encourage patients and healthcare providers to talk about CAM usage (44). Further exploration of patient communication training programmes focused on CAM would be productive.

RQ6: What is the added benefit of patient communication training to programmes with provider communication training?

The establishment of valid patient communication training programmes that demonstrate key patient outcomes ultimately leads to the ability to examine the interaction of patient communication training with physician communication training. One design can be thought of as a 2×2 design, where physicians are either trained or untrained and their patients are either trained or untrained. Using some of the outcomes described above, such research could begin to examine the relative efficacy of training either or both parties in the physician–patient communication dyad.

Conclusion

Physician–patient communication is a dynamic, socially-constructed process that requires competent communication on both sides in order to be effective. Although work in training physicians has, and continues to be, critical, we need to expand our thinking to include how to best prepare patients to participate in consultations in ways that will lead to concordance. There is a paucity of published reports of comprehensive patient communication training interventions that move beyond question asking to include other important skills. Growing this area of training and research will contribute in significant and vital ways to scholarship on physician–patient communication and to patients' experiences.

References

1. Parker PA, Davison BJ, Tishelman C, *et al.* What do we know about facilitating patient communication in the cancer care setting? *Psycho-Oncology* 2005; **14**: 848–858.
2. Street R. Communication in medical encounters: an ecological perspective. In: Thompson T, Dorsey AM, Miller KI, *et al.*, editors. *Handbook of Health Communication*. Mahwah, NJ: Lawrence Erlbaum Associates; 2003.
3. Roter DL, Stewart M, Putnam SM, *et al.* Communication patterns of primary care physicians. *Journal of the American Medical Association* 1997; **277**(4): 350–356.
4. Marvel MK, Epstein RM, Flowers K, *et al.* Soliciting the patient's agenda: Have we improved? *Journal of the American Medical Association* 1999; **281**(3): 283–287.

5. Bylund CL, Makoul G. Examining empathy in medical encounters: an observational study using the Empathic Communication Coding System. *Health Communication* 2005; **18**(2): 123–140.

6. Chewning BA, Wiederholt JB. Concordance in cancer medication management. *Patient Education and Counseling* 2003; **50**: 75–78.

7. Brown RF, Butow PN, Dunn SM, *et al.* Promoting patient participation and shortening cancer consultations; a randomised trial. *British Journal of Cancer* 2001; **85**: 1273–1279.

8. Butow PN, Brown RF, Cogar S, *et al.* Oncologists' reactions to cancer patients verbal cues. *Psycho-Oncology* 2002; **11**: 47–58.

9. Cegala DJ, McClure L, Marinelli TM, *et al.* The effects of communication skills training on patients' participation during medical interviews. *Patient Education and Counseling* 2000; **41**(2): 209–22.

10. Golin CE, DiMatteo MR, Gelberg L. The role of patient participation in the doctor visit: Implications for adherence to diabetes care. *Diabetes Care* 1996; **19**: 1153–1164.

11. Brown RF, Butow PN, Boyer MJ, *et al.* Promoting patient participation in the cancer consultation; evaluation of a prompt sheet and coaching in question asking. *British Journal of Cancer* 1999; **80**(1/2): 242–248.

12. Cegala DJ, Marinelli T, Post D. The effects of patient communication skills training on compliance. *Archives of Family Medicine* 2000; **9**(1): 57–64.

13. Cegala DJ, Post DM, McClure L. The effects of patient communication skills training on the discourse of older patients during a primary care interview. *Journal of the American Geriatric Society* 2001; **49**(11): 1505–1511.

14. Post DM, Cegala DJ, Marinelli TM. Teaching patients to communicate with physicians: the impact of race. *Journal of the National Medical Association* 2001; **93**(1): 6–12.

15. Tran AN, Haidet P, Street RL, Jr. O'Malley KJ, Martin F, Ashton CM. Empowering communication: a community-based intervention for patients. *Patient Education and Counseling* 2004; **52**: 113–121.

16. Fisch M, Cohen MZ, Rutledge C, *et al.* Teaching patients how to improve communication with their healthcare providers: a unique workshop experience. *Journal of Cancer Education* 2003; **18**: 18–193.

17. Towle A, Godolphin W, Manklow J, *et al.* Patient perceptions that limit a community-based intervention to promote participation. *Patient Education and Counseling* 2003; **50**(3): 231–3.

18. Cegala DJ. *Communicating with your doctor: the PACE system.* 2000. Available from: **http: //patcom. jcomm.ohio-state.edu/index.htm**

19. Brown RF, Bylund CL. Communication skills training: describing a new conceptual model. *Academic Medicine* 2008; **83**(1): 37–44.

20.. Brown RF, Butow PN, Boyle F, Tattersall MH. Seeking informed consent to cancer clinical trials; evaluating the efficacy of doctor communication skills training. *Psycho-Oncology* 2007; **16**(6): 507–516.

21. RPSGB. *From Compliance to Concordance: achieving shared goals in medicine taking.* 1997 (cited 08.15.08). Available from: **http: //www.concordance.org**

22. Shah B, Chewning B. Conceptualizing and measuring pharmacist-patient communication: a review of published studies. *Research in Social and Adminstrative Pharmacy* 2006; **2**(2): 153–185.

23. Pollock K. *Concordance in Medical Consultations: a Critical Review.* Abingdon: Radcliffe Publishing Ltd; 2005.

24. Chewning B, Sleath B, Shah BK, *et al.* Concordance in medication decisions for reheumatoid arthritis: patient-provider discussion pathways. In: *European Association for Healthcare Communication.* Basle, Switzerland; September 2006.

25. Chewning B, Sleath B, Shah BK, *et al.* Comparing patient interviews to a concordance observational coding tool of the medication decision process. In: *International Conference on Communication in Healthcare.* Charleston, South Carolina; October 2007.

26. Hermansen-Kobulnicky CJ, Widerholdt JB, Chewning B. Adverse effect monitoring: opportunity for patient care and pharmacy practice. *Journal of the American Pharmacological Association* 2003: **44** (1): 75–86.

27. Hermansen-Kobulnicky CJ, Chewning, B. Teaching cancer patients to monitor side effects: An exploratory test ot increase shared decision making. In *European Conference on Communication in Healthcare*. Warwick, England; June 2002.

28. Wiederholt JB The patient: our teacher and friend. *American Journal of Pharmaceutical Education* 1997; **61**: 415–23.

29. Epstein RM, Street RL. Patient-centered communication in cancer care: promoting healing and reducing suffering. *National Cancer Institute, NIH Publication No. 07–6225. Bethesda, MD* 2007.

30. Kurtz S, Silverman J, Draper J. *Teaching and Learning Communication Skills in Medicine*. Abingdon: Radcliffe Medical Press Ltd; 1998.

31. Maly RC, Frank JC, Marshall GN, DiMatteo MR, Reuben DB. Perceived efficacy in patient-physician interactions (PEPPI): validation of an instrucment in older persons . *Journal of the American Geriatric Society* 1998; **46** (7) 889–94.

32. Wolf MS, Change CH, Davis T, Makoul G. Development and validation of the communication and attitudinal self-efficacy scale for cancer (CASE-cancer). *Patient Education and Counseling* 2005; **57**(3): 333–41.

33. Post DM, Cegala DJ, Marinelli TM. Teaching patients to communicate with physicians: the impact of race. *Journal of the National Medical Association* 2001; **93**(1): 6–12.

34. Like R, Zyzanski SJ. Patient requests in family practice: a focal point for clinical negotiations. *Family Practice* 1986; **3**(4): 216–228.

35. Brown RF, Hill C, Burant CJ, *et al.* Satisfaction of early breast cancer patients with discussions during initial oncology consultations with a medical oncologist. *Psycho-Oncology* 2009; **18**(1): 42–49.

36. Fogarty LA, Curbow JR, McDonnell K, *et al.* Can 40 seconds of compassion reduce patient anxiety? *Journal of Clinical Oncology* 1999; **17**: 371–379.

37. Broom A. Medical specialists' accounts of the impact of the Internet on the doctor/patient relationship. *Health (London)* 2005; **9**(3): 319–338.

38. Sabel MS, Strecher VJ, Schwartz JL, Wang TS, Karimipour DJ, Orringer JS, et al. Patterns of internet use and impact on patients with melanoma. *Journal of the American Academy of Dermatology* 2005: **52** (5): 779–85.

39. Helft PR, Eckles RE, Johnson-Calley CS, Daugherty CK. Use of the internet to obtain cancer information among cancer patients at an urban county hospital. *Journal of Clinical Oncology* 2005; **23** (22); 4954–62.

40. Fleisher L, Bass S, Ruzek SB, McKeown-Conn N. Relationships among internet health information use, patient behavior and self efficacy in newly diagnosed cancer patients who contact that National Cancer Institute's NCI Atlantic Region Cancer Information Service (CIS). *Proc AMIA Symp.* 2002: 260–264.

41. Imes R, Bylund CL, Routsong T, *et al.* Patients' reasons for refraining from discussing internet health information with their healthcare providers. *Health Communication* 2008.; **23**: 538–547.

42. Bylund CL, Sabee CM, Imes RS, *et al.* Exploration of the construct of reliance among patients who talk with their providers about internet information. *Journal of Health Communication* 2007; **12**(1): 17–28.

43. Richardson MA, Masse LC, Nanny K, Sanders C. Discrepant views of oncologists and cancer patients on complementary/alternative medicine. *Supportive Care in Cancer* 2004; **12** (11): 797–804.

44 NCCAM. Time To Talk. 2007. Available from: **http://nccam.nih.gov/timetotalk/**

Section F

International initiatives in communication training

Section editor: Barry D Bultz

This section demonstrates the efforts of leaders in communication training to advance programmes in their various jurisdictions and provides the reader with an opportunity to view a broad array of perspectives. In this section, training strategies and programmes from the United States, Switzerland, Australia, the United Kingdom, and Belgium are described in detail. These evidence-based communication training programmes offer insight into programme development and effective training procedures. Programme evaluation highlights the lessons learned and provides direction for moving forward with communication training programmes.

Chapter 54

The Oncotalk model

Robert M Arnold, Anthony T Back, Walter F Baile,
Kelly Fryer-Edwards, and James A Tulsky

In 2002, we received funding from the National Cancer Institute to develop a new teaching model for communication skills at the end of life, aimed at medical oncology fellows. Using this model, called Oncotalk, we have taught roughly 10% of the oncology fellows trained in the United States over a 5-year period. In developing the programme, we utilized key educational principles, some of which had been used in other communication skills training, others of which evolved as a result of the unique demands of the teaching context. Given our primary audience of oncology fellows, we paid particular attention to how we structured the programme in order to ground the learning in practical, patient care challenges that reflected their clinical experiences. Throughout the course of development, implementation, and evaluation of this project, we learned important lessons not previously discussed in the literature that can be taken up and tested further by other communication skills educators (1). Using our Oncotalk experience, this chapter will describe common evidence-based principles used in developing an advanced communication skills programme; identify unique aspects of the learning context within an intensive retreat structure, and illustrate the lessons learned that can be tested in other settings. The aim is to provide tools and frameworks to facilitate teaching communication skills within oncology and other clinical training programmes that prepare clinicians to work with seriously ill patients.

Why have Oncotalk?

A variety of studies document shortcomings in communication between physicians and patients with advanced cancer (2). First, the literature suggests that oncologists do not often talk to patients with advanced cancer about palliative care (3). Even when discussions occur, poor quality frequently undermines their usefulness. Tulsky *et al.* found that physicians who do talk about advanced care planning focus largely on treatments, rarely give patients enough information to make informed decisions, and neglect more general values and goals (4, 5).

Deficiencies in communication are common. For example, a variety of studies have shown that oncologists rarely discuss issues surrounding quality of life with patients who have advanced cancer (6). It is, therefore, no surprise that most oncologists are inaccurate in their assessment of patient's emotional distress (7).When patients express negative emotions, their doctors typically respond by changing the subject, by providing reassurance, or by providing cognitive information (8).

Oncologists' communication skills are likely sub-optimal because, until recently, they have received little training in this area. A survey of over 3200 American Society of Clinical Oncology members found that few had formal training in end-of-life care or communication skills (9). More recently, fellows revealed that only 15% had any exposure to communication skills training (10). While the American Council of Graduate Medical Education includes communication skills as a core competency for all oncology fellows, little of this education relates to communication with patients having advanced cancer (11). Oncology fellows reported in one study that they felt more capable talking about chemotherapy side-effects than discussing ending chemotherapy and focusing on quality of life (12). While fellows routinely have difficult conversations with seriously ill patients, only 56% of them report being observed and getting feedback on these conversations by their attending physicians (12).

A number of important organizations have called for improved communication skills at the end of life. The National Cancer Institute designated cancer communication as an 'extraordinary scientific priority' in 2002, and developed a Health Communication and Informatics Research Branch. An Institute of Medicine report entitled *Ensuring Quality Cancer Care* recommended that cancer treatment discussions should represent shared decision-making between oncologist and patient, which requires that the oncologist have excellent communication skills (13). Finally, the National Institute of Health State of the Science in End of Life Care summary statement concluded that 'effective communication is critical' to improving outcomes in end-of-life care (14). This combination of empirical data and institutional reports led to broad support for developing a centralized training programme like Oncotalk.

Evidence-based principles for teaching communication skills

A Cochrane systematic review of communication skills training for healthcare providers working with cancer patients and their families conclude that: communication skills do not reliably improve with experience alone; and training programmes using appropriate educational techniques are effective in improving skills (18). Studies of oncologists, internists and family medicine physicians demonstrate that after communication skills training, doctors discuss more psychosocial issues, use more open-ended questions, are better able to elicit patients' values and feelings, and attend to distress (15–17).

A theory of teaching communication skills

At the centre of the Oncotalk design for both intervention and evaluation is self-efficacy theory (19). In self-efficacy theory, the impetus for change resides in the individual's efficacy expectations. These expectations reflect the learner's beliefs about his/her ability to perform the task. Efficacy expectations are acquired from four sources: performance accomplishments, vicarious experience, verbal persuasion, and emotional state (18, 20, 21, 22).

Based on this theoretic model and the Cochrane review, we chose the following design features for the Oncotalk intervention:

1. Brief didactic sessions to provide specific communication models. A systematic review of continuing medical education indicates that traditional lecture-based conferences have little direct effect on changing physician performance. That being said, it is still necessary to provide a cognitive map for the upcoming skill practice. Didactics are minimized and focus on both rationale for, and demonstration of, specific skills. Thus, Oncotalk limits didactics to thirty minute blocks in which specific skills were identified and illustrated.

2. Skill practice with group feedback. Previous studies indicate that demonstration of new skills is not sufficient. Successful programmes have the participant try new behaviours and receive immediate feedback on their performance. Oncotalk focused over 75% of its time on skill practice within a small group of fellows, allowing them to receive immediate feedback from their peers and see how other fellows interacted with patients.

3. Use of simulated patients. The use of simulated patients allows the participant to learn, in an environment approximating clinical practice, the exact skills that they will use in clinical

practice. In addition, using simulated patients allows the participant to rewind and try the same scenario in different ways. Finally, simulated patients can be trained to provide immediate feedback on his or her experience of the participant's behaviour. Oncotalk uses five simulated patient cases in which the patient story unfolds over four visits, allowing the learners to give bad news, negotiate treatment goals, and talk about end-of-life issues.

4. Focusing on the participant's needs. Allowing the participants open time to focus on self-identified skills and challenges is key. Research in adult learning indicates that learning must be relevant to a valued task, immediately transferable, and participant-centred. Didactics and structured skill practice can target participant goals, but some open space should be utilized to address unique participant challenges. Oncotalk did this in two ways. First, participants were asked to identify their learning goals before every practice session. Second, open sessions, in which fellows role-played their most difficult patients, were scheduled to allow fellows to name and work on encounters that were particularly important and challenging to them.

5. Attend to participants' attitudes and emotions. Successful courses address physician attitudes and emotions, as well as knowledge and skill deficits. Caring for oncology patients, particularly dying patients, can elicit strong feelings in the physician. Most courses spend some time focusing on emotional issues, either by integrated discussion within the skill practice sessions or as a separate reflective session on specific emotional issues. In addition to talking about fellows' emotions during practice sessions, Oncotalk included specific reflective exercises to help fellows think about their professional identity and to consider what might be possible for their clinical practice going forward.

6. Because of the complexity of the teaching and the challenging nature of the learning, we chose an intensive retreat as the primary educational intervention for teaching communication skills. While possible to do in shorter sessions over a longer time period within the healthcare setting, removing fellows from their daily work routine allowed them to leave their pagers behind and encouraged them to focus on learning. Oncotalk is scheduled in an intense three-and-a-half day block of time.

These basic teaching and learning components of the Oncotalk programme are then populated with specific core content (23).

Core cognitive maps in end-of-life communication

While details in the literature on communication skills in end-of-life care vary, we identified a core set of common communication skills. Our objective in the didactic sessions was to provide the fellows with a cognitive overview of these core skills. Then in the skills practice session, they could practice the skills, including skill practice for when predictable and unpredictable challenges arise.

We emphasized a foundation with three basic skills in our first session. 'Ask tell ask' requires that participants assess the patient's experience prior to giving information and then inquire about what the patient heard. Second, encouraging the patient to tell the story was taught using open-ended questions and phrases such as, 'Tell me more.' Finally, we provided several tools for responding with empathy using the acronym NURSE: **N**ame the emotion, show that you **U**nderstand the emotion, **R**espect the patient's experience, use **S**upportive statements, and **E**xplore the patient's experience (24).

The foundational skills were repeated throughout the task-specific communication skills. Following a trajectory of illness, we began with the task-specific skill of giving bad news. We teach this skill using the SPIKES (Setting, Preparation, Information, Knowledge, Empathy, Strategy) acronym (9). Participants find this acronym helpful as it gives them a structured way to think about an emotionally difficult task. This acronym relies heavily on the core skills taught in the first session as it suggests:

(1) asking the patient's perception before given the bad news; and

(2) empathizing with the patient's emotional reaction before going on to make a plan.

Giving bad news is central to talking about transitioning from curative to palliative goals of care. Talking about transitions requires that an oncologist be able to give bad news and then help the patient come up with other goals in the time that they have remaining. This requires skills such as first recognizing the transitions discussion as a bad-news discussion, then employing specific communication strategies, such as hoping for the best, preparing for the worst (25), and attending to loss, and the shift in expectations using wish statements (26).

Finally, like most clinicians who work with seriously ill patients, oncologists have to learn to talk about dying in an explicit fashion. Talking about dying requires the learners to integrate the skills outlined above, including: the ability to integrate giving bad news while attending to strong emotions, and to assess the patient's fears, concerns, and hopes. We explicitly speak about how these skills integrate to achieve two new communication challenges: talking about code status (DNR) and saying goodbye to a patient (27).

Teaching using simulated patients

One of the ways we emphasize the developmental aspects of skills is to use a simulated patient case study. Each patient's story unfolds over five sessions and the participant is given a specific task at each (see Table 54.1). Using the time-series case studies has many advantages. First, by working with the same patient over an illness trajectory, it allows the participants to develop a relationship with the patient, making the emotional work more realistic. Second, because each day focuses on a specific skill in a specific order, participants learn basic skills before moving on to complex ones. Finally, by having five distinct patients we can ensure that the participants experience (either directly or vicariously) a diverse set of patients. For example, the patients responded to bad news with different emotional responses—anger, sadness, disbelief, frustration, and overwhelmed—each of which required a different response from the participant.

Table 54.1 Communication skills curriculum based on illness trajectory

Session	Content focus	Skills practice with simulated patient
1	Developing a relationship. Dealing with uncertainty.	47 Female with breast cancer after lumpectomy, chemotherapy, radiation 1 year ago seen for routine surveillance, notes some back pain.
2	Giving bad news.	1 week later: bone scan ordered last visit shows multiple metastases; CT shows liver metastases.
3	Transition to palliative care.	3 years later: now having received multiple chemotherapy regimens, with disease progression on therapy.
4	Discussing do-not-resuscitate orders.	2 months later: at home with hospice, told nurse she 'wants everything'.

From reference 28.

The Oncotalk experience[1]

Between April 2002 and June 2007, 180 medical oncology fellows, mostly in the 2nd and 3rd years of their fellowship, were asked to participate in three-and-a-half day intensive communication skills retreats. We ran two courses a year and had 20 participants per retreat, allowing us to run small groups with a 5:1 faculty to participant ratio. Based on our sample sized calculations, evaluative data were collected on 120 participants, distributed in training programmes across the United States (28).

The programme evaluation includes both self-evaluation measures of competence and satisfaction, as well as a comparison of pre-retreat and post-retreat encounters with standardized patients (see 26 for a complete description of the methods). Each participant completed two pre-retreat and two post-retreat simulations—one focusing on giving bad news and the other on transitioning to palliative care. The evaluative standardized patient encounters were audio-taped and were analysed for behaviour change by independent and blind coders. The investigators developed a coding instrument consisting of a set of observable behaviours for each communication task. The codes were intended to represent best practice communication behaviours that could be recognized by coders with adequate inter-rater reliability. The task-specific codes for bad news, for example, were based on the literature and the SPIKES acronym. Finally, as part of the audio-tape evaluation, we asked the coders to guess whether the tape they were listening to was done pre- or post-intervention.

The participants' evaluations of Oncotalk have been overwhelmingly enthusiastic. For example, they rated the statement, 'I would recommend this training to other fellows' (mean = 4.95 on a 5-point Likert scale). All components of the retreat were highly rated.

Respondents clearly learned skills that they did not know prior to the retreat. For example, of the participants who, prior to the retreat, did not respond empathically after giving bad news, 73% did so after the retreat. In response to the required standardized patient statement, 'I'm really scared', 100% of the participants who had not responded empathically to this cue in the pre-test were able to do so post-retreat. We also measured whether participants were able to use empathic statements. Post-retreat, both the number and the types of empathic responses markedly increased. Participants acquired a median of six new communication skills related to giving bad news.

Similar improvements were found in participants' skill in discussing transitions to palliative care. In post-retreat encounters, participants demonstrated statistically significant skill acquisition in the following skills: assessing understanding, discussing the overall clinical picture, responding to emotion, and asking about worries, fears, and concerns. Again a large number of participants improved their skills. For example, when the standardized patient hears that palliative chemotherapy is no longer working and asks 'Isn't there anything more you can do?', 92% of the participants pre-retreat did not include an empathic or an 'I wish' statement in their response. Post-retreat, approximately a third of these participants used one of these responses.

Finally, blinded coders were able to correctly identify pre- or post-retreat participants in 91% of the bad news and 70% of the transition audio-recordings (28).

What we learned from Oncotalk

In developing and implementing Oncotalk, we learned a number of important and somewhat unexpected lessons about how to teach communication skills. First, we learned about the

---

1. Portions of this section are modified from reference 28.

importance of trust in the small group. In early renditions of Oncotalk, we had participants spend time in both small groups of five, where they did skills practice, and larger groups of ten, where they did their reflective exercises. Participants felt more comfortable talking about their emotions and worries in the small groups because they had spent time as a cohort and had taken risks together. In our follow-up teaching sessions, we have paid more attention to the importance of trust within the group. Now, all teaching, reflective exercises and follow-ups take place in the same five-person small groups.

Second, in teaching these sessions, we began to see a common developmental learning process. Participants have to first recognize an emotion in the encounter (the patient seems emotional), then name this emotion (the patient's emotion is sadness), and finally they need to be able to respond empathically to the patient's emotion ('You seem really sad'). While many communication skills programmes emphasize the words to say to patients, developing a sense for the learning trajectory helped us target our feedback and learning experiences to move a participant towards responding genuinely to a patient's needs. Different insights will move participants along the trajectory at a different pace. Some insights are instrumental, meaning that the conversation can move forward after responding to a patient's emotion in a genuine way; others involve a shift in how the participants come to see their responsibility to develop a therapeutic alliance with the patient. Either insight helps move them forward toward recognizing and responding to emotions.

Third, we were impressed by the importance of participants' own emotions in learning communication skills. Most of the participants knew how to give bad news and they could quickly tell you the cognitive steps involved in SPIKES. However, in the process of having to give the news, even to standardized patients, they got tripped up by their own emotions. Sadness led them to hedge or to provide false reassurance, or their anxiety led them to move quickly into a treatment plan before the patient was ready to hear it. It was critical for us to acknowledge the participant's sadness and the powerlessness in preventing the progression of cancer. Once faculty attended to the participant's own sadness, they were better able to cope with the patient's sadness. To a certain degree, we were role modelling how to be empathetic regarding emotion. Moreover, by normalizing their emotions, we allowed them to be more comfortable in feeling emotions when talking about death and dying. Finally, some participants worried about being overwhelmed by the patient's emotions and thus blocked discussion of difficult topics. The use of simulated patients allowed us to take a time-out for discussion, if the participant seemed overwhelmed.

Fourth, our Oncotalk experience helped teach us the importance of positive feedback and reflection. For decades sociologists have commented on the punitive and negative teaching methods used in medical education. To a certain degree, the participants came to Oncotalk wanting to learn what 'they did wrong'. This meant that they did not appreciate their strengths in communicating with patients and, therefore, could not make a conscious effort to use them when stuck. Once a participant saw that they were viewed by others as calm and empathic, they could be more intentional in using these skills when a patient got upset. In addition, once the participants recognized their strengths, they were more willing to self-identify their weaknesses.

This lesson of emphasizing the positive occurred in the other sessions, as well as within the skill practice sessions. For example, initially in the didactics we role-played bad encounters and asked the participants to comment on what could have been done differently. Based on the feedback, we realized that many of the participants had never had the skills of a good communication encounter described. They needed a positive role model to demonstrate and name each of the skills that one uses in a difficult discussion. We, therefore, modified the curriculum and focused on role-plays that illustrated how the encounters should go.

The reflective sessions also changed over time to emphasize positive experiences. In the initial Oncotalk retreats, our reflective sessions dealt with loss or participants' most difficult encounters. These sessions elicited little discussion and received the most negative feedback of the entire retreat. Therefore, about half-way through the sessions, we changed the exercises to focus on the positive aspects of healing. For example, rather than have them talk about the most difficult death, we asked them to talk about the last time they felt like a healer. By focusing on the positive aspects of communication, the participants got in touch with why they went into oncology in the first place and how they could utilize their clinical skills to promote more healing. Following this change, the sessions received better participant evaluations.

Finally, Oncotalk helped us see the importance of skills practice that enables participants to experience success. Participants often want to practice in the hardest possible situation, what we called 'cases from hell'. The problem in these situations is that it is very hard to experience success. Regardless of what the participant does, the case goes badly, decreasing self-efficacy and confidence. We, therefore, focused on helping the participant identify their 'learning edge' (i.e. work that would be challenging for the participant, but not overwhelming). The goal was to encourage the participant to choose to work on a skill on which they have yet to achieve competency, but not one where they are unlikely to succeed. By succeeding they learned how the new skills positively impacted the simulated patient, which in turn, encouraged them to try the skills again.

These teaching skills helped us envision the process of oncology communication skill learning as a series of steps resulting in a positive feedback loop:

◆ the participant hears feedback about strengths from the group;

◆ the participant identifies a salient skill that requires work;

◆ the participant practices these skills in a small group with trusted colleagues;

◆ the participant achieves some success in learning the new skill; and

◆ the participant reflects on their progress and revises their learning goal based on the session (1).

Conclusion

Over a 5-year period, we trained 10% of America's oncology fellows. Oncotalk represents a successful model of a residential communication skills course, and given the behaviour change outcomes, represents a benchmark for this kind of teaching model.

Oncotalk, however, is only the first step. A number of factors need to be addressed before oncological communication training can be scaled up to serve more healthcare professionals. The first factor is the most difficult: faculty teaching capacity. There are few oncology faculty with training in the facilitation and communication skills required to conduct this teaching. Given this, we have begun a follow-up project entitled Oncotalk Teach, designed to begin training a cohort of oncology faculty who can use Oncotalk principles in communication teaching done at their home institutions, using real-time clinical encounters. The other factors, while notable, are not quite as difficult: the course is relatively expensive, requires time off from clinical respon-sibilities, and requires the commitment from training programmes to prioritize this aspect of education for oncologists in training. However, the advantage of training a cadre of local com-munication experts is that communication can be integrated into fellows' clinical training, much like other important educational objectives.

Oncotalk has shown that we can improve fellows' communication skills. The next genera-tion of courses needs to build on this success in order to ensure that all oncologists are skilled in communicating with their cancer patients.

References

1. Edwards-Fryer K, Arnold RM, Baile W, *et al.* Teaching communication skills: a qualitative study of reflective teaching practices. *Academic Medicine.* 2006; **81**: 638–644.

2. Barclay JS, Blackhall LJ, Tulsky JA. Communication strategies and cultural issues in the delivery of bad news. *J Palliat Med.* 2007; **10**(4): 958–977.

3. Gattellari M, Voigt KJ, Butow PN, *et al.* (2002). When the treatment goal is not cure: are cancer patients equipped to make informed decisions? *J Clin Oncol.* 2002; **20**(2): 503–513.

4. Tulsky JA, Fischer GS, Rose MR, *et al.* Opening the black box: How do physicians communicate about advance directives? *Ann Int Med.* 1998; **129**(6): 441–449.

5. Roter DL, Larson S, Fischer GS, *et al.* Experts practice what they preach: a descriptive study of best and normative practices in end-of-life discussion. *Arch Int Med.* 2000; **160**: 13477–13485.

6. Detmar SB, Muller MJ, Wever LD. The patient–physician relationship; patient–physician communication during outpatient palliative treatment visits: an observational study. *JAMA.* 2001; **285**(10): 1351–1357.

7. Ford S, Fallowfield L, Lewis S. Can oncologists detect distress in their out-patients and how satisfied are they with their performance during bad news consultations? *Br J Cancer.* 1994; **70**(4): 767–770.

8. Pollak KI, Arnold RM, Jeffreys A, *et al.* Oncologist communication about emotion during visits with advanced cancer patients. *J Clin Onc.* 2007; **25**: 5748–5752.

9. Baile WF, Buckman R, Lenzi R, *et al.* SPIKES-A six-step protocol for delivering bad news: application to the patient with cancer. *Oncologist.* 2000; **5**(4): 302–311.

10. Hoffman M, Ferri J, Sison C, *et al.* Teaching communication skillsL an AACE survey of oncology training programmes. *J Cancer Ed.* 2004: **19**(4): 220–224.

11. Weissman DE, Block SD. ACGME requirements for end-of-life training in selected residency and fellowship programmes: a status report. *Acad Med.* 2002; **77**: 299–304.

12. Buss M, Lessen DS, Sullivan AM, *et al.* A study of oncology fellows' training in end-of-life care. *J Supp Onc.* 2007: **5**(5): 237–245.

13. Hewih M, Simme JV, eds. *Ensuring Quality Cancer Care.* Washington D.C.: National Academy Press, 1999.

14. State of the Science Conference Statement. *Improving End-of-Life Care.* National Institutes of Health, 2004. Available from: http: //**consensus.nih.gov/2004/2004EndOfLifeCareSOS024html.htm**

15. Roter DL, Hall JA, Kern DE, *et al.* Improving physicians' interviewing skills and reducing patients' emotional distress. A randomized clinical trial. *Arch Intern Med.* 1995; **155**(17): 1877–1884.

16. Fallowfield L, Jenkins V, *et al.* Efficacy of a Cancer Research UK communication skills training model for oncologists: a randomized controlled trial. *Lancet.* 2002; **359**(9307): 650–656.

17. Delvaux N, Merckaert I, Marchal S, *et al.* Physician communication with a cancer patient and a relative: a randomized study assessing the effects of consolidation workshops. *Cancer.* 2005; **103**(11): 2397–2411.

18. Fellowes D, Wilkinson S, Moore P. Communication skills training for health care professionals working with cancer patients, their families and/or careers. *Cochrane Database Syst Rev* (2) 2004: CD003751.

19. Bandura A. Self-efficacy mechanism in human agency. *Am Psychol.* 1982; **37**: 122–147.

20. Maguire P, Faulkner A. Improve the counseling skills of doctors and nurses in cancer care. *Br Med J.* 1988; **297**: 847–849.

21. Kurtz S, Silverman J, Draper J. *Teaching and Learning Communication Skills in Medicine,* 2nd edition. Radcliffe Medical Press; 2005.

22. Carroll JG, Lipkin M, Nachtigall L, *et al.* (eds.) *A Developmental Awareness for Teaching Doctor–Patient Communication Skills. The Medical Interview.* New York: Springer; 1995: 388–396.

23. Back A, Arnold RM, Tulsky J, *et al.* Teaching communication skills to medical oncology fellows. *J Clin Onc.* 2003; **21**(12): 2433–2436.

24. Smith RC, Hoppe RB. The patient's story: integrating the patient-and physician-centered approaches to interviewing. *Ann Intern Med.* 1991; **115**(6): 470–47.

25. Evans W, Tulsky J, Back A, *et al.* Communication at times of transitions: how to help patients cope with loss and re-define hope. *The Cancer Journal.* 2006; **12**(5): 417–424.

26. Back, A, Arnold RM, Quill T. Hoping for the best, preparing for the worst. *Ann Int Med.* 2003; **138**(5): 439–444.

27. Back AL, Arnold RM, Tulsky JA, *et al.* On saying goodbye: acknowledging the end of the patient-physician relationship with patients who are near death. *Ann Intern Med.* 2004 **142**(8); 682–685.

28. Back AL, Arnold RM, Baile WF, *et al.* Efficacy of communication skills training based on illness trajectory for medical oncology fellows. *Arch Int Med.* 2007; **167**: 453–50.

Chapter 55

The Swiss model

Stiefel F, Bernhard J, Bianchi G, Dietrich L, Hürny Ch, Kiss A and Wössmer B

The Swiss Communication Skills Training (CST) for oncology clinicians was initiated in 1998 by the Swiss Cancer League (SCL), who mandated a national task force[1] to elaborate a concept for a CST for oncology physicians and nurses (1). In order to learn about key elements of existing CST, the task force, together with the SCL, organized a meeting with three invited experts—Leslie Fallowfield and Peter Maguire from the United Kingdom, and Darius Razavi from Belgium—who presented their models by means of interactive workshops; chiefs of service and head nurses from different oncology centres participated in this meeting. Based on these experiences, the task force developed a concept for a national CST for oncology clinicians.

Initially, a train the trainers' course was organized for the members of the task force allowing them to experience the CST as participants and to gain insight into its dynamics. Following a pilot CST, organized in the German, French, and Italian parts of Switzerland for local chiefs of oncology services and head nurses, the Swiss CST was implemented; it was officially endorsed by the Swiss Society of Medical Oncology (SSMO), and sponsored by two pharmaceutical companies who were willing to financially support this training during the first years.

In 2001, the SSMO declared this CST to be mandatory for physicians specializing in oncology. By the end of 2007, about four hundred physicians and nurses working with cancer patients had participated in this training.

Setting of the Swiss CST

Several times a year, a CST for up to ten participants is organized by two of the trainers. The trainers have extensive experience in psycho-oncology; their professional background is psychiatry, psychology, internal medicine and nursing, and all of them have been trained in psychoanalytic, systemic or cognitive-behavioural psychotherapy or in psychosomatic medicine and supervision. The CST starts with a 2-day course, followed by four to six individual supervisions and ends with a half-day course 6 months later. The training is based on case discussions, role-plays, and video-analyses of participants' interviews with a patient simulated by an actor (each participant is filmed at the beginning and the end of the training). The Swiss CST provides only a very limited amount of theory; it is mainly based on interactivity and practical exercises by means of case presentations, role-plays, analyses of video sequences, and guided imagery.

---

1. The initial task force consisted of: M Andrey, J Bernhard, A Bischoff, L Dietrich, Ch Hürny, A Kesselring, A Kiss, F Stiefel, M Tomamichel and B Wössmer.

Objectives of the Swiss CST

The training focuses on four elements of communication: (1) structure, (2) exchange of information, (3) emotions and (4) relational aspects. While these elements are interdependent and occur simultaneously, for didactic reasons they will be discussed separately and illustrated by examples.

Structure

The training aims to raise participants' awareness of structural elements of the consultation, such as the setting (time, space, participants, etc.), negotiation of the patient's and clinician's agenda, announcement of transitions to new topics during the interview and regular intermediate syntheses of what has been discussed. The example in Box 55.1, taken from a CST, illustrates the difficulty of a nurse to follow a coherent structure, changing topics rapidly and without announcing the transitions.

Exchange of information

Participants of the training learn that different types of questions (closed, open and leading questions) have different functions within a consultation. They also learn that non-verbal expression of time pressure can hamper exchange of information, while a concentrated interest in the patient can facilitate the exchange of information. Training also focuses on using language that can be understood by the patient; limiting the amount of information provided; checking patient comprehension; and identifying anxiety or other sources of a diminished capacity, which may affect patient retention of information. Box 55.2 illustrates an exchange of information characterized by medical jargon, which may not be understood by the patient.

Emotions

The CST teaches how emotions of the patient can be perceived (verbal and non-verbal expression) and how they can be contained in an empathic manner. Participants learn to distinguish between a cognitive expression (communicating information) and an emotional expression (communicating a feeling), and learn how to respond accordingly. Box 55.3 illustrates the failure of a clinician to recognize this distinction and then responds with a cognitive, medical answer, instead of providing empathic support.

Box 55.1 Structure—chaotic and transitions not announced

Nurse: Before you receive chemotherapy, we will give you a medication to help with the nausea.

Patient: …good.

Nurse: Chemotherapy is not always associated with nausea, but we would like to prevent it, that's why we prescribe you this medication…. Where do you work?

Patient: I own a small factory…

Nurse: The chemotherapy should be well tolerated; we only give you this medication as a precaution.

Patient: OK.

Box 55.2 Exchange of information—jargon, lack of checking

Physician: You describe what sounds like a paraneoplastic phenomenon.

Patient: Can't we do something, where does it come from?

Physician: Paraneoplastic syndromes have different origins. It is difficult to treat.

Patient: But I thought that I have only cancer…

Physician: Paraneoplastic symptoms may be related to immunological responses induced by your cancer.

Patient: Immunological responses?

Physician: Yes, immunological responses, leading to paraneoplastic syndromes induced by cancer, very rare…

Relational aspects

Relational aspects of the interview are important, but difficult for participants to perceive. Relational aspects are discussed by viewing and analysing selected video sequences and role-plays. Sequences characterized by abrupt transitions from one topic to another; an escalation of an underlying relational dynamic; inadequate non-verbal expressions or stagnation in a topic, are used to illustrate relational aspects of communication. Participants recognize that effective communication is not concerned with the question 'who is right?' and are trained to let the patients express their views and to accept that different views can coexist. Box 55.4 illustrates how the anxiety of a clinician, projected on to the patient, leads to the proposition of a consultant instead of first clarifying the patient's needs.

Box 55.3 Emotions (deception)—failure to let the patient develop his perspective and failure to provide empathic support

Physician: To summarize, the results show that the cancer has come back.

Patient: But I thought that I was cured!

Physician: I told you two years ago…

Patient: That doesn't make sense, I don't want any further treatment.

Physician: I would suggest a new chemotherapy…

Patient: With the same results?

Physician: Chemotherapy may reduce the tumour mass and prolong your life.

Patient: I don't know; this is so unexpected.

Physician: Palliative chemotherapy could have a positive impact.

> ## Box 55.4 Relational aspects—projection of anxiety and introduction of a consultant without clarifying concerns
>
> Patient: I do understand. The operation was only partly successful and now chemotherapy seems necessary?
>
> Physician: That's correct.
>
> Patient: (sighs) My kids are still small and...
>
> Physician: We do have psycho-oncologists, they could be of help.
>
> Patient: I would like first to think about everything.
>
> Physician: I just thought that maybe you feel lonely and the kids...
>
> Patient: No, my husband is very supportive.

While improvements with the first three elements (structure, exchange of information and containing emotions) can be obtained within the first two days of the training, relational aspects are more easily discussed in individual supervision.

Observations from the Swiss CST

Communication difficulties in the video-taped interviews are identified by an unbalanced focus on medical issues, a predominance of closed questions, abrupt transitions from one topic to another, interruptions of the patient, premature or inadequate comforting or avoidance of patients' concerns. For each participant, different sequences of their filmed interviews are selected and discussed.

With regard to the different elements of the interview, we observe the following difficulties during the training. Interviews are 'under-structured' (e.g. when talking to anxious patients) or 'over-structured', with the consequence that the patient is deprived of the possibility to exist as an individual. Information is not adapted to the patient's needs: clinicians show difficulties distinguishing between cognitive and emotional expressions of the patient; questions are answered without clarifying underlying concerns; and the comprehension of the provided information is not checked. Emotions of the patient are not identified or are avoided, and helplessness exists as to how to respond to an irritated, anxious or sad patient. Inadequate relational reactions from clinicians are linked to specific situations, such as the limits of medical treatment, transition between curative and palliative treatment or the patient's refusal to comply with prescriptions; in such moments, clinicians are subjected to pressure and may lose the capacity to continue to support the patient and respond with empathy.

Specificities of the Swiss model: interdisciplinary training, individual supervision and mandatory training

Interdisciplinary training is a key element of the Swiss CST. Working with both nurses and physicians allows the opportunity to, not only to practise interdisciplinary communication, which is often a major problem in daily clinical care, but also the opportunity to recognize the specific challenges and responsibilities of each profession through the case discussions and video-taped interviews.

We have observed differences between professions with regard to communication skills. In general, physicians have a good capacity to structure the interview, to adequately provide medical information and to assume leadership during the consultation. On the other hand, physicians sometimes structure the interview in a way that hinders the discussion of certain topics, such as prognosis of the disease; they forget to check if the information has been understood by the patient; and have difficulties perceiving the emotional climate, and may react with irritation when confronted with 'difficult' patients. Nurses usually show a good capacity to obtain sensitive information, to facilitate emotional expression and to contain patients who are angry, anxious or depressed. On the other hand, they sometimes loose leadership during the interview, have difficulties changing back to the medical agenda or to end a consultation, and are inclined to take the blame when the patient is irritated by the disease, its treatments or the physicians.

However, working with participants of different professional backgrounds also has disadvantages. If, for example, a professional group is over-represented, specific topics of the minority may be neglected and some participants may feel inhibited to discuss sensitive issues in front of the other profession.

After the initial 2-day training, participants attended four to six individual supervisions over the next 6 months. In the French part of Switzerland, supervision is provided either in the trainer's office or, more rarely, in the oncologist's office. In other parts of Switzerland, supervision is conducted over the phone due to geographical distances. Participants wish to discuss very different issues in the supervision; some like to work on audio- or video-taped consultations, others demand to reflect on difficult cases or ask for 'live supervision', with the supervisor being present in the medical consultation.

Often participants present a 'difficult patient' and then, through supervision, recognize that the problem they encounter is related to their own communicational difficulties. For example, a young oncologist who worked in a palliative care unit presented the case of a 55-year-old man with brain metastases who asked for another MRI. After the oncologist replied that 'this was not necessary any more', the patient refused to speak to him for three days. During supervision, the oncologist recognized that instead of clarifying the underlying concerns of the patient's question, he had responded with a 'medically correct', but empathically inadequate, answer.

Sometimes supervision may also lead to a reflection on a participant's personal issues that are affecting communication. For example, an oncologist presented the case of an elderly patient suffering from advanced breast cancer, who complained about pain but at the same time refused analgesic treatment; the oncologist became so angry that he started shouting at her. During supervision, the clinician first realized that this 'unreasonable behaviour' of the patient may have had a hidden meaning (preservation of autonomy, fears associated with pain medication, etc.). Once the clinician realized these possible sources of the patient's behaviour, he was able to reflect on his own strong emotional reaction. He reported that he not only felt angry, but also very anxious when he shouted at the patient, and linked his reaction to his own medical history of melanoma three years ago: 'I would certainly not be alive any more if I had not followed the doctor's advice and someone not following medical advice had certainly provoked this great deal of anxiety'. During follow-up supervisions he became more and more aware of how his own medical history affected his psychological state and interfered, as in the case he presented, with his clinical work. The presented case was finally understood as a collusion (a reaction of the clinician, which is shaped by an unconscious and unresolved problem he shares with the patient): both were struggling with dependency/independency issues, manifested in the patient by the refusal to accept pain medication and in the physician by the refusal to integrate that he had recently been himself a patient. These insights and the experience of the supervision with a mental health professional motivated this oncologist to enter psychotherapy.

The 'narcissistic deconstruction' that participants experience when confronted with their filmed interview in CST often leads to a crisis situation, which stimulates a reflection on (professional) identity. In individual supervision, participants start to discuss sensitive issues and some of them link their own (biographical) elements with difficulties in daily clinical work. Individual supervision is, therefore, a cornerstone for the identification and analysis of relational aspects of communication and allows one to recognize that communication is a co-construction, which demands not only technical skills, but also the willingness to reflect on oneself and one's own relational patterns. The confronting experience in CST is certainly a key element for change and improvement of skills; for some participants, however, it represents too much of a challenge to face. We have observed on rare occasions that participants experienced great difficulties in the training and were left quite distressed. While most of the vulnerable participants seem to benefit from training, for a minority, the experience can be counterproductive. However, up to now we lack a procedure to exclude these clinicians from CST and to offer them an adequate alternative.

Until the decision of the SSMO to declare CST as mandatory for specialization in oncology, participation was voluntary. Since then, some of the clinicians enter the training with ambivalent feelings and sometimes explicitly declare that they are only motivated by the fact that CST has become mandatory. However, even these ambivalent participants generally engage actively in the CST and we observe that defensive oncologists quite often turn from passive resistance to motivated participation, and then benefit a great deal from training. The fact that the CST is mandatory, therefore, allows otherwise refractory physicians to gain a more constructive perspective with regards to communication in cancer care. It also provides a powerful signal of the SSMO to the medical community, to the patients and to society as the whole, that communication matters for oncology clinicians. We are, therefore, very grateful to the SSMO for their support and the trust by declaring this CST as mandatory for oncology physicians.

Research

The evaluation of the CST by the participants (2), effectuated by the SCL, was very positive with regard to the perception of different skills improvements, the various contents of the model and the trainers, confirming the impression of the task force that the training is appreciated.

The Swiss CST in oncology has been investigated by means of three scientific projects, all financially supported by Oncosuisse (**www.oncosuisse.ch**). The first project (3) evaluated the videos before and after CST, and focused on clinician–patient interactions. The videos of the 258 nurses and physicians who participated in the Swiss CST were analysed with the Roter Interaction Analyses System (RIAS), which yields categories under which patient and professional utterances can be summarized. Furthermore, it reports on the emotional climate of the interview, using global ratings. Interviews were also analysed with the Observing Patient Involvement Scale (OPTION), which assesses to what extent professionals involve patients in decision-making. A total of 54,692 utterances were analysed; the largest part of the interviews consisted of the exchange of information (36,677 utterances). The following results were observed: nurses showed a significant increase in the proportion of empathic statements (1.6% versus 3.2%) and of reassuring statements (2.3% versus 3.4%), a decrease in medical information given (17.8% to 13.3%) and an increase in closed and open questions concerning psychosocial information (2.8% to 4.0%); (simulated) patients speaking with the nurses showed a decrease of medical information provided and an increase of reported life-style information (8.1% versus 6.7%; 3.3% versus 5.7%). In physicians, an increase in checking/summarizing utterances (1.8% versus 2.3%) and an increase in patients' explicit agreement statements (3.6% versus 4.7%) were observed. In addition, after training, the length of patients' speech without being interrupted by the nurses increased (3.7 to 4.3 utterances), but not when speaking with physicians (2.8 versus 2.9 utterances). The authors concluded that there were many significant improvements in nurses on various dependent variables, but for the physicians the outcome was more limited.

The second project focused on psychodynamic aspects of CST (4, 5). The aim was to investigate if clinicians' defence mechanisms are modified by CST, based on the hypothesis that this is the underlying process of skills improvement. Operating without conscious effort and triggered by anxiety-provoking situations, defences contribute to the individual's adaptation to, and protection from, stress (6). Usually described in patients (for example, as denial when facing threatening news), defences operate also in any individual and thus also in clinicians under distress. In patients, different types of defence mechanisms have been described (7) and classified depending on their degree of adaptation to, or distorting of, reality, ranging from 'immature defences', such as projection or denial, to 'mature defences', such as displacement or intellectualization (7, 8). While patient's defence mechanisms have been studied extensively in psychotherapy research (9), they have never been investigated in clinicians, not even in psychiatrists or psychotherapists (4, 5). As in patients, clinicians' defences diminish their ability to integrate all aspects of a given situation, and thus may hamper the working alliance with the patient and the recognition of patient's needs. Especially when immature defences are triggered, a clinician might then be perceived by the patient as detached and less empathic. After CST, most clinicians felt more secure (or less anxious) when facing patients in interviews and, therefore, less defensive, they were better prepared to encounter the patient, to perceive their emotions, and to respond empathically. In a first step of this project, a sample of 114 videos (57 videos pre- and 57 videos post-CST) were compared to 112 videos of a control group (56 videos using the same actors and the same scenarios as in the CST group, 56 videos 6 months later, no training). The videos were evaluated with the Clinician Defence Mechanism Rating Scale (DMRS-C) (9), which identifies a total of 30 defence mechanisms assigned to seven hierarchical levels: mature, obsessional, other neurotic, narcissistic, disavowal, borderline and action defences. Each level includes three to eight individual defences, which can be weighted according to its level of maturity and summed up to an overall defensive functioning score (ODF). Results showed:

(1) a high number (mean = 16, SD = 6) and a high variety (all hierarchical levels were observed) of defences triggered by the 15-minutes interviews;

(2) no evolution difference (ODF) with regard to defences between groups; but

(3) an increase of mature defences after CST for clinicians with an initial higher level of defensive functioning.

A follow-up project (10) aims to evaluate if levels of defences correlate with CST outcome, as measured by traditional measurements of skills improvement, such as the RIAS.

The third, ongoing project (11) is a linguistic investigation of CST, which aims to analyse the aforementioned sample (communication skills group and control group) from a linguistic perspective. This project aims to identify various quantitative and qualitative linguistic indicators of change of communicational competences. Furthermore, the data will also be evaluated with regard to socio-linguistic links between language and social identities, such as age, gender and professional background (physicians, nurses).

Ultimately, such research might allow the conceptualization of a broader offer of CST, which integrate relational and linguistic aspects in the training and which eventually might correspond more adequately to the individual needs of participating clinicians (12).

Acknowledgement

We would like to express our gratitude to Maya Andrey, former head of the Division of Psycho-Social Issues of the Swiss Cancer League, for her initiative and support in the development and organization of this Swiss CST.

References

1. Kiss A. Communication skills training in oncology: a position paper. *Ann Onco*1999; **10**: 899–901.
2. Navarra S. Communication skills training: réjouissante evaluation. *Schweizer Krebs Bulletin* 2001; **4**: 183.
3. Langewitz W, Szirt L, Nübling M, *et al. Evaluation of the Swiss Cancer League Communication Skills Program for Oncologists and Oncology Nurses.* Final Report, OncoSuisse 2003.
4. Favre N, Despland JN, De Roten Y, *et al.* Psychodynamic aspects of communication skills training: a pilot study. *Support Care Cancer* 2007; **15**: 333–337.
5. Bernard M, de Roten Y, Despland JN *et al. Communication Skills Training and Clinicians' Defences in Oncology: An Exploratory, Controlled Study.* Psycho-Oncology 2009.
6. Perry JC. A pilot study of defences in psychotherapy of personality disorders entering psychotherapy. *Journal of Nervous and Mental Diseases* 2001; **189**: 651–660.
7. Vaillant GE. *Ego Mechanisms of Defence.* Washington, American Psychiatric Press, 1992.
8. Perry JC, Cooper S. An empirical study of defence mechanisms: I clinical interview and life vignette ratings. *Archives of General Psychiatry* 1989; **46**: 444–452.
9. Despland JN, Bernard M, Favre N, *et al.* Clinicians' defences: an empirical study. *Psychology and Psychotheraphy: Theory, Research and Practice,* 2009; **82**: 73–81.
10. Stiefel F, de Roten Y, Despland JN, *et al.* Effects of communication skills training on working alliance and oncology clinicians' defence mechanisms and communication styles. *Oncosuisse;* Glant 1595-08-2004.
11. Stiefel F, Singy P. Linguistic aspects of Communication Skills Training. *Oncosuisse;* Grant 02035-02-2007
12. Stiefel F (ed). *Communication in Cancer Care. Recent Results in Cancer Research.* Springer Verlag, Berlin, Heidelberg 2006.

Chapter 56

The Australian model

Caroline Nehill and Alison Evans

Introduction

In Australia, one in three men and one in four women will be diagnosed with cancer in their life-time (1). Management of these cancer patients occurs along a continuum starting with screening and diagnosis, through treatment and supportive care, to follow-up, and, in some cases, palliative and end-of-life care, with services provided in both tertiary and primary settings. This process is further complicated by Australia's diverse geography and mix of public and private service delivery settings. As a result, over the course of their journey, patients with cancer will come into contact with a wide range of health professionals in different service-delivery settings, often in different geographic locations. The potential for confused messages, duplication of information, and a sense of isolation and confusion for patients navigating this system is enormous, adding to the fear and anxiety caused by their diagnosis. This complex system underscores the importance of effective and sensitive communication with the patient, their carers and family, and with the other members of the treatment team.

Communication skills training for health professionals involved in cancer care is available in Australia through a number of avenues. Courses and workshops are provided through professional colleges representing different disciplines involved in cancer care, cancer organizations, and local service providers, in both the public and private sectors. While the importance of communication skills is introduced to undergraduate students in medical schools and is part of The Cancer Council Australia's *Ideal Oncology Curriculum for Medical Schools* (2), the majority of formal communication skills training occurs at the postgraduate level, primarily in the form of interactive workshops implemented by one or more trained facilitators.

This chapter describes current approaches to communication skills training for oncology health professionals in Australia, including the benefits and limitations of the current model, as well as future directions and priorities. To provide some context, the chapter starts with a brief discussion of current Australian policy relating to communication skills training for oncology health professionals.

Communication skills in Australia: policy

The importance of communication skills training for oncology health professionals is emphasized in a number of Australian frameworks, reports, and clinical practice guidelines. A consultative report developed by key national cancer bodies in 2003 (3) highlighted consumer and healthcare provider views of the need for formal training and retraining in communication skills for health professionals working in a cancer care setting, including general practitioners. This view is reiterated in the National Service Improvement Framework for Cancer (4) and is formalized in the *Clinical Practice Guidelines for the Psychosocial Care of Adults with Cancer* (5).

While communication skills training is becoming more common across Australia, it has been proposed that its routine implementation will only be universally applied through inclusion in a formal accreditation or credentialing framework (3). An Australian model framework for cancer services standards proposed in 2005 (6) includes participation in regular communication skills training as a component. In 2005, a Senate Community Affairs Committee Inquiry into services and treatment options for persons with cancer, proposed that enhanced communication skills training is required at undergraduate and postgraduate levels, and that professional colleges representing the various disciplines involved in cancer care should undertake a more active role in the provision of such training for their members (7). As a first step towards formalizing this requirement, participation in communication skills training has been included as one of a set of *Indicators for Psychosocial Care of Adults with Cancer* (8) developed and currently being trialled in an effort to provide a way for services to measure whether cancer teams and services are delivering psychosocial care in accordance with best practice.

The level of support for ongoing communication skills training provided by professional medical organizations, varies. A number of colleges and professional bodies include the need for graduates to demonstrate effective communication skills as a principle or aim of training (e.g. Royal Australian College of General Practitioners, Royal Australian and New Zealand College of Radiologists), while only a few include communication skills training as a compulsory element (e.g. Royal Australian and New Zealand College of Obstetricians and Gynaecologists, Medical Oncology Group of Australia and the Australasian Chapter of Palliative Medicine). A larger number include attendance at communication skills workshops in their continuing professional development programmes (e.g. Royal Australasian College of Surgeons, Royal Australasian College of Physicians).

In 2007, the Cancer Council Australia published an *Ideal Oncology Curriculum for Medical Schools* (2), which includes the need to demonstrate a range of communication skills, including breaking bad news, tailoring information, providing supportive counselling, and explaining the risks and benefits of treatments. While this has been adopted by many Australian medical schools, it is important to acknowledge that preparing medical students for the clinical challenges that occur in oncology practice can be difficult. For this reason the major focus for communication skills training for oncology health professionals in Australia is in the postgraduate setting.

Approaches to communication skills training in Australia

Undergraduate training

The importance of effective communication skills and introductory training is introduced to medical and allied health students in Australia at the undergraduate level, and communication skills training is increasingly becoming a core component of the curriculum of many universities. However, practical application of skills comes only with experience. Thus, while the undergraduate setting provides an ideal opportunity to introduce the concept of communication skills, it is essential that skills development is recognized as an integral part of ongoing professional development and a compulsory competence for professional registration.

Postgraduate training

At a postgraduate level, communication skills training in Australia generally takes the form of intensive small-group workshops or larger seminar-style presentations. Workshops are the more common approach and typically use facilitators from psycho-oncology and appropriate clinical backgrounds, with actors playing the role of patients where relevant. Workshops are based around a particular issue to be communicated with a range of modules currently available. Box 56.1 provides

> ## Box 56.1 List of communication skills modules provided through the National Breast and Ovarian Cancer Centre*
>
> - General interactional skills.
> - Breaking bad news.
> - Eliciting and responding to emotional cues
> - Effectively communicating prognosis in cancer care.
> - Improving communication within the multidisciplinary team.**
> - Discussing the transition from curative care to palliative care.
> - Addressing the needs of younger women with breast cancer.
> - Communication skills training for radiographers performing mammography.
> - Effectively discussing a diagnosis of ductal carcinoma *in situ.*
> - Effectively discussing complementary therapies.
>
> * Resources available through the National Breast and Ovarian Cancer Centre.
>
> **Module developed jointly by the National Breast and Ovarian Cancer Centre and the Pam McLean Cancer Communication Centre.

a list of modules available through the National Breast and Ovarian Cancer Centre. Other modules are also provided through other organizations. The majority of modules focus on interactions between the health professional and the patient; however, a module that is proving to be increasingly popular is one that focuses on improving communication between members of a multidisciplinary team.

Module development

Several groups and organizations in Australia are involved in the development of communication skills workshop modules and the implementation of workshops. In general, all follow a similar approach. Workshop modules are developed using a rigorous evidence-based methodology. An expert group commissioned to develop the module performs a literature review, which is used to inform a series of recommendations about optimal communication techniques for the particular topic. These recommendations may also be used as the basis for a checklist provided to workshop participants as an ongoing reminder of the communication techniques they learn in the workshops. PowerPoint slides are used to highlight key messages and evidence points as a primer at the beginning of the workshop. For each module, a set of clinical scenarios is also developed that form the basis for discussion and skills training within the workshop. Prior to finalizing the module, a targeted external review process is conducted, using national and, where appropriate, international experts to ensure relevance and currency of the information.

Small-group workshops

Reviews of research have shown that communication skills workshops are most effective when they are interactive, encourage participation, allow skills to be practised, and allow participants to receive feedback on their performance (9). A combination of these strategies is ideal and can lead to improvements in communication skills. Small-group, facilitated, interactive workshops give health professionals the opportunity to practice communication techniques in a safe and supportive environment.

Small-group workshops typically run for 3–4 hours and include a short presentation of the background information and learning points, tailored by the facilitators to the needs of the audience. This is followed by the introduction of the patient to the group, with information about his or her circumstances and a description of the information to be communicated. A series of role-play interactions then follows, with participants being invited to take the role of the health professional. Interactions can be stopped at any time through a time-out by the facilitator or the participant, providing the opportunity for discussion of the interaction and allowing alternative strategies to be played out in a safe environment.

Historically, these workshops have focused mainly on specialist clinicians, and have been run in association with annual scientific meetings or congresses. Workshop participation is generally coordinated through a voluntary response to promotional mailers or newsletter articles. More recently this approach has been broadened to target other disciplines, with cancer nurses and allied health professionals voicing a keen interest in participating in training workshops. One successful approach has been to partner with a relevant organization or body to broaden the reach of the programme beyond a one-off event. For example, a partnership between National Breast and Ovarian Cancer Centre and the State/Territory-based programmes of the national mammographic screening service BreastScreen Australia, resulted in a series of national workshops that successfully targeted over 200 radiographers performing mammographic screening.

Workshop facilitation

The development of the module and supporting resources represents only one component in the delivery of an effective communication skills workshop. Successful implementation of the module is dependent on skilled and experienced facilitators who are able to use the information provided as the basis for a tailored and interactive learning experience for workshop participants. This requires an understanding of the subject matter of the module and training in presentation and facilitation skills. The optimal model used in the majority of workshops in Australia involves two facilitators: a psycho-oncologist who is familiar with a broad range of communication techniques and the implications of different approaches to communication, and a specialist in the particular discipline being targeted by the workshop who can frame the information in terms most relevant to the participants.

Australia is fortunate to have a number of international experts in communication skills training who are able to not only facilitate workshops, but also teach and mentor new facilitators. Successful facilitator training identifies new trainers, provides ongoing support, and allows opportunities to practice skills and to receive feedback. However, this is an intensive exercise requiring adequate resourcing. Furthermore, experience has shown that merely inviting interested individuals to participate in a facilitator training course is not sufficient to ensure an ongoing commitment to undertake training workshops. Clarification and agreement of expectations from the outset is important, as is identifying individuals who have expressed a specific interest and commitment to communication skills training. For example, as part of National Breast and Ovarian Cancer Centre's National Communication Skills Training Initiative, facilitators undergo an intensive 2-day training course, and are then asked to co-facilitate at least two workshops with an experienced facilitator before being given the opportunity to take the role of lead facilitator. If deemed necessary by the mentor, additional co-facilitation opportunities are provided before the trainee is given lead facilitation status.

Actor training

Actors who play the role of patient in communication skills training workshops also require an intensive period of training. In order to provide a realistic portrayal of the patient's feelings and emotions in a particular scenario, the actor must understand the possible ramifications of different diagnoses and treatments, as well as the background information about the individual case being portrayed. Typically, an actor will be trained in one or more patient cases, which can then be adapted to incorporate different scenarios according to the workshop being undertaken. For example, the case of a 42-year-old woman with breast cancer may be adapted to be used in a *Breaking Bad News* workshop or in a workshop relating to *Responding to Emotional Cues*. In Australia, the Pam McLean Cancer Communication Centre provides training for professional actors including training on the clinical and psychosocial aspects of specific cases. Actors are also trained to provide in-role feedback to workshop participants.

Alternative approaches

A range of approaches to communication skills training based on the small workshop model have been implemented in Australia. These include 1–2 day seminars providing training relevant to all stages of the cancer journey, as well as the inclusion of workshops as part of annual conferences for professional colleges and organizations. These approaches have been implemented to varying degrees of success; the common barrier being the challenge of incorporating training into current work commitments.

A number of alternative approaches have been suggested, such as integrating training into the daily routine of health professionals, one-on-one assessment, and mentoring. Research into these methods is currently being explored in order to ensure evidence-based training.

Training for general practitioners has tended to be linked to a risk management approach, with courses being run primarily to reduce litigation. In 2007–08 National Breast and Ovarian Cancer Centre trialled an alternative approach for training general practitioners based on the traditional small-workshop model. A series of DVD-based case scenarios were developed and used as the basis of workshops rolled out through the Australian General Practice Network as part of ongoing continuing professional development programmes for general practitioners. The DVD is designed to mimic the interactive workshops, with a range of scenarios and approaches to communication, which are presented to stimulate discussion amongst workshop attendees. Such an approach may also lend itself to a distance-learning programme for individual practitioners unable to attend a group session. Immediate post-workshop evaluation has indicated that the workshop format was successful in achieving its objectives and that the format was acceptable to general practitioners. Long-term evaluation is being undertaken to determine the impact of the training on participants' confidence levels and communication styles.

Benefits and limitations of current model

The interactive workshop approach has a number of benefits and limitations. The small-group nature of the workshops (typically four to six participants) means that participants receive a personalized training experience. Scenarios can be tailored to address particular issues that participants have experienced and all participants have the opportunity to practice new techniques and approaches in a safe and supportive environment. However, the small-group, interactive nature of the workshops is seen by some as threatening, and anecdotal feedback, as well as feedback in a small handful of evaluation forms completed by workshop participants, indicates that not everyone feels comfortable with role-play in a group setting. Alternative approaches, such as using DVD-based scenarios to initiate discussion, are currently being trialled; however, it remains to be seen whether this approach achieves the same level of participant understanding and skill in the long term.

A major limitation of the current approach is that it is resource intensive. Training for facilitators and actors requires ongoing funding and support, and workshop coordination requires extensive administrative support. While efforts are being made to build capacity across Australia for locally run workshops, the current small pool of experienced facilitators means that there are often considerable travel costs associated with running a workshop.

Reliance on voluntary registration for workshop attendance is another limitation of the current model. Targeting those individuals who may have a high need for training but do not recognize this need, or those who are averse to training in a group setting, is an ongoing issue. As mentioned previously, some proposed models include a one-on-one assessment and mentoring approach with individuals identified by supervisors or mentors rather than simply relying on voluntary registration. However, such resource-intensive models are likely to be unsustainable in the long-term and may only have utility for the occasional case.

Evaluation of workshop outcomes

While post-workshop evaluation and anecdotal feedback suggests that interactive workshops are viewed positively by both participants and facilitators, there is little evidence demonstrating improvements in communication skills. For the majority of workshops, evaluation is currently limited to a pre-/post-workshop questionnaire exploring the participant's level of understanding and confidence communicating in a particular scenario and their satisfaction with the workshop format. In response to a recommendation from a think-tank of national and international experts held in 2005, a national workshop was held in 2006 to explore approaches to coding and evaluating communication skills interactions in the research setting. However, even without a formal approach to coding, the use of a follow-up survey weeks or months post-workshop may provide insight into skill retention and implementation. There are some small studies emerging that explore health professional participants' psychosocial beliefs about patient care, confidence, and practice behaviour before workshops and six weeks after participation in a workshop (10). While early results have shown significant improvements in the confidence levels of participants and in participant communication with patients, further investigation is required to determine the impact on clinical practice.

National Communication Skills Training Initiative

The National Breast and Ovarian Cancer Centre is Australia's independent authority and information source on breast and ovarian cancer. Funded by the Australian Government, the National Breast and Ovarian Cancer Centre works in partnership with health professionals, cancer organizations, researchers, governments, and patients to improve outcomes in breast and ovarian cancer. Since 1997, the National Breast and Ovarian Cancer Centre has implemented a National Communication Skills Training Initiative through a partnership with a number of other organizations and individuals. This initiative started with the aim of providing training for health professionals involved in the care of patients with breast cancer. However, the commonality in issues for other cancer types, along with the increased awareness of the need for communication skills training has led to a broadening to other cancers in recent years. The initiative is overseen by a multidisciplinary steering committee, which includes representation from psycho-oncology, nursing, medical oncology, and surgical disciplines, as well as consumer representation. The steering committee meets on a quarterly basis to discuss the progress of the initiative, review resources, and identify new opportunities. The steering committee members are also integral to the implementation of workshops and facilitator training.

The aims of the National Communication Skills Training Initiative are:

- to ensure that high-quality communication skills training is available to health professionals treating people with cancer by:
  - developing standardized communication skills training modules and recommendations for best practice;
  - building capacity to implement communication skills training through facilitator training;
  - supporting the implementation of local interactive training workshops for health professionals that use a best practice approach;
- to ensure that all individuals providing communication skills training have access to information about new research, resources, and other programmes across Australia;
- to ensure that all organizations wishing to co-ordinate communication skills training have access to information about available programmes and best practice standards;
- to promote communication skills training as a compulsory professional competence for all health professionals.

Coordination of the initiative is managed through project staff at the National Breast and Ovarian Cancer Centre. This includes commissioning and coordinating reviews of new modules, planning and coordinating workshops, and coordinating facilitator training and ongoing mentoring. The National Breast and Ovarian Cancer Centre also acts as a central hub for sharing ideas with other groups involved in communication skills training. The recent development of a central website allows not only the dissemination of information about the National Communication Skills Training Initiative, but also the promotion of initiatives conducted by State-based groups. This national hub aims to reduce replication of activity and to promote resource sharing, recognizing that much of the development work has already been undertaken and that the emphasis should now be on maximizing efforts to implement communication skills training.

A current focus for the National Communication Skills Training Initiative is to build local capacity to implement communication skills training. This is accomplished by making modules available to other organizations wishing to implement training workshops, providing grants to allow groups to hold local workshops, providing funding to facilitate the training of actors in each State to support workshops, and coordinating facilitator training courses and ongoing mentoring opportunities.

Other training providers

In Australia, communication skills training for oncology health professionals is implemented by a number of organizations across a wide range of settings. Examples include:

- an integrated hospital-based programme at the Peter MacCallum Cancer Centre in Victoria; launched in 2007, all clinical staff at this comprehensive cancer centre are provided with the opportunity to attend facility based interactive workshops;
- a State-based programme delivered through the Cancer Council Victoria's, Victorian Cancer Clinicians Communication Program, providing structured workshops to all health-care professionals throughout the State;
- development and delivery of a range of tailor-made communication skills training programmes, as well as actor and facilitator training through the Pam McLean Cancer Communication Centre, Australia's only dedicated communication skills service provider.

Future directions

Much progress has been made in the implementation of communication skills training in Australia, with the importance of communication skills training now recognized in cancer frameworks, clinical practice guidelines, and in oncology curricula. However, there is more that could be done to ensure that all oncology health professionals undertake training and retraining. Whether this will truly be achieved without some form of accreditation or credentialing programme to ensure uptake, remains to be seen. In the meantime, the lessons learned from the activities of the past 10 years can certainly be used to build a more cohesive and universal approach to training that will ensure that all health professionals have the basic skills to be able to communicate effectively and sensitively with patients and their carers.

The future lies in developing a sustainable model that balances the delivery of a high-quality and relevant educational experience with the need for a cost-effective approach. The focus is now on building capacity, utilizing existing evidence-based resources, and trialling and evaluating innovative delivery methods in partnership with national and international researchers. Collaborations between existing national and State-based cancer organizations, service providers, researchers, and funding bodies are required to extend the current reach and ensure sustainability of training. There is also an urgent need to broaden responsibility for implementation to organizations outside those currently involved whilst maintaining the high-quality evidence-based approach.

The recent advent of national cancer educational programmes for oncology health professionals in Australia provides the opportunity for a formalized national approach to the implementation and evaluation of communication skills training across Australia. The potential for collaboration between cancer organizations and State and Federal Government bodies, represents an exciting opportunity to develop a model that addresses Australia's unique geographical and health service delivery characteristics, providing access to relevant training for all health professionals. The development of a successful training framework will ensure not only the sustainability of training in Australia but will facilitate the implementation of new and innovative approaches to communication skills training for all health professionals working in cancer.

References

1. Australian Institute of Health and Welfare (AIHW) and Australasian Association of Cancer Registries (AACR) (2007). *Cancer in Australia: an overview, 2006.* Cancer series no. 37. Cat. no. CAN 32. Canberra: AIHW.

2. Oncology Education Committee (1999). *Ideal Oncology Curriculum for Medical Schools.* The Cancer Council Australia, Sydney, NSW.

3. Clinical Oncology Society of Australia (2002). The Cancer Council Australia and the National Cancer Control Initiative. *Optimising Cancer Care in Australia.* National Cancer Control Initiative, Melbourne, VIC.

4. National Health Priority Council (2004). *National Service Improvement Framework for Cancer.* Commonwealth of Australia, Canberra, ACT.

5. National Breast Cancer Centre and National Cancer Control Initiative (2003). *Clinical Practice Guidelines for the Psychosocial Care of Adults with Cancer.* National Breast Cancer Centre, Camperdown, NSW.

6. The Cancer Council Australia, Australian Cancer Network and the National Breast Cancer Centre (2005). *A Core Strategy for Cancer Care Accreditation of Cancer Services – a Discussion Paper.* National Breast Cancer Centre, Camperdown, NSW.

7. Senate Community Affairs Reference Committee (2005). *The Cancer Journey: Informing Choice.* Commonwealth of Australia, Canberra, ACT

8. National Breast Cancer Centre (2007). *Indicators for Psychosocial Care of Adults with Cancer.* National Breast Cancer Centre, Camperdown, NSW.

9. Razavi D, Merckaert I, Marchal S, *et al.* (2003). How to optimise physicians' communication skills in cancer care: results of a randomised study assessing the usefulness of post-training consolidation workshops. *Journal of Clinical Oncology* **2**(26): 3141–3149.

10. Sutherland G, Hegarty S, White V, *et al.* (2007). Development and evaluation of a brief, peer-led communication skills training programme for cancer clinicians. *Asia-Pac J Clin Oncol* **3**: 207–213.

Chapter 57

The United Kingdom general practitioner and palliative care model

Simon Noble, Nicola Pease, and Ilora Finlay

Introduction

Within the United Kingdom (UK), the general practitioner (GP) will manage the care of the majority of patients with life-limiting and terminal disease. Even those patients with complex problems requiring specialist palliative care involvement, are likely to receive the majority of their care at home or within the community healthcare system, with their GP as key healthcare worker. The consultation is at the heart of general practice and communication skills, underpining the UK General Practitioner Vocational Training Scheme (GPVTS). To attain membership of the Royal College of General Practitioners (RCGP), trainees are required to undertake learning methods during their training programme as outlined in the RCGP Curriculum (1), which include:

- video analysis of consultations;
- random case analysis of a selection of consultations;
- sitting in with GPs and other healthcare professionals in practice to observe different consulting styles;
- GP trainer to sit in with specialty registrar to give formative feedback;
- patients' feedback on consultations, using satisfaction questionnaires or tools.

Whilst the GPVTS offers exposure opportunities to develop generic communication skills within the primary care setting, the breadth of possible consultations and clinical scenarios will only offer limited depth of experience with respect to specific specialties. Furthermore, the time restraints in the primary care consultation encourage brevity and such skills developed for GP settings may not be transferable to specialist palliative care.

Cardiff university model

Since its development in 1987, the Cardiff University Post Graduate Course has offered specialist palliative care education to meet the needs of specialists and of GPs with a developing specialist interest. It has evolved to become an internationally recognized and quotable qualification, with alumni in over thirty countries. In recognition of the needs of children with life-limiting illness, a paediatric option has also been developed. The course utilizes a web-based portfolio e-learning system and is available to physicians, nurses, pharmacists, social workers, physiotherapists, occupational therapists, pastoral workers, dieticians and other allied healthcare professionals, reflecting the multi-professional approach to learning and patient care.

Communication skills training makes up an integral part of the course that initially requires close supervision and support. For this reason the course includes two 'face-to-face' residential modules to address the fundamentals of communication skills before empowering the adult learner to further progress their skills through self-directed learning. Combinations of interactive teaching experiences are used in communication skills training, where the evidence, rationale, and 'toolkit' for good communication can be explained. This is followed by an opportunity to explore and practice such tools in a safe, learning environment using role-play. The outline for the teaching programme is discussed below and consists of five core sections:

◆ Introduction to the process of communication.
◆ Analysis of the consultation.
◆ The Cardiff six-point toolkit.
◆ Role-play.
◆ Reflection on real world experience/portfolio learning.

Introduction to the process

The introduction occurs early within the course as part of the first residential module and is given as an interactive lecture. Participants will need sufficient time prior to the course to reflect on relevant pre-course material and an opportunity for facilitators to address any concerns that are raised. For many participants, the communication skills component of the course is the one that gives them most cause for concern; an interactive lecture engaging the whole class can be reassuring for candidates to see that their concerns are shared by others.

The importance of good communication should be discussed and participants may wish to explore the consequences of a bad consultation. Various aspects of healthcare-related communication can, and should, be discussed including: the consent process; the role of communication in advanced care planning (for adults and children); the identification and exploration of psychosocial issues; written communication, either to the patient, other healthcare professionals, or carers; and information leaflets including a discussion on their limitations.

The Cardiff six-point toolkit

The Cardiff six-point toolkit developed in recognition of the fact that many participants have limited experience with role-play and find the experience quite stressful. The tool kit attempts to break down the bare essentials of the palliative consultation. It offers six key techniques or tools that should be applied to any consultation and developed as individual skills to improve the role-play and real-world consultation. These are listed below and discussed in further detail after:

◆ listening;
◆ reflection;
◆ summarizing;
◆ question style;
◆ comfort;
◆ language.

Depending upon the experience and confidence of the individual, and at the discretion of facilitator, participants may focus on several tools in one role-play scenario. For the less confident individual, a role-play that has the objective of focusing on only one of the tools can still produce significant developments. This is most marked when focusing on tools 1, 2, and 3.

Tool 1: listening/use of silence

One of the key tools that can be used in teaching communication skills is the appropriate use of silence which will facilitate active listening. Silence is a valuable tool in communicating. It helps by:

+ allowing the patient time to assimilate news;
+ demonstrating that the patient is being listened to;
+ giving the patient time to react;
+ giving the patient time to ask questions.

Communication studies suggest that doctors do not listen to their patients enough and interrupt patients' dialogue early, thus creating a barrier to communication. In addition, early interruption may result in relevant facts being missed from the patient's history (2, 3).

In the initial stages of the consultation participants should be encouraged to:

+ Allow the patient to talk. This is best achieved by the role-play facilitator, instructing the participant to avoid interrupting the patient and allowing them to tell the whole story.
+ Engage in active listening. This involves the avoidance of interrupting and the continuation of dialogue with short words of encouragement such as 'I see', 'Yes', 'Go on', or merely by maintaining eye contact and using appropriate body language such as nodding. Scenarios that can be used to explore the use of listening skills may include breaking bad news, dealing with anger, or managing the distressed patient.

  If you give a patient bad news or a lot of difficult information, it is inevitable that there will be silence. You will hear silence, but for the patient opposite you there is nothing but noise. It's just all internal. They need a bit of time to sort it out in their head and if you talk too soon during the silence, it will interrupt them. (4)

The judicious use of silence can allow the patient to feel more in control of the consultation, and to set the pace and direction of the topics to be covered. As a general rule, the patient should have about 80% of the consultation time to talk with the doctor or nurse speaking for about 20% of the time. Unfortunately, the reverse is often seen in practice, with the healthcare professional dominating the conversation and not allowing the patient time to say whatever is uppermost on their mind.

Tool 2: reflection

Good use of reflection is important. It really makes the patient feel you are listening to them. (4)

This technique is particularly useful for participants new to communication skills training, who get stuck and do not know what to say next. Reflecting back what a patient has just said may help and will encourage the patient to proceed with their story. It also demonstrates that they are being listened to and helps to develop rapport. In addition, it is a technique that can be used to encourage dialogue at times when the patient may be finding it difficult to go on because of their feelings. Reflection can also be used to pick up on key words said by a patient and signal that they are being followed up on.

Tool 3: summarizing/recapping

Another technique that can be practiced is summarizing. It is useful to encourage candidates to do this, especially when they are unsure where to go with the consultation or if their mind goes blank.

> Just by recapping with: 'So what you're saying is…' makes you feel that you are being taken seriously. (4)

Going back over the patient's story with them demonstrates to the patient that they have been listened to. It also offers them a chance to clarify anything that may have been missed. Often, they will then pick up on something and direct the consultation towards their agenda.

Tool 4: question style

The question style is crucially important. As a general rule, the more open the question the greater the amount of information obtained. So the open questions, such as 'How have things been?', allows the patient to tell the doctor anything at all about what has been happening—ranging from medical details of the condition to social catastrophes, other family illness, and so on. Focused questions do just as the name describes, they focus down onto a particular area and then explore it further: 'Can you tell me more about your pain?'; then further direct questions may have a place such as: 'Does the skin over the area feel very sensitive?'. Of course, the style of question must fit the occasion—using focused or direct questions too early leaves the patient feeling interrogated, but unable to express the real issues that are troublesome.

Multiple questions (double-barrelled questions) and leading question styles are best avoided in all consultation settings. Multiple questions, as their name suggests, are a series of questions asked in one statement, they are often confusing for the patient, as they are not sure which part to answer first. For example: 'The pain that you mentioned, is that a new pain or has it been there for some time? Do the pain killers make it any better?'. Leading questions often direct the consultation to the wrong answer, thereby providing misinformation to the healthcare professional. For example: 'On the new pain killers, how much better is your pain?'.

Tool 5: comfort

The concept of comfort encompasses many facets to the effective consultation. First and foremost, it reminds participants of the importance of preparation for the consultation. The more they develop their communication skills, the more comfortable they will be in communicating.

It also highlights the importance of the setting in which communication occurs. Experienced communicators will recognize that a sensitive consultation needs to take place in a quiet place, free from interruptions and disturbances. The physical environment of the consultation should avoid barriers, such as a desk or computer, between the doctor and patient; should avoid sitting the patient in the glare of bright light from a window or lamp; and should ensure that the patient has as comfortable a chair as the healthcare professional.

Participants must also be encouraged to understand that discussing upsetting or bad news is likely to evoke strong emotions. Bad news by definition it is going to upset the receiver. Participants may feel guilty that they have made the patient cry and may feel compelled to say something to 'make it better'. However, such remarks often come across as banal and patronizing, just as a mother says 'There there, don't cry' to a child.

Such words provide false reassurance; they may stem the flow of tears and distress in the immediate term but will lead to further problems later, such as mistrust or lack of confidence in physicians. In general, 'jollying along' makes the professional feel better but blocks the patient's ability to communicate.

Tool 6: language

When discussing language, it is often considered under the broad categories of verbal and non-verbal language. Every person communicates a great deal by the way they look, their expression, their body posture and their overall demeanour—indeed it is said that about 80% of communication is non-verbal (5). The remainder is made up of the language used to speak, whether that language is spoken, written or in another form. In the context of a consultation it is verbal communication that often receives most attention, with relatively little attention being paid to the non-verbal.

All healthcare professionals must guard against using jargon and remain aware of the settings in which they are most likely to use it:

◆ tacit vocabulary;
◆ fear of causing distress;
◆ as a barrier.

Tacit vocabulary

The majority of medical education is conducted solely amongst clinical peers, and complex medical words or abbreviations become commonplace in their vocabulary. Sometimes when professionals relax in a consultation, they find themselves using jargon, which they no longer consider abnormal or specialist. Exercises that encourage candidates to focus on using vocabulary raised by the patient can help to develop insight into the way that everyday speech of a professional can be quite incomprehensible to a patient.

Fear of causing distress

People are sometimes worried about using words such as 'cancer' and may be tempted to use euphemisms to avoid causing distress. Once again, this may avoid immediate distress but leads to problems later on.

Patients require uncomplicated words brought sympathetically, which is something that participants can explore within the context of role-play and reflection.

As a barrier

Jargon and complex words are frequently used as a barrier to further communication between doctor and patient. By using medical words, doctors establish that they have a greater knowledge and expertise, thereby exerting their position of superiority over the patient. When professionals become nervous or unsure, they often resort to the communication style in which they feel most comfortable.

Role-play

Role-play using either actors or colleagues as patients, has long been a useful tool for developing communication skills (6). Within the Cardiff model, it is done as a small group of learners with one trained facilitator and the participants playing the role of patients. Small numbers of participants promote a cohesive group, help students feel safe, and ensure that everyone has the opportunity to role-play. Students generally become supportive and constructive and view their 'turns' at role-play as an opportunity to develop further. Discussions of difficult issues/encounters lead to personal growth and adjustment. The learning and teaching becomes increasingly learner-centred and increasingly complex communication situations can be introduced without the risk of the student feeling overwhelmed or inadequate (7).

Role-play allows people to be prepared for situations that they rarely encounter; the skills for breaking bad news or dealing with anger are best learned prior to such an encounter in practice. Role-play affords the learner the luxury of a second try at a difficult encounter and the group process often enhances learning.

There are several basic principles that should underpin any such learning session:

- clearly established rules of role-play;
- strict adherence to confidentiality;
- safe environment;
- avoidance of role-playing situations that are potentially distressing for learners in the initial learning sessions;
- option to call 'time-out' at any point;
- opportunity for all learners to participate;
- non-confrontational feedback;
- time for those involved to 'come out of role' after a session;
- review of learning points and de-brief at end of each session.

A formative learning approach is useful during the role-play sessions as it helps focus both participants and observers on to the principles and techniques of communication. Establishing learning needs and outcomes with the group is a useful way of planning the session. When learning needs are being defined, it is helpful for the student to think about the activities and skills that need to be improved and then to write the learning outcomes in these terms. This will help the learner to be able to demonstrate that learning has occurred—a process that is becoming increasingly important in the current climate of revalidation of professional groups in some countries, such as the USA and the UK. An example of some learning outcomes for communication skills teaching are given in Box 57.1.

Box 57.1 Cardiff course communication learning outcomes

At the end of the module the students will be able to:
- demonstrate non-verbal ways of:
  —facilitating a patient feeling comfortable and safe;
  —opening up a communication;
  —helping a patient to disclose their problems;
- demonstrate the use of open questions;
- demonstrate the use of focused questions;
- demonstrate the process of checking that a patient has understood information;
- apply the process of closure of a consultation;
- demonstrate a stepwise approach to breaking bad news;
- demonstrate respect of the patient and the patient's concerns;
- list potential barriers to communication with patients, with patients' families and with colleagues;
- suggest ways to overcome barriers to communication;
- reflect on their own communication style;
- analyse the processes they use in a consultation.

It should be noted that the assessment schedule for a simulated consultation covers many of these areas, so the assessment is explicitly matched to the learning outcomes.

Within the role-play setting, facilitators must be prepared to give feedback and, where appropriate, feedback can also be given by other observers. Pendleton's method is one of the safest ways to give feedback singly or involving other participants. It involves the application of four enquiries (8):

- Asking the learner what went they felt they did well or were particularly happy with.
- Asking other learners what they observed to be done well.
- Asking the learner what they felt could be improved.
- Asking the other learners what they felt could be improved.

This approach to feedback has the merit of first highlighting what was done well, thereby reinforcing good practice and offering positive suggestions for improvement. Those members of the group who are not role-playing should take an active part in the appraisal system to observe and learn from peers. More recently the Calgary–Cambridge approach to communication skills teaching has been developed as a facilitation tool (9). It encourages a far more agenda-led approach to communication skills, encouraging learners to focus on those specific areas of the consultation that they otherwise avoid through lack of confidence.

The skills to facilitate such sessions are very sophisticated, so training the trainers is strongly recommended before embarking on this teaching style. Most learning of value will occur from the role-play itself and the feedback session, but summative assessment can highlight particular areas of weakness. Selected video-taped consultations can complement role-play. Box 57.2 illustrates

---

Box 57.2 Summative marking schedule for palliative care consultation*

1. Puts patient at ease.
2. Establishes problems sufficiently to erect hypothesis.
3. Prioritizes problems/hypothesis.
4. Checks back on problem list agreement.
5. Elicits fears/concerns.
6. Elicits beliefs/concepts/attitudes.
7. Establishes physical/psychosocial relationship of complaints.
8. Explores physical issues appropriately.
9. Evolves plan acceptable to patient.
10. Checks back that plan is understood/agreed.
11. Overall non-verbals facilitate.
12. Overall verbals appropriate.
13. Overall patient appears comfortable/safe.
14. Overall respects patient's pace.
15. Overall closes interview well.

*Marks are given in each section out of ten, five being a pass mark.

© Cardiff University.

a suggested marking scheme for the palliative care consultation—it is used in the Cardiff diploma/masters course in palliative medicine.

Reflective practice/portfolio learning

An opportunity to explore and practice such tools within the safe confines of a learning environment is invaluable prior to bringing these skills to the real world. Within the Cardiff model, participants are required to submit two video-recordings of consultations from their own practice. The first, submitted in the year one of study, should feature a real patient from their day-to-day practice. The following year requires a more complex consultation reflecting the progress made over the year. The consultation should cover one of the following scenarios: collusion, denial, handling uncertainty, or inter-professional relations. In view of the complexities of such scenarios and the logistics of recoding such an encounter, candidates are allowed to use an actor patient for this consultation.

Candidates are required to provide a critique of their own consultation using the form shown in Table 57.2. Examiner's marks take into account the views of the participants in identifying whether they have identified their own learning needs and have been able to achieve them through the self-critique of the video-recording. This process is essential if the training given on the course is to successfully promote life-long learning. It is not enough to train people in communication skills, they must be trained to continue to further develop and hone how they talk with patients and their families throughout their career. The self-critique has developed from the self-directed portfolio learning model, which relies heavily on reflective practice.

Portfolio learning is now widely recognized as a valuable learning tool as it provides a record of learning and also acts as a stimulus to reflection. Portfolio learning is designed to provide

---

Box 57.3 Successful portfolios consist of the following elements (10)

- Factual case histories around which the learning usually occurs.
- References to items that have influenced the clinical decision-making process and have been foci of learning.
- References to diverse sources (e.g. text-book reading, literature search, lay press, conversations with colleagues).
- A record of the clinician's own decision-making processes, including details of decisions made and how the student came to them.
- Documentation of how the student felt at the time: sources of stress or doubts are as useful as the outcome, since the personal feelings of the learner will influence how they were able to approach a problem.
- Ethical considerations.
- Illustrative items such as photographs, drawings, quotations, poetry, etc., may clarify points being made.
- Some form of indexing is important, so the learner and supervisor can follow the learning process and refer to specific items at a later date

a chronological record of the learning process of the student. The learning process is self-directed; the learner chooses the areas within a subject of particular interest. In the context of adult learners, this enables each participant to meet their own individual learning objectives. Those unaccustomed to this learning style often require gentle support and supervision, as it differs greatly from their previous technical-rational learning experiences. The beauty and simplicity of a reflective portfolio, which allows the learner to determine format, learning objectives and emphasis to the learner, may be seen by some as too unstructured and challenging. Most physicians are new to the relative lack of prescribed formal structure in the portfolio. Depending upon the experience of the educational supervisor, even the method of presenting the portfolio can be relaxed if the reasons are clear. The learner should be encouraged to develop the portfolio in a similar way to an artist's portfolio, reflecting their freedom of creativity in presentation. Most successful portfolios consist of the elements described in Box 57.3.

Within the realms of self-directed learning, the portfolio will act both as a tool for learning and as evidence to the supervisor that learning has taken place. It is important that adult learners have feedback on their progress. This can sometimes be difficult with portfolio marking, since the scope and form of portfolios may differ greatly. Formative assessment between the supervisor and student, in an informal setting, is essential; it enables the supervisor to give constructive feedback to the student and provide support, especially to those new to the concept of portfolio learning. The supervisor will need to identify those students who require more frequent feedback sessions and extra support. Summative assessment can help the student identify areas of learning that they may wish to consider in the future. Examples of a mark schedule, as used at Cardiff university for a general portfolio are given in Table 57.1.

A suggested framework for participants to formulate a critique around their video-consultation is outlined in Table 57.2. In addition, Table 57.3 contextualizes the consultation for the course examiner to better enable them to understand the background to the video recording.

Table 57.1 Summative portfolio mark schedule

	Score
Contextual description of case	5%
Biological issues of the case	5%
Individual issues of the case	5%
Team-working	10%
Clarity of presentation	10%
Decision-making logic	20%
Attribution of evidence	20%
Critical analysis	15%
Index and discretionary marks	10%
Total	**100%**
© Cardiff University.	

Table 57.2 Reflective critique form

Part	Content
1	Your previous knowledge, reflections and experience in consultations of this type
	(10 marks)
2	Key learning areas identified from the critique of this consultation
	(10 marks)
3	How will your clinical practice change as a result of this learning?
	(10 marks)
4	The resources used to reflect on the communication style within this consultation and explain of how they have influenced practice
	(10 marks)

© Cardiff University.

Table 57.3 Background to consultation

Reason for consultation
Relevant background information (e.g. previous consultations with this patient or information from a referral letter).
Explain the presence of anyone else present (if not stated on the video).
Physical findings relevant to profession, if any.
Working diagnosis (if relevant to profession).
Management plan (provide information regarding any prescription given, test ordered or other action taken that is not made completely clear from the tape).
Overview (in approximately 50 words outline the setting of the consultation, what was achieved, and what issues may arise later).

Conclusions

Over the coming years, United Kingdom GPs will be responsible for more patients with advanced cancer and terminal disease. In addition to medical developments and advances in healthcare, GPs will need to engage in an ongoing development of their communication skills, in particular with respect to difficult scenarios around end-of-life care. The models described above deliver an evidence-based template of training, supported by a simple toolkit with which to empower GPs to enhance their communication skills throughout their professional careers.

References

1. Royal College of General Practitioners (2002) *The General Practice Consultation*. RCGP London.
2. Beckman HB, Frankel RM. The effect of physician behaviour on the collection of data. *Ann Intern Med* 1984; **101**: 692–6.
3. Fletcher C. Listening and talking to patients. I: The problem. *Br Med J* 1980; **27**: 281 (6244): 845–7.
4. Dalton HR, Noble SIR. *Communication Skills for Final MB: A Guide to Success in the OSCE*. Churchill Livingstone; 2005; 6, 7, 20.
5. Finlay IG, Sarangi S. *Oral Medical Discourse, Communication Skills and Terminally Ill Patients*. Encyclopaedia of Language and Linguistics, 2nd edition. Elsevier Oxford.
6. Mansfield F. Supervised role-play in the teaching of the process of consultation. *Med Educ* 1991; **25**: 485–90.
7. Lipkin M. Jr. Williamson P. Teaching interviewing using direct observation and discussion of actual interviews (chapter 35). In: Lipkin M Jr Putnam SM, Lazare A (eds) (1995) *The Medical Interview. Clinical Care, Education and Research*. New York: Springer-Verlag.
8. Pendleton D, Schofield T *et al*. *The consultation: an approach to learning and teaching*. Oxford University Press Oxford; 1984.
9. Kurtz S, Silverman J, Draper J. *Teaching and Learning Communication Skills in Medicine*. Radcliffe Medical Press, Oxford; 1988.
10. Finlay IG, Stott NCH, Marsh HM. Portfolio learning in palliative medicine. *Eur J Cancer Care* 1993; **2**: 41–3.

Chapter 58

Communication skills training and research: the Brussels experience

Isabelle Merckaert, Yves Libert, and Darius Razavi

Introduction

In the last two decades, communication skills training programmes, designed for healthcare professionals working in cancer care, have been the focus of several research endeavours of the Brussels research group. The efficacy of these programmes has been tested in studies using a controlled design. Studies varied in the type of healthcare professional, the type of teaching method, the length of training, and the outcome measures. These programmes aimed to determine which training techniques and programme duration promoted the transfer of learned skills to the clinical practice. As a result, research efforts have focused on communication skills to be taught and on training techniques to be used.

Training programmes

The aim of the randomized, controlled trials was to determine the optimal duration of a training programme in order to ensure training effects. The duration of each training programme was chosen according to recommendations made at the time of the development of the programme and according to results of the programmes developed previously. In the first study, the impact of a 12-hour training programme on healthcare professionals' attitudes was assessed (1, 2). Results revealed the very limited efficacy of this 12-hour training programme in changing healthcare professional attitudes. In another study, a longer 24-hour design was used to assess the impact of communication skills training on nurses' attitudes, occupational stress, and communication skills used in simulated interviews (3). The results indicated that the 24-hour communication skills training programme was efficacious, but also that there was a need to consolidate the skills acquired by regular post-training sessions. A 105-hour communication skills training programme was, therefore, designed to further increase efficacy of the training programme and to test the transfer of learned skills in clinical practice. This amount of time allowed each nurse enough time to test the proposed communication strategies in the role plays. The efficacy of this programme was confirmed by a randomized, controlled design measuring changes in attitudes, professional stress, and communication skills used in simulated and in actual patient interviews (4).

Another line of studies involved physicians working in cancer care. The aim of the first of these studies was to assess the impact on physicians' communication skills of a 40-hour communication skills training programme, utilizing a 2½-day basic training programme followed by six 3-hour consolidation workshops (5, 6). The duration of the basic training programme was chosen according to the results of previous studies that showed the usefulness of short training programmes designed for physicians (7, 8). The design of the workshops was chosen because it had been suggested that consolidation follow-up sessions were required to facilitate maintenance of newly acquired skills and transfer into the clinical practice (9). The aim of the second, outgoing, study is to assess the efficacy of a training programme designed for residents (10).

Designs and samples

All of the studies used a randomized, pre-post design. With regard to samples, the first was aimed at different types of healthcare professionals (nurses, social workers, and occupational therapists), the second at nurses, and the third at specialist physicians dealing with cancer patients. The rationale behind the samples included in the successive randomized studies was based on the investigators' wish to determine the threshold of training programme efficacy, not only as regards improvements in communication skills but also as regards improvements in participants' attitudes and stress levels, and in patients' satisfaction. The issue of the efficacy of the training programmes designed for nurses was chosen to be raised first for feasibility reasons and was then followed by the programmes designed for physicians.

The first topic to be considered concerns participant recruitment. It should be emphasized that recruitment of participants was difficult for both nurses and physicians. Different strategies were used: recruitment was done either by contacting the participants' workplace or the participants themselves. As regards recruitment through the workplace, the results of our studies show that many hospitals are unwilling to free up the requisite time for the training programme. Once given the opportunity by their workplaces, a majority of healthcare professionals agreed to participate. As regards recruitment through contacting the participant themselves, our experience shows that contacting them directly by phone or by organizing information sessions is a more productive recruitment strategy compared to invitation mailings.

Interventions

The training programmes developed by our group were based on adult theory for complex learning. They were learner-centred, skills-focused, practice-oriented, and tailored to participants' needs. Training was organized in small groups of up to 12 participants in the nurse study and was reduced to 6 participants in the physician study. Organizing training in smaller groups allowed participants to more intensively practice the learned skills in the role plays. Training included a cognitive, a behavioural, and a modeling component.

The cognitive component of learning focused on the provision of lectures and handouts providing evidence of current needs in healthcare professional communication skills and reasons for these. For example, the 105-hour nurse training programme included 30 hours of theoretical information about basic communication components, psycho-social dimensions associated with cancer diagnosis and treatments, coping with patients' and their relatives' uncertainties and distress, detecting psychopathologic reactions, and discussing death and euthanasia (legal in Belgium). The physician training programme included a 2-hour plenary session focusing on theoretical information. The first lecture covered the aims, functions, and specificity of communication in cancer care, the second focused on how to handle cancer patient's distress.

The rationale underlying the inclusion of a focus on distress is based on the fact that between 10 and 50% of cancer patients experience high levels of distress (11–13). Studies have shown that oncologists often fail to recognize distress in their patients and tend to underestimate the level of distress that they experience (14–18). Our hypothesis was that the acquisition of some knowledge about distress through this lecture, coupled with learning to use communication skills promoting disclosure of concerns, could improve physicians' detection of distress.

The decision was made to focus part of the training programme on the issue of communication with a patient when one of his or her relatives is present because three-person interviews are frequent in cancer care but the communication skills used by physicians in this particular context had not been studied specifically before. Previous studies indicate that relatives are often present in 'difficult' situations or when patients are 'vulnerable' (19–21). Relatives are more likely to be present when the patient is older and has a poorer performance status, or at specific time points in the course of the disease: for initial visits, immediately after cancer recurrence, and in the terminal phase of the disease. Relatives mainly accompany the patient to provide support or to serve as the patient's advocate. Accompanying relatives are, moreover, sometimes also the patient's primary caregiver. As the patient's caregiver, they may influence the patient's compliance with treatment and may experience emotional distress.

The behavioural component was based on role-plays. Role-plays allow participants to practice the suggested skills in a protected environment where trials are encouraged and errors are experienced. In the 105-hour nurse training programme, every participant had the opportunity to participate in four role-plays. These role-plays were video-taped and feedback was delivered from the video-recordings (4). While this type of role-play allows viewing and reviewing the sequence of interactions, it does not allow the participant the opportunity to try the suggested skill(s). Skill trial had to be planned for one of the next role-play sessions. In the study directed at specialist physicians working in oncology, role-plays with immediate feedback were used (5). Such role-plays allowed physicians to immediately test the suggested skills in the 'protected' environment of the role-play. During the first sessions, physicians practiced the communication tasks discussed in the lectures through pre-defined role-plays with immediate feedback led by experienced facilitators. The next sessions focused on role-plays based on clinical problems brought up by the participants. In all studies, participants were asked to play the role of the patient in at least one session. This was done in order to allow them the opportunity to experience the emotional impact of communication skills used by colleagues. The bimonthly consolidation workshops were spread over a 3-month period to allow physicians to test their newly acquired skills in their everyday practice and to report any difficulties encountered in their implementation.

Modelling was achieved through nurses' and physicians' observation of the skills used by their colleagues in the role-plays. This allowed them to observe the positive and negative consequences of using specific communication skills for patients and healthcare professionals.

Taught skills

The choice of the skills taught was based on results of studies indicating the positive impact of using specific communication skills on patients' disclosure of concerns (22). Communication skills promoting patients' disclosure of concerns are important because they allow healthcare professionals to respond to patients' concerns and needs in terms of information and support that can be provided. They are also the basis of a patient-centred communication. Though there are many different definitions, patient-centredness can be defined as healthcare professionals' behaviours that enable the patient to express his/her perspective on illness, treatment, and health-related behaviour, his/her symptoms, concerns, ideas, and expectations (23, 24). Healthcare professionals should use facilitating behaviours—behaviours that aim to elucidate the patient's perspective on illness and treatment, such as assessment skills (open and open-directive questions, assessing, checking, summarizing), information skills (appropriate information), and supportive skills (acknowledging, appropriate reassurance giving, empathy, or educated guesses). They should also avoid inhibiting or blocking behaviours—behaviours that restrain the patient from expressing his or her view, such as leading or multiple questions, premature information or reassurance (25).

Outcome measures

Three different approaches have been used for measuring changes in participant communication behaviours: measuring participant-based outcomes; assessing behavioural changes in the use of communication skills; and measuring patient-based outcomes.

Participant-based outcomes can be proximal measures directly related to healthcare professionals' behaviour in the observed consultation (i.e. increased confidence, comfort in interaction, reported use of specific skills) or distal measures concerning the more general functioning of healthcare professionals (e.g. attitudes, burnout, stress). In terms of participant-based outcomes, we decided in our studies to focus on changes in distal measures, such as participants' attitudes, stress, and burnout. This allowed us to observe the impact of the training programmes on the general functioning of healthcare professionals. In the physician study we also assessed physicians' ability to detect patients' distress (26, 27). Indeed, research suggests that physicians have a limited ability to detect patient distress and often tend to under-estimate the level of distress that they experience (14–18).

The behavioural assessments of communication skills rely on audio- or video-recordings of medical interviews (whether actual or simulated patient interviews) before and after training, and on the objective coding of behaviours using an interaction analysis system. Our studies used the Cancer Research Campaign Workshop Evaluation Manual (CRCWEM) (28), which is an utterance-by-utterance analysis assessment tool. Raters were blind to the trained or untrained status of the physicians and to the assessment time. The CRCWEM (28) rates the form, function, content, and emotional level of each utterance from transcripts of audio- or video-taped consultations. In the physician study a new coding (coders identified whether the utterance was addressed to the patient, the relative, or to both) was added in order to analyze three-person interviews (6). Raters were specifically trained to ensure concordance of ratings. Training included reading the manual, doing rating exercises, and being supervised by the rater coordinator. Before beginning to rate, raters had to reach a certain level of concordance that was measured through a validating test. Moreover, to ensure a quality control and to avoid rating conflicts, raters were systematically supervised by the rater coordinator. This was done through regular sessions where rating problems were discussed. Finally, a computer program was designed to detect potential rating inconsistencies of the raters. The nurse study also used a computer assisted content analysis program called PROTocol ANalyser (PROTAN) (29), which allows the researcher to count the number of words corresponding to word categories defined by dictionaries. PROTAN was used to tag both patients and nurses emotional words found in the transcripts of audio-recorded simulated and actual patient interviews (30). Behavioural analysis is a time-consuming and cost-intensive process, however, it is required in order to ascertain training effects in an objective, non-self report fashion.

The third approach involves measuring patient-based outcomes, which can be proximal measures (such as patient perception of physician behaviour or patient satisfaction with the interview) or distal measures (such as compliance with treatment, anxiety, quality of life, or general health) (31). As far as we know, studies have mainly focused on proximal measures and few programmes to date have included patient-based distal measures. In terms of patient-based outcomes, our studies focused on proximal measures: patient perception of, and satisfaction with, nurses' and physicians' behaviour (5, 4, 6). Changes in anxiety pre-post interview are another proximal measure that has been considered in our physician study (32, 33).

Interaction analyses are objective observational measures of nurse or physician behaviours, while patient perception of nurse or physician behaviours reflects the effects of those communication skills on patients. The two types of measures are thus complementary as they allow evaluating the effect of communication skills training programmes at different levels.

Training effects

First of all, it should be noted that retention of participants in the different studies was high. This may be due to the fact that the programme contents matched the participants' needs (role-plays brought up by the participants or pre-defined and based on realistic clinical cases) and/or to the fact that healthcare professionals engaging in such a long training programme were highly motivated.

In terms of participant-based outcomes, the first 12-hour training programme produced a positive shift in participant attitudes; however, this improvement only concerned the healthcare professionals who reported more negative attitudes at baseline. Post-training changes, moreover, were short-lived, as they were no more noticeable after one year (1, 2). The longer 24-hour communication skills training programme reported a significant training effect on nurses' attitudes, especially on those related to self-concept, and on the level of occupational stress related to inadequate training (3). However, two months after training, this study also found a loss of these training effects. The 105-hour communication skills training programme using the same design and tools as the previous two led to more improvements on nurses' attitudes and stress, and these improvements lasted over time (4).

Results of the physician study, showed no statistically significant time and group-by-time effects on physicians' level of burnout (34). Finally, and interestingly, in terms of participant-based outcomes, with regard to physicians' detection of distress of the patient and their relatives, results were mixed. Regardless of whether physicians attended the basic training programme or the basic training programme followed by the consolidation workshops, no change was observed in physicians' ability to detect their patients' distress in two-person interviews. However, physicians' detection of patients' distress in three-person interviews showed a positive training effect when compared to physicians in the wait list group (26, 27). Interestingly, these two studies showed that physicians' use of assessment skills focusing on psychological concerns and supportive skills are associated with an improvement in detection of distress. These results indicate that a certain degree of mastery in assessment and supportive skills is probably needed to allow accurate distress detection.

In terms of behavioural changes, the 24-hour communication skills training programme reported limited changes regarding nurses' communication skills used post-training (3). By contrast, the 105-hour communication skills training programme showed significant improvements in nurses' communication skills both in simulated and in actual patient interviews (most improvements were observed in simulated interviews). Just after training, and 3 months later, facilitative behaviours (open questions, evaluative functions) significantly increased and inhibiting behaviours (statements and responses, information without investigation, false reassurance, and blocking) significantly decreased. In actual patient interviews, trained nurses used more educated guesses, alerting to reality, and confronting utterances (4). Training effects were also observed in an increase in the number of emotional words (distress words) used by nurses in simulated and actual patient interviews (30).

Results of the physician study showed that physicians participating in the basic training programme improved their communication skills over time in two-person interviews and that the emotional level of the interviews increased. Physicians who participated in the post-consolidation workshop, moreover, used more strategies promoting patients' disclosure of concerns (respectively more open and open directive questions in simulated interviews and more acknowledgements, empathic statements, educated guesses, and negotiations in actual patient interviews) and less communication behaviours inhibiting disclosure of concerns (fewer premature reassurances in simulated interviews) (5). Finally, the six 3-hour bimonthly consolidation workshops following the 2½-day basic training, improved communication skills addressed to patients and relatives in three-person interviews. More precisely, those who participated in the post-consolidation workshop addressed the patient using more strategies promoting patients' disclosure of concerns both in simulated and in actual patient interviews. Results of this study show a transfer of learned skills to clinical practice. This study also shows that the transfer of learned skills to clinical practice is difficult when a relative is present (6).

In terms of patient-based outcomes, results of the 105-hour communication skills training programme on patient satisfaction should be stressed. Patients interacting with trained nurses reported a higher level of satisfaction with several dimensions of nurses' communication behaviours (introduction, concern clarification, information, and reassurance). This result is interesting in that no studies have reported an impact of training on patients' satisfaction. As it is often observed in studies, patients' levels of satisfaction are at ceiling already at baseline. The use in our study of a scale based on the three functions of communication (evaluation, information, and support) has allowed us to highlight changes in dimensions of patients' satisfaction.

Two main measures were used to assess the impact of the training programme devoted to physicians on patient-based outcomes: the patients' and relatives' satisfaction and the evolution of patients' and relatives' anxiety following interview. Although our intensive training programme did not lead to an increase in patient satisfaction in two-person interviews as such, for physicians who attended the consolidation workshops, patients reported that their physician had a better perception of their understanding of the disease (5). In three-person interviews, however, patients who interacted with physicians, who had been randomized to the consolidation workshops, reported a higher degree of satisfaction with physicians' performance. Interestingly, a higher degree of satisfaction with physicians' performance was not found for relatives (6). Finally, no statistically significant difference was observed in the evolution of patients' anxiety following a two-person interview, whether physicians attended the basic training programme or the basic training programme followed by the consolidation workshops (32). No statistically significant change in patients' and relatives' anxiety following a three-person interview was found either (33). It is interesting to note that on average anxiety decreased following the interview, whether a relative was present or not.

Results of these studies show the influence of some physicians' communication skills on the evolution of patients' anxiety. In particular, the more physicians used screening questions like 'have you any other concerns or questions' or 'what else', the more patients' anxiety decreased following the consultation.

Finally, another important issue in communication skills training is the identification of factors that could mitigate the impact of learning. In our physician study, we assessed the predictive value of one characteristic of physicians on their ability to learn new communication skills. It is widely recognized that educational interventions may be more effective for people with an 'internal' Locus of Control (LOC) (who believe that life outcomes are controlled by their own characteristics or actions) compared to people with an 'external' Locus of Control (who believe that life outcomes are controlled by external forces such as luck, fate, or others). Therefore, we tested the hypothesis that physicians with an 'internal' LOC would demonstrate communication skills acquisition to a greater degree than those with an 'external' LOC (35). As it was expected, learned communication skills are more frequent among physicians with an 'internal' LOC compared to the frequency of learned skills among physicians with an 'external' LOC either in two-person or three-person simulated interviews.

Conclusion

In the last two decades, several communication skills training programmes, designed for healthcare professionals working in oncology, have been tested in Brussels. The first line of studies involved different types of healthcare professionals (nurses, social workers, and occupational therapists), the second line of studies involved nurses, and the third line of studies involved physicians working with cancer patients. The main aim of the training programmes in these different lines of studies was to promote the knowledge and use of communication skills to improve patient care. Results of these studies have allowed us to draw some conclusions with regards to intervention techniques and training effects.

As in most efficacy studies, one of the difficulties of our investigations was the recruitment of healthcare professionals. Few studies have reported the recruitment strategies utilized, thus, comparison between recruitment strategies is difficult. Recruitment could be facilitated by better strategies to inform hospital managers about the professional benefits of these training programmes for their workers. Another way to increase participation would be to build smaller group sessions (two to three participants) at the workplace or to design training programmes tailored for each team of healthcare professionals.

It is not surprising that a dose-effect was found for training on communication skills. Moreover, the transfer of some skills—for example, skills addressing relatives' concerns and needs—are limited, even after a long training programme. Training programmes focusing on patient-centred communication skills acquisition seem to produce little change in specific participant-based outcomes, such as detection of distress or burnout, or on patient-based outcomes, such as satisfaction and anxiety. Two perspectives could be drawn from these results. First, future studies should explore why some participant-based outcomes or patient-based outcomes that are complementary in theory are not linked empirically. Second, future studies should further assess the impact of specific training modules on some participant-based outcomes and/or on some patient-based outcomes. Such specific training modules should in theory follow training programmes, including consolidation sessions following a basic training in order to ensure transfer of learned skills to clinical practice.

Our techniques were learner-centred, skills-focused, practice-oriented, and tailored to the participants' needs. In particular, the use of role-plays based on clinical cases brought up by the participants and the use of immediate feed-back appears to be effective. This could be due to the fact that these techniques allowed healthcare professionals to receive feedback about their communication difficulties. Trainers should, therefore, be able to provide such feedback to each participant.

Assessment tools used in our studies led to solid conclusions about behavioural changes but were very expensive. In particular, the use of interaction-process analyses was cost-intensive. A first way to reduce this cost could be to use speech-recognition technology to facilitate transcription and to develop computer-assisted systems of interaction analyses. Such a system has been developed for French transcripts (36). Another positive impact of such systems could be to provide healthcare professionals with an annotated feedback, which may further facilitate communication skills learning.

Some results of our communication skills training programmes on the patient should be stressed. In the 105-hours study, patients interacting with trained nurses reported a higher level of satisfaction with some dimensions of nurses' communication skills (concern clarification, information, and reassurance), despite the small number of facilitative communication skills changes observed in actual patient interviews. In the physician study, in three-person interviews, patients interacting with physicians who benefited from consolidation workshops reported higher satisfaction scores. These impacts highlight that cancer patients may be able to perceive and appreciate their healthcare professionals' communication skills. This type of result validates the usefulness of communication skills training programmes for healthcare professionals.

Finally, one of our studies shows that the Locus of Control is a psychological characteristic associated with a learning style (35). This type of study indicates the importance of taking into account participant characteristics that may predict optimal versus suboptimal learning. Other potential predictors may be attitudes, beliefs, outcome expectancies, self-efficacy, and coping style. Taking into account such predictors in designing the content of future training may further increase training efficacy. Also, it may be possible to tailor communication skills training programmes to the participant.

Results of our studies confirm the usefulness of communication skills training programmes for healthcare professionals working in cancer care. To be effective, training should include learner-centred, skills-focused, and practice-oriented techniques; be organized in small group; and be at least 20-hours long. The development of communication skills training programmes designed for nurses and physicians can thus be recommended to all healthcare professionals working regularly with cancer patients and their families.

References

1. Razavi D, Delvaux N, Farvacques C, *et al.* Immediate effectiveness of brief psychological training for health professionals dealing with terminally ill cancer patients: a controlled study. *Soc Sci Med*, 1988; **27**(4): 369–75.

2. Razavi D, Delvaux N, Farvacques C, *et al.* Brief psychological training for healthcare professionals dealing with cancer patients: a one-year assessment. *Gon Mosp Psychiatry*, 1991; **13**(4): 253–60.

3. Razavi D, Delvaux N, Marchal S, *et al.* The effects of a 24-h psychological training programme on attitudes, communication skills and occupational stress in oncology: a randomised study. *Eur J Cancer*, 1993; **29A**(13): 1858–63.

4. Delvaux N, Razavi D, Marchal S, *et al.* Effects of a 105 hours psychological training programme on attitudes, communication skills and occupational stress in oncology: a randomised study. *Br J Cancer*, 2004; **90**(1): 106–14.

5. Razavi D, Merckaert I, Marchal S, *et al.* How to optimize physicians' communication skills in cancer care: results of a randomized study assessing the usefulness of posttraining consolidation workshops. *J Clin Oncol*, 2003; **21**(16): 3141–9.

6. Delvaux N, Merckaert I, Marchal S, *et al.* Physicians' communication with a cancer patient and a relative: a randomized study assessing the efficacy of consolidation workshops. *Cancer*, 2005; **103**(11): 2397–411.

7. Levinson W, Roter D. The effects of two continuing medical education programmes on communication skills of practicing primary care physicians. *J Gen Intern Med*, 1993; **8**(6): 318–24.

8. Maguire P, Booth K, Elliott C, *et al.* Helping health professionals involved in cancer care acquire key interviewing skills—the impact of workshops. *Eur J Cancer* 1996; **32A**(9): 1486–9.

9. Parle M, Maguire P, Heaven C. The development of a training model to improve health professionals' skills, self-efficacy and outcome expectancies when communicating with cancer patients. *Soc Sci Med*, 1997; **44**(2): 231–40.

10. Bragard I, Razavi D, Marchal S, *et al.* Teaching communication and stress management skills to junior physicians dealing with cancer patients: a Belgian Interuniversity Curriculum. *Support Care Cancer*, 2006; **14**(5): 454–61.

11. Derogatis LR, Morrow GR, Fetting J, *et al.* The prevalence of psychiatric disorders among cancer patients. *JAMA*, 1983; **249**(6): 751–7.

12. Chochinov HM, Wilson KG, Enns M, *et al.* Prevalence of depression in the terminally ill: effects of diagnostic criteria and symptom threshold judgments. *Am J Psychiatry*, 1994; **151**(4): 537–40.

13. Zabora J, BrintzenhofeSzoc K, Curbow B, *et al.* The prevalence of psychological distress by cancer site. *Psycho-Oncology*, 2001; **10**(1): 19–28.

14. Ford S, Fallowfield L, Lewis S. Can oncologists detect distress in their out-patients and how satisfied are they with their performance during bad news consultations? *Br J Cancer*, 1994; **70**(4): 767–70.

15. Newell S, Sanson-Fisher RW, Girgis A, *et al.* How well do medical oncologists' perceptions reflect their patients' reported physical and psychosocial problems? Data from a survey of five oncologists. *Cancer,* 1998; **83**(8): 1640–51.

16. Passik SD, Dugan W, McDonald MV, *et al.* Oncologists' recognition of depression in their patients with cancer. *J Clin Onol,* 1998; **16**(4): 1594–600.

17. Fallowfield L, Ratcliffe D, Jenkins V, *et al.* Psychiatric morbidity and its recognition by doctors in patients with cancer. *Br J Cancer,* 2001; **84**(8): 1011–5.

18. Sollner W, DeVries A, Steixner E, *et al.* How successful are oncologists in identifying patient distress, perceived social support, and need for psychosocial counselling? *Br J Cancer,* 2001; **84**(2): 179–85.

19. Adelman RD, Greene MG, Charon R. The physician–elderly patient-companion triad in the medical encounter—the development of a conceptual-framework and research agenda. *Gerontologist* 1987; **27**(6): 729–34.

20. Labrecque MS, Blanchard CG, Ruckdeschel JC, *et al.* The impact of family presence on the physician cancer-patient interaction. *Soc Sci Med* 1991; **33**(11): 1253–61.

21. Beisecker AE, Moore WP. Oncologists' perceptions of the effects of cancer patients' companions on physician-patient interactions. *J Psychosoc Oncol,* 1994; **12**(1/2): 23–39.

22. Maguire P, Faulkner A, Booth K, *et al.* Helping cancer patients disclose their concerns. *Eur J Cancer,* 1996; **32A**(1): 78–81.

23. Levenstein JH, McCracken EC, McWhinney IR, *et al.* The patient-centred clinical method. 1. A model for the doctor-patient interaction in family medicine. *Fan Pract,* 1986; **3**(1): 24–30.

24. Smith RC, Hoppe RB. The patient's story: integrating the patient- and physician-centered approaches to interviewing. *Ann Intern Med,* 1991; **115**(6): 470–7.

25. Zandbelt LC, Smets EM, Oort FJ, *et al.* Patient participation in the medical specialist encounter: does physicians' patient-centred communication matter? *Patient Educ Couns,* 2007; **65**(3): 396–406.

26. Merckaert I, Libert Y, Delvaux N, *et al.* Factors that influence physicians' detection of distress in patients with cancer: can a communication skills training programme improve physicians' detection? *Cancer,* 2005; **104**(2): 411–21.

27. Merckaert I, Libert Y, Delvaux N, *et al.* Factors influencing physicians' detection of cancer patients' and relatives' distress: can a communication skills training programme improve physicians' detection? *Psycho-Oncology,* 2008; **17**(3): 260–9.

28. Booth C, Maguire P. *Development of a rating system to assess interaction between cancer patients and health professionals.* London: Report to Cancer Research Campaign; 1991.

29. Hogenraad R, Daubies C, Bestgen Y. *Une théorie et une méthode générale d'analyse textuelle assistée par ordinateur: le Système PROTAN (PROTocol ANalyser).* Computer programme manual. Unpublished document. Louvain-la-Neuve: Université Catholique de Louvain, Psychology Department; 1995.

30. Razavi D, Delvaux N, Marchal S, *et al.* Does training increase the use of more emotionally laden words by nurses when talking with cancer patients? A randomised study. *Br J Cancer,* 2002; **87**(1): 1–7.

31. Hulsman RL, Ros WFG, Winnubst JAM, *et al.* Teaching clinically experienced physicians communication skills. A review of evaluation studies. *Med Educ* 1999; **33**(9): 655–668.

32. Lienard A, Merckaert I, Libert Y, *et al.* Factors that influence cancer patients' anxiety following a medical consultation: impact of a communication skills training programmeme for physicians. *Ann Oncol,* 2006; **17**(9): 1450–8.

33. Lienard A, Merckaert I, Libert Y, *et al.* Factors that influence cancer patients' and relatives' anxiety following a three-person medical consultation: impact of a communication skills training programme for physicians. *Psycho-Oncology,* 2007.

34. Bragard I, Libert Y, Etienne AM, *et al*. Impact of communication skills training programmes on physicians' level of burnout: results derived from a randomized controlled study. Submitted to *Med Educ*.

35. Libert Y, Merckaert I, Reynaert C, *et al*. Physicians are different when they learn communication skills: influence of the locus of control. *Psycho-Oncology*, 2007; 16(6): 553–62.

36. Razavi D, Durieux JF, Moucheux A, *et al*. LaComm: a French medical communication analysis software. *Psycho-Oncology*, 2006; **15**(2): S192-S192 Meeting Abstract 450 Suppl. S.

Section G

Research in cancer communication

Section editor: Barry D Bultz

It is fitting that research in cancer communication training closes this comprehensive textbook. Asking key questions through research provides the catalyst for change in programme development and implementation. This concluding section highlights evaluation methods for communication training programmes and participants. Quantitative and qualitative methodologies that probe the subtleties of communication training are described in detail. Through the use of these evaluation techniques, participants gain insight into strengths and weaknesses, while programme developers identify shortcomings of extant programmes. This section provides tools for further efforts to advance research in the field of communication training evaluation.

Chapter 59

Evaluating communication skills training courses

Lyuba Konopasek, Marcy Rosenbaum, John Encandela, and Kathy Cole-Kelly

Introduction

Across the continuum of medical education the focus is shifting from the teacher and the curriculum to the learner and the evaluation of educational outcomes. In the field of communication skills training, educators are now carefully examining the outcomes of their programmes. While the effect of many communication skills training programmes have been measured exclusively with questionnaire surveys of learner satisfaction, a number of other outcome measures are essential to consider in planning effective evaluation strategies. These include surveys of self-efficacy, demonstration of skills, patient satisfaction surveys, and health outcomes. In this chapter we will identify assessment strategies used for communication skills training, describe how to design an effective evaluation methodology, and consider how outcomes have been measured in the oncology communication skills training literature.

Evaluation is broadly defined as the use of social research methods to systematically investigate the quality and effects of an intervention, activity, or programme (1). In education, the object of evaluation may be individual learners, educational interventions, or educational policy and other social structures affecting education. For the sake of this chapter, we will concentrate on evaluation of learners and interventions.

Educational interventions to be evaluated can be a single instructional or training activity (e.g. a lecture or training demonstration to teach a clinical skill), a set of such activities (e.g. all educational endeavours that occur within a clinical rotation), or an entire curriculum or training programme (e.g. the medical education curriculum or residency programme). Each of these levels of activity depends on the same set of social research methods that help determine how and how well the intervention has been implemented (a focus on process) and how and how well it has achieved its intended results (a focus on outcomes). The most effective approach to determine how well an educational intervention has attained its desired outcomes is to consider the aggregate results of individual-learner evaluations. In this way, evaluations of individuals can be useful in both providing feedback to individual learners and providing feedback to educators about the effects of the programme on a cumulative set of learners.

Evaluation data can also be used to answer research questions; however, it is important to draw a distinction between evaluation and research. Evaluation is an ongoing process that occurs in conjunction with the curriculum in order to address the efficacy of the training programme and its learners. On the other hand, the purpose of research on a particular educational intervention is to answer a specific question and produce generalizable results, which can be used in promoting dissemination of this intervention (2). In both instances it is necessary to use reliable and valid tools for measuring outcomes and, in fact, the results of programme evaluation can be used for research projects.

Evaluation of communications training programmes should follow standards and guidelines familiar in other types of research. For instance, assessment of training should produce data that are valid and reliable. The validity of a measure or assessment is the extent to which it measures what is intended to be measured. For example, faculty ratings of learners' skills to communicate with patients provide a valid measure to the extent that these ratings actually reflect how well learners communicate with patients. If these ratings merely reflect raters' behaviours (e.g. using a 5-point scale, faculty raters may habitually assign 4s to all junior residents and 5s to all senior residents) then these ratings are not valid measures of learners' communication skills. Moreover, if the interest is in whether a measure provides a valid assessment of the training intervention's effect on learners, evaluators would need to make certain that the measure reflects the interventions' desired outcomes for learners. For instance, a measure of the effectiveness of a communication skills training may be thought to be valid if the measure is able to detect changes in learners' communication skills from pre-intervention to post-intervention periods.

Similarly, evaluation of training should meet standards of reliability. In brief, an assessment approach is reliable when it yields 'consistent results regardless of when it is used, who uses it, and which item or case is assessed' (3). Though new measures or instruments may be available, it is typically recommended that educators locate reliable measures already existing for assessing communication skills. As a precaution, the assessment tool should be implemented under conditions that are similar to the conditions in which the tool was initially tested.

It is also important that assessment approaches be feasible, especially given the resource and time constraints that confront medical educational programmes. To be feasible, an assessment approach should require a reasonable amount of time, training, materials or technology, and financial cost. To determine feasibility, the cost of implementation—especially the amount of time it will take trainers and trainees to conduct the assessment—must be weighed against the potential benefit of assessment data.

Perhaps most important, assessments should yield information that will be useful to the trainees and to programmes as a whole. A good test of usefulness is asking these questions of any evaluation:

1. Will learners know how well they perform and what they need to do to improve as a result of assessment findings?
2. Will trainers know how to improve training and curriculum as a result of the findings?

Assessment methods and evaluation system design

The design of a programme evaluation system should be considered at the beginning of planning for a curriculum or teaching module. Rather than being an after-thought, the development of the evaluation system should proceed in parallel with curricular planning and design. Evaluation should also be closely linked to the content, the learning objectives, the process, and the instructional methodology.

Other issues to consider when developing a programme assessment plan include use of control groups, recruitment and randomization of participants, method of observation, blinding of subjects and raters, use of validated instruments, and timing of assessment. A 2002 Cochrane review of communication skills training for healthcare professionals working with cancer patients, their families, and/or caregivers found that most studies measured changes in physician attitudes and/or knowledge rather than actual behaviour. Butow similarly points out that most physician evaluations use self-report methods, and also states that patients are rarely asked about impact (4). Furthermore, while there are some randomized controlled trials (RCTs) on the effect of communication skills training in oncology (5–9), most reports do not use control groups. Also, in the majority of studies, subjects have self-selected to attend the training, thus, personal motivation may be a confounding factor. It is difficult to double-blind the study subjects to allocation in behavioural interventions such as communication skills training (10). The blinding of raters is possible, although not always done. Finally, the sustainability of training effect needs to be considered. In most studies, the impact of the intervention is generally measured immediately after training. Some authors have also measured effects one to 6 months (5), and up to 12 months later (11).

One way of assuring that many of the above evaluation standards are met is to closely align evaluation plans with corresponding curriculum and programme plans. A useful tool in helping to build such congruence is the logic model, which is a graphic depiction of the basic programme or curriculum organization (12). A logic model consists of related components:

- *Inputs* or resources that are needed in order to implement a programme or curriculum. Inputs commonly consist of funding, materials, equipment, and programme or instructional staffing.

- *Activities* are the actual instructional and programme processes that are implemented. These can be workshops, classes, special training events, etc.

- *Outputs* are the immediate results or products of activities as experienced by participants of these activities, such as the trainees of a communications training programme.

- *Outcomes* are the desired results or changes in knowledge, attitudes, behaviours, or skills among participants or trainees that should come about as a result of taking part in the programme or curriculum.

Sketching out exactly how a programme or curriculum will operate by using a set of inputs to deliver activities and outputs, and how these will influence desired outcomes among trainees, provides a framework for evaluating the total curriculum/programme and its results. An example of a communications training logic model and its corresponding evaluation plan is shown in Fig. 59.1.

Desired outcome measurements need to be considered explicitly in developing an evaluation system. Kirkpatrick has defined four levels of evaluation related to educational interventions and ways to assess their impact (13) (see Fig. 59.2). These levels progress from Level 1, measuring learner reactions; to Level 2, measuring learning as indicated by change in attitudes, knowledge, and/or skills; to Level 3, measuring changes in learner behaviours; and finally to Level 4, measuring the intervention's impact on society (e.g. the effect on healthcare outcomes, such as adherence and patient satisfaction). For purposes of this chapter, we will examine each of these evaluation levels, examples of types of measures used for each level in specific relation to communication skills training, advantages and disadvantages of types of measures for each level, and will present some examples of evaluation studies using multiple levels.

Kirkpatrick's Level 1

In Level 1, the learner's reaction to the training is evaluated. These types of measures examine participants' views on the learning experience, its organization, presentation, content, teaching methods, and quality of instruction. In other words, did the participants like the training? Instruments that measure at this level have often been called 'smile sheets' and are the focus of many communication skills programme evaluations (14). They often take the form of Likert scales focused on different aspects of training programme content and organization, supplemented with opportunities for open-ended comments.

Advantages of using this type of assessment method include identification of learners' perceptions of what did and did not work in terms of training method and content with minimal effort in developing and implementing evaluation instruments. Assessment of trainee reactions can be

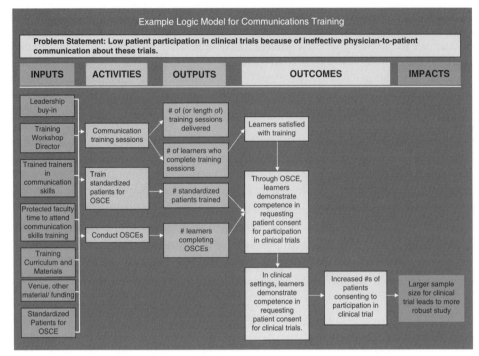

Figure 59.1 Sample logic model

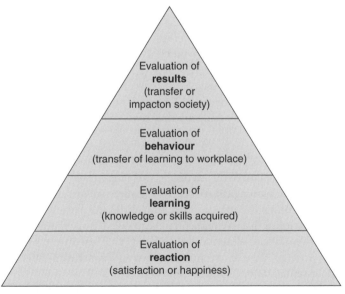

Figure 59.2 Kirkpatrick's triangle

easily conducted using paper-based surveys at the end of a training programme or paper and/ or web-based surveys administered at some point after training has been completed. Delayed administration of this type of programme evaluation until days, weeks, or months after completion of training allows for an assessment of trainees longer term satisfaction with programme content and structure. A major disadvantage of relying solely on trainee reaction for evaluation is that the report that learners liked an educational intervention does not tell what they learned. For example, an entertaining trainer may yield extremely high satisfaction ratings but may not be particularly adept at ensuring any learning. Satisfaction ratings can also be influenced by the selection criteria for participants. Participants volunteer for many communication skills training programmes described in the literature. Measures of satisfaction by participants who want to learn a particular subject may not be generalizable. A final limitation is that smile sheets focus attention on evaluation of the teacher and instructional methods rather than on the learner and impact on learning. Thus, while they are easy to administer, give the instructor immediate feedback, and look valid because quantifiable data is generated, Level 1 evaluations should not be the only measure of a module's impact.

Kirkpatrick's Level 2

Level 2 addresses changes in learner's attitudes, knowledge, and/or skills, as measured both through self-assessment and paper-based assessment of knowledge and skills. Steinert and others have adapted Kirkpatrick's model to distinguish between changes in attitudes (Level 2A) and changes in knowledge and/or skills (Level 2B) (15).

Level 2A

Level 2A evaluations focus on learners' self-efficacy and changes in attitudes towards learning or using a specific skill. Self-efficacy is assessed by asking learners if they perceive a change in specific knowledge or skill domains following training. For example, Baile evaluated two half-day communication skills workshops with satisfaction questionnaires (Level 1), as well as Level 2A self-efficacy measures (16). In addition to finding that participants were satisfied with the workshops, Baile found that participants felt that learning objectives were met, and that they had greater confidence in communicating bad news. Use of these types of measures prior to and after training allow for comparison, lending added strength to these self-assessments. Self-efficacy can also be measured using a retrospective pre-test and post-test survey, where participants are asked to compare their skills prior to the training with skills after the training (17). Level 2A evaluations can also measure attitudes toward communication skills; for example, learners' perceptions of the importance of a particular communication skill, as well as plans to use this skill (18). Parle asserted that attitudes, such as self-efficacy and outcome expectancy towards skills, are essential to the maintenance and development of communication skills (19). By measuring ratings of confidence in key communication areas immediately after an intervention and again three months later, Fallowfield demonstrated that these types of changes in attitude of senior clinicians who complete a training course can be sustained over a 3-month period (20). Thus, advantages of this type of evaluation include understanding the learner's attitude towards a new skill, which is an important pre-requisite to actually applying it in clinical practice. The limitation is that this level of evaluation does not assess actual knowledge, skills, or behaviours.

Level 2B

Level 2B evaluations include measurement of knowledge and skill level through paper exams and/ or observed simulated patient encounters with standardized checklists, i.e. Objective Structured Clinical Exams (OSCEs). When viewed in aggregate, data on individual learner performance can yield valuable information for programme evaluation. As with all Level 2B evaluations, this is only a measure of the impact of an educational intervention if pre- and post-intervention measurements of knowledge or skills are compared. While paper exams can provide information on achievement of certain stated learning objectives related to knowledge, such as learning a new conceptual framework for a communication skill, observed encounters with simulated patients are considered a high-fidelity method for measuring the skills related to communication (21). The OSCE format allows for behaviours to be observed, measured, and analysed (22), identifying learners' ability to put content into practice in a simulated situation. OSCEs also allow for control of variables that cannot be controlled in actual clinical encounters. This is especially important in programme evaluation in which OSCEs are used to measure specific tasks that have been taught. While many OSCE stations are designed to focus primarily on the process of communication and interpersonal skills, it is possible to challenge learners with increasingly complex content. Hodges (23) demonstrated that OSCE stations with more challenging content, such as difficult emotional situations, can be created with acceptable reliability. Most programmes have used single, focused, simulated patient (SP) encounters to test specific skills before and after the training (6, 24). A potential limitation of relying on only one patient interaction to measure the effect of an educational intervention is case specificity (interaction with one patient cannot reliably predict performance) (25). Multiple station OSCEs control better for case specificity. Disadvantages of using SPs include labour and cost intensity, the challenge of rater reliability, and the potential for trainees' perception that they are less realistic than actual encounters. Also, while this level of evaluation may measure what a learner is capable of achieving, either in a written exam or a simulated patient exam, it does not measure actual behaviour change in clinical practice (26).

Back's evaluation of Oncotalk, a communication skills retreat workshop for oncology fellows, is an excellent example of the use of SPs for measuring the efficacy of training (27). Participant communication skills were measured before and after a training intervention by analysing audio-taped, standardized, patient encounters. The audio-tapes were assessed by blinded coders using a validated coding system. Back's decision to not use a separate cohort of individuals as a control was informed by a number of studies, which demonstrated that communication skills do not improve in control arms (28, 7, 29). Back's study clearly demonstrated an increase in the use of taught skills with simulated patients, but stopped short of evaluating the impact of the workshops on physician behaviour in the live clinical encounter.

Kirkpatrick's Level 3

Level 3 evaluation assesses the actual change in communication behaviours in the context of patient care. As communication is a behavioural skill, assessment of actual communication behaviour is considered one of the most accurate measures of the impact of training programmes. A variety of approaches have been used to assess changes in communication behaviours related to cancer care: observation of encounters with patients by others (live, audio-taped, or video-taped), use of unannounced patients to assess behaviours, and use of real patients to assess behaviours. Disadvantages of assessing communication skills in patient encounters include costs and logistical challenges associated with gathering this type of data, inability to standardize the encounter to assure certain communication challenges and opportunities, and the additional time required to systematically analyse the data. Observing 5–9 different patient encounters per measurement time can help solve the problem of variability in these interviews (30).

Kirkpatrick's Level 4

Level 4 evaluations measure change in patient care outcomes related to the education intervention. Approaches to measuring the impact of training on healthcare outcomes include changes in patient satisfaction and changes in healthcare outcomes measured by chart review. Patient surveys have been used in several settings, including following a hospital or outpatient office visit. The American Board of Internal Medicine uses these surveys as part of their recertification modules and some healthcare plans utilize them as a component of accreditation. The surveys ask real patients about their experiences with the physician's communication skills. Many authors have suggested that patients' responses on these surveys are a more accurate reflection of the physicians' skills than observed encounters with skills checklists. It must be noted, however, that these surveys have been conducted primarily with physicians in practice versus with medical students or residents. The surveys also have some other complicating factors, such as a possible confusion between what the patient reports as being done well versus what really occurred in the encounter. Exploring further use of patient surveys for medical students and residents is certainly worth consideration. The importance of looking beyond changes in behaviour to patient outcomes is illustrated by Brown's study in which a one-day experiential workshop on seeking informed consent for cancer clinical trials led to some changes in physician behaviour, as measured by audio-taped patient interviews (31). These changes, while statistically significant, did not lead to any significant patient outcomes.

Planning for Assessment

In planning for assessment, it is also critical to select appropriate instruments for measuring programme effect. Skills checklists of observed behaviours in interactions with peers, simulated patients, or real patients are essential for assessing communication and interpersonal skills explicitly in level 2B, level 3, and even some level 4 evaluations. Checklists can be standard observation instruments, examining general communication skills, or study-specific instruments, which focus on the behaviours taught in the training programme (30). Examples of standard observation instruments include the Medical Interaction Process System (MIPS) (32, 11) and Roter's Interaction Analysis System (RIAS) (33). In programme evaluation, skills checklists should link closely with learning objectives and the conceptual communication skills framework that is being taught. In a review of the communication objectives and behaviours addressed in the communication skills literature, Cegala (34) found that many studies did not specify behaviours taught, and in several studies there was a mismatch between objectives and instruments used. Checklists generally describe a skill and are linked to an evaluation component that is either a numeric (Likert) scale of ratings for low to high ratings or merely headings (e.g. done, not done, or does not apply). Some checklists include anchoring statements to help the observer best define the numeric rating. Many checklists provide space for a brief narrative or general comments. Some checklist forms request respondents to record the time the skill was done or could have been done (e.g. an empathic opportunity), so that when the learner observes his/her interview, the specific time when that skill was done or could have been done is apparent. The rater of the checklist may be a peer, a senior learner, a faculty member, a trained simulated patient, or a real patient. Makoul's Communication Assessment Tool is an example of a checklist that has been validated as an instrument for patients' assessment of physicians in live encounters (35). Observations used for coding may be live, video-taped, or audio-taped. Analysing audio-taped encounters is limited by inability to assess non-verbal cues. Ensuring familiarity and comfort in using the scale, and inter-rater reliability are critically important if it is to serve as the basis for programme evaluation. Of note, in a review of 14 evaluation studies of communication skills training programmes for clinically experienced physicians, Hulsman found positive training effects in only half or less of observed behaviours (30). Positive training effects may also be obscured by high performance levels prior to the training, another potential bias for self-selected participants (30). An additional potential limitation is that many checklists emphasize thoroughness and, therefore, present long lists of questions or items; thus, experienced clinicians whose approach is more focused may actually receive a lower score because they have not asked all of the questions on the list, even if they have communicated effectively (25).

As we have described, Kirkpatrick's model can be useful for guiding evaluation of training programmes. While the model is not meant to be hierarchical, the rigor of the information gleaned in general increases as we move up the levels. In addition, the labour and cost intensity of different levels appears to increase as we move up the levels, with smile sheets being easiest to implement, while measurement of actual behaviour and patient outcomes is more intense. Many programme evaluations report using a combination of assessments at different levels to develop an overall picture of the reactions to training plus impact of training on knowledge, attitudes, behaviour, and outcome. Several studies described below illustrate assessment strategies that employ multiple Kirkpatrick levels and thus yield different kinds of information to inform programme efficacy and development.

Butow's 2008 study of the effect of a communication skills programme to increase oncologists' skills in eliciting and responding to emotional cues, is an RCT that demonstrates evaluation at multiple levels (5). It assessed doctor behaviour through video-taped SP encounters and evaluated physician burnout and satisfaction through questionnaires as secondary outcome measures. Burnout was studied as a secondary measure because difficulties with communication have been shown to be associated with increased physician stress and burnout. An acceptability survey was completed six months after the intervention and was very positive, with all doctors utilizing the patient information, believing that the training provided them with useful information, and finding that practicing skills was useful. However, the SP data revealed no significant change in the number of behaviours demonstrated. Further, the physicians' surveys were also unchanged in terms of burnout. Thus, while the physicians' high level of acceptability is certainly important for intended behaviour change, it does not guarantee it. This study illustrates the need to evaluate at multiple levels.

Delavaux's randomized study on the effect of additional training on physician communication skills in the three-person interview, is another excellent example of using multiple evaluation levels, and also illustrates the importance of examining the perceptions of all participants in the interview (6). In this study, physicians, patients, and family members all completed surveys assessing perceptions of the physician's behaviours. The physicians were evaluated in both SP and in live patient encounters. Of note, the assessment yielded valuable aggregate data describing which skills improved and which skills required more focus in future training. While physician perception and patient satisfaction were positive, there was no change in the family members' satisfaction, indicating a need for further training in this domain.

Fallowfield's study of the effect of a 3-day course and written feedback on communication skills included ratings made by researchers, doctors, and patients and evaluations on multiple Kirkpatrick levels (7, 11). Oncologists applied to join the course, so there was an element of self-selection in the trial. They were then all video-taped in 6–10 encounters in the clinical setting and randomly assigned to one of four study groups. All groups, including the controls, were video-taped at baseline, as described, and again 3 months after the training intervention, at the same time as the intervention groups. One of two raters analysed each of the videos using a validated instrument. Measured outcomes addressed several of Kirkpatrick's levels: physician satisfaction (enjoyment, relevance to practice) and confidence (Level 1), ratings of observed behaviours in practice (Level 3), and patient satisfaction (Level 4). One limitation of her study was that in using live unscripted patients, not all behaviours taught could be observed or evaluated, especially if the circumstances for using them are rare and not likely to occur over just 6–10 encounters. Furthermore, if the behaviours are not observed both before and after the intervention, it is difficult to assess if there has been a change as a result of the programme.

Summary and implications

This chapter has provided an overview of approaches to evaluating communication skills training programmes. This review has several important implications for future design of communication skills training evaluation. First, the majority of training evaluations reported in the literature have tended to limit measures to Kirkpatrick's Levels 1 and 2, likely reflecting the relatively lower cost required in these types of evaluations. Evaluators should be encouraged to consider how to better measure the impact of training programmes on actual behaviour and/or healthcare outcomes for a more rigorous understanding of both the shorter and longer term impacts of the educational programme. Second, choice of evaluation methods should be based on overall curriculum design and objectives. For example, if the objective of the training is to change attitudes, a pencil and paper measure of attitudes may suffice; however, if the objective is to change learner behaviour, the impact of training is best measured using SP or actual patient encounter observations. Third, use of methods that measure impact of training on more than one level can provide a more in-depth picture of the effects of training on attitudes, knowledge, behaviour, and skill. Fourth, while we have emphasized the importance of learner and programme evaluation for assessing the impact of training, evaluation also serves the purpose of increasing learners' and practitioners' perceptions of the value and importance of the skills being assessed. As an example, the incorporation of explicit assessment of learner communication skills through OSCEs as part of high stakes national licensing exams in Canada, the UK, the US, and other countries, has stimulated an increased emphasis on the importance of these skills among learners, educators, and practitioners. Evaluation measures can also provide essential feedback for individual learners on how they can improve their communication skills and can provide feedback to help guide curriculum development and revision. Finally, evaluation of communication training interventions can provide the basis for scholarship that can be disseminated to academic colleagues interested in designing, assessing, and improving their own communication skills training programmes. Designers and implementers of communication skills training programmes should be encouraged to use rigorous programme evaluations and to disseminate their results in the literature.

References

1. Rossi PH, Lipsey MW, Freeman HE. *Evaluation: a systematic approach*, 7th edn. Thousand Oaks,CA: Sage; 2004.
2. Morrison J. Evaluation. *BMJ* 2003; **326**: 385–7.
3. Lynch DC, Swing SR. Key considerations for selecting assessment tools and implementing assessment systems [online] [cited 2008 March 9]. Accreditation Council for Graduate Medical Education Website: **http: //www.acgme.org/outcome/assess/refList_archive.asp**
4. Butow P. Commentary on developing communication competency in the context of cancer: a critical interpretive analysis of provider training programmes. *Psychooncology* 2005; **14**: 873–4.
5. Butow P, Cockburn J, Girgis A, *et al.* Increasing oncologist's skills in eliciting and responding to emotional cues: evaluation of a communication skills training programme. *Psychooncology* 2008; **17**(3): 209–18.
6. Delvaux N, Merckaert I, Marchal S, *et al.* Physician's communication with cancer patient and relative: a randomized study assessing the efficacy of consolidation workshops. *Cancer* 2005; **103**(11): 2397–411.
7. Fallowfield L, Jenkins V, Farewell V, *et al.* Efficacy of a cancer research UK communication skills training model for oncologists: a randomized controlled study. *Lancet* 2002; **359**(9307): 650–6.

8. Razavi D, Delvaux N, Marchal S, *et al.* The effects of a 24-h psychological training programme on attitudes, communication skill and occupational stress in oncology: a randomized study. *Eur J Cancer* 1993; **29**A(13): 1858–63.

9. Razavi D, Delvaux N, Marchal S, *et al.* Does training increase the use of more emotionally laden words by nurses when talking with cancer patients? A randomized study. *Br J Cancer* 2002; **87**: 1–7.

10. Smith S, Hanson JL, Tewksbury LR, *et al.* Teaching patient communication skills to medical students: a review of randomized controlled trails. *Eval Health Prof* 2007; **30**: 3–21.

11. Fallowfield L, Jenkins V, Farewell V, *et al.* Enduring impact of communication skills training: results of a 12-month follow-up. *Br J Cancer* 2003; 89: 1445–9.

12. WK Kellogg Foundation. *Using logic models to bring together planning, evaluation, and action: logic model development guide.* Battle Creek (MI): WK Kellogg Foundation; 2004.

13. Hutchinson L. Evaluating and researching the effectiveness of educational interventions. *BMJ* 1999; **318**: 1267–9.

14. Rosenbaum ME, Ferguson KJ, Lobas JG. Teaching medical students and residents skills delivering bad news: a review of strategies. *Acad Med* 2004; **79**(2): 107–17.

15. Steinert Y, Mann K, Centeno A, *et al.* A systematic review of faculty development initiatives designed to improve teaching effectiveness in medical education. BEME Guide No 8. Medical Teacher 2006; **28**: 497–526

16. Baile WF, Kudelka AP, Beale E, *et al.* Communication skills training in oncology: description and preliminary outcomes of workshops on breaking bad news and managing patients reactions to illness. *Cancer* 1999; 86(5): 887–97.

17. Skeff KM, Stratos GA, Berman J, *et al.* Improving clinical teaching: evaluation of a national dissemination programme. *Arch Intern Med* 1992; **152**: 1156–61.

18. Jenkins V, Fallowfield L. Can communication skills training alter physicians' beliefs and behaviour in clinic? *J Clin Oncol* 2002; **20**(3): 765–9.

19. Parle M, Maguire P, Heaven C. The development of a training model to improve health professionals' skills, self-efficacy and outcome expectancies when communicating with cancer patients. *Soc Sci Med* 1997; **44**: 231–40.

20. Fallowfield L, Lipkin M, Hall A. Teaching senior oncologists communication skills: results from phase 1 of a comprehensive longitudinal programme in the United Kingdom. *J Clin Oncol* 1998; **16**(5): 1961–8.

21. Duffy FD, Gordon GH, Whelan G, *et al.* Assessing competence in communication and interpersonal skills: the Kalamzoo II report. *Acad Med* 2004; **279**: 495–507.

22. Adamo G. Simulated and standardized patients in OSCEs: achievements and challenges 1992–2003. *Med Teach* 2003; **25**(3): 262–70.

23. Hodges B, Turnbull J, Cohen R, *et al.* Evaluating communication skills in the OSCE format: reliability and generalizability. *Med Educ* 1996; **30**: 38–43.

24. Maguire P, Booth K, Elliot C, *et al.* Helping health professionals involved in cancer care acquire key interviewing skills—the impact of workshops. *Eur J Cancer* 1996; **32**(9): 1486–9.

25. Smee S. Skill based assessment. *BMJ* 2003; **326**: 703–6.

26. Maguire P. Improving communication with cancer patients. *Eur J Cancer* 1999; **35**(14): 2058–65.

27. Back AL, Arnold RM, Baile WF, *et al.* Efficacy of communication skills training for giving bad news and discussing transitions to palliative care. *Arch Int Med* 2007; **167**: 453–60.

28. Levinson W, Roter D. The effects of two continuing medical education programmes on communication skills of practicing primary care physicians. *J Gen Int Med* 1993; **8**: 318–24.

29. Fellowes D, Wilkinson S, Moore P. Communications skills training for healthcare professionals working with cancer patients, their families, and/or caregivers. *Cochrane Data Base of Systematic Reviews* 2004, Issue 2: CD 003751.

30. Hulsman RL, Ros WJ, Winnubst JA, *et al*. Teaching clinically experienced physicians communication skills. A review of evaluation studies. *Med Educ* 1999; **33**: 655–68.

31. Brown RF, Butow PN, Boyle F, *et al*. Seeking informed consent to cancer clinical trials; evaluating the efficacy of doctor communication skill training. *Psycho-Oncology* 2007; **16**: 507–16.

32. Ford S, Hall A, Ratcliffe D, Fallowfield L. The Medical interaction process system (MIPS): an instrument for analysing interviews of oncologists and patients with cancer. *Soc Sci Med* 2000; **50**(4): 553–66.

33. Roter D, Larson S. The Roter interaction analysis system (RIAS): utility and flexibility for analysis of medical interactions. *Patient Educ Couns* Apr 2002; **46**(4): 243–51.

34. Cegala DJ, Broz SL. Physician communication skills training: a review of theoretical backgrounds, objectives, and skills. *Med Educ* 2002; **36**: 1004–16.

35. Makoul G, Krupat E, Chang CH. Measuring patient views of physician communication skills: development and testing of the communication assessment tool. *Pat Educ Couns* 2007; **67**: 333–42.

Chapter 60

Qualitative approaches to clinician–patient communication

Felicia Roberts

In *The Country Doctor*, Kafka's central character laments that writing a prescription is easy, but coming to an understanding with people is hard.[1] If the practice of medicine were as simple as sending a clear message, then the practitioner's job would be reduced to correctly formulating the right words. The reality, however, is that patient care is not simply about message transmission, it is about a dynamic interplay of information, emotions, expertise, goals, beliefs, and so on. To study the artful management of the complexities of healthcare communication, qualitative approaches can be highly productive and can stimulate new insight: 'how' may be a more relevant question to begin with than 'how much'.

In oncology and palliative care, as in any medical domain, both physicians and patients have concerns, though perhaps somewhat different ones, regarding preferred trajectories and outcomes of the medical visit. Whether or not these preferences are realized during a consultation, patients come away with information about the nature and course of their illness, as well as with recommendations on how, or whether, to proceed with treatment. Physicians, from their side, face the tension of maintaining the delicate balance between informative yet hopeful communication (1). They deftly navigate the line between recommending treatment and avoiding guarantees (2). For those concerned with understanding these kinds of communication tensions in the practice of medicine, the inductive and interpretive approaches presented in this chapter may prove useful. The methods outlined here have particular relevance for face-to-face communication, though reference will also be made to studies in the wider healthcare setting. The final sections of the chapter reflect on the special ethical challenges facing researchers engaged in field-based studies, and a brief discussion is offered concerning the trade-offs between reliability and validity in qualitative research.

Unique contribution of qualitative methods for studying clinician–patient communication

Engaging in health communication research presumes a wide range of goals: to discover something new or to understand a phenomenon more fully; to make the world better in some way; or to advocate for a position in a manner that is acceptable to a community of practitioners, scholars, or policy makers. Regardless of the research goal, each person engaged in the process brings preconceptions of how the world works, what constitutes knowledge, and what is the most appropriate way to find answers to his or her individual questions. The trade-offs between

---

1. This is a close paraphrase from a translation by Willa and Edwin Muir in *Selected Short Stories of Franz Kafka*, New York, NY: Random House, 1952, p.152.

quantitative and qualitative approaches have been extensively debated—see Heritage and Maynard (3) for a brief review in the context of medical encounters—but there is no *best* way to study clinician–patient interaction. If, however, one determines that a qualitative approach is most appropriate for his/her research goals—see Silverman (4) for guidance in this regard—then one is embarking on a project that demands close attention to participant orientations and understandings of their own activities.

What distinguishes the qualitative study is its commitment to understanding lived experience by privileging the dialogic nature of human life. From this vantage point, understanding is created in concert with others; it is not the result of a correct message being sent down a correct channel. Hence the lament of Kafka's country doctor who recognizes that it is our discursive involvement with others that produces the challenges of everyday life. For doctors, as for all of us, meaning is created socially; we cannot produce understanding in isolation. But, it is that very essence of creating meanings through talk that can also lead to misunderstanding. If it were as simple as writing prescriptions, medical visits would be much shorter.

Although there is agreement that talk is at the centre of the social, diagnostic, and therapeutic work of medicine, approaches for understanding face-to-face communication vary substantially. The process of coding interactions into countable units can help to establish the basis for standardized comparisons, but there is the risk of turning participants' communicative acts (the talk) into a by-product of the physician–patient relationship (5). Those quantitative approaches that centre on unitizing the countable verbal and non-verbal elements of an interaction, introduce a level of abstraction that can compromise a transactional understanding of the nature of communication. The talk and embodied action are no longer viewed as dynamically constructing meaning and the researcher can lose sight of how understanding is constructed as an ongoing process.

It may go without saying, but is worth repeating, that just because a strategy for data collection is observational does not mean that the method is qualitative. Loosely structured observation of lived activity, highly structured interviews, and electronic recording of interaction are simply ways of corralling and making manageable the study of the seamless processes of human interaction. For example, focus groups are often included in discussions of qualitative methods even though there is nothing qualitative, per se, about a focus group; it is simply a technique for eliciting stories, beliefs, conversations, and so on. These could be quantified (coded and counted) or, conversely, qualitatively examined. Taking a qualitative approach, the researcher is committed to being reflexively aware of his or her own meanings as an analysis emerges of the participants' orientations. The aim is to reconstruct the sense-making practices of the participants, not necessarily to confirm a theoretical concern of the researcher.

In addition to providing rich interactional detail, which can be an end in itself, qualitative approaches can also serve as groundwork for further exploration. For example, Garant (6) provides an informal report of her experience as a psychiatric nurse who, in the course of her work (though not as a formal study) asked patients what it means to have cancer. Several conceptualizations emerged concerning impediments to the coping process (e.g. fear of incapacitation, alienation, contagion), which could be followed up in additional studies, whether qualitative or quantitative. Thus, field techniques, such as observation, interviews, and recordings can provide data for qualitative analysis of participant orientations or they can provide the necessary rich grounding for informed development of testable hypotheses.

Representative approaches and relevant empirical studies

In this section, data collection techniques and interpretive approaches are discussed with examples from relevant empirical healthcare research. The goal is to present a variety of frameworks that share grounding in terms of basic field techniques for data collection (observation, interviews, recordings) but which differ in scope, focus, or fundamental philosophy. First, field-based frameworks are presented that draw on a traditional scientific approach of observing and describing real entities. Gubrium and Holstein (7) have termed this the 'naturalist idiom' in qualitative research because it adheres to a belief in a discoverable truth, one which will 'truly' represent participant lives. Included here are ethnography, grounded theory, conversation analysis, and ethnography of communication.

In contrast to these naturalistic approaches, postmodernism is also presented because it offers a different philosophical basis, one which highlights paradoxes, thus disrupting the traditional sense of a shared or monolithic truth that can be captured and represented. The value of this form of scholarship is that it can provide openings for new insight. Healthcare researchers need not shy away from postmodern philosophy just because it seems to lack the traditional notions of shared or observable reality. On the contrary, a postmodern approach may well offer a way into understanding the healthcare setting that would be inconceivable from more traditional vantage points.

Whatever the philosophical grounding (e.g. naturalist vs. postmodern) researchers using these approaches are generally interested in patients' and practitioners' beliefs, practices, and understandings of health and illness. They are attempting to derive participants' understandings from the researcher's detailed observation, description, and analysis of behaviour and artefacts. For a comprehensive discussion and critique of the philosophical grounding and practical implementation of these research approaches, see Gubrium and Holstein (7).

Ethnography

'Ethnographic methods' has become an umbrella term for a wide array of procedures for data collection, analysis, and description of findings. Under this heading, interviewing and focus groups will be discussed, though these techniques are not unique to ethnographic studies.

Steeped in an anthropological tradition, ethnographic description can evoke contrasting impulses: on the one hand, there is the risk of treating individuals and groups as 'exotic', while on the other hand, there is a sincere concern with understanding participant viewpoints. This tension provides a productive dialectic in which to explore the world of health and healthcare. For studies of medical interaction, an ethnographic approach can provide a wide scope, taking in a setting as large as an oncology unit within a hospital (e.g. Germain, 8) as though it were a unique culture, or studies can be more focused on particular segments of a culture. For example, Linnard-Palmer and Kools (9) examined nurses' attitudes and interactions in the context of paediatric oncology. In this study, thematic analysis of field interviews and observations addressed the ethical complexities embedded in nurses' interactions with parents who refuse treatment for their children. These sorts of studies provide descriptive and empirical detail as a basis for deeper understanding of lived patterns of activity as well as for participants' understanding of their own and others' actions.

Engaging in ethnographic research has traditionally entailed extensive (up to, and beyond, a year) participant observation in a particular group or organization. The goal has been to minimize presuppositions about the group, giving rich descriptions and analyses that provide some sense of what 'really' goes on at the level of daily practice. This analytic stance, to capture reality in the quotidian, is probably 'the predominant language of qualitative research' (7, p.6) and is most characteristically embodied in ethnographic studies. A classic study in medical anthropology, the description of medical student life in the freshman and clinical years (10), is presented almost as if the medical students were an isolated group in a far-off land, yet another early ethnographic study contributed tremendously to our conceptualization of 'hospitalized dying' (11, p.xii) as an orchestrated process. These classical approaches to ethnographic research in medical settings provide an overview of particular cultures or segments of the culture in a way that is primarily intended to suggest the cognitive contours of the participants' experience (12).

Other forms of naturalistic inquiry move beyond description of knowledge and beliefs to paint participants' experiences in their 'full emotional colour' (7, p.9). There is still use of the same fieldwork and data-collection techniques (establishing rapport, building trust, observing, and interviewing), but analysis is focused on feelings as opposed to beliefs. The representation of these emotionalist studies can draw on unconventional formats, such as poetry and drama. While this may seem at odds with a scientific orientation, it could provide an interesting avenue for clinician researchers who may wish to delve into the complexity of emotions in their field, perhaps allowing them to better address their own as well as their patients' needs.

Technological advances have brought audio- and video-recording into the researcher's toolkit. While early medical field studies also used recordings (e.g. Glaser and Strauss; 11, 13) the effort was primarily to record interviews with participants, not necessarily the medical visit itself. Nonetheless, using recording technologies, the traditional immersion approach of the ethnographer can be supplemented by the close analysis of participant activities as recorded by an electronic device. In this way, the observer can reconstitute meaning through detailed description as well as analyze how participants manage and create meaning in the process of actual interaction (see below, Conversation analysis).

Interviewing

In many field-based approaches, interviewing is a core technique; it is a conversation with a purpose, but one that primarily benefits the researcher, not the participant (14). From an ethical standpoint, and in terms of informed consent, it is important to recognize the different types of interviews because not all of them lend themselves easily to the consent process.

Interview types are delineated based on the depth and range of the conversation and the type of relationship one has with the participant (15). 'Ethnographic interviews' are those conversations that can just happen when the researcher is in the study setting and something serendipitously prompts a question related to the research project. There is nothing purposive about this type of interview; the researcher simply makes use of the moment to elaborate on some point of interest. In contrast, 'informant interviews' are designed with a purpose. Participants comment on their experiences and may be contacted several times to discuss various topics of interest to the researcher. These can be open-ended conversations, but they are entered into with a general purpose in mind. Further along the continuum, 'respondent interviews' are brief, stand-alone interactions that generally have pre-set questions in a particular order. These are the least naturalistic and are likely to provide superficial, even socially desirable, responses that do not reflect actual attitudes and behaviours.

Focus groups

Focus groups provide an excellent format for understanding the world of the patient or the practitioner through their own stories, accounts, and experiences. For example, Zimmerman and Applegate (16) use this technique to examine the ways in which hospice teams communicate. In contrast to individual interviews, and contrary to conventional assumptions, focus groups provide a setting in which people are more likely to disclose their health or professional concerns (see Wilkinson for a review, 17). This group activity can stimulate deeper thinking and participants may reveal a broader spectrum of meanings. Whereas an individual may be reluctant to disclose deeper feelings to a researcher who does not share their experience, the focus group encourages people to share in a supportive atmosphere.

Focus groups have been used in a wide variety of health research and allow researchers to observe, if not wholly natural and spontaneous discussions, then at least the process of how beliefs are presented and possibly altered in concert with others (17, p.338). In addition to promoting greater disclosure, focus-group data can also foreground ways of speaking that are natural to the participants. Since the focus-group participants often share some health or professional concern, this approach can help researchers get deeper and more detailed insight into meanings that might otherwise be missed in individual interviews.

Grounded theory

Grounded theory is a research strategy for inductively developing concepts and theories. Glaser and Strauss (11, 13), who developed this approach, were among the first to use field observations and in-depth interviews in order to 'grasp the actor's viewpoint' (18, p.6) in the medical setting. Triggered by an interest in medical sociology, Glaser and Strauss first attempted to describe and understand the process of dying as it occurred in a hospital setting (11, 13).

In grounded theory, analysis proceeds as a coding process that is intended to open up an initial understanding and allow core categories to emerge. The purpose is not to deconstruct an interaction into countable units, but to understand and integrate what is available from interviews and observations. As analysis proceeds, there is a movement away from literal meanings and toward the relationships among concepts (18). It should be noted that grounded theory has evolved in two directions: one characterized by a more agnostic stance towards data (19) and the other by a more question or theory-driven approach (20). Regardless of the strand that one follows in a grounded theory approach, the focus is always on discovery as opposed to hypothesis testing. While the notion of 'hypothesis' is used in an informal way in grounded theory, it develops in terms of plausibility, not testability.

Clair (21) used this approach to study the end of life among oncology patients in a hospital setting. From data collected in the oncology unit, Clair inductively generated the concept of 'regressive intervention', demonstrating how physicians withdraw, whether abruptly or gradually, once the patient has been re-cast, by the physician's diagnosis, from the sick role to the dying role. While medical staff are still expected to maintain humane, palliative treatment, the patient relies less and less on medical staff and families become more accountable for the patient's activities. Using recordings of interactions along with observations, this study demonstrates a grounded theory approach in that analysis is used to develop theory rather than to verify a theory.

Conversation analysis

Conversation analysis (CA) is one among many approaches for the study of spoken discourse. (See Schiffrin and Titsch et al. for introductions to the wide and complex variety of methods referred to as 'discourse analysis'; 22–23.) CA, like several other approaches to the study of face-to-face interaction, requires recorded interactions as the form of data for analysis. Unlike ethnographic and grounded theory approaches, however, which can be based on field observations and interviews, CA is predicated on capturing naturally occurring interactions in real time. This technical requirement, which initially was just a way to 'keep a grip' on the social world (24, p.235), is nonetheless grounded in the philosophical and sociological traditions that undergird this particular form of discourse analysis (24–25).

In contrast to other methods outlined in this chapter, researchers using a CA approach are not engaged in describing contexts or in deriving concepts and theories through inductive coding; nor is conversation analysis a critical approach, though it can be used to uncover members' orientations to dominant ideologies. Unlike most other approaches to the study of discourse, which treat context as an external phenomenon, CA treats context as something shaped through participant talk and action (26–28). This concern with participant agency is a central tenet of this qualitative approach and is, therefore, highly useful for discerning patient and clinician perspectives as evidenced through their embodied actions.

Through close transcription of recorded materials (29–30) the conversation analyst attends to the details of verbal and non-verbal behaviour to see how the participants create meanings. It is thus possible to observe what themes or roles the participants make relevant (or not) and how they accomplish that work through face-to-face interaction. This allows researchers to closely view and describe the visible processes of 'coming to an understanding' (in Kafka's terms).

It is clear from conversation analytic studies in oncology settings that health practitioners risk meeting with resistance from their clients when there is a failure to properly justify the advice or recommendation (31–32). Indeed, the final formulation of a treatment recommendation can be accounted for by the conversational actions of both participants, including the shaping that occurs when patients subtly resist an initial formulation (33). In other words, recommendations are not unidirectional forms of communication. Additionally, patients' poor understanding of the risks and benefits of cancer treatment (34–35) has been explained by an examination of the inherently equivocal nature of those recommendations (2). An unavoidable tension persists between oncologists' presentation of recommendations and their avoidance of guarantees. Moreover, it has been suggested that oncologists' talk about clinical trials is shaped in such a way that it may contribute to differing rates of enrolment (36).

Also important for oncology and palliative care is Maynard's work (37) on bad news delivery. This line of research has demonstrated how acceptance of, or resistance to, bad news is interactionally achieved. When practitioners are able to draw out a client's point of view and can find ways to incorporate that into the news delivery, there can be a smoother transition to acceptance of bad news. Maynard thus recommends eliciting the patient's perspective before delivering news. By connecting bad news to what patients have already expressed to the practitioner about what they know and believe, medical news will be in relation to that, rather than simply being dropped into the conversation as a confusing surprise. Maynard also highlights how news itself is neutral, perhaps a key point for clinicians to remember. The valence of news as 'good' or 'bad' is dependent on the participant's reception of it. While we assume, for example, that a prognosis with a short horizon is bad news, if a patient has been preparing for death, it may be a relief to know that the end will arrive soon.

Ethnography of communication

In contrast to conversation analysis, which comprises a micro-analytic stance toward interaction and which focuses on recorded face-to-face communication, ethnography of communication takes a wider view. Similar to a traditional ethnographic approach, the aim is to describe and explain values, actions, and norms within broader structures of cultural knowledge and behaviour. The focus is more concentrated, however, on language practices: what is said, where it is said, by whom, in what manner, through what channel, for what goals, and according to which norms (38, pp.52–71). Findings are based on field observations and interviews, collection of artifacts (e.g. documents), and similar to grounded theory, a process of tracking back and forth in a 'dialectic interplay' between description, analysis, and development of theoretical explanations (23). This method generates a wide angle view of settings, but keeps a spotlight on speech events, taking into account observable activities as well as participants' accounts of their behaviours.

Fisher (39) uses this framework to explain differing rates of treatment of cervical dysplasia in two separate clinics. The differences, which could not be easily explained on medical or socio-demographic grounds, are discerned qualitatively by highlighting strategic uses of language that may represent the physicians' attitudes toward different patients.

Postmodernism

Postmodernist and critical modernist scholarship, like other interpretive approaches, emphasizes the discursive or social construction of reality. Data-collection techniques, such as examination of texts, participant observation, and interviews, are shared with other qualitative approaches. However, in postmodern scholarship, the underlying assumption is that there is no single, observable truth. Although pain and illness certainly exist as biological realities, they are understood as socioculturally experienced. In other words, a patient's experience of disease is shaped as much by belief systems and cultural norms as by physical reality. As reviewed and evaluated in Lupton (40), the value of postmodern and critical modernist approaches for understanding healthcare is their insistence on examining paradoxes and problems. Variant truths are highlighted and can, therefore, be compared and contrasted. The emancipatory impulse in critical modernist scholarship allows for exposure of inequalities as well as the possibility for negotiation and change (41, p.14).

Postmodernist and critical modernist research primarily uses the analytic tools of literary criticism (e.g. discernment of metaphor, tropes, and themes). For example, the military and sports metaphors that predominate in Western medicine (41–43), along with a belief in the individual will for overcoming adversity, clearly shapes the practice of informing patients. The dominant ideology is for patients to 'fight' their disease (44); however, some research suggests that doctors were still not fully and clearly disclosing cancer diagnoses (45). This raises a paradox: the ideology of the individual's ability to overcome adversity through their own effort is at odds with a choice to shield patients from discouraging news that might somehow constrict their ability to fight. On the flip side of the metaphor that indicates 'fighting' for life, is that cancer patients may experience being at war with themselves, which has implications for the patient's sense of rationality (46, p.27).

As spotlighted in postmodern and critical research, contradictory ideologies and explorations of metaphor provide points of departure for thinking about the ways in which attitudes, behaviours, and even the experience of pain and illness, are communicatively shaped. Through thematic and rhetorical analysis of textual, observational, and interview data, scholars in the postmodern and critical modernist traditions examine the cultural and personal paradoxes forming webs of meaning within which patients and clinicians strive to make sense of health and illness.

Ethical issues in field-based qualitative research

Because much of the qualitative research in medical settings relies upon observations, interviews, and recordings of interaction, studies can be intrusive and lengthy. And, since there is an ongoing and interactive relationship between the researcher and the setting's participants, issues of rapport, confidentiality, and consent can be particularly delicate matters. Thus, the ethical challenges faced in field-based studies can be unique in that they are emergent and unpredictable. Some have even argued that covert research of difficult to reach populations (e.g. the homeless) should be allowed without the constraints of informed consent and voluntary participation (47–49). This position is untenable in the healthcare context, where the biomedical and social overlap seamlessly.

Fine (50) argues that ethnographers are socialized to accept an idea of themselves as empathetic, honest, and accurate; however, the necessities of maintaining good relations for ongoing field observations actually may entail everything from minor interpersonal deceptions to highly suspect and intentional shaping of events. In other words, as Lindlof and Taylor (15) argue, the danger for the field observer or interviewer is in 'assuming that attainment [of ethical ideals] is easy' (p.140). Punch (51) acknowledges the inevitability of deception at some minor level, but exhorts the researcher to continually monitor and reflect upon his/her practices. Seeing documents or overhearing conversations that might otherwise have been guarded by participants, presents ethical challenges that are bound to occur in busy, public domains. These gray areas (52) can be particularly sensitive in medical settings where, perhaps naively, staff believe they are doing a good job of protecting patient confidentiality.

The sensitive nature of medical settings also raises the critical question of the incorporation of follow-up with participants who may have been observed or interviewed at vulnerable moments. Polit and Hungler (53) address this dilemma in the context of how parents cope with a child's terminal illness. Since such a study would require a potentially painful probing of parents' emotional states, the researcher must consider not only whether the benefit of such knowledge would assist in the design of effective strategies for helping parents, but also what the long-term result of making such demands on parents would be. Once the child has died, what is the researcher's responsibility to the parents? Protection of subjects must, therefore, be broadly construed and considered integral to follow-up as well as to implementation.

An additional complexity of field research in medical settings is that social and medical settings are permeable; people who were not expected, and, therefore, were not part of a consent process, can enter a scene. Thus, the ability to easily obtain informed consent is undermined (54). In envisioning projects, researchers should consider the possibility of such contingencies and plan accordingly. Post hoc consent may be possible, but is often untenable. Furthermore, some locations are considered public (e.g. corridors) and would be exempt from consent procedures, while others (e.g. patient rooms) may be considered private. For those collecting audio- or video-recorded data, an additional consent form is warranted that outlines possible uses of the recorded data beyond research team meetings (e.g. for use in classrooms, at conferences, in electronic journals). Participants should initial those uses to which they consent; this would constitute full and open disclosure concerning the use of recordings. Clearly, the complexities of attaining informed consent are many, and must be balanced against the potential social and scientific benefits to be gained.

Finally, though not an ethical issue at first glance, researchers must 'consider the possible consequences of their culturally ascribed identities for the ethics and politics of conducting research' (15, pp.141–2). The physical characteristics, social attributes, and degree of insider knowledge are among the 'ambiguous gifts' that fieldworkers can carry unwittingly into a scene and which will therefore 'establish axes of difference and similarity' with other participants (15, pp.141–2). Again, the researcher's reflection and monitoring of these dimensions both in planning and implementation are necessary for considering the ethical challenges of field-based studies.

For those interested in healthcare communication research in cyberspace, Jones (55) lays out ethical issues that are relevant for that medium where what is considered public, private, and deceptive becomes even more challenging for research.

Validity and reliability

Scholars differ in their opinions of whether or not reliability and validity are relevant concepts for qualitative research. From a social constructionist perspective, the argument is that the transient and contingent nature of human interaction renders any concern for reliability irrelevant. Validity is probably more relevant, since a particular interaction or event may be accurately analysed, but rare enough that it would be hard to find another just like it for comparison. Although the process of collecting instances and comparing them provides for a grounded claim about a particular action or behaviour, it is also the case that 'one' is a number and that analysis of a particular case holds value (56) and can be built upon for developing further insights.

However, Silverman (57) warns that if qualitative researchers are not mindful of issues of reliability and validity then they are at risk of engaging in the romanticism of nineteenth-century thinkers and chroniclers. In that tradition, observers may have selected data for its dramatic or exotic qualities, or because it fit an idealized pre-conception of the culture being studied. Therefore, Silverman suggests formulating hypotheses and testing assumptions through triangulation and checking for participant validation.

Conclusion

Misunderstandings, whatever their root-cause, can haunt patients and practitioners as they strive to make sense of a complicated interpersonal world within the medical organization. The value of qualitative and interpretive methods for studying medical communication resides precisely in the ability of the researcher to discern practices and beliefs that may give rise to misunderstandings. These participant orientations and behaviours are not necessarily available at a conscious level and may only be available through systematic observation and interpretive analysis. In addition to gathering patient and clinician narratives about their experiences and beliefs (through interviews and focus groups), a great deal can be learned from systematic observation and recording of actual interactions (ethnographic and conversation analytic approaches), which can capture details of the dynamic, transactional nature of (mis)understanding. Greater attention to theory development that is grounded in inductive analysis and interpretive procedures (such as grounded theory) can bring to light the inter-dependent relationship of practitioner and patient in terms of the larger social context. Critical and postmodernist approaches help to uncover paradoxes and power dynamics that can bring to the surface the webs of social and cultural meaning in which we manoeuver with little awareness.

To better understand patient–clinician communication is to better understand the ongoing, situated processes that constitute communication. How are recommendations made, how is advice given and received, how do both parties participate in the construction of the medical moment? These kinds of questions imply understanding of the communication process, not just its outcomes. By definition a process is a series of activities, but in human terms, these activities rarely have discreet, discernable boundaries. Qualitative methods lend themselves especially well to understanding this fluid, socially constructed process of communication.

References

1. Helft PR. An intimate collaboration: prognostic communication with advanced cancer patients. *J Clin Ethics*. 2006; **17**: 110–21.

2. Roberts F. *Talking about treatment: recommendations for breast cancer adjuvant therapy*. New York: Oxford University Press; 1999.

3. Heritage J, Maynard DW. *Communication in medical care*. Cambridge (UK): Cambridge University Press; 2006.

4. Silverman D. *Doing qualitative research: a practical handbook*. Thousand Oaks (CA): Sage; 2005.

5. West C. *Routine complications: troubles with talk between doctors and patients*. Bloomington (IN): Indiana University Press; 1984.

6. Garant C. Stalls in the therapeutic process. *Am J Nurs*. 1980; **80**: 2166–7.

7. Gubrium JF, Holstein JA. *The new language of qualitative method*. New York: Oxford University Press; 1997.

8. Germain CP. *The cancer unit: an ethnography*. Wakefield (MA): Nursing Resources, Inc.; 1979.

9. Linnard-Palmer L, Kools S. Parents' refusal of medical treatment for cultural or religious beliefs: an ethnographic study of health care professionals' experiences. *J Pediatr Oncol Nurs*. 2005; **22**: 48–57.

10. Becker H, Geer B, Hughes E, *et al. Boys in white*. Chicago: University Press; 1961.

11. Glaser WA, Strauss MR. *Awareness of dying*. Chicago: Aldine Publishing; 1965.

12. Johnson JM. *Doing field research*. New York: Free Press; 1975.

13. Glaser WA, Strauss MR. *Time for dying*. Chicago: Aldine Publishing; 1968.

14. Bingham WVD, Moore BV. *How to interview*, 4th edn. New York: Harper and Row; 1959.

15. Lindlof TR, Taylor BC. *Qualitative communication research*, 2nd edn. Thousand Oaks (CA): Sage; 2002.

16. Zimmerman S, Applegate JL. Person centered comforting in the hospice interdisciplinary team. *Commun Res*. 1992; **19**: 240–63.

17. Wilkinson S. Focus groups in health research: exploring the meanings of health and illness. *J Health Psychol*. 1998; **3**: 329–48.

18. Strauss AL. *Qualitative analysis for social scientists*. Cambridge (UK): Cambridge University Press; 1987.

19. Glaser BG. *Emergence vs. forcing: advances in the methodology of Grounded Theory*. Mill Valley (CA): Sociology Press; 1992.

20. Strauss MR, Corbin J. *Basics of qualitative research*. Thousand Oaks (CA): Sage; 1990.

21. Clair JM. Regressive intervention: the discourse of medicine during terminal encounters. *Adv Med Sociol*. 1990; **1**: 57–97.

22. Schiffrin D. *Approaches to discourse*. Malden (MA): Blackwell Publishing; 1994.

23. Titsch S, Meyer M, Wodak R, *et al. Methods of text and discourse analysis*. London: Sage; 2000.

24. Heritage J. *Garfinkel and ethnomethodology*. Cambridge (UK): Polity Press; 1984.

25. Silverman D. *Harvey Sacks: social science and conversation analysis*. New York: Oxford University Press; 1998.

26. Pomerantz A, Fehr BJ. Conversation analysis: an approach to the study of social action as sense making. In: Van Dijk TA, editor. *Discourse as social interaction*. London: Sage; 1997, pp.64–91.

27. Schegloff EA. On talk and its institutional occasions. In: Drew P, Heritage, J, editors. *Talk at work: interactions in institutional settings*. Cambridge (UK): Cambridge University Press; 1992, pp.101–134.

28. Schegloff EA. Whose text? Whose context? *Discourse and Society*. 1997; **8**(2): 165–87.

29. Roberts F. Transcribing and transcription. In: Donsbach W, editor. *International encyclopedia of communication*. Vol. 11. Oxford (UK) and Malden (MA): Wiley-Blackwell; 2008, pp.5161–65.

30. Roberts F, Robinson JR. Interobserver agreement on first-stage conversation analytic transcription. *Hum Commun Res*. 2004; **30**: 376–410.

31. Heritage J, Sefi S. Dilemmas of advice: aspects of the delivery and reception of advice in interactions between health visitors and first-time mothers. In: Drew P, Heritage J, editors. *Talk at work: interaction in institutional settings*. Cambridge (UK): Cambridge University Press; 1992, pp.359–417.

32. Silverman D, Bor R, Miller R, *et al*. Obviously the advice is then to keep to safer sex: advice-giving and advice reception in AIDS counseling. In: Aggleton P, Davies P, Hart G, editors. *AIDS: rights, risk, and reason*. Bristol (PA): Taylor and Francis, Falmer Press; 1991, pp.174–191.

33. Costello BA, Roberts F. Medical recommendations as joint social practice. *Health Commun*. 2001; **13**: 241–60.

34. Siminoff LA. Description and correlates of breast cancer adjuvant treatment decisions [dissertation]. Baltimore (MD): Johns Hopkins Univ; 1987.

35. Siminoff LA, Fetting JH, Abeloff MD. Doctor–patient communication about breast cancer adjuvant therapy. *J Clin Oncol*. 1989; **7**(9): 1192–1200.

36. Roberts F. Qualitative differences among cancer clinical trial explanations. *Soc Sci Med*. 2002; **55**: 1947–55.

37. Maynard D. *Bad news, good news: conversational order in everyday talk and clinical settings.* Chicago: University of Chicago Press; 2003.

38. Hymes D. Models of the interaction of language and social life. In: Gumperz J, Hymes D, editors. *Directions in sociolinguistics: the ethnography of communication.* New York: Holt, Rinehart and Winston, Inc.; 1972, pp.35–71.

39. Fisher S. Doctor talk/patient talk: how treatment decisions are negotiated in doctor-patient communication. In: Fisher S, Todd AD, editors. *The social organization of doctor–patient communication.* Washington (DC): Centre for Applied Linguistics; 1983, pp.135–157.

40. Lupton D. *Medicine as culture,* 2nd edn. London: Sage; 2003.

41. Erwin D. The militarization of cancer treatment in American society. In: Baer H, editor. *Encounters with biomedicine: case studies in medical anthropology.* New York: Gordon and Breach; 1987, pp.201–27.

42. Clarke J, Robinson J. Testicular cancer: medicine and machismo in the media (1980–94). *Health.* 1999; **3**; 263–82.

43. Seale C. Sporting cancer: struggle language in news reports of people with cancer. *Sociol Health Illn.* 2001; **23**: 308–29.

44. Goode MJ, Good B, Schaffer C, *et al.* American oncology and the discourse on hope. *Cult Med Psychiatry.* 1990; **14**: 59–79.

45. Taylor K. Physicians and the disclosure of undesirable information. In: Lock M, Gordon D, editors. *Biomedicine examined.* Dordrecht: Kluewer; 1988, pp.441–63.

46. Pinell P. How do cancer patients express their points of view? *Sociol Health Illn.* 1987; **9**: 25–44.

47. Berg BL. *Qualitative research methods for the social sciences,* 6th edn. Boston: Allyn and Bacon; 2007.

48. Miller JM. Covert participant observation: reconsidering the least used method. *J Contemp Crim Justice.* 1995; **11**: 97–105.

49. Miller JM, Tewksbury R. *Extreme methods: innovative approaches to social science research.* Boston: Allyn and Bacon; 2001.

50. Fine GF. Ten lies of ethnography: moral dilemmas of field research. *J Contemp Ethnography.* 1993; **22**: 267–94.

51. Punch M. *The politics and ethics of fieldwork.* Beverly Hills (CA): Sage; 1986.

52. Shulman D. Dirty data and investigative methods: some lessons from private detective work. *J Contemp Ethnography.* 1994; **23**: 214–53.

53. Polit DF, Hungler B. *Nursing research: principles and methods.* Philadelphia: Lippincott; 1995.

54. Fluehr-Lobban C. Informed consent in anthropological research: we are not exempt. *Hum Organ.* 1994; **53**: 1–10.

55. Jones RA. The ethics of research in cyberspace. *Internet Res.* 1994; **4**: 30–5.

56. Schegloff EA. Reflections on quantification in the study of conversation. *Res Lang Soc Interact.* 1993; **26**(1): 99–128.

57. Silverman D. *Interpreting qualitative data: methods for analyzing talk, text and interaction.* Thousand Oaks (CA): Sage; 1993.

Chapter 61

Issues in Coding Cancer Consultations: interaction analysis systems

Phyllis N Butow and Sarah Ford

Introduction

It is now well accepted that communication between the health-professional and the patient is a critical component of quality patient care and that poor communication can adversely affect both patient and health professional outcomes. However, audits of doctor and nurse communication with patients have consistently revealed deficits, prompting the growth of communication skills training for both junior and senior clinicians, and the publication of communication guidelines for various challenging situations. Such training and resources should optimally be evidence-based; recommending communication practices that have been clearly shown to produce improved patient and doctor outcomes. Furthermore, the efficacy of such training, and the extent to which guidelines are implemented in routine clinical practice, should be demonstrated. These goals require valid and reliable methods for documenting how patients and health professionals communicate with each other.

Coding health-professional-patient encounters

Interaction analysis systems (IAS) enable the analysis of communication between the doctor, patient, family, and other health professionals in a qualitative and quantitative fashion. Two types of IAS can be identified: 'content' systems, which describe task-oriented behaviour, and 'process' systems, which measure socio-emotional behaviour (although most combine the two in varying degrees). Besides this distinction, IAS differ with regard to their clinical relevance (e.g. specific to general practice or to a particular specialty), extent of coverage (whole consultation or specific behaviours only), and communication modes encoded (verbal, non-verbal, or both) (1). Which IAS is best for a particular situation depends on a number of factors, including the research or clinical question being explored, the communication model or theory utilized and the resources available for analysis. In this chapter, we will explore some of the advantages and disadvantages of different IAS systems in different settings.

Interaction analysis systems

Ong et al. (1) conducted a systematic review of the literature in this area in 1995 and identified twelve whole consultation IAS systems. A search of the more recent literature revealed only two new systems: CN-LOGIT (later re-named CANCODE) (2) and The Medical Interaction Process System (MIPS) (3). The most commonly applied system is the Roter Interaction Analysis System (RIAS), developed by Roter et al. (4). Seven of the interaction analysis systems have been applied in the cancer setting (2–8). Only the RIAS, MIPS, and CANCODE have been assessed for both reliability and validity. These systems are described in some detail below.

RIAS

The RIAS is derived loosely from social exchange theories related to interpersonal influence, problem-solving, and reciprocity. The RIAS codes every doctor and patient utterance into one of 37 mutually-exclusive and exhaustive categories. In the RIAS, utterances are defined as the smallest distinguishable speech segment to which a classification may be assigned. The unit may vary in length from a single word to a lengthy sentence. The RIAS captures socio-emotional behaviours, including social behaviour, agreement, paraphrasing, showing concern, reassurance, reflection, and disagreement; and task-oriented behaviours, including giving directions, asking for clarification, asking medical/therapeutic questions, asking life-style/feelings-related questions, giving medical/therapeutic information, giving life-style/feelings-related information, medical/therapeutic counseling, life-style/feelings-related counselling, and other. These categories can be combined to reflect the total amount of talk in broader categories. Additionally, global ratings of anger, anxiety, dominance, interest, responsiveness, and warmth are allocated (9, 10). This system was first applied in the general practice environment (11, 12), then in other areas such as the cancer setting (4, 13).

The RIAS has a number of advantages. It is widely used and, therefore, there is a plethora of comparative data available. It has been shown to be reliable and valid, with training, in a variety of medical settings (4). The RIAS has a strong focus on socio-emotional information which may be appropriate for some research/clinical goals, but not others. It records number of events, not time spent and, therefore, does not fully reflect the balance between different components in the consultation (although it is perfectly possible to time speech units and this was demonstrated recently in a study which used the computer software The Observer Base Package and Observer Video Analysis to both time and apply sequence analysis to RIAS data; 14). Other disadvantages of the RIAS are that it allows only one code per unit of speech, therefore, multidimensional aspects of the same communication behaviour are lost, and it does not code non-verbal behaviour. Furthermore, by necessity, the RIAS picks up very general aspects of the consultation. Codes are limited, and focus on general communication skills. If the researcher, educator, or clinician is seeking to capture or provide feedback about specific communication behaviours (such as the provision of particular information items, or responses to individual emotional cues) the RIAS will not be helpful. For more information on the RIAS see Chapter 62.

MIPS

The Medical Interaction Process System (MIPS) is a coding system adapted from the RIAS, designed specifically for the cancer setting. The system incorporates the content and process of an interaction and takes account of information transfer on multiple levels. It captures not just the linguistic (syntax) level, but also the paralinguistic (e.g. tone of voice) and kinesic (e.g. body language) levels of behaviour. Video-tape was chosen as the primary method of observation for the MIPS because it encapsulates all levels of behaviours exhibited in face-to-face interaction. However, this does not prevent the use of the system for coding audio-taped interviews.

The MIPS draws upon the biopsychosocial model and utilizes a patient-centred approach (i.e. it views patients as providing cues to their feelings and fears, which, if responded to appropriately, will lead to their disclosure). The system classifies doctor–patient interactions in terms of modes of exchange and content (thus incorporating process and content). Like the RAIS, the basic coding unit is the utterance. A separate utterance is coded for each independent and non-restrictive dependent clause of a sentence. Each utterance is assigned one content code and one mode of exchange, and may either be doctor or patient initiated. Content categories reflect the topics being addressed in each utterance (e.g. cancer treatment, diagnostic tests, psychological issues).

Modes refer to the process or function of an utterance (e.g. giving information or asking questions). Paralinguistic elements are encompassed by 12 affective categories. Kinesic behaviour can be captured by 11 global body language ratings, such as shoulder position (twisted versus square) and posture (closed versus open), alongside the main coding system.

The design of the MIPS coding sheet allows the recording of affective information that can be coded in addition to content and mode categories. The coding format allows consultations to be coded in sequence for detailed analysis and individual feedback. Each unit is numbered so that specific sequences can be isolated for in-depth analysis. For example, coders can record the number of emotional cues exhibited by patients and a clinician's inclination to either address or ignore these. The coding sheet also allows the examination of behaviour sequences (e.g. the number of patients' responses to open and focused-open questions compared to other forms of less efficient questioning styles). In addition to the main coding sheet, an Interview profile sheet provides a snap-shot of the consultation by allowing a coder to view the main categories of information contributed by doctor and patient.

However, the time taken to code each tape (three and a half times the total length) makes the system less desirable to use than, for example, a more simple communication skills checklist. Once coded, the MIPS data is entered into a spreadsheet that totals the numbers of utterances according to each specific category. Coding tends to be a tedious and lengthy process requiring meticulous care from the coder; therefore, it is still a relatively labour-intensive method of coding medical interactions. Unlike most simple checklists, the MIPS system has the potential to be applied for the dual purpose of providing feedback for use during the teaching of communication skills and serving as a tool for empirical process-outcome research. The two major advantages of the MIPS over other coding systems are that: first, the system allows for parallel coding, thus avoiding major coding conflicts; and, second, the design of the coding sheet results in a multidimensional view of the consultation and prevents data loss. It is also a flexible instrument that allows both the micro- and macro-analysis of doctor–patient interactions.

The MIPS has demonstrated good results in terms of convergent validity, inter-coder reliability (3), and criterion validity (15), and is a useful tool for evaluating the enduring impact of communication skills training (16). However, the global affective and non-verbal ratings are less reliable than the verbal frequency categories, and in this respect represent a weakness in the system (15). Non-verbal behaviours are extremely difficult to rate unless labour intensive methods are used whereby behaviours are recorded at frequently timed intervals throughout an encounter. Furthermore, global ratings tend to be influenced by the subjective impressions of the raters, which can result in poor reliability coefficients.

CANCODE

CANCODE is a computer-based method composed of three parts:

(1) micro-level analysis in real time, retaining the sequence of events;

(2) event counts; and

(3) macro-level analysis of consultation style and affect.

The consultation is divided into units of speech, which change when a person stops speaking or changes speech content. Whilst listening to the audio-tape and looking at the transcript, the coder gives each unit of speech four codes:

(1) *source* (doctor, patient, or third party);

(2) *process* (open and closed questions, initiated statements, and responses to questions);

(3) *content* (diagnosis, prognosis, treatment, medical history and presenting symptoms, other medical matters, social matters, and other);

(4) *emotional tone* (friendly/warm, tense/anxious, sad/depressed, frustrated/angry, or matter of fact).

The coder enters the codes by keyboard into a specially designed software package, while listening to the audio-tape in real time. The computer calculates the time spent for each individual code, combination of codes, and the total consultation, as well as the number of times each code or combination of codes appears. Thus, the computer sums the data into higher order categories (e.g. all codes for diagnosis regardless of process). The CANCODE system is able to process the resultant data sheet automatically to a spreadsheet in the Statistical Package for the Social Sciences (SPSS) for further analysis. A number of consultations can be coded under a project name and then transferred to the same large database. CANCODE has the ability to record the frequency as well as time length for a particular code. Given that event sequence is retained, information about sequence patterns could be utilized in interaction analysis; however, this has not yet been attempted. This interaction analysis system was shown to be valid and to have good inter- and intra-rater reliability (2, 17, 18).

CANCODE has a number of advantages. For use in analysing cancer interactions, it is likely to have greater specificity and sensitivity than the RIAS because it was developed specifically for this setting. It has been shown to be reliable and valid in the cancer setting, with appropriate training. It is multidimensional, allowing the capture of multiple aspects of a single communication behaviour and it allows time to be captured, as well as the number of exchanges. However, CANCODE, like RIAS and MIPS, is resource intensive, requiring a significant time investment from coders. It does not code non-verbal behaviour and, like RIAS and MIPS, it does not capture specific behaviours beyond the general coding within its system.

The characteristics and utility of the three whole-consultation interaction analysis systems (RIAS, MIPS and CANCODE) are summarized in Table 61.1.

Specific behavioural coding systems

A number of coding systems have been developed that endeavour to capture specific behaviours. These coding systems do not code the entire consultation, but rather look for particular target behaviours and rate them as present or absent. Sometimes a qualitative rating is also applied (such as basic/extended, or poor/good). Specific coding systems have been developed to capture many aspects of the consultation, including: response to emotion (19), information giving (20), shared decision-making (21, 22), and conversation about alternative therapies (23). Some of these are described below.

Butow *et al.* (19), developed a system for coding the emergence of, and response to, emotional cues in oncology consultations, which was further refined by Duric and colleagues (24). Transcripts of audio-taped consultations were read to identify emotional cues. Cues were coded for *emotion:* (depression, anger, grief, denial, guilt, and other feeling/psycho-social issue), intensity (weak, moderate, and strong), and *consultation context* (history, diagnosis, prognosis, treatment, other medical, psychosocial, social exchange, and other/non-specific). The doctor's behaviour directly before and after the cue was coded in terms of *form* (open question, minimal encourager, and statement), *content* (psychosocial, and not psychosocial), and *level of empathy* (ignores or delays, responds to content only, responds to feeling, and invites elaboration). Inter- and intra-rater reliability of the coding system was high (most elements, >90%). This system was applied in genetic counselling consultations and the analysis showed that more emotional cues of distress occurred

TABLE 61.1 Comparison of RIAS, MIPS and CANCODE

Interaction Analysis System	Interaction Type/ Interview Situation	Observational Medium	Coding Flexibility	Communication Levels	Usefulness as a teaching tool	Usefulness as a research tool
Roter Interaction Analysis System (RIAS) (9).	Originally developed for doctor–patient interaction in general practice, but applicable to the cancer consultation.	Traditionally direct coding of audiotapes, but sequential coding of videotape possible using The Observer Base Package (14).	One code per utterance. Records number of events, but not necessarily in sequence unless computer package used. Coding conflicts more likely.	Socio-emotional, and task focused categories at the linguistic and, paralinguistic levels with global affective ratings. No non-verbal.	Content items are very broad with only general communication categories and in this respect the system is less useful as a teaching tool.	Proven reliability and validity. Widely used in process outcome research in a range of settings with a resulting large volume of comparable research data.
Medical Interaction Process System (MIPS) (3).	Specifically developed for the analysis of doctor–patient interactions in the oncology consultation.	Sequentially coded from videotapes and/ or audiotapes using specially designed coding sheet.	System allows for parallel coding of utterances and incorporates the content and process of an interaction. Each unit assigned at least one content code and one mode.	Linguistic, para-linguistic, affective and limited global non-verbal. Specific interviewing behaviour items.	Items relate to specific interviewing skills including responses to patients' cues thus providing useful information for teaching purposes and individual feedback.	Good reliability and validity. Useful tool for evaluating the impact of UK communication skills workshops. Increasingly being used for cancer specific communication research in Canada.
CANCODE (formerly CN-LOGIT) (2).	Computer-based interaction analysis system developed purposefully for coding the cancer consultation.	Sequentially coded in real time from audio or videotape directly into a computer software program.	Each unit of speech has four codes: source, process, content and emotional tone. Can record frequency as well as time length for particular codes.	Micro-level analysis, event counts and macro-level analysis of the consultation. Linguistic, affective and paralinguistic. No non-verbal.	In general a good evaluation tool, but more specific communication skills and narrower content categories would be useful.	Reliability and validity good in the cancer setting. Used successfully in studies to describe and characterise the Australian cancer consultation and promote patient participation.

when the consultant responded empathetically to the first cue of distress, and post-consultation depression scores were significantly reduced if more empathic responses were given (24).

Koedoot and colleagues (20) developed a coding system to capture the adequacy of information given by oncologists to cancer patients when proposing palliative chemotherapy. Twenty-six items of information within six categories were coded as *issue not mentioned, issue just mentioned once,* or *issue explained more extensively.* Applying this system, they found that medical oncologists mentioned or explained the disease course (53%), symptoms (35%), and prognosis (39%) to some patients. Most patients were told about the absence of cure (84%). Watchful-waiting was mentioned to only half of the patients, either in one sentence (23%) or explained more extensively (27%). The authors concluded that patients were currently inadequately informed of their treatment options.

Elwyn and colleagues (21) developed OPTION, a coding system designed to measure the extent to which health professionals involve patients in treatment decisions. It was created for the GP setting, but is certainly applicable to the oncology setting. Twelve items are rated on a 5-point scale, (0 = the item is not observed; 1 = a minimal attempt is made to exhibit the behaviour; 2 = the behaviour is observed and a minimal skill level achieved; 3 = the behaviour is exhibited to a good standard; 4 = the behaviour is exhibited to a very high standard). OPTION has been shown to have good inter- and intra-rater reliability and to be sensitive and specific (21, 25). It has been used to demonstrate the impact of communication skills training in involving patients in decision-making (25) and has recently been shown to have good validity in an Italian setting (26).

Discourse analysis

A final approach to interaction analysis is provided by the proponents of discourse analysis. Discourse analysis aims to contribute to the understanding and evaluation of the text of interest, by revealing the meanings behind what is said and not said in the text. At the more sophisticated level of evaluation, linguistic discourse analysis reveals why the text is or is not effective for its own purposes. Analysis at the evaluative levels requires interpretation, not only of the text itself but also of the context from which the text is drawn, and of the systematic relationship between context and text (27). A number of different approaches to discourse analysis exist, but all attempt to move beyond counting behaviours to understanding language as a whole, including what is not said.

The advantages of discourse analysis is that it captures much more subtle aspects of communication, such as power plays, systematic avoidance of certain topics, or discussion of issues such as prognosis only for certain purposes (such as to assist a treatment decision) and not others (such as to assist with existential crises). However, it is even more time-consuming than other approaches and can generally be applied only to a small number of texts, which limits generalizability.

The impact of visual input on communication coding

All IAS require considerable resources to code large-study samples. Thus, it is not surprising that most of the systems described above use the more cost-effective audio-tape, as opposed to video-recordings. However, visual cues may increase the sensitivity and validity of verbal codes, and non-verbal behaviour itself is known to play a highly significant role in communication. Only 7% of emotional communication (how the person is feeling) is thought to be conveyed verbally, 22% is thought to be provided by voice tone, and 55% by visual cues like eye contact and body positioning (28). Several studies have reported that emotional information is the dimension of communication most associated with the patient outcomes of satisfaction and quality of life (28, 30). That is, patients' ratings of satisfaction and quality of life are influenced more by their perception of the emotional support being communicated by their health providers, than by the information communicated. The cancer consultation is particularly emotionally laden and anxiety provoking for many patients (31). As a consequence, patients may look for cues to find out what they ought to be feeling or thinking. Furthermore, many actively search for details about their disease, and non-verbal communication leaks (kinesic leakages) can unintentionally convey ambiguous information that causes them further anxiety (32). Patients are very sensitive to these issues, and to inconsistencies between physician's verbal and non-verbal communication (33). Thus, non-verbal behaviours, including visual cues, are likely to be significant in this context.

Using audio-tape, an IAS is only capable of capturing emotional content conveyed verbally by voice tone, possibly missing up to 55% of other emotional information as mentioned above. With CANCODE, some difficulty has been encountered recording emotional content expressed by a doctor and to a lesser degree by the patient. Across a sample of some 300 consultations with 10 doctors, emotional tone was most commonly coded as emotion category matter of fact, likely reflecting the doctor's consistent clinical manner and the patient's attempt to behave in a socially acceptable manner. The RIAS captures affect, based on voice tone by using global ratings (9, 10), which may be more sensitive and valid.

A recent study (18) compared CANCODE coding based on audio- versus video-tape recordings of the same consultations. Intra-rater reliability scores for audio-to-audio coding were very similar to those for audio-to-video coding. This suggests that video-tape did not substantially change coding of verbal elements. Similar findings were reported by Weingarten and colleagues (34) who compared the coding of patient-centredness, first using only the audio track, and then by using both the audio and video tracks. They found excellent agreement between the two coding methods and concluded that less than 5% of the information was lost by using only audio-data. However, Dent and colleagues (18) also found that purely non-verbal codes, using Mehrabian's classification (35), were as sensitive, if not more sensitive, than verbal measures to doctor response to different patient types. Thus, it is probably worthwhile to use both verbal and non-verbal coding if possible.

Summary

The preceding examples demonstrate some of the various types of interaction analysis systems for examining health professional–patient encounters. The RIAS, MIPS, and CANCODE have proven reliability and validity in the cancer setting. Whereas the RIAS was originally developed for use in general practice consultations, the MIPS and CANCODE were specifically designed for coding interactions in the cancer setting, and in this respect are likely to have greater specificity and sensitivity than the RIAS. However, the RIAS is probably the most widely used system of interaction process; therefore, a much larger pool of comparative data have accumulated for this system. Unlike the RIAS, the design of the MIPS allows a multidimensional view of the consultation, as parallel coding is possible. However, unlike the CANCODE that has a specially designed software package, the MIPS does not record the consultation in real time.

Each system has merits; therefore, researchers must choose a system that is most suited to achieving their objectives. There are several considerations to be taken into account such as: the type of encounter being studied (e.g. initial bad news interview, oncology follow-up consultation, genetic counselling session); the categories of behaviours being measured (e.g. verbal versus non-verbal, specific interviewing skills such as cue detection/question style, the level of patient involvement); and the purpose of the analysis (e.g. the evaluation of communication skills teaching and/or general process-outcome research). For all systems the coding of non-verbal (kinesic) behaviour has yet to be perfected and the issue of whether it is more effective to code from video-tape versus audio-tape is still to be resolved. In sum, no single system of interaction process analysis can hope to capture every behavioural aspect of an encounter, but some may be more useful than others depending on the task at hand.

References

1. Ong LML, De Haes JCJM, Hoos AM, *et al.* Doctor–patient communication: a review of the literature. *Soc Sc Med* 1995; **40**: 903–18.

2. Butow PN, Dunn SM, Tattersall MHN, *et al.* Computer-based interaction analysis of the cancer consultation. *Br J Cancer* 1995; **71**: 1115–21.

3. Ford S, Hall A, Ratcliffe D, *et al.* The medical interaction process system (MIPS): an instrument for analysing interviews of oncologists and patients with cancer. *Soc Sci Med* 2000; **50**: 553–66.

4. Ong LML, Visser MRM, Kruyver IPM, *et al.* The Roter interaction analysis system (RIAS) in oncological consultations: psychometric properties. *Psycho-Oncology* 1998; **7**: 387–401.

5. Maguire P, Fairbairn S, Fletcher C. Consultation skills of young doctors. Benefits of feedback training in interviewing as students persist. *Br Med J* 1986; **292**: 1573.

6. Weston WW, Brown JB, Stewart MA. Patient-centered interviewing. Part I. Understanding patient's experiences. *Can Family Physician* 1989; **35**.

7. Blanchard CG, Ruckdeschel JC, Fletcher BA, *et al.* The impact of oncologists' behaviours on patient satisfaction with morning rounds. *Cancer* 1986; **58**(2): 387–93.

8. Eussen G, Borgers M, Visser A. Een observatiesysteem Voor de analyse van de inhoud van de communicatie tussen kankerpatienten en specialisten. *Gedrag en Gezonheid* 1992; **20**(2).

9. Roter D, Larson S. The Roter interaction analysis system (RIAS): utility and flexibility for analysis of medical interactions. *Pt Educ Counsel* 2002; **46**: 243–51.

10. Hall JA, Roter DL, Rand CS. Communication of affect between patient and physician. *J Health Social Behav* 1981; **22**: 18–30.

11. Levinson W, Roter DL, Mullooly JP, *et al.* Physician–patient communication: the relationship with malpractice claims among primary care physicians and surgeons. *JAMA* 1997; **277**(7): 553–9.

12. Roter D, Rosenbaum J, de Negri B, *et al.* The effects of a continuing medical education programme in interpersonal communication skills on doctor practice and patient satisfaction in Trinidad and Tobago. *Med Educ* 1998; **32**(2): 181–9.

13. Ford S, Fallowfield L, Lewis S. Doctor–patient interactions in oncology. *Soc Sci Med* 1996; **42**: 1511–9.

14. Eide H, Quera V, Graugaard P, *et al.* Physician–patient dialogue surrounding patients' expression of concern: applying sequence analysis to RIAS. (Comparative Study. Journal Article. Research Support, Non-U.S. Gov't) *Soci Sci Med* 59(1): 145–55, 2004

15. Ford S, Hall A. Communication behaviours of skilled and less skilled oncologists: a validation study of the Medical Interaction Process System (MIPS). *Patient Educ Couns* 2004; 54: 275–82.

16. Fallowfield L, Jenkins V, Farewell V, *et al.* Enduring impact of communication skills training: results of a 12-month follow-up. *Br J Cancer* 2003; **89**(8): 1445–9.

17. Brown RF, Butow PN, Dunn SM, *et al.* Promoting patient participation and shortening cancer consultations: a randomised trial. *Br J Cancer* 2001; **85**: 1273–9.

18. Dent E, Butow P, Brown R, *et al.* The Cancode interaction analysis system in the oncological setting: Reliability and validity of video and audio tape coding. *Patient Education and Counseling.* 2005; **56**(1): 35–44.

19. Butow PN, Brown RF, Cogar S, *et al.* Oncologists' reactions to cancer patients' verbal cues. *Psycho-oncology* 2002; **11**(1): 47–58.

20. Koedoot CG, Oort FJ, de Haan RJ, *et al.* The content and amount of information given by medical oncologists when telling patients with advanced cancer what their treatment options are. palliative chemotherapy and watchful-waiting. (Journal Article. Research Support, Non-U.S. Gov't) *Euro J Cancer* 2004; **40**(2): 225–35, Goss C.

21. Elwyn G, Hutchings H, Edwards A, *et al.* The OPTION scale: measuring the extent that clinicians involve patients in decision-making tasks. (Journal Article) *Hlth Expectas* 2005; **8**(1): 34–42.

22. Guimond P, Bunn H, O'Connor AM, *et al.* Validation of a tool to assess health practitioners' decision support and communication skills. (Clinical Trial. Journal Article. Randomized Controlled Trial. Validation Studies) *Pt Edu Counsel* 2003; **50**(3): 235–45.

23. Schofield PE, Juraskova I, Butow PN. How oncologists discuss complementary therapy use with their patients: an audio-tape audit. *Supp Care Cance* 2003; **11**(6): 348–55.

24. Duric V, Butow P, Sharpe L, *et al.* Reducing psychological distress in a genetic counseling consultation for breast cancer. *J Genet Counsel* 2003; **12**(3): 243–64.

25. Elwyn G, Edwards A, Hood K, *et al.* Study Steering Group. Achieving involvement: process outcomes from a cluster randomized trial of shared decision-making skill development and use of risk communication aids in general practice. (Clinical Trial. Journal Article. Randomized Controlled Trial. Research Support, Non-U.S. Gov't) *Fam Practice* 2004; **21**(4): 337–46.

26. Fontanesi S, Mazzi MA, Del Piccolo L, *et al.* Shared decision-making: the reliability of the OPTION scale in Italy. *Pt Educa Counsel* 2007; **66**(3): 296–302.

27. Eggins S. *An Introduction to Systemic Functional Linguistics.* London: Printer Publishers, 1994.

28. Bensing J. Doctor–patient communication and the quality of care. *Soc Sci Med* 1991; **32**: 1301–10.

29. Ong LML, Visser MRM, Lammes FB, *et al.* Doctor patient communication and Cancer patients' quality of life and satisfaction. *Patient Education and Counseling* 2000; **41**: 145–56.

30. Larsen KM, Smith CK. Assessment of nonverbal communication in the patient–physician interview. *J Family Pract* 1981; **12**: 481–8.

31. Holland JC. Psycho-oncology: overview, obstacles and opportunities. *Psycho-oncology* 1992; **1**: 1–13.

32. DiMatteo MR, Taranta A, Friedman HS, *et al.* Predictingpatient satisfaction from physicians' nonverbal communication skills. *Med Care* 1980; **18**(4): 376–88.

33. Friedman HS. Nonverbal communication between patients and medical practitioners. *J Social Sci* 1979; **35**(1), 82.

34. Weingarten MA, Yaphe J, Blumenthal D, *et al.* A comparison of videotape and audio-tape assessment of patient-centredness in family physician's consultations. *Patient Educ Counsel* 2001; **45**: 107–10.

35. Merhabian A. *Scoring Criteria for some categories of nonverbal and implicit verbal behavior in Nonverbal Behavior*, 1972: Aldine & Atnerton, Inc-Chicago.

Chapter 62

The Roter Interaction Analysis System (RIAS): applicability within the context of cancer and palliative care

Debra Roter

Introduction

While references to the physician–patient relationship are evident from the time of the Greeks, systematic study of the medical dialogue is a modern phenomenon. Technological advances have made the observation and analysis of large numbers of medical visits feasible, and indeed, the number of empirical studies of doctor–patient communication has grown markedly over the last three decades. The Roter Interaction Analysis System (RIAS) has emerged over this period as the single most widely used system of medical interaction assessment worldwide. It has been used in over 150 communication studies conducted in North America, Europe, Asia, Africa, and Latin America. These studies have described communication across a spectrum of medical specialties and healthcare settings, including adult and paediatric primary care, emergency medicine, obstetrics and gynaecology, surgery, nursing, podiatry, genetic counselling, family planning services, dentistry, and veterinarian practice, as well as cancer and palliative care.

The purpose of this chapter is to provide a broad overview of the characteristics of RIAS and to illustrate its contribution to the field of cancer communication by reviewing a body of cancer and palliative care studies in which the RIAS has been used.

Conceptual foundations of the RIAS

The RIAS is derived loosely from social exchange theories related to interpersonal influence, problem-solving, and empowerment (1, 2). It is a tool well-suited for viewing the dynamics of resource exchange between patients and providers through the medical dialogue. The social exchange orientation is consistent with health education and empowerment perspectives that view the medical encounter as a 'meeting between experts' through which dialogue shapes the therapeutic relationship and reflects patient and provider roles and obligations (3). Conceptually, the communication categories can be broadly viewed as reflecting socio-emotional and task-focused elements of medical exchange (4). Physicians' task-focused behaviours are defined as technically-based skills used in problem-solving that comprise the base of the 'expertness' acquired through professional medical education and for which a physician is consulted. From a communication perspective, physicians' task behaviours include those related to performance of medical functions, such as data gathering, tests and procedures, the physical exam, and patient education and counselling. The affective dimension of physician behaviour includes those exchanges with explicit socio-emotional content related to the building of social and emotional rapport; for instance, the use of social amenities, empathy, concern, or reassurance. These are not generally regarded as behaviours that have been acquired in medical school.

In many ways, patients' communication may be viewed in a parallel fashion. In this regard, Engle's insight into the dual nature of patient motivation for seeking a doctor's care is illuminating; the 'the need to know and understand' can be viewed in task-focused terms, while the 'need to feel known and understood' may be better understood in socio-emotional terms (5). Task-focused communication is reflected largely in patient question asking and information giving, while the socio-emotional domain includes the expression of concern, optimism, empathy, laughter and joking, and social chit-chat. Within this theoretical grounding, the RIAS provides a framework of mutually exclusive and exhaustive categories, whereby the contributions to the medical dialogue of both patients and providers may be richly elaborated and finely detailed.

The RIAS is applied to the smallest unit of expression or statement to which a meaningful code can be assigned, generally a complete thought expressed by each speaker in the medical dialogue. These units are assigned to 40 mutually exclusive and exhaustive categories that reflect the content and form of the medical dialogue. Form distinguishes statements that are primarily informative (information giving), persuasive (counselling), interrogative (closed and open-ended questions), affective (social, positive, negative, and emotional), and process-oriented (partnership building, orientations, and transitions). In addition to form, content areas are specified for exchanges about medical condition and history, therapeutic regimen, life-style behaviours, and psychosocial topics relating to social relations, feelings, and emotions. The majority of code categories are equally applicable to both physician and patient speakers; however, six categories are physician-specific (i.e. asking for patient opinion or self disclosure) and two categories are patient-specific (i.e. requesting service or medication and disclosing psychosocial information).

In addition to the verbal categories of exchange, coders rate each speaker separately on a six-point scale reflecting the affective and emotional tone of the exchange. The affective dimensions rated include: anger, anxiety, dominance, interest, friendliness, engagement, sympathy, and hurry. Sadness and emotional distress are also rated but are patient-only categories. The global ratings are largely independent of the literal (verbal) content and can be considered a marker of nonverbal communication conveyed through voice tone (6).

The unit of analysis is the smallest unit of expression to which a meaningful code can be assigned, which is defined as a single thought expressed as a simple sentence, a sentence fragment or clause, or single word. The codes are mutually exclusive and exhaustive. RIAS codes can be used individually or combined to summarize the dialogue in a variety of ways. For instance, medical questions and psychosocial questions can be separately tallied, subclassified as open or closed, combined to form superordinate categories, or made into ratios (e.g. open to closed questions, biomedical to psychosocial questions, etc.). Similar groupings can be derived from information-giving and counselling categories. Other variable combinations represent composites of partnership building, positive and negative talk, emotional expression, and orientations and instructions. Patient-centredness scores can be computed using a variety of formulas by which the relationship of variables reflecting physician versus patient communication control are explored (7).

Codes also mark five visit phases: opening, history, physical exam, counselling and discussion, and closing. As a result, the specific communication codes falling within each of these segments of the visit can be analysed and summarized separately. While the phases of the visit are not directly parallel to the functions of the visit, they capture a functional dynamic that cues both patients and providers to normative expectations for particular communication behaviours. For instance, the opening is useful in attending to social amenities and greetings, as well as establishing the visit agenda and probing the full spectrum of patient concerns. The history segment presents the primary opportunity for patients to tell their story and present details regarding their concerns and expectations, while physicians probe symptoms and medical history. The exam segment is dedicated to technical procedures, and perhaps the opportunity for 'laying-on of hands'. The closing is the time for summary and planning for follow-up, as well as the time that patients sometimes convey a 'foot out the door' problem that had not been addressed earlier in the visit (8).

A useful framework for organizing the many individual coding categories is the Four-Function Communication Model (9). This framework is a variant of the widely used 'Three Function Model' of physician communication (10) with the integration of patient communication behaviours into visit functions and the identification of a distinct activation and engagement function. In brief, question-asking and information giving facilitate performance of two medical interview functions: 'Data Gathering' to understand the illness experience and 'Education and Counselling' to provide information and motivation to adhere to drug and life-style recommendations. The third medical interview function 'Emotional Expression and Responsiveness' includes emotional statements of both patients and physicians.

The fourth function, 'Partnership Building and Activation' is reflected in the verbal strategies that help patients integrate, synthesize, and translate between the biomedical and psychosocial paradigms of the therapeutic dialogue. These include verbal engagement strategies, such as explicitly asking if meaning is clear and checking understanding by paraphrase and interpretation. Physicians can facilitate this function by asking the patient for their opinion and preferences, and by encouraging the patient to speak through verbal and nonverbal signals of attentiveness.

Table 62.1 displays the four-function framework with physician and patient dialogue examples for each RIAS code. (The RIAS coding manual and detailed descriptions and examples for each code can be found at http://www.rias.org along with a full annotated bibliography of RIAS studies.)

Cancer, palliative care, and end of life

The bulk of RIAS studies to date have been in primary care; however, there is a rapidly growing body of studies relevant to cancer communication. A review of this literature has identified 32 papers published over the past decade in which RIAS has been applied to cancer-related medical care contexts (11–42). The studies are varied in regard to country and language of encounter, clinical setting, study participant characteristics, and study objectives and design. A detailed analysis of these studies is beyond the scope of the current review, however, a selected review follows to highlight the diversity and contribution of this body of work and to illustrate key coding elements of the RIAS.

Cross-cultural and linguistic adaptation

The Netherlands has contributed the lion's share of cancer communication studies (11, 12, 25, 26, 28–33, 38–42), followed by the US (34–37, 17–20, 27), Norway (13–16, 22), Japan (23, 25), and the UK (21). The process of non-English coding has varied from country to country, but almost always begins with RIAS training before a translation of the American English RIAS codebook is undertaken. During the training, meaning and nuance of the code categories are discussed in light of semantic, cultural, and emotive language characteristics relevant to verbal and non-verbal (voice tone) communication. The success of multiple language adaptation of the system is in no small part due to the use of local language examples for all code categories based on actual visit recordings and transcripts. Part of this translation process goes beyond simply judging the content of explicit statements to a consideration of vocal qualities that convey affective cues that are pertinent to assigning a code classification.

Table 62.1 Functions, Code Definitions, and Dialogue Examples of RIAS Codes

Medical Interview Functions	Specific RIAS Codes (patient and physician)	Physician Dialogue Examples	Patient Dialogue Examples
Data Gathering	Open-ended questions re: medical condition/symptoms therapeutic regimen lifestyle and self-care psychosocial topics	What can you tell me about pain? How are the meds working? What are you doing to keep yourself healthy? What's happening with his father?	What can I expect in terms of pain? How would I know if the treatment is working? What else will I be able to do to keep healthy? How do kids handle this kind of thing?
	Closed-ended question re: medical condition/symptoms therapeutic regimen lifestyle and self-care psychosocial topics	Does it hurt now? Do you take your meds? Are you still smoking? Is your wife back?	Will the rash get worse? Will this med make me sleepy? Is there a walking group? Is it ok if my wife calls you?
Information Exchange	Biomedical information re: medical condition and symptoms therapeutic regimen	The medication may make you drowsy. You need to take it for 10 days.	I think the medication is making me feel drowsy. I took it for 3 days and stopped.
	Lifestyle and self-care information	Getting plenty of exercise is always a good idea. I can give you some tips on quitting.	I try to get out to walk every day.
	Psychosocial exchange (including problems of daily living, issues about social relations, feelings, emotions)	It's important to get out and do something daily. The community center is good for company.	I spend more time alone than I would like.
Emotional Expression and Responsiveness	Positive talk (specific categories) agreements Jokes/laughter Compliments/approvals	Yes, that's right. You will think I'm a vampire—I need blood again. You look fantastic, you are doing great.	Ok, I'll do that. I don't think I have any more blood Thank you for being such a great doctor.
	Negative talk (specific categories) Disapproval (direct) Criticisms (of others not involved in the visit)	No, stop that it won't help at all. They never have enough openings in that center.	That med was a waste of money. The receptionist at that center was so rude.
Emotional Expression and Responsiveness	Social talk (non-medical, chit-chat)	How about them O's last night?	I'm more of a Colts fan.
	Emotional talk (specific categories) concerns reassurance/optimism empathy partnership legitimation	I'm worried about that. I'm sure it will get better. You seem very angry. We'll get through this together. Anyone would feel that way in your situation.	I'm worried about that. I'm sure it will get better. I can see how harried you are. I know we'll get through this together. I bet everyone reacts this way.

Table 62.1 (continued) Functions, Code Definitions, and Dialogue Examples of RIAS Codes

Medical Interview Functions	Specific RIAS Codes (patient and physician)	Physician Dialogue Examples	Patient Dialogue Examples
Partnership Building and Activation	Facilitation (specific categories) asking for patient opinion asking for understanding, checking for understanding back-channels and cues of interest	What do you think is going on? Do you follow me? Let me make sure I've got it right. Uh-huh, right, go on, hmm.	Do you follow me? Let me make sure I've got it right. Uh-huh, right, go on, hmm.
	Orientation ((specific categories) Directions/instructions Transitions and fragments	I'd like to do a physical now. Get up on the table. Now we'll check your back. So—ok, ..	I am going to ask my list of questions now. So,...

Sensitivity to medical context

Aside from language adaptability, sensitivity of the system to variations in medical contexts is critical to its utility. In this regard, an important study designed to explore the ability of RIAS to distinguish communication patterns of cancer consultations from those of primary care was undertaken by Ong and colleagues a decade ago (28). In this primarily psychometric study, the application of the RIAS (in Dutch) to a sample of primary care and oncology consultation audio-tapes were compared along a number of communication dimensions. The investigators found that oncologists were more verbally dominant, more informative, more attentive, and more expressive of concern to patients than were general practitioners. The study also found that the oncologists were less likely to engage in social exchanges or in persuasive counselling with their patients than the generalists. Inasmuch as these differences were anticipated, considering the nature of an oncology consultation, the findings were interpreted as a validation of the system's discriminatory power and sensitivity to context.

Utility in addressing a range of study objectives

The RIAS has been used in a variety of oncology-related contexts to address descriptive, predictive, and evaluative communication objectives. Many of the studies were designed to provide a broad quantitative description of the communication experience of cancer patients in ways not previously investigated. For instance, communication dynamics associated with the first delivery of bad news (21), curative and palliative care within the context of chemotherapy or radiotherapy (11, 39), or distinctions between initial visits and later visits (22). Other descriptive studies addressed the contribution of patient and consultation characteristics to the cancer dialogue (24, 37). Studies reporting associations between RIAS-based communication codes and patient outcomes can be viewed as indicators of the system's predictive validity and measurement sensitivity. A variety of outcomes were assessed in the reviewed studies, with measures of patient satisfaction, comprehension or understanding, or aspects of decision making most commonly related to communication elements (13, 22, 23, 30, 33, 35–37, 42). Similarly pointing to predictive validity and measurement sensitivity of the RIAS, are three evaluative studies of communication training interventions. Notably, these training interventions were directed to very different provider targets, including cancer ward nurses (25), radiation oncologists (40), and genetic counselling providers (32).

Coding multiple speakers

The system has the ability to distinguish the contribution of multiple speakers, including family members accompanying the patient and medical team members consulting with the treating physician. Most of the descriptive literature reflecting medical exchange is dyadic (patient and provider); however, it is common for additional participants to be present and to contribute to the conversation of medical visits. This is especially true when bad news is anticipated, important treatment transitions and decisions are contemplated, when the patient's cognitive abilities are compromised, when medical procedures are to be administered, or when a consultant or other health professionals are brought into the encounter. These circumstances are all found in the oncology context, introducing the challenge of capturing the verbal contributions of three, four, or even more participants. The third party may represent a patient proxy who largely speaks for the patient or someone who contributes to the conversation in a minor way providing support to the patient. A third party may also be a health provider (e.g. a consultant, supervisor, nurse, or social worker) called to the consultation room to assist the physician, the patient, or the patient's family.

The genetic counselling studies in the US and in the Netherlands (17, 31) illustrate the use of this function by accounting for both patient and patient–companion participation in counselling sessions. The analysis by Verhaak and colleagues (42) similarly distinguished the dialogue contribution of patients and patient proxies to informed consent exchanges in radiotherapy consultations.

Use of visit segments

Few studies have taken advantage of the ability of the RIAS coding software to specify five phases of the visit. Only one study included in this review explored this aspect of visit exchange, although in a somewhat abbreviated manner. The study by Eide and colleagues (13) used a three-segment visit approach (history, exam, and counselling) to explore differences in predictors of patient satisfaction. The investigators found that social talk was a positive correlate during the history segment and psychosocial discussion was a negative correlate of satisfaction, if present during the physical exam.

Adaptation of the RIAS to specific context: genetic counselling

An emerging area of cancer-related communication is the field of cancer genetics and genetic counselling. Two studies in this area were conducted almost simultaneously in the Netherlands (31) and in the US (35). The adaptations of the RIAS that were developed for these studies to assure capture of specific genetic-counselling content are noteworthy. In the US study, clinical information given about the genetic marker and cancer risks was specified as either general and population-based (e.g. 'overall one in nine women develop breast cancer') or personalized (e.g. 'based on your family history, your risk of having the genetic mutation is about 20%'). The adaptation also included subcategories designed to distinguish information about testing and treatment that is generalized (e.g. 'there are some tests that identify genes but no one really knows what they mean in terms of disease risk') from testing information that is personalized (e.g. 'the test you would have is very specific and if the mutation is found it means you are at higher risk than other women to develop breast cancer').

The Dutch researchers also subdivided several categories in their genetic counselling adaptation. For instance, questions, information, and counselling related to screening/prophylactic surgery, family pedigree, and communication within the family (among several other categories) were distinguished from other larger blocks of questions, information, and counselling (31).

Some studies compliment RIAS coding with an assessment of clinical proficiency, usually through the use of gold-standard criteria set by experts in the field or a review of the literature. For example, in the study of end-of-life discussions, a 21-item checklist reflecting important skill areas, such as probing and eliciting the patient's values and experience, and providing support for decision-making was used to assess specific skills alongside general communication style (34). In a similar vein, Pieterse and colleagues (31) developed an 11-topic checklist to assess the comprehensiveness of genetic counselling.

Use within hospital settings

Virtually all of the RIAS studies have been in the outpatient context, with the exception of the nursing communication studies by Kruijver and colleagues (25, 26). In this work, the investigators explored communication dynamics in simulated hospital admissions interviews between ward nurses and newly diagnosed cancer patients. This study is also notable in that it is among the few studies in the cancer study database to use patient simulations, along with the US genetic counselling study (34) and the Dutch medical student study (12).

Explorations in secondary analysis

Secondary analysis of the cancer-related RIAS databases produced a variety of novel methodological applications. Especially evident in this arena are several studies by Eide and colleagues exploring communication sequence and correlates surrounding empathic exchange (14) and use of the RIAS to triangulate qualitative coding of empathy (15, 16). Also noteworthy are novel methodological explorations of psycho-physiological correlates of cancer communication. In the Dutch study in this area, the physiological effects evident among medical students undertaking a bad news communication task were explored (12), while the US study explored the physiological impact on analogue clients viewing cancer genetic counselling segments (20).

Implications for future research, training and clinical practice

As is evident from the RIAS-based oncology studies described above, the system is highly adaptable and can be tailored to capture unique contextual dimensions associated with the nature of the medical situation and circumstance being studied. The resource-conservative nature of RIAS makes it logistically possible to conduct research on the large number of encounters that are needed to adequately power intervention studies. Since RIAS coders work directly from the spoken record, an audio- or video-tape, it eliminates the very resource-intensive effort necessary for accurate and full transcription. Transcription conventions designed to capture linguistic properties of speech, for instance, those suggested by Jefferson, are estimated to take many hours of painstaking preparation for each hour of recorded conversation (43). Not only does RIAS avoid the burden of transcript preparation but it is enriched by incorporating voice tone and phrasing cues into coding decisions. High levels of reliability and reasonable coding speed are usually achieved by coders within six to eight weeks of practice. A well trained RIAS coder can complete basic coding of a medical encounter in approximately four times real time duration of the session.

Considering the differences in national health systems, the linguistic demands of translation and adaptation, and the cultural diversity represented in so many different national settings, the advantages and challenges of a common language-based measurement tool are considerable. As previously discussed, the RIAS is sufficiently broad so as to capture core elements common to cancer communication, regardless of national or linguistic context, and is sensitive enough to be used in descriptive, predictive, and concurrent validity studies across a variety of healthcare contexts.

Note

Our website **RIAS.ORG** welcomes visitors interested in posting RIAS-related studies and abstracts, sharing experience in using and adapting the RIAS, and to view the coding manual. Also available on the website is information regarding our software, training, and bibliographic abstracts of studies that have used the RIAS.

References

1. Bales RF. *Interaction process analysis.* Cambridge: Addison-Wesley, 1950.
2. Freire P. *Pedagogy of the oppressed.* New York: Seabury Press, 1970.
3. Tuckett D, Boulton M, Olson C, *et al.* Meetings between experts. *Health Educ Q*, 1985; **15**: 379–394.
4. Ben-Sira, Z Affective and instrumental components in the physician–patient relationship: An additional dimension of interaction theory. *J Health Soc Behv* 1980; **21**: 170–181.
5. Engel GL. How much longer must medicine's science be bound by a seventeenth century world view? In White K (ed.) *The task of medicine.* Menlo Park, California: The Henri J. Kaiser Family Foundation, 1988.
6. Hall J, Roter D, Rand C. Communication of affect between patients and physicians. *Journal Health & Social Behaviour* 1981; **11**: 18–30.
7. Roter DL, Hall JA. Physician gender and patient-centered communication: a critical review of empirical research. *Annual Review of Public Health* 2004; **25**: 497–519.
8. Roter DL, Hall JA. *Doctors talking with patients/patients talking with doctors: improving communication in medical visits,* 2nd edition. Westport, CT: Praeger Publishing, 2006.
9. Roter DL. The enduring and evolving nature of the patient-physician relationship. *Patient Educ Couns* 2000; **39**: 5–15.
10. Cohen-Cole, S. *The medical interview: the three function approach.* St. Louis, MO: Mosby, 1991.
11. Detmar SB, Muller MJ, Wever LD, *et al.* The patient–physician relationship. Patient–physician communication during outpatient palliative treatment visits: an observational study. *JAMA* 2001 Mar 14; **285**(10): 1351–1357.
12. van Dulmen S, Tromp F, Grosfeld F, *et al.* The impact of assessing simulated bad news consultations on medical students' stress response and communication performance. *Psychoneuroendocrinology* 2007 Sep–Nov; **32**(8–10): 943–950.
13. Eide H, Graugaard P, Holgersen K, *et al.* Physician communication in different phases of a consultation at an oncology outpatient clinic related to patient satisfaction. *Patient Educ Couns* 2003 Nov; **51**(3): 259–266.
14. Eide H, Quera V, Finset A. Exploring rare patient behaviour with sequential analysis: an illustration. *Epidemiol Psichiatr Soc* 2003 Apr–Jun; **12**(2): 109–114.
15. Eide H, Frankel R, Haaversen AC, *et al.* Listening for feelings: identifying and coding empathic and potential empathic opportunities in medical dialogues. *Patient Educ Couns* 2004 Sep; **54**(3): 291–297.
16. Eide H, Quera V, Graugaard P, *et al.* Physician–patient dialogue surrounding patients' expression of concern: applying sequence analysis to RIAS. *Soc Sci Med* 2004 Jul; **59**(1): 145–55.
17. Ellington L, Roter D, Dudley WN, *et al.* Communication analysis of BRCA1 genetic counselling. *J Genet Couns* 2005; **14**: 377–386.

18. Ellington L, Maxwel A, Baty BJ, *et al.* Genetic counselling communication with an African American BRCA1 kindred. *Soc Sci Med* 2007 Feb; **64**(3): 724–734.

19. Ellington L, Baty BJ, McDonald J, *et al.* Exploring genetic counselling communication patterns: the role of teaching and counselling approaches. *J Genet Couns* 2006 Jun; **15**(3): 179–89.

20. Ellington, Matwin, Uchino, *et al.* The Body's Response to Healthcare Provider Communication: The Impact of Dominant versus Facilitative Styles. JABR. Forthcoming.

21. Ford S, Fallowfield L, Lewis S. Doctor –patient interactions in oncology. *Soc Sci Med* 1996 **42**(11): 1511–1519.

22. Graugaard PK, Holgersen K, Eide H, *et al.* Changes in physician–patient communication from initial to return visits: a prospective study in a haematology outpatient clinic. *Patient Educ Couns* 2005 Apr; **57**(1): 22–29.

23. Ishikawa H, Takayama T, Yamazaki Y, *et al.* Physician–patient communication and patient satisfaction in Japanese cancer consultations. *Soc Sci Med* 2002 Jul; **55**(2): 301–311.

24. Ishikawa H, Takayama T, Yamazaki Y, *et al.* The interaction between physician and patient communication behaviours in Japanese cancer consultations and the influence of personal and consultation characteristics. *Patient Educ Couns* 2002 Apr; **46**(4): 277–285.

25. Kruijver IP, Kerkstra A, Bensing JM, *et al.* Communication skills of nurses during interactions with simulated cancer patients. *J Adv Nurs* 2001 Jun; **34**(6): 772–779.

26. Kruijver IP, Kerkstra A, Kerssens JJ, *et al.* Communication between nurses and simulated patients with cancer: evaluation of a communication training programme. *European J Onc Nurs* 2001; **5**(3): 140–150.

27. Nelson EL, Spaulding R. Adapting the Roter interaction analysis system for telemedicine: lessons from four specialty clinics. *J Telemed Telecare* 2005; **11** Suppl 1: 105–107.

28. Ong LM, Visser MR, Kruyver IPM, *et al.* The Roter Interaction Analysis System (RIAS) in oncological consultations: psychometric properties. *Psycho-Oncology* 1998; **7**: 387–401.

29. Ong LM, Visser MR, van Zuren F, *et al.* Cancer patients coping styles and doctor-patient communication. *Psycho-Oncology* 1999, **8**: 155–166.

30. Ong LM, Visser MR, Lammes FB, *et al.* Doctor–patient communication and cancer patients' quality of life and satisfaction. *Patient Educ Couns* 2000 Sep; **41**(2): 145–156.

31. Pieterse AH, van Dulmen AM, Ausems MG, *et al.* Communication in cancer genetic counselling: does it reflect counselees' previsit needs and preferences? *British Journal of Cancer* 2005 May 9; **92**(9): 1671–1678.

32. Pieterse AH, van Dulmen AM, Beemer FA, *et al.* Tailoring communication in cancer genetic counselling through individual video-supported feedback: a controlled pretest-posttest design. *Patient Educ Couns* 2006 Mar; **60**(3): 326–335.

33. Pieterse AH, van Dulmen AM, Beemer FA, *et al.* Cancer genetic counselling: communication and counselees' post-visit satisfaction, cognitions, anxiety, and needs fulfillment. *J Genet Couns* 2007 Feb; **16**(1): 85–96.

34. Roter D, Ellington L, Erby LH, *et al.* The Genetic Counselling Video Project (GCVP): models of practice. *Am J Med Genet C Semin Med Genet* 2006 Nov 15; **142**(4): 209–220.

35. Roter DL, Larson S, Fischer CS, *et al.* Experts practice what they preach: A descriptive study of best and normative practices in end of life discussions. *Arch Intern Med* 2000; **160**: 3477–3485.

36. Siminoff LA, Ravdin P, Colabianchi N, *et al.* Doctor –patient communication patterns in breast cancer adjuvant therapy discussions. *Health Expect* 2000 Mar; **3**(1): 26–36.

37. Siminoff LA, Graham GC, Gordon NH. Cancer communication patterns and the influence of patient characteristics: disparities in information-giving and affective behaviours. *Patient Educ Couns* 2006 Sep; **62**(3): 355–360. Epub 2006 Jul 24.

38. Timmermans LM, van der Maazen RW, Verhaak CM, *et al.* Patient participation in discussing palliative radiotherapy. *Patient Educ Couns* 2005 Apr; **57**(1): 53–61.

39. Timmermans LM, van der Maazen RW, Leer JW, *et al.* Palliative or curative treatment intent affects communication in radiation therapy consultations. *Psychooncology* 2006 Aug; **15**(8): 713–725.

40. Timmermans LM, van der Maazen RW, van Spaendonck KP, *et al.* Enhancing patient participation by training radiation oncologists. *Patient Educ Couns* 2006 Oct; **63**(1–2): 55–63.

41. Timmermans LM, van Zuuren FJ, van der Maazen RW, *et al.* Monitoring and blunting in palliative and curative radiotherapy consultations. *Psychooncology* 2007 Dec; **16**(12): 1111–1120.

42. Verhaak CM, Kraaimaat FW, Staps AC, *et al.* Informed consent in palliative radiotherapy: participation of patients and proxies in treatment decisions. *Patient Educ Couns* 2000 Aug; **41**(1): 63–71

43. Jefferson G. Transcription notation. In Atkinson JM, Heritage J (eds) *Structures of social action* (pp.ix –xvi). Cambridge, England: Cambridge University Press, 1984.

Index